Concise Human Physiology

EDITED BY

M.Y. SUKKAR

MB, BS (Khartoum), PhD (Edinburgh)
Professor of Physiology
Faculty of Medicine and Allied Sciences
King Abdulaziz University
Jeddah, Saudi Arabia

H.A. EL-MUNSHID

MB, BS (Khartoum), PhD (Newcastle), MD (Lund)
Professor of Physiology
College of Medicine and Medical Sciences
King Faisal University
Dammam, Saudi Arabia

M.S.M. ARDAWI

BMedSc, MA, DPhil (Oxford), FACB (USA), FRCPath (UK)
Professor of Clinical Biochemistry and Immunology
Department of Clinical Biochemistry
Faculty of Medicine and Allied Sciences
King Abdulaziz University
Jeddah, Saudi Arabia

SECOND EDITION

T0181951

Blackwell
Publishing

©1993, 2000
Blackwell Science Ltd
Editorial Offices:
9600 Garsington Road, Oxford OX4 2DQ
23 Ainslie Place, Edinburgh EH3 6AJ
350 Main Street, Malden
  MA 02148 5020, USA
54 University Street, Carlton
  Victoria 3053, Australia

Other Editorial Offices:
Blackwell Wissenschafts-Verlag GmbH
Kurfürstendamm 57
10707 Berlin, Germany

Blackwell Science KK
MG Kodenmacho Building
7–10 Kodenmacho Nihombashi
Chuo-ku, Tokyo 104, Japan

First published 1993
Second Edition 2000
2   2006

A catalogue record for this title
is available from the British Library

ISBN 978-0-632-05586-9

Library of Congress
Cataloging-in-Publication Data

Concise human physiology/edited by
M.Y. Sukkar,
H.A. El-Munshid, M.S.M.
  Ardawi.–2nd ed.
      p. cm.
Includes bibliographical references and
index.
ISBN 978-0-632-05586-9
1. Human physiology.
2. Human physiology–Study and
teaching–Developing countries.
I. Sukkar, Mohamed Yousif.
II. El-Munshid, H.A.
III. Ardawi, M.S.M.

QP34.5.C66 2000
612–dc21   99-053652

DISTRIBUTORS

Marston Book Services Ltd
PO Box 269
Abingdon, Oxon OX14 4YN
(Orders: Tel: 01235 465500
          Fax: 01235 465555)

USA
  Blackwell Science, Inc.
  Commerce Place
  350 Main Street
  Malden, MA 02148-5020
  (Orders: Tel: 800 759 6102
                 781 388 8250
            Fax: 781 388 8255)

Canada
  Login Brothers Book Company
  324 Saulteaux Crescent
  Winnipeg, Manitoba R3J 3T2
  (Orders: Tel: 204 837 2987)

Australia
  Blackwell Science Pty Ltd
  54 University Street
  Carlton, Victoria 3053
  (Orders: Tel: 3 9347 0300
            Fax: 3 9347 5001)

For further information on
Blackwell Publishing, visit our website:
www.blackwellpublishing.com

Contents

Contributors

A.M. ABDUL GADER MB, BS (Khartoum), PhD (Dundee), FRCP (Edinburgh). *Professor of Physiology, Faculty of Medicine, King Saud University, Riyadh, Kingdom of Saudi Arabia. (Formerly Associate Professor, Faculty of Medicine, University of Khartoum, Khartoum, Sudan.)*

T.S. AHMED MB, BS (Khartoum), PhD (Bristol). *Associate Professor, Department of Physiology, Faculty of Medicine, University of Khartoum, Khartoum, Sudan, at present on secondment to King Saud University, Riyadh, Kingdom of Saudi Arabia.*

M.S.M. ARDAWI BMedSc (Oxford), MA (Oxford), DPhil (Oxford), FACB (USA), FRCPath (UK). *Professor of Clinical Biochemistry and Immunology, Department of Clinical Biochemistry, Faculty of Medicine and Allied Sciences, King Abdulaziz University, Jeddah, Kingdom of Saudi Arabia.*

M.A. BALLAL MB, BS (Khartoum), PhD (Nottingham). *Associate Professor, Department of Physiology, Faculty of Medicine, University of Khartoum, Khartoum, Sudan, at present on secondment to King Saud University, Riyadh, Kingdom of Saudi Arabia.*

H.A. EL-MUNSHID MB, BS (Khartoum), PhD (Newcastle), MD (Lund). *Professor of Physiology, College of Medicine and Medical Sciences, King Faisal University, Dammam, Kingdom of Saudi Arabia. (Formerly Associate Professor, Faculty of Medicine, University of Khartoum, Khartoum, Sudan.)*

M.O. HASSAN MB, BS (Khartoum), PhD (Glasgow), FRCP. *Professor of Physiology, College of Medicine, Sultan Qaboos University, Muscat, PO Box 32485, Al-Khod, Sultanate of Oman. (Formerly Chairman, Department of Physiology, Faculty of Medicine, King Abdulaziz University, Jeddah, Kingdom of Saudi Arabia.)*

M.M. KARDASH MB, BS (Khartoum), FCCP, PhD (Leeds). *Consultant Cardiologist, Assir Central Hospital, Abha, Kingdom of Saudi Arabia.*

N.A. MAHMOUD MB, BS (Khartoum), PhD (Edinburgh). *Professor of Physiology, Faculty of Medicine, University of Khartoum, Khartoum, Sudan. (Formerly Professor of Physiology, Faculty of Medicine, University of Kuwait, Kuwait.)*

H.A. NASRAT MB, BCh (Cairo), MRCOG (London), FRCS (Edinburgh). *Consultant, King Abdulaziz University Hospital, and Assistant Professor, Department of Obstetrics and Gynaecology, Faculty of Medicine, King Abdulaziz University, Jeddah, Kingdom of Saudi Arabia.*

M.Y. SUKKAR MB, BS (Khartoum), PhD (Edinburgh). *Professor of Physiology, Department of Physiology, Faculty of Medicine and Allied Sciences, King Abdulaziz University, Jedda, Kingdom of Saudi Arabia. (Formerly Professor of Physiology, Faculty of Medicine, University of Khartoum, Khartoum, Sudan.)*

A.M. ZIADA MB, BS (Khartoum), PhD (Birmingham). *Assistant Professor, Department of Physiology, Faculty of Medicine, King Abdulaziz University, Jeddah, Kingdom of Saudi Arabia.*

Preface to Second Edition

Since the first edition of *Concise Human Physiology* went into print we have received a considerable amount of feedback from over seven countries in the Middle East, Southern Asia and Africa. We also had the opportunity to meet students who had used the text. Their satisfaction was most gratifying and their suggestions for improvement were most welcome. In particular we were pleased to hear that students had appreciated the text's simple, flowing style and the abundance of information within a concise format. Specific constructive comments from teachers and students were taken into account in the second edition, but, alas, we cannot respond to the introduction of colour for reasons of economy. For the same reason we had to omit Chapter 2 (The Social Environment) and Chapter 19 (An Introduction to Statistics). We apologize to those readers who had found them useful.

In the second edition, the length and style of the text has been kept very much the same. A greater effort was made to further simplify the English and to clarify the explanation of important concepts. All chapters have been thoroughly revised and updated, and some new diagrams added. Chapter 1 has a new section on cell physiology, made necessary by the rapid growth of knowledge in the field of molecular biology. Parts of Chapters 5, 6, 8 and 16 have been completely rewritten to give a more coherent view of newer concepts and more up-to-date information.

While the book still aims at a well defined scope and depth of core human physiology, it is highly desirable that students and medical schools, where possible, reinforce textbook studies by the use of now available computer assisted learning. CD programs offer marvellous opportunities for exciting and enjoyable learning. These provide colour, sound, animation and interactive learning which are highly effective.

The editors would like to take this opportunity to express their gratitude and appreciation to all the contributors who have worked on this edition and to those who, for various reasons, have not continued to contribute. Thanks are also due to the Department of Physiology at King Abdulaziz University for support and to the King Fahad Medical Research Centre for services provided in the preparation of the manuscript. Special thanks are due to Mrs Helen Khoja for her patient and competent secretarial support. Last, but by no means least, we would like to extend our hearty appreciation to the students and teachers whose comments we have found most useful and whose appreciation of this book has made our effort very much worthwhile.

M.Y.S.
H.A.E.
M.S.M.A.

Preface to First Edition

During the last 15 years more colleges of medicine and allied health sciences have been established in the developing countries than ever before. The special needs of students in these institutions are inadequately met by available textbooks, which have been written primarily for medical students in Europe and the United States—more often than not for a wide readership which includes science and postgraduate students. This textbook aims to address the special needs of students in developing countries, in both content and presentation. For this purpose, there are four main features which make this book different from all others.

The first of these features is the language. Most of the colleges in developing countries use the English language as the medium of instruction. Most countries have started to use their own languages as the medium of instruction in pre-university education. For this reason, most students find it difficult to use existing textbooks of basic medical sciences.

This textbook sets out to use as simple language as possible through the use of simple vocabulary and sentence structure. It is anticipated that the student will be helped in three ways: (i) comprehension of the basic concepts of human physiology; (ii) economic utilization of the learner's time; and (iii) a smooth introduction to the use of the scientific textbook by avoiding the frustration that goes with the absence of the above two.

The second feature addresses the selection of content. During the last two decades the medical curriculum has witnessed two apparently contradictory phenomena. On the one hand, there has been a tremendous growth in the amount of knowledge in basic medical sciences. This has resulted in overcrowding of the curricula and the growth in size of almost all known textbooks. On the other hand, recent developments in curriculum design have brought into focus the need for integration of basic sciences with the clinical disciplines. One way to achieve this is the introduction of clinical sciences in the early years of the programme. Thus, pathology, microbiology and pharmacology have crept back into the medical curriculum. Consequently, the time allocated for learning basic medical sciences has decreased.

Under these conditions selection of content presents a challenge to both the student and the teacher. This textbook aims to present the basic principles and concepts of human physiology required for the study and practice of medicine and to present these within a reasonable length. Two ways have been adopted to solve this problem: (i) the contents have been selected to give adequate scope and depth relevant to the study of medicine; and (ii) experimental evidence and descriptions of animal experiments have been cut down to a minimum. Except where such experiments help to reinforce the scientific method, such content has been totally eliminated. It is realized, however, that some students will find the time to consult other reference works. A bibliography drawn upon in the selection of contents is provided. Some special titles are also recommended for further reading at the end of each chapter.

The third feature of this book is its orientation to the tropical environment with its characteristic health problems. The populations to be served by the graduates largely consist of women and children. The health problems of pregnant women and small children present the majority of cases seen in primary health care. Thus, separate chapters on nutrition and on pregnancy and perinatal physiology have been included. Most of the graduates will practise medicine as general practitioners in a tropical and largely rural environment. The special physiological mechanisms invoked in the adaptation of the individual and the community to the tropical environment have been given special attention. Nutrition is presented as a basic science which calls upon the biochemical and physiological mechanisms concerned with the utilization of nutrients. The orientation of nutritional information focuses on the use of locally available foods and the prevention of malnutrition. This also serves as a unique opportunity to introduce basic community medicine concepts at an early stage of the curriculum.

The fourth feature is the selection of authors, all of whom have had significant experience in teaching medicine and allied health science students in developing countries. Each has contributed to areas in which they have special interest and published research. The focus of editing was to harmonize the treatment and style of presentation in the various chapters.

We would like to express our appreciation of the co-operation of all the contributors without whose support this work would not have been possible. We would like to thank all those who have helped in the making of this textbook, especially the members of the Department of Physiology, Faculty of Medicine, King Abdulaziz University, for their continuous support and advice during the preparation of the manuscript. Special thanks go to Mrs Kay Gari for excellent secretarial help and for the preparation of the final manuscript. The credit for preparation of the illustrative material goes to Mr Mannan Azmi of the King Fahad Medical Research Centre, King Abdulaziz University. Last, but not least, we would like to thank our families for their patience in bearing with us during the lengthy period of the preparation of this textbook.

We hope the product will be found useful by students and teachers. The editors will be delighted to receive comments and suggestions from experienced teachers and from students for the purpose of improving future editions.

M.Y.S.
H.A.E.
M.S.M.A.

1 / An Introduction to Human Physiology

Objectives

On completion of the study of this chapter, the student should be able to:

1 Appreciate the relationship between humans and their environment so as to identify the place of human physiology in the study of medicine as a health and social science.

2 Comprehend the functional organization of the organ systems of the human body in order to develop a holistic approach to the study of medicine.

3 Understand the concepts of the internal environment and its constancy as an important condition for normal health.

4 Acquire basic information on body composition so as to interpret changes which occur in disease processes, such as dehydration, oedema, hyper- and hypo-osmolality and acid–base disturbances.

5 Describe the major components and properties of control systems so as to explain the physiological mechanisms encountered in the study of the organ systems.

6 Describe and explain the functions of the molecular components of a typical cell.

7 Explain the various mechanisms of intercellular communication.

Humans and the environment

The human individual can be viewed as an integral part of the community and the environment in which he/she lives. Human physiology is a science which analyses the body functions and their interaction with the environment. In so doing, we seek to understand the mechanisms whereby these interactions take place. The study of human physiology is an essential prerequisite to the practice of preventive and curative medicine.

Humans, as living organisms, are influenced by the environment in which they live. This *external environment* has its physical, chemical and biological as well as its psychosocial components. The human individual interacts with the climate of the environment, thrives on the air, water and foods available in it, and becomes victim to the pathogenic organisms and other hazards prevalent in his/her surroundings. Humans are also influenced by the customs, beliefs and values which shape the psychosocial structure of their community. The major environmental factors with which the human organism interacts can be summarized as oxygen, water, food, physical environment, social environment,

microorganisms and parasites (Fig. 1.1). Some of these components are the main life support. The human body uses or adjusts to these components throughout life. Most of the concerns of medicine attempt to maintain the balance of this interaction in favour of humans. Social and preventive medicine attempt to maintain the equilibrium of the individual, the family and the community with their environment. Curative medicine helps to readjust the equilibrium of the human body when it is disturbed by disease.

The human physiologist is concerned with the following aspects of this system:

1 The way in which the human body is functionally equipped to interact with its environment.

2 The mechanisms by which the individual adjusts to the environment.

3 The maintenance of internal balance, normal function and, therefore, the health of the body and mind.

4 The functions of physical and mental work and productivity.

Through the following discussion, each of the above statements will be analysed and explained.

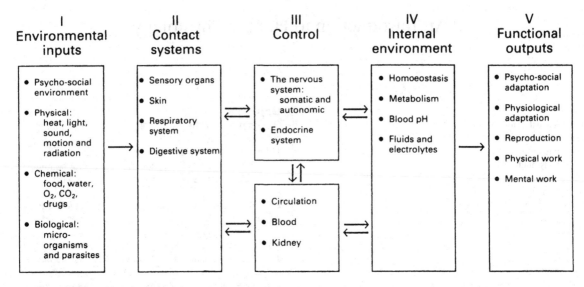

Fig. 1.1 A schematic representation of the functional relationships of body systems.

In the first place, the human body interacts with its external environment through the systems listed in the second column in Fig. 1.1. These have been labelled the *contact systems* because they come into direct contact with the external environment. The respiratory system is in contact with the atmospheric air. The digestive system is in contact with food and drink. The skin comes into close contact with and senses the objects, materials and temperature of the environment. The sensory organs help us to smell, taste, hear or see the various components of our surroundings. The contact systems differ from all the other functional divisions of the human body in this respect, i.e. direct contact with the outside world. It is not surprising, therefore, that many of the defence and protection mechanisms are found in these systems. It is also not surprising that hypersensitivity (allergy) occurs mainly in the skin (allergic skin conditions), respiratory system (asthma and allergic rhinitis) and the gastrointestinal tract (allergic diarrhoea and colitis).

The internal environment and homoeostasis

To adjust to the changes which take place in the external environment, many detectors and sensory mechanisms are involved. These send messages to the systems responsible for control of body functions, i.e. the nervous system and the endocrine glands. These organs will initiate and control the processes by which the body adjusts to changes in the external environment. They also respond to changes which take place inside the body, such as the ingestion and absorption of food and water, the change in composition and pH of the body fluids and the accumulation of products of metabolism. These two systems can be called the organs of control (Fig. 1.1). Together or singly, they provide the mechanisms of communication and adjustment of the *internal environment*. This is the second concern of human physiology. These adjustments in body functions are required to meet external variations, such as heat and cold, and internal changes due to various activities, such as muscular exercise or absorption of nutrients from the gastrointestinal tract. The nervous system and the endocrine glands provide a means of communication between the various parts of the body. The nervous system works by means of electrical signals, which travel in the nerves, and the endocrine glands release hormones, which are transported in the blood to the target organs.

The internal environment

The human body, like other complex living organisms, consists of organs and tissues, which, in turn, are made up of cells. The smallest unit of life in this complex structure is the cell. The cells of the body live in a fluid environment. It is this tissue fluid (i.e. **interstitial fluid**) which represents the **internal environment**. The function of all the organ systems of the body is to ensure that the physical and chemical characteristics of the tissue fluid remain constant within narrow limits. Thus, the temperature, the pH and the concentration of chemical components of the internal environment are precisely regulated by physiological processes

Fig. 1.2 The compartments and volumes of body fluids.

collectively described as **homoeostatic mechanisms**. This is the third and major concern of human physiologists. The concept of 'internal environment' was introduced by the French physiologist Claude Bernard in 1857. He stated that all the life processes have but one goal, that of maintaining the constancy of the internal milieu (environment), and that the fixity of this internal milieu was the necessary condition for free existence.

The body fluids
The body of a 65 kg man contains about 40 litres of water. The distribution of this water can be measured by special methods, which are discussed later in this chapter. It has been found that about 25 litres are found inside the cells (**intracellular**) and 15 litres are outside the cells (**extracellular**). Figure 1.2 shows the main compartments of body fluids.

The extracellular fluid can be further subdivided into a part which is found within the vascular system of the circulation (**intravascular**) and one which lies between the cells (**interstitial**). The interstitial fluid volume includes lymph, which cannot be measured separately.

There is a third component of extracellular fluid, which is referred to as **transcellular fluid**. This is fluid secreted by epithelial linings, e.g. cerebrospinal fluid (CSF), fluid in transit in the gastrointestinal tract and urinary system, and fluid in potential spaces such as the joint cavities and in the pleural and peritoneal spaces. The total amount of transcellular fluid is normally small. However, large volumes can be formed in disease states, such as pleural effusion and collection of fluid in the peritoneal cavity (*ascites*). Large losses of gastrointestinal secretions occur in diarrhoea and vomiting, which lead to dehydration and electrolyte disturbances.

Homoeostasis
The constancy of the internal environment (**homoeostasis**) is achieved in spite of changes in the surroundings. It is also possible to maintain the steady state during changes of body function, e.g. increased muscular activity, which generates heat, CO_2 and other metabolic products. **Homoeostatic mechanisms**, therefore, are all the automatic reactions which take place in the body in response to changes in the external or internal environments and which tend to correct all deviations from normal.

The internal equilibrium is assisted by the blood and circulatory systems. Efficient distribution of heat and nourishment is achieved through the bloodstream and lymphatic drainage. These systems also remove the waste products of metabolism and normal wear and tear of tissues. These are carried to the kidneys, where waste products such as urea and acids (H^+) are excreted in the urine, and to the lungs, where CO_2 is removed. The kidneys have many important functions which maintain the chemical composition of the internal environment. It should be noted that these functions are carried out under the close control of the nervous system and the endocrine glands.

Energy supplies, protein, minerals and vitamins maintain normal nutrition and balanced metabolism. Equilibrium exists among intake, storage and metabolism. Metabolic processes are also homoeostatically controlled by the endocrine system (see column IV, Fig. 1.1).

It appears from the above discussion that the organ systems listed in column III of Fig. 1.1 serve the all-important tasks of maintaining internal equilibrium. This is essential both for normal physiological functions for manual and mental work and for healthy psychosocial interactions in the community. Once these adjustments are made, then the person can lead a productive life. The body can then be said to be healthy, i.e. in a state of physical and mental well-being. The United Nations World Health Organization (WHO) gives an extended definition of health to include the environment in which people live. Health is defined as 'a state of complete physical, social and mental well-being' and not merely as the absence of disease or infirmity.

The physiologist is also concerned with the functions required for physical and mental productivity (column V, Fig. 1.1). Skeletal muscles undergo physical and chemical changes in order to do work. They use chemical energy and are therefore able to convert it into mechanical work.

It goes without saying that the maintenance of adequate supplies and a stable internal environment allows the higher functions of the brain (such as learning and creative thinking) to work. For these functions to flourish, a conducive socio-economic environment is required, which further emphasizes the wisdom of the above definition of health.

Adaptation

The functional outputs (Fig. 1.1, column V) also refer to the adaptation of the individual to the physical and social environments. Unlike homoeostasis, adaptation is concerned with the long-term adjustments required for a 'normal' life. Adaptation to the environment can be considered successful when the relationship of the human individual or community is in a state of balance and productivity. The practice of **community medicine** (social and preventive medicine) aims to enhance this process through environmental health, health education and other promotional and supportive health measures. Thus, immunization of children against prevalent diseases makes them more adapted to survive in health in a particular locality.

Examples of **physical adaptation** are seen in the body shape, body composition and skin colour of people who live under different climatic conditions. Cold climates favour deposition of fat, a short stature and white skin (e.g. the Inuit of North Canada). Hot climates favour a lean and tall body frame as well as the formation of protective pigment in the skin (e.g. the Dinka of southern Sudan and the Masai of Kenya). The density of skin pigment varies directly with the amount of sunshine and protects the body from a harmful excess of ultraviolet rays. The body shape tends to be related to the ability to lose and conserve heat. A more or less spherical shape has a small surface area proportional to mass and favours heat conservation. On the other hand, a long cylindrical body shape has a greater surface area proportional to mass and therefore favours heat loss.

There are also **physiological adaptations** which maintain body functions under extremes of environmental conditions. For instance, people living at high altitudes make more red blood cells and haemoglobin so as to be able to live and work at a lower oxygen pressure. Similarly, people living in cold environments increase their thyroid function so as to generate more heat in the body through a higher rate of metabolism.

Psychosocial adaptations take place under a variety of conditions. People who migrate to different countries will acquire behaviour and habits more acceptable to the new society. Individuals who make new partnerships in business or in friendship have to adjust to the new partner by understanding, developing new concepts or giving up old ones. Marriage is an excellent example where each of the partners adjusts to the attitudes and behaviour of the other so as to build a home and to raise a family. The discipline of social and preventive medicine considers the individual as a member of a family and the family as a unit of the community. These subdivisions have profound effects in the determination of health and the patterns of prevailing disease.

Decisions taken by the physician, whether diagnostic, preventive or curative, will have to take into account the family and the social environment as well as the various physical, chemical and biological factors referred to in column I of Fig. 1.1.

In conclusion, it seems that the doctor is dealing with a complex situation. Disease is basically an expression of the failure of body mechanisms to maintain homoeostasis in the face of challenge, which may take many forms, e.g. hereditary defects, infection, injury, neoplasms and degenerative conditions. In simple terms, the doctor tries to help the body maintain the *internal environment* through curative medicine practices. He/she also tries to help the process of physical and social adaptation in his/her practice of community medicine and **primary health care**, which endeavour to take health to the community rather than wait for the individual to become sick and to seek treatment.

The composition of the human body

Body water

The human body is made mainly of water, which constitutes about 60% of body-weight in the adult. However, the amount of body water varies with age. The newborn have about 82% of body-weight as water at birth and the elderly about 52% (Table 1.1). Loss of body water is a common cause of death in children who suffer from dehydration in developing countries.

Table 1.1 Variation of total body water with age and sex expressed as a percentage of body-weight.

	Male (%)	Female (%)
At birth	82	82
Children and adolescents	70	70
18–20 years	59	57
20–40 years	61	51
40–60 years	55	47
Over 60 years	52	46

Table 1.2 Water content of plasma and various tissues.

Plasma	90–92%
Muscle	72–78%
Bone	45%
Adipose tissue	13%
Enamel	5%

Table 1.3 Body composition of a 70 kg man.

	Weight (kg)	Body-weight (%)	Lean mass (%)
Water	42.0	60	75
Protein	12.6	18	20
Fat	12.6	18	—
Minerals	2.8	4	5
Total	70.0	100	100

Table 1.4 The concentrations of major cations and anions in body fluids (mmol/l).

	Extracellular fluid		Intracellular fluid
	Plasma	Interstitial	
Cations (mmol/l)			
Na^+	145	140	10
K^+	4	4	145
Ca^{2+}	5	5	1
Mg^{2+}	2	2	40
Total (+)	156	151	196
Anions (mmol/l)			
Cl^-	105	110	3
HCO_3^-	28	31	10
Protein	17	4	45
HPO_4^{2-}	6	6	138
Total (−)	156	151	196

The amount of water in the body is affected by the quantity of body fat. Lean subjects have a higher percentage of water than those with more body fat. This is because adipose tissue contains far less water than muscle, skin and other soft tissues (Table 1.2). Women have more fat than men; therefore, as expected, they have a lower percentage of body water than men (Table 1.1).

Protein

Protein is the second largest component in the human body. Protein is found in the structure of all tissues, but by far the largest amount is found in skeletal muscle.

Fat

The next largest component in lean individuals is fat. This is found in the form of triacylglycerol in adipose tissue, which constitutes the main energy store of the body (Table 1.3). These stores are found around abdominal viscera and in subcutaneous tissues. Normally, men have less fat than women. In women, fat distribution represents one of the secondary sex characteristics. It gives the female body its typical feminine configuration. Fats, in the form of phospholipids, are found in the structure of cell membranes. An appreciable part of the structure of the central nervous system (CNS) is fat.

Minerals

The minerals are present in the human body in relatively small quantities with the exception of calcium. The total body calcium is about 1.2 kg in a young adult, the bulk of which is found in the bones. Minute, but functionally significant, amounts of calcium are found in body fluids.

In adults the total amount of iron is about 3 to 4 g, 70% of which is the haem parts of haemoglobin and myoglobin. These proteins are associated with carriage of oxygen. Iron is also found in iron stores, in transport forms and in iron-containing enzymes (e.g. cytochrome oxidase).

Other minerals and electrolytes are found in the body fluids in minute concentrations, which are closely regulated to maintain the composition of the internal environment. Their concentrations in the intracellular fluid are different from those in extracellular fluid (Table 1.4). This difference depends on the permeability of the cell membrane and on active transport at the living cell membrane. Passive equilibrium is also attained by means of physical factors such as concentration gradients and electrical charge distribution (see Chapter 3).

The body fluids

Measurement of body fluids

The volumes of the various compartments of the body fluids can be measured using well-known techniques employing the **dilution principle**. If a known quantity of a substance is dissolved in an unknown volume of fluid, we can calculate the volume from the following relationship:

$$V = \frac{Q}{C}$$

where V = volume; Q = quantity of substance; and C = final concentration of substance after even mixing in the fluid to be measured.

The substance chosen is injected into the bloodstream. The choice of substance for measurement of a certain compartment of body fluid, e.g. extracellular fluid (ECF), should take into consideration that the substance should distribute itself only in the ECF and should not enter the cells. Other prerequisites are that the substance should distribute itself uniformly in all parts of the fluid to be measured and that it should not be rapidly excreted or metabolized. The method for measurement of its concentrations should not provide practical difficulties. Obviously, if a substance is to be administered into a patient, it should not be toxic.

If a small amount of the substance is metabolized or excreted during the period of mixing, this amount must be subtracted from the total amount administered before dividing by the final concentration.

Total body water

The total body water is measured by injection of a substance which will diffuse freely in all the fluid compartments. Examples of suitable substances are **deuterium oxide (D_2O)**, **tritiated water (^3H_2O)**, **antipyrin** and **amino-antipyrin**. A sample of plasma is obtained for measurement of the concentration (C) of the substance used. The total body water can be obtained by calculating Q/C. Slightly different results are obtained depending on the characteristics of the substance used.

Extracellular fluid

Two types of substances are used for measurement of ECF: (i) **saccharides**, e.g. inulin, sucrose, raffinose and mannitol (an alcohol derived from mannose); and (ii) diffusible ions, e.g. **sulphate**, **thiosulphate**, **thiocyanate**, chloride, bromide and sodium. The saccharides give lower volumes because they enter some compartments rather slowly (especially the CSF). They are also excreted in the urine. The ions, however, tend to give higher results because small amounts penetrate the intracellular compartment. Radio-isotopes, especially (^{35}S) sulphate, have been used with good results. Because of errors due to using different substances, it is advisable to qualify the result, e.g. sulphate space, thiocyanate space, etc.

The volume of *intracellular* fluid can be determined by subtraction of ECF from total body water.

Plasma volume

In the case of plasma volume, the dilution method uses a dye which binds itself to plasma albumin, such as **Evans' blue**. Radioactively labelled **albumin** using iodine (^{131}I) has also been used. These substrates give a measurement of plasma volume. The **blood volume** can be calculated from the measured volume of plasma. First, the haematocrit or packed-cell volume (PCV) is measured by centrifugation of a sample of blood. The **haematocrit** is the proportion of blood volume occupied by red blood cells expressed as a percentage. The blood volume is given by the formula:

$$\frac{\text{Blood}}{\text{volume}} = \text{Plasma volume} \times \frac{100}{100 - \text{Haematocrit}}$$

Thus, if the haematocrit is 45%, the proportion of plasma would be 55% of the blood volume:

$$\text{Blood volume} = \text{Plasma volume} \times \frac{100}{55}$$

If red blood cells labelled with radioactive chromium (^{51}Cr) are used, then a direct value of the blood volume is obtained.

When plasma volume is subtracted from the volume of ECF, the volume of *interstitial fluid* including lymph is obtained.

Tissue fluid exchange

The intravascular fluid consists of the blood plasma. The interstitial fluid is similar to plasma in composition except for its low content of protein. These two parts of the extracellular fluid are in constant exchange. The circulation renews the tissue fluid and maintains its constancy by supplying materials needed by the cells and removing those produced by cellular metabolism. Exchange of fluid between the capillary blood and the interstitial compartment takes place continuously. It is estimated that about 150 litres of fluid diffuse out of the blood capillaries and re-enter again every hour.

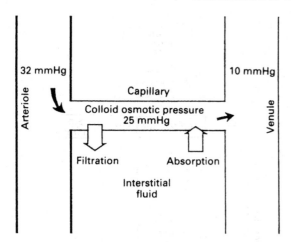

Fig. 1.3 Diagrammatic representation of the forces responsible for exchange of fluids across the blood capillary membrane. The hydrostatic pressure and the colloid osmotic pressure of the interstitial fluid have been omitted for simplification.

The forces which govern this exchange of fluid between the plasma and the interstitial fluid are: (i) **hydrostatic pressure** due to fluid tension within the circulation (the blood pressure); and (ii) the **colloid osmotic pressure** of the plasma proteins, also known as oncotic pressure (see Fig. 1.3).

The hydrostatic pressure is much higher in the capillaries than in the tissue spaces and tends to drive fluid out of the capillaries by **filtration**. The colloid osmotic pressure is much higher in the blood plasma than in the interstitial fluid because the plasma proteins are retained inside the capillaries. This tends to draw water into the capillaries by **osmosis**. These two forces act in opposite directions. While the colloid osmotic pressure is uniform throughout the capillary length, the hydrostatic pressure falls from the arteriolar to the venular end. At the arteriolar end of the capillary, the hydrostatic pressure is greater than the colloid osmotic pressure and therefore fluid tends to pass to the outside of the capillaries. At the venous end of the capillaries, the hydrostatic pressure is less than the colloid osmotic pressure and therefore water is *reabsorbed* into the capillaries at this end (Fig. 1.3). It is important to note that, in the lungs, capillary hydrostatic pressure is uniformly less than the colloid osmotic pressure and therefore there is no filtration. The alveoli are kept dry. In the glomerular capillaries of the kidney, the hydrostatic pressure is much higher than the colloid osmotic pressure. Therefore, filtration takes place without reabsorption.

Starling's hypothesis states that there exists an equilibrium between the colloid osmotic pressure and the hydrostatic pressure so that about 90% of the fluid which passes into the interstitial space goes back into the circulation at the venular end of the capillaries. The remaining 10% is drained via the **lymph vessels**, which start blindly in the interstitial space.

The colloid osmotic pressure in the interstitial fluid is about 5 mmHg, while the hydrostatic pressure is usually of the order of a few mmHg negative or positive and varies in the different body tissues. These two forces tend to cancel each other and therefore play a minor role under normal conditions. Small amounts of albumin normally pass into the interstitial spaces, but these are constantly removed via the lymphatics and returned to the bloodstream, together with some of the interstitial fluid formed.

Applied physiology of tissue fluid exchange

Oedema

Oedema is defined as the abnormal collection of fluid in the interstitial spaces. There are three main causes which occur frequently in clinical practice:

1 *Increased capillary hydrostatic pressure.* This is usually due to obstruction of blood in the venous system. Failure of the right ventricle (as in congestive heart failure) results in a rise in the central venous pressure in the great veins near the heart and consequently a rise in capillary hydrostatic pressure. This causes increased filtration and if pressure at the venular end becomes close to or exceeds the value of the colloid osmotic pressure (normally about 25 mmHg), then the return of fluid by osmosis will be opposed and accumulation of fluid in the interstitial space results.

2 *A decrease in the plasma colloid osmotic pressure.* This is either due to excessive loss of albumin in the urine (as in kidney disease) or deficiency of albumin production (as in chronic liver disease or malnutrition). The fall in plasma albumin results in failure of reabsorption of water and therefore accumulation of fluid in the interstitial space.

3 *Obstruction of lymph vessels.* This results in accumulation of albumin in the interstitial space, which is normally cleared away by the lymphatics. Thus, a significant rise in the colloid osmotic pressure of the interstitial fluid results in oedema.

The forces which govern fluid exchange across the capillary wall are delicately balanced. This allows a continuous flow of fluid through the tissue spaces, so that equilibrium with the blood plasma is ensured and transport of nutrients and removal of waste products are achieved.

Control mechanisms

The functions of the different systems of the body are
closely monitored and adjusted to meet the demands of
the body, which change with various activities, e.g. intake
of food and water, running or doing heavy manual work.
The adjustments also respond to changes in the external
environment to which the body is exposed at any given
time, e.g. sitting in a hot room or going out into the cold
night air.

Control theory

When a system is described as controlled, this means that
its variables are kept within a prescribed range. Control
theory deals with the analysis of the whole system, so that
the relationships between inputs and outputs are defined.
In engineering science, these relationships are expressed
in mathematical terms. In biological systems, mathematical
models have been used in analysing and studying biological phenomena.

Example:

$$\text{Arterial blood pressure} = \frac{\text{Cardiac output (flow)}}{\text{Resistance to flow}}$$

In the control of arterial blood pressure, variables such
as the cardiac output and arteriolar resistance are adjusted
so as to maintain arterial blood pressure within the normal
range. The purpose of control is to maintain the variables
of a system within the range of reference or standard
values.

Control systems

A control system can be analysed into various components
for the purpose of understanding the relationships between
them. The model in Fig. 1.4 shows a simplified control system divided into four major components:

1 *A receptor*, or sensing device, sensitive to the changes
which take place in the internal environment. These receptors are usually specialized and will respond to change in
one variable, e.g. blood pressure, oxygen, body temperature, osmotic pressure, etc.

2 *A controller*. The controller in biological systems is
usually in the central nervous system, where receptor
signals are received, analysed and compared with reference
values or set norms. After comparison, an error signal is
sent out. The appropriate response is given by the controlled system.

3 *The controlled system*. This represents one or more
effector organs, which are responsible for the functions

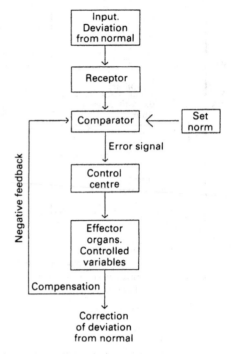

Fig. 1.4 The major components of a negative feedback control
system in simple form.

involved. In the above example, the heart and blood-
vessels represent the controlled systems responsible for
the function of regulation of blood pressure.

4 *Regulated variable*. The blood pressure is the regulated
variable in this case. However, it can be further analysed
into subsidiary variables which may affect the blood pressure, such as the heart rate and the strength of cardiac muscle
contraction (together these two determine the output of
the heart). Another subsidiary variable is the diameter of
blood-vessels, which determines the resistance to blood
flow to the tissues. The regulated variable is monitored
by the sensing device. Therefore, a **feedback mechanism**
exists between the output and the input.

Examples of homoeostatic mechanisms

The homoeostatic mechanisms described below are everyday life examples selected to illustrate the control systems
outlined above:

1 *Core body temperature* in humans is maintained within a
fraction of a degree on both sides of 37°C. If this temperature starts to rise, even by a small fraction of a degree,
homoeostatic regulation is immediately called for and the
error in body temperature is immediately corrected.

The temperature rise is measured by means of sensitive

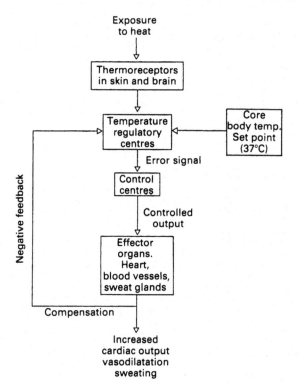

Fig. 1.5 The control of body temperature used to illustrate the interrelations of the components of a control system.

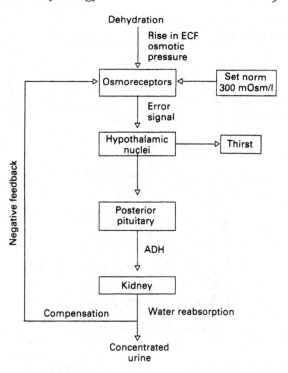

Fig. 1.6 The control of water excretion through a control system involving the osmotic pressure of extracellular fluid (ECF). ADH, antidiuretic hormone.

receptors situated in the skin and at the base of the brain (in the hypothalamus). These receptors send signals to the heat-regulatory centres in the hypothalamus. Here the receptor signals are compared with the set normal temperature. The output of the control centres, e.g. those controlling skin blood-vessels and the sweat glands, is adjusted accordingly. The responses promote heat loss, for example: (i) more blood flows to the skin so that heat can be lost from the surface of the body by radiation; and (ii) production of sweat, which evaporates from the surface of the skin, producing a cooling effect (Fig. 1.5).

The temperature receptors continue to monitor the compensation of body temperature and keep the hypothalamus informed through a feedback mechanism so that excessive heat loss does not occur, thus completing the control system of receptor, comparator, control centre, controlled variables and feedback.

2 *Control of water intake and water loss.* The body water is maintained within narrow limits. Changes in the content of body water occur when we go without drinking, as in fasting or being lost in the desert. Changes can also occur when we become dehydrated through loss of

water in sweating, vomiting and diarrhoea. Conversely, a large intake of fluid by mouth or through intravenous infusion can produce changes in body water in the opposite direction.

These physiological and pathological changes call for immediate responses. The normal osmotic pressure of plasma is 290 mosmol/litre. Any change is detected by receptors in the hypothalamus of the brain. These receptors are called *osmoreceptors*. Signals are sent in the form of electric impulses to other parts of the hypothalamus (thirst centre) and we feel thirsty and therefore seek water to drink (Fig. 1.6). At the same time signals are sent to the posterior pituitary gland just below the hypothalamus. A hormone is released in the circulation, which is called antidiuretic hormone (ADH) because it acts on the kidney to produce a low volume of more concentrated urine by decreasing water loss.

This approach to the analysis of homoeostatic control provides a model suitable for studying and describing all physiological regulatory mechanisms. A large number of such mechanisms will be encountered in the study of body functions in the following chapters.

(a)

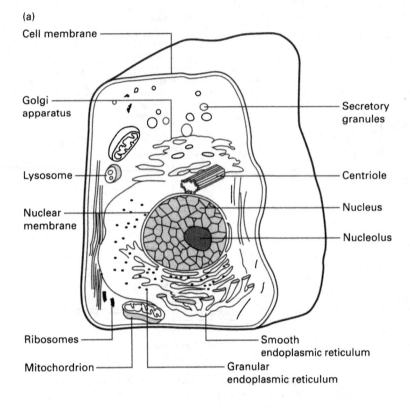

Cell membrane

Golgi apparatus

Lysosome

Nuclear membrane

Ribosomes

Mitochordrion

Secretory granules

Centriole

Nucleus

Nucleolus

Smooth endoplasmic reticulum

Granular endoplasmic reticulum

(b)

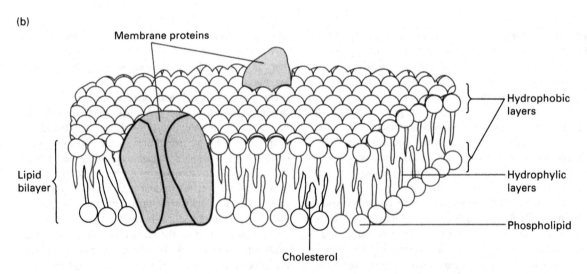

Membrane proteins

Lipid bilayer

Hydrophobic layers

Hydrophylic layers

Phospholipid

Cholesterol

Fig. 1.7 (a) A diagrammatic representation of a typical cell showing various intracellular organelles. (b) The cell membrane showing the lipid bilayer and membrane proteins.

Table 1.5 Function of cell organelles.

Endoplasmic reticulum	1 Provide tubules and vesicles which conduct substances formed in one part of the cell to other parts 2 Provide a large surface area for attachment of enzyme systems on its membrane 3 Provide attachment for ribosomes composed of RNA molecules essential for protein synthesis 4 Space within endoplasmic reticulum connects to that between the two layers of the nuclear membrane
Mitochondria	These are responsible for utilization of energy found in the nutrients and oxygen
Golgi apparatus	This is a prominent structure in secreting cells. It takes up endoplasmic reticulum vesicles and processes their contents to form lysosomes and secretory vesicles and other components of the cytoplasm
Ribosomes	1 These contain many proteins and several ribonucleic acids (three at least) 2 Protein synthesis takes place in the ribosomes, e.g. hormones, enzymes and the proteins of other cell components
Lysosomes	Provide intracellular digestion of substances or particles of debris from damaged organelles or ingested food substances and pathogenic organisms
Secretory vescicles	Secretory substances are formed in the cytoplasmic reticulum, processed by the Golgi apparatus to form secretory vesicles or granules which can be secreted either into the bloodstream or in specialized duct systems
Peroxisomes	These are vesicles containing oxidizing enzymes which oxidize alcohol and other toxic substances

Cell physiology

In the previous parts of this chapter, we considered the human body as a whole and emphasized its integration within the ecology of its surroundings, be they biological, chemical, physical or psychosocial. We also discussed macrosystems of control which involve one or more organ systems. However, it is now possible to study cellular, intercellular and intracellular processes of regulation of tissue and organ functions. Although most of such processes lie within the realm of medical biochemistry and molecular biology, it is necessary to develop an awareness of their important contributions to the understanding of physiological mechanisms.

The cell

Detailed structural descriptions of the cell and its contents are outside the scope of this book. The following will explain the functions common to all cells. Special attention will be given to the cell membrane structures, which play important roles in the control of membrane permeability and therefore transport and excitation.

Figure 1.7(a) shows the structure of a typical cell. The **nucleus** of the cell is the control house of cell functions. It contains the deoxyribonucleic acid (DNA), which is the genetic material required for control of the synthesis of the cell proteins, especially the cell enzymes and secretions. The DNA also replicates so as to reproduce new cells. The nuclear membrane is a double membrane separated by a space continuous with that of the endoplasmic reticulum. These two membranes are also traversed by pores, which allow the passage of molecules from the cytoplasm to the inside of the nucleus, e.g. some hormone complexes which influence protein synthesis. The nucleolus, found within the nucleus, is a dense structure which contains ribonucleic acid (RNA) similar to that of ribosomes. It becomes larger when there is active protein synthesis. Table 1.5 gives a brief description of the functions of the cell organelles.

Molecular considerations of cell physiology

The cell membrane

This consists of a bilayer of phospholipid molecules. The phosphate hydrophilic ends of the molecules of the outer layer face the water of the ECF and those of the inner layer point towards the cytoplasm (Fig. 1.7b). The hydrophobic hydrocarbon ends of the two layers face each other inside the membrane. This arrangement does not allow the passage of polar molecules, such as amino acids, sugars and ions, across the membrane. Transport of these molecules is achieved through specialized protein molecules embedded in the lipid bilayer.

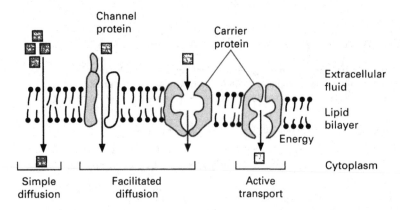

Fig. 1.8 Types of transport across the cell membrane. Channel and carrier proteins are shown as integral parts of the membrane.

Membrane proteins. The membrane is in fact a mosaic of phospholipids and protein. **Extrinsic (or peripheral) proteins** are those which are loosely bound by electrostatic forces to the cell wall exterior or interior. Examples are antigens and cell enzymes. **Intrinsic (or integral) proteins** are those which are more closely associated with the phospholipid molecules. These protein molecules are large and may extend across the whole thickness of the lipid bilayer. Projecting portions of some of these proteins may have carbohydrate chains attached to them; thus they are called *glycoproteins*.

The intrinsic proteins serve several functions. **Transport proteins** serve as **channels** or as **carrier proteins** with specific solute transport functions (Fig. 1.8). In muscle fibres, **anchoring proteins** are the receptors which attach the end-plates of contractile proteins to the cell membrane. Some transport proteins are attached to one side of the cell membrane, e.g. luminal or basal side, e.g. gastrointestinal or renal tubular epithelial tissues.

Membrane channels. These are membrane pores or 'tubes' made of one or more membrane protein that travel the whole thickness of the membrane. The inside of the tube is a lining of hydrophilic groups, while the outside facing the phospholipids has numerous hydrophobic groups. This arrangement allows the tube to be filled with water and can therefore allow the diffusion of ions in aqueous solution.

Channels are structurally specialized to allow passage of different ions. Thus there are Na^+, K^+ and Ca^{2+} channels. While Na^+ channels have a strong negative charge inside, K^+ channels are not charged. Some can open and close spontaneously, others are *gated channels*, whose opening and closing can be regulated by chemical messengers—*chemical gated*—or by change in the membrane potential—*voltage gated*.

Membrane carrier proteins. Some carrier proteins can be activated by concentration gradient; for others adenosine triphosphate (ATP) provides the driving force. The sodium–potassium pump, found in all cell membranes, is a good example. It is also known as Na^+-K^+ adenosine triphosphatase (ATPase). The conformation of this carrier protein can change in different phases of its activity. It can be closed to the ECF and open to the cytoplasm and vice versa. When it is open to the cytoplasm it takes up Na^+. Then the pump hydrolyses ATP to phosphorylate a specific site on the protein carrier and thus changes its conformation. As a result, the carrier loses its affinity for Na^+, which is thrown out of the cell, and takes up K^+ from the ECF. The binding of the K^+ ions causes the phosphate to dissociate and this reverses the configuration, so that K^+ ions are released to the cytoplasm (Fig. 1.9). The rate of the Na^+-K^+ pump is regulated by the intracellular Na^+ concentration so that accumulation of Na^+ does not occur.

Cotransport is a term given to carrier systems which utilize the concentration gradient of one solute as a driving force for transporting another solute against the concentration gradient (Fig. 1.10). An example of this system is the absorption of glucose from the intestine, which uses the Na^+ concentration gradient at the luminal side of the membrane to transport glucose into the cell. The glucose can therefore be absorbed irrespective of its concentration.

Intercellular communication

Communication between cells takes place in most cases by means of **chemical messengers**. There are three main types of these: (i) **chemical transmitters** are released by nerve endings in the synaptic gaps (e.g. acetylcholine, noradrenaline [norepinephrine]); (ii) **hormones** are released by endocrine cells into the extracellular fluid, enter the capillaries and therefore circulate in the blood. They act on

Extracellular fluid

Lipid bilayer

ATP

ADP

Intracellular fluid

Fig. 1.9 The Na^+–K^+ transport protein showing binding sites. Both ions are transported against concentration gradients using energy from ATP.

Extracellular fluid

Amino acid

Glucose

Lipid bilayer

Cytoplasm

Fig. 1.10 Cotransport. Some cells utilize the sodium gradient in the extracellular fluid (or intestinal lumen) for transporting glucose and amino acids.

distant tissues (e.g. insulin, cortisol and thyroid hormones); and (iii) the third type are **paracrine hormones**, which are released into the interstitial fluid but which act locally on neighbouring cells (e.g. somatostatin). It is noteworthy that one substance may play different roles in different organs, e.g. noradrenaline (norepinephrine) is a neurotransmitter in the CNS and in autonomic nerves, but it is also a hormone when secreted into the blood by the adrenal medulla. In general, chemical messengers act by combining with or activating specific receptors found on the cell surface or intracellularly.

Cell membrane receptors

These structures are protein molecules, which have now been isolated, characterized and assayed. They are not fixed features of the cell membrane because their numbers can increase (up-regulation) or decrease (down-regulation). Combination of a chemical messenger or **ligand** with its receptor serves as a triggering mechanism for various changes to take place inside the cells.

Based on the way they work, there are three categories of surface receptors: (i) channel-linked receptors; (ii) catalytic receptors; and (iii) G-protein-linked receptors. A **channel-linked** receptor binds to its chemical messenger and causes a specific ion channel to open or close. These receptors therefore control the influx or efflux of ions across the cell membrane. This type of receptor is found mainly in the central nervous system and at neuromuscular junctions. When the appropriate ligand binds to a **catalytic** receptor the latter acts as a **protein kinase**, which mediates the transfer of phosphate groups from ATP or guanosine triphosphate (GTP) to proteins. Therefore they influence the functions of intracellular proteins. **G-protein-linked** receptors bind to specific ligands and activate a G protein located on the cytoplasmic surface of the cell membrane. The activated G protein then brings about the activation of other enzymes or ion channels.

Second messengers

Most membrane receptors act through the generation of a second messenger inside the cell. The most common second messengers (or intracellular mediators) are cyclic adenosine monophosphate (cAMP), Ca^{2+} and inositol triphosphates, e.g. IP_3 (see Table 1.6).

Cyclic AMP is an important intracellular mediator, formed from ATP when **adenylate cyclase** located in the cell membrane is activated. Calcium acts as a second messenger in response to the activation of many surface receptors. The intracellular Ca^{2+} concentration is increased either due to opening to Ca^{2+} channels or to the release of

Ligand	Second messenger
Acetylcholine	Ca^{2+}, inositol triphosphates
Catecholamines (α_1 receptors)	Ca^{2+}, inositol triphosphates
Catecholamines (β receptors)	cAMP
Follicle-stimulating hormone	cAMP
Glucagon	cAMP
Histamine (H_2 receptors)	cAMP
Luteinizing hormone	cAMP
Parathyroid hormone	cAMP
Thyrotrophin	cAMP
Vasopressin (V_1 receptors)	Ca^{2+}, inositol triphosphates
Vasopressin (V_2 receptors)	cAMP

Table 1.6 Examples of some ligands and their second messengers.

bound Ca^{2+} inside the cell from the endoplasmic reticulum and other organelles. Receptors linked to G protein stimulate a membrane enzyme, phospholipase C (PLC), resulting in the hydrolysis of a membrane phospholipid to give inositol triphosphate (IP_3). IP_3 acts as the main second messenger which releases Ca^{2+} from the endoplasmic reticulum.

Intracellular receptors

Some ligands are lipid-soluble and therefore can pass through the cell membranes. They bind to receptors in the cytoplasm or on the nucleus. Activated receptors act on the nuclear DNA to stimulate transcription of messenger RNA (mRNA), which is translated in the ribosomes, resulting in protein synthesis. These proteins are mainly enzymes, which alter the cell function in the direction of the general effect of the hormone or ligand. Examples of intracellular receptors are those described for steroid and thyroid hormones. Different types of receptors for each hormone may be found in different cells. This explains the wide variety of effects these hormones have.

Growth factors

A system of extracellular ligands known as growth factors (GF) regulate cell replication in response to injury and to replace normal wear and tear. These factors are also important in the inhibition of unwanted growth. At present more than 40 growth factors have been identified. Examples of the growth factors are the platelet-derived growth factor (PDGF), epidermal growth factor (EGF) and insulin-like growth factor I (IGF-I). The growth factors are protein or polypeptide molecules that bind the membrane receptors on their target cells. A cell that produces a growth factor does not have the receptor; otherwise it would stimulate its own growth. However, some of the factors have been implicated in the causation of cancer.

Further reading

1 Guyton, A.C. & Hall, J.E. (1991) Functional organisation of the human body and control of the internal environment. In: *Textbook of Medical Physiology*, 8th edn, pp. 1–8. Saunders, Philadelphia.
2 Sherwood, L.L. (1996) Cellular physiology: In: *Human Physiology*, 3rd edn, pp. 17–45. Wadsworth, Bemont, California.

2 / The Blood

Objectives

On completion of the study of this chapter, the student should be able to:

1 Understand the processes involved in blood cell formation and their requirements so as to explain the causes of defects in haemopoiesis.

2 Describe the morphology and functions of different types of cells found in the blood so as to recognize abnormalities such as anaemias and leukaemias.

3 Explain the basic mechanisms of the immune system.

4 Enumerate the types of plasma proteins and describe their origins, concentrations and functions so as to recognize disturbances of their kinetics.

5 Describe the basis of blood group classification and its application in blood transfusion.

6 Understand the mechanisms of haemostasis so as to explain the causes of excessive bleeding and intravascular clotting.

Introduction

Blood is classified as a connective tissue with an excessive and complex liquid intercellular material, the plasma, in which the blood cells or formed elements are suspended. The proportion of plasma to cells can easily be determined by spinning a sample of blood in a centrifuge tube. The percentage volume of whole blood occupied by packed red cells, i.e. packed-cell volume or the haematocrit, is 37–47% in males and slightly less in females. Blood may be obtained easily from the superficial veins of the body and its analysis may give a good idea of the status of body functions.

Functions of the blood

Blood is the main transportation vehicle of the body. It carries oxygen and nutrients to tissues and waste products of metabolism, e.g. carbon dioxide and urea, to the lungs and kidneys. Most of the hormones are also carried from the endocrine glands to target organs. Blood also has important homoeostatic functions exemplified in the following. Blood circulation helps to distribute heat around the body from metabolically active and warmer organs, e.g. liver and gut, to peripheral organs, thereby helping to maintain an even body temperature. Buffers in the blood, like haemoglobin, plasma proteins, bicarbonate and others, help to keep the hydrogen concentration of the extracellular fluid constant at a pH of 7.4. Blood plays a vital protective function against infection by virtue of its leucocytes and antibodies (immunoglobulins) in the plasma. Furthermore, injury to blood-vessels is followed by blood clotting, which stops further loss of this vital fluid.

Composition of the blood

Blood consists of:
1 Formed elements (blood cells), of which there are three types:
   (a) red cells—erythrocytes;
   (b) white cells—leucocytes;
   (c) platelets—thrombocytes.
2 Plasma.

Formation of blood (haemopoiesis)

Definitions

Erythropoiesis: formation of erythrocytes.
Leucopoiesis: formation of leucocytes.
Thrombopoiesis: formation of thrombocytes (platelets).

Sites of blood formation

1 *In the fetus*:
   (a) *The yolk sac* is the only site of blood formation in the first 3 months of life. Thereafter, haemopoiesis starts in the liver and spleen and continues until the 7th month of intrauterine life.
   (b) *Bone marrow*. Blood formation in the bone marrow commences in the 4th month of intrauterine life and from the 7th month of intrauterine life until birth it becomes the only haemopoietic organ.

2 *After delivery and throughout life*. Bone marrow (red marrow) fills all the bone cavities throughout childhood but it is gradually replaced by fatty yellow marrow. This is particularly noticed in long bones, where red marrow shrinks towards the ends (epiphyses), leaving the shaft cavity (diaphysis) to be filled by yellow marrow. In addition and throughout life, red marrow continues to occupy the cavities of flat bones, e.g. skull, iliac bones, sternum, ribs and scapula, as well as vertebrae and small bones of the hands and feet. Twenty-five per cent of the cells in red marrow are erythrocyte precursors, while the remaining 75% are leucocyte precursors. This is perhaps due to the longer survival time of erythrocytes—120 days as compared with only a few days for leucocytes; therefore, the need to produce red cells is less pressing than producing the short-lived leucocytes. In certain blood diseases, e.g. chronic anaemias in children, spleen and liver resume their fetal haemopoietic function and start producing blood cells. This is referred to as **extramedullary haemopoiesis**.

Red blood cells (erythrocytes)

Development

The production of erythrocytes starts from the primitive haemopoietic stem cell, which becomes successively a **proerythroblast**; **early, intermediate** and **late normoblast**; **reticulocyte**; and finally an erythrocyte or mature red cell. In the early stages of this production line, there is mitotic multiplication of developing cells, followed later by maturation, i.e. the development of both functional and structural cell characters, and finally release into the bloodstream. The process of maturation involves reduction in size, shrinkage and disappearance of the nucleus and the acquisition of the vital red pigment haemoglobin. The appearance of **reticulocytes** in peripheral blood indicates rapid production of erythrocytes, which is a sign of good response to treatment of anaemia.

Structure

The erythrocyte is a non-nucleated cell shaped like a flat biconcave disc. Its dimensions are shown in Fig. 2.1. It is made of a framework of protein (**stromatin**) containing a concentrated solution of **haemoglobin**. The red cell is

Fig. 2.1 Outline and dimensions of a typical red blood cell.

flexible and can easily be distorted during its passage in capillaries.

Red cell membrane
The red cell membrane is 75 Å (7.5 nm) thick and is composed of phospholipid and protein. It is semipermeable, allowing controlled movement of water but maintaining a potassium/sodium ratio as found in the intracellular/extracellular fluid compartments.

Chemical composition
Red blood cells consist of 60% water and 40% solids (90% haemoglobin and 10% stromatin). The cytoplasm contains adenosine triphosphate (ATP), which is generated mainly by the process of glycolysis.

Lifespan
Red cells live for about 120 days, i.e. 1/120 circulating erythrocytes is renewed daily and the total number of erythrocytes is renewed once every 3 to 4 months.

Red blood cell count in peripheral blood:
Males   4.8–5.8 million cells/mm^3
Females   4.2–5.2 million cells/mm^3

It is estimated that about 3 million red blood cells are normally broken down every second and, since in a normal healthy person the total number of red cells remains within normal limits, about 3 million red cells must be produced per second. When this balance is disturbed, i.e. production is decreased or destruction increased, the red cell count and haemoglobin level drop, resulting in anaemia.

Destruction and removal of red cells occur in the **reticuloendothelial system**. Ageing cells become progressively deficient in the enzymes needed for deriving energy from glucose and therefore it becomes difficult for the cell to maintain its integrity. The cells then burst or succumb to osmotic lysis, fragmentation and erythrophagocytosis by reticuloendothelial cells. The components of the destroyed cells are dealt with in the following manner: iron is reused in haemoglobin synthesis, globin is degraded and its amino acids are returned to the amino acid pool of the body, and the **pigment**, **haem**, is ultimately converted to **bilirubin**, which is excreted in bile.

Functions
By virtue of their content of haemoglobin, the function of red cells is the transport of oxygen from lungs to tissues and carbon dioxide from tissues to the lungs for excretion. The biconcave discoidal shape of mature erythrocytes is well adapted to its function of gas transport; the surface area of the red blood cell is larger than the minimal area needed to enclose its volume which would be provided if the cell were a simple sphere. Furthermore, in the narrow channels of the microcirculation where O_2 is given up, more red cells can be accommodated in a given volume of blood than would be possible if red cells were spherical in shape. Lastly, the red cell membrane, being elastic and distortable, facilitates the movement of these cells through the 4 μm wide terminal capillaries where oxygen is delivered and carbon dioxide removed.

Metabolism
The erythrocyte is metabolically active and gets its energy through breakdown of glucose (glycolysis). Knowledge of red cell metabolism is essential to the clear understanding of methods used in red cell preservation in blood banks, where blood is collected in an anticoagulant solution containing glucose (dextrose) as a source of energy. Blood is then stored in the cold (temperatures of 4°C) to reduce the metabolic rate of erythrocytes; consumption of energy (i.e. ATP) at 4°C is 30 times slower than at 37°C.

Nutritional requirements for red cell production
Most of the substances required for erythropoiesis are available from the metabolic pool of the body. However, the following substances are described as 'essential' for normal **erythropoiesis** since deficiency of any of them results in detectable changes in the blood:
1 *Amino acids.* The supply of proteins in the diet provides the amino acids needed for the synthesis of the **globin** of **haemoglobin**. It is known that haemoglobin, being a vital pigment, has a high priority for the available protein and therefore, in humans, protein deficiency must be very severe before haemoglobin synthesis is impaired. In kwashiorkor, a hypoplastic anaemia develops which disappears spontaneously on feeding. This anaemia is

characterized by a reduction in the cellularity of the bone marrow (hence the name hypoplastic).

2 *Iron*. This is dealt with in detail at a later stage in this chapter. Iron deficiency causes **microcytic hypochromic anaemia**, i.e. smaller than normal red cells with reduction in the haemoglobin content.

3 *Vitamins*. There are several vitamins essential for normal haemopoiesis:

(a) Vitamin B_{12} (**cyanocobalamin**) and **folic acid** play an important role in the synthesis of **nucleoproteins**. The deficiency of either leads to a disturbance of deoxyribonucleic acid (DNA) metabolism in developing nucleated red cell precursors. The result is megaloblastic (mega = large) erythropoiesis and megaloblastic (**macrocytic**) anaemia (**pernicious anaemia**).

(b) As a reducing agent, *vitamin C* (ascorbic acid) facilitates iron absorption in the gut by helping to keep iron in the reduced (ferrous, Fe^{2+}) state. Ascorbic acid is also involved in the normal metabolism of *cyanocobalamin* and *folic acid*. Diets deficient in vitamin C are likely to be deficient in folic acid. Both vitamins are present in vegetable foods and both are heat-labile and therefore deficiency of both vitamins is common. The result can be normocytic, macrocytic or microcytic anaemia with normochromic or hypochromic red cells.

(c) *Pyridoxine* (B_6) is essential for haem and nucleoprotein production. Its deficiency in infants causes hypochromic microcytic anaemia which does not respond to iron therapy but only to pyridoxine.

(d) Riboflavin, nicotinic acid, pantothenic acid, biotin and thiamine are B vitamins that are involved in various intermediary metabolic processes. It is more common to find multiple deficiencies of these vitamins than deficiencies of one member. When deficiency occurs, the result is almost always a normochromic normocytic anaemia which can be cured by administering the missing vitamin.

(e) Recently, *vitamin E* has been reported to be essential for the normal synthesis of erythrocyte membrane in infants and, when deficient, it may cause haemolytic anaemia due to excessive haemolysis, i.e. destruction of red cells.

4 *Trace elements*. Copper, cobalt, zinc, manganese, nickel and other minerals are present in the erythrocyte. There is no clear evidence in humans to suggest that deficiency of any of these elements produces anaemia, but it is of interest to note that cobalt stimulates the formation of erythropoietin and, if given in quantities in excess of the normal dietary needs, results in the development of polycythaemia (increased number of circulating red cells).

Control of erythropoiesis

Erythropoietin

Oxygen deprivation (hypoxia) or blood loss triggers the formation of the hormone *erythropoietin*, which acts on the bone marrow to stimulate erythropoiesis.

Chemistry

Erythropoietin is a glycoprotein (24% carbohydrate and 76% protein) with a molecular weight of about 34 000. Its protein is made of a single chain of about 165 amino acids.

Sources

Most of the hormone erythropoeitin (90%) is produced in the peritubular cells of the renal cortex and outer medulla; the rest is secreted by the liver. The stimulus to erythropoietin production is hypoxia, caused either by anaemia or by other forms of impaired oxygen delivery to the kidney. The half-life of erythropoietin is 6.7 hours and the principal site of its degradation is in the liver.

Action

Erythropoietin stimulates the early **stem cell** (otherwise called the erythropoietin-sensitive stem cell or erythrocyte-committed stem cell) to differentiate into a proerythroblast. Erythropoietin seems to trigger the processes which eventually lead to haemoglobin synthesis. In addition, it also stimulates self-replication and proliferation of the erythropoietin-sensitive stem cells. Erythropoietin does not seem to influence the maturation stages in the erythrocyte production line.

Erythropoietin can be detected in the plasma and urine of normal persons and this is taken as evidence that the hormone is needed for normal erythropoiesis. But high levels occur in anaemia (not anaemia of renal failure) and in hypoxia due to living at high altitudes or as a result of heart or lung disease. In the latter situation, high levels of erythropoietin result in increased production of erythrocytes and consequently an increased number of circulating cells (erythrocytosis, polycythaemia) (Fig. 2.2).

In conclusion, erythropoiesis is determined by the rate of erythropoietin formation, which, in turn, is controlled by the relation of oxygen supply to oxygen demand. When oxygen supply does not meet demand, e.g. hypoxia, erythropoietin formation and thus erythropoiesis are increased, more red cells are produced and this corrects the decrease in oxygen supply to the tissues.

Fig. 2.2 The mechanism of production of erythropoietin.

Androgens, thyroid hormones, cortisol and growth hormone

Deficiency of any of these hormones usually results in anaemia, mostly normochromic or normocytic, which may be corrected by giving the missing hormone. This has been taken to support the importance of these hormones in normal erythropoiesis.

Iron metabolism

Distribution of iron in the body

The total amount of iron in the body of a healthy adult is 3–5 g distributed as follows:

1 *Haemoglobin*. Most of the iron in the body (65–75%, average: 3000 mg) is present in haemoglobin (in the red blood cells, 1 g haemoglobin contains 3.4 mg iron).

2 *Storage (available) iron*. Twenty per cent of the total body iron (average: 1 g) is present as the protein–iron compound **ferritin** in the liver, spleen and bone marrow.

3 *Cellular or tissue (non-available) iron*. This is the iron (average 150 mg) which is present in body cells as a major component of oxidative enzyme systems, e.g. **cytochrome**, and as part of myoglobin.

4 *Transport or plasma iron*. A very small amount of iron (3–4 mg) is found in the plasma in combination with a β-globulin, transferrin. This iron is being transferred from one point of use to another. A very minute amount of iron is present in blood in the form of ferritin. Measurement of **serum ferritin** is a reliable indicator of the level of iron stores in the body. Figure 2.3 shows a diagrammatic representation of iron metabolism.

Iron in food

The average diet provides 10–20 mg iron/day. Liver, being an important storage organ for iron, is the richest dietary

Fig. 2.3 Iron metabolism.

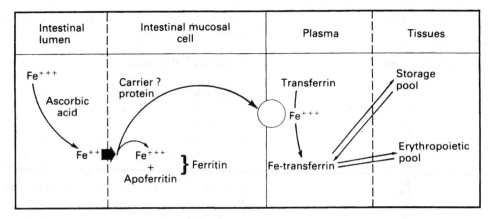

Fig. 2.4 The phases of iron absorption, its transport in plasma and its fate in the tissues.

source. Other good sources include: beef, mutton, fish, egg yolk, cereals, beans, lentils and green leafy vegetables. When food is cooked in iron utensils, some iron is added from the utensils.

Forms of iron in food

1 *Organic porphyrin* (haem) iron is the iron present in animal protein foods such as meats, fish and egg yolk.
2 *Inorganic (non-haem) iron* is the iron present in foods of vegetable origin.

Absorption

Most of the iron in food is in the oxidized *ferric (Fe^{3+})* state; however, it is absorbed better when it is in the reduced *ferrous (Fe^{2+})* state. This reduction is facilitated by gastric acidity and the presence of reducing agents in the diet, especially vitamin C and protein –SH groups. The maximal absorption of iron occurs in the upper parts of the small intestine, especially the duodenum. Ferrous ions are carried into the mucosal cell by active transport. Once iron is inside the cell, it becomes attached to a **non-ferritin protein carrier**. Iron is then either transferred across the serosal border of the cells, where it is picked up by **transferrin** and carried to various sites in the body, or it remains within the cell, where it stimulates **ferritin** formation by combining with an intracellular protein, **apoferritin**, to form **ferritin**, which is deposited in the mucosal cell (Fig. 2.4).

Normally, 10–15% of the ingested iron is absorbed, i.e. 1–2 mg/day. Absorption depends on two important factors: the size of iron stores and the rate of erythropoiesis. If the former is small or the latter is high, then the rate of absorp-

tion will be increased. In addition, absorption of iron can be decreased by several factors: (i) the presence of phosphates, phytates or oxalates in the diet, as these anions bind and deposit iron in the gut and therefore iron will not be available in the free state for absorption; (ii) surgical removal of the stomach (gastrectomy) or achlorhydria (lack of hydrochloric acid), which decreases iron reduction; and (iii) malabsorption syndromes or any disease that causes steatorrhoea or chronic diarrhoea, which results in decreased absorption of iron.

Transport and storage

When the absorbed iron reaches the plasma it is converted back to the ferric (Fe^{3+}) state. It then combines with a specific iron-binding β-globulin called **transferrin** to form a ferric–protein complex which is the plasma transport form of iron. Transferrin conveys iron to the various body cells for storage or utilization.

Transferrin is a globular protein (molecular weight 86 000) and is normally 30–40% saturated with iron; the remaining 60–70% forms the unsaturated latent iron-binding capacity. The plasma iron level is normally 100–130 μg/100 ml. However, when the transferrin is fully saturated with iron the plasma iron level will be about 300 μg/100 ml. This is called the total iron-binding capacity (TIBC) of plasma (Fig. 2.3).

Iron is stored in the reticuloendothelial cells in the main storage organs for iron, which are the liver, spleen and bone marrow. Iron is stored in two forms: **ferritin** and **haemosiderin**. Ferritin consists of a protein shell of 24 subunits (apoferritin) formed of identical polypeptide chains arranged to form a hollow shell around a central cavity, which contains a variable amount of ferric iron (about 2500 atoms), principally as hydrous ferric oxide-phosphate. Haemosiderin is believed to be an aggregate of ferritin molecules. In iron storage organs, there is always a predominance of ferritin (65%) over haemosiderin (35%) molecules.

Excretion and daily requirements

The body conserves iron very well and, under normal circumstances, little iron is lost. Total daily losses in men are 0.5–1.0 mg and these occur through several routes:

1 *Faeces*. Other than unabsorbed ingested iron, faecal iron comes from desquamated intestinal epithelial cells in addition to small amounts found in bile and saliva.

2 *Skin*. Skin loss consists of desquamated cells, lost hairs and nails and traces of iron in sweat.

3 *Urine*. Urinary loss of iron is negligible.

In women, the monthly menstrual losses are about 15–28 mg iron, i.e. an additional 0.5–1 mg iron/day compared with men. About 400–900 mg of iron are lost by women during pregnancy and childbirth, i.e. approximately an extra 1–2 mg iron/day.

The daily requirements for iron are the amounts of iron needed to be absorbed to meet these losses, bearing in mind that women always have higher requirements than men due to menstruation, pregnancy and childbirth. Periods of growth during infancy, childhood and adolescence involve enlargement of the blood volume to maintain blood flow to the new tissues. During such periods the increased requirements for iron are met by increased absorption of iron from the intestine.

Haemoglobin

Oxygen and some carbon dioxide transport depends almost totally on the presence of the red respiratory pigment haemoglobin in the erythrocytes. Haemoglobin increases the ability of the blood to carry oxygen by 60-fold. Plasma carries 0.3 ml O_2/100 ml while whole blood carries 20 ml/100 ml. This vital function makes haemoglobin one of the most important constituents of higher organisms.

Structure

Haemoglobin (haem + globin) is a conjugated protein with a globular molecule (molecular weight 64 000) composed of four subunits (two α and two β chains); each unit contains a red **iron–porphyrin** or **haem** group bound to a polypeptide chain. The iron in the haem is in the divalent (ferrous, Fe^{2+}) state and can combine reversibly with

oxygen to form oxyhaemoglobin without change in the valency of iron. The polypeptide chains are collectively called **globin**.

Types of normal haemoglobin

Adult haemoglobin (HbA)

All haemoglobins have one pair of amino acid chains in common, alpha (α) chains, each made up of 141 amino acids. In HbA, α chains are paired with beta (β) chains of 146 amino acids each. HbA constitutes 98% of the haemoglobin in healthy adults.

Haemoglobin A_2 (HbA$_2$)

In HbA$_2$ the globin moiety is composed of two α and two δ chains. The δ chains consist of 146 amino acids, 10 of which are different from those of the β chain in HbA (hence the name delta chain). HbA$_2$ is present in very small amounts at birth and reaches the adult level of about 2% during the first year of life.

Haemoglobin F (HbF)

This is the major respiratory pigment during intrauterine life. It has two α chains and two gamma (γ) chains. Like the β chains, the γ chains are made up of 146 amino acids each. However, 37 amino acid residues are different from those of the β chain. At birth, 80–90% of the total haemoglobin is haemoglobin F. It then falls rapidly to about 5% at 6 months being replaced by HbA. A level of 1% may be detected at puberty and adulthood.

Functions

1 *Carriage of oxygen* is the most important property of haemoglobin. When haemoglobin is exposed to oxygen, two atoms of oxygen are taken up by each subunit molecule of haemoglobin to form oxyhaemoglobin.

2 *Carriage of carbon dioxide*. Reduced haemoglobin combines reversibly with carbon dioxide to form carbaminohaemoglobin:

$$Hb + CO_2 \rightleftharpoons HbCO_2$$

3 *Buffer*. Haemoglobin, being a protein, acts as one of the buffers in blood, accounting for about 70% of its buffering power.

Haemoglobin can also combine with gases other than oxygen and carbon dioxide. For example, Hb has greater (250 times) affinity to carbon monoxide than to oxygen. Treatment of carbon monoxide poisoning is to give pure O_2 at high pressure (hyperbaric oxygen).

Smokers of tobacco are reported to have about 5% of the haemoglobin or more combined with carbon monoxide.

Breakdown

The life of the haemoglobin molecule ends with the end of the lifespan of erythrocytes. Haemoglobin is broken down into its components—globin and haem.

Fate of the haem group

After the extrusion of iron, the rest of the molecule is converted to **biliverdin**, which undergoes reduction to **bilirubin**. Both substances are named **bile pigments**, as they are excreted in bile. Bilirubin is poorly soluble in water. Once it is released from the reticuloendothelial system into the plasma, it is bound to albumin, which greatly increases its solubility, and in the bound form bilirubin is carried to the liver. It is conjugated with glucuronic acid in the liver cells and this step renders bilirubin water-soluble. It is then excreted in bile into the small intestine, where it is converted by bacterial action to **urobilinogen**. Some of the urobilinogen remains in the small intestine and gives the stool its characteristic orange-brown colour. The rest is absorbed into the bloodstream and is eventually excreted by the kidneys in urine.

Jaundice

Jaundice is a yellowish colour of the skin, sclera and other tissues due to the accumulation of excess bilirubin in the plasma and tissue fluids. The normal adult total plasma bilirubin range is 0.5–1.0 mg/100 ml. The yellow pigmentation is not obvious until the plasma concentration of bilirubin exceeds 2 mg/100 ml.

An excess of bilirubin in the plasma can result from three causes:
1 Excessive breakdown of erythrocytes—haemolytic jaundice (prehepatic).
2 Infective or toxic damage to the liver—hepatic jaundice.
3 Obstruction to the outflow of bile from the liver—obstructive jaundice (posthepatic).

Anaemia

Anaemia is defined as a decrease in the concentration of haemoglobin in the blood below the normal level for the same sex and age. Accordingly, anaemia may occur if the number of red cells (red cell count) falls below the normal level or if the erythrocyte count is normal but their load of haemoglobin (mean corpuscular haemoglobin (MCH)) is less than normal. A patient suffering from anaemia usually complains of tiredness and easy fatigability on minor physical effort. These and other symptoms of anaemia are due to the decrease in the oxygen supply to the tissues.

Causes and classification of anaemia

1 *Blood loss*, whether acute, as in haemorrhage following a car accident, or chronic, which occurs in chronic bleeding in the gastrointestinal tract, e.g. piles, peptic ulcer or the presence of worms, particularly hookworms, in the intestine.

2 *Diminished red cell production by the bone marrow.* This may occur in the following situations:

(a) Deficiency of a nutritional substance(s) required for erythropoiesis (nutritional anaemia). Iron deficiency causes the marrow to produce cells smaller in size than normal (microcytes) and with a small load of haemoglobin, since iron is an integral component of the haemoglobin molecule. The cells therefore have a lighter red colour than normal (hypochromic). Iron-deficiency anaemia is described as **microcytic hypochromic** anaemia. It is the commonest type of anaemia in the developing countries and is mainly due to a deficiency of iron in the diet or blood loss. It is particularly likely to occur in children and adolescents due to the demands of growth, and in women of child-bearing age due to blood losses during menstruation and childbirth.

Deficiencies of vitamin B_{12} and folic acid cause megaloblastic anaemia. Dietary deficiency is almost unknown. However, deficiency occurs as a result of malabsorption (see Chapter 8). Folic acid deficiency in the diet is also common in tropical countries, where the resulting anaemia is prevalent in malnourished children and in women during pregnancy, when the general body requirements for folic acid increase.

(b) Diminished red cell production may occur when the bone marrow space is occupied by secondary cancer cells or fibrous tissues, as in myelosclerosis, or as a result of destruction by radiation or drugs (**aplastic anaemia**).

3 *Excessive destruction of red cells (haemolytic anaemia).* The factors causing destruction may be within the red cells, e.g. presence of an abnormal haemoglobin such as HbS, due to which the cells take a sickle or crescent shape when exposed to low oxygen tension. These sickle cells have a short lifespan as they are readily broken down and removed by the reticuloendothelial system. **Sickle-cell anaemia** is very common in the tropics particularly in people of West African origin.

The cause of haemolysis may come from outside the red cells, e.g. blood group incompatibility, where an antibody may react with a blood group antigen present in the red cell membrane, resulting in agglutination and haemolysis of red cells.

Polycythaemia

Polycythaemia is an increase in the number of red blood cells per unit volume of blood.

Classification

1 *True or absolute polycythaemia*, characterized by an increase in the total number of circulating red cells (red cell mass). It is of two types:

(a) *Primary or polycythaemia rubra vera*, where bone marrow continues to produce red cells with no regard to the normal physiological negative feedback mechanism of the hormone erythropoietin.

(b) *Secondary polycythaemia*, due to hypoxia, as in high altitudes and chronic respiratory or cardiac disease. This type of polycythaemia is characterized by high levels of **erythropoietin** released in response to hypoxia.

2 *Relative polycythaemia* occurs in cases of dehydration due to excessive fluid loss (vomiting or sweating) or decreased water intake. Plasma volume is decreased and consequently the red cells are concentrated (haemoconcentration). Thus, there is no increase in the red cell mass but the ratio of cells to plasma is high.

Leucocytes

Classification

The blood leucocytes (white blood cells) are a heterogeneous population of nucleated cells lacking haemoglobin. There are five distinct morphological types classified into two groups on the basis of the presence or absence of granules in their cytoplasm:

1 **Granulocytes** (with cytoplasmic granules): these are the neutrophils, eosinophils and basophils.

2 **Agranulocytes** (without cytoplasmic granules): these are the monocytes and lymphoctyes.

Figure 2.5 gives the dimensions and morphological characteristics of the leucocytes.

Neutrophil 40–60%	Eosinophil 0.5–1%	Basophil 0.5–1%	Monocyte 6–10%	Lymphocyte 20–40%
Morphological features:				
Diameter 10–16μm	Diameter 12–18μm	Diameter 10–14μm	Diameter 15–20μm	Diameter 5–8μm (small lymphocyte) 9–15μg (medium and large lymphocyte)
Nucleus: Lobulated (2–5 lobes) connected by chromatin strands. Nucleus is made of dense masses which take the purple stain	Made usually of 2 lobes – stains less deeply than neutrophil	Rarely segmented and its margins are usually obscured by the overlying cytoplasmic granules	Usually kidney shaped. Nuclear chromatin made of interwoven threads which are without compact blocks. Stains faintly	Rounded or slightly indented. Nuclear chromatin is clumped in the form of dark masses
Cytoplasm: Contains fine granules which stain purplish	Contains the characteristic large spherical bright red granules	Contains large coarse rounded or oval dark deeply staining granules which overlie the nucleus	Grey-blue giving a ground glass appearance with fine reddish azurphilic granules	Large lymphocyte has abundant cytoplasm which usually takes pale blue stain and may contain fine reddish granules

Small lymphocyte has a very scanty cytoplasm forming a small rim around the nucleus |

Fig. 2.5 The shapes, dimensions and special morphological features of the various types of leucocytes.

Formation of leucocytes (leucopoiesis)

Sites of formation

1 **Granulocytes**: bone marrow.
2 **Lymphocytes**: bone marrow, thymus, lymph nodes and other collections of lymphoid tissues, e.g. wall of the intestine.
3 **Monocytes**: bone marrow.

Formation of granulocytes (granulopoiesis)

The life history of the granulocytes begins in the bone marrow, where there is progressive division and maturation from the earliest cell, the stem cell, successively through the cell types myeloblast, promyelocyte, myelocyte, metamyelocyte, band neutrophil and segmented neutrophil. The myeloblasts, promyelocytes and myelocytes are capable of mitotic division and cell replication; hence, these are collectively called the **proliferating granulocyte pool**. From the metamyelocyte stage onwards, no cell division occurs and therefore the metamyelocytes, band neutrophils and segmented neutrophils are together referred to as the **maturation pool**. Maturation takes the form of biochemical and morphological changes in both the nucleus and the cytoplasm. The nucleus becomes condensed and broken up into lobes. In addition, fine neutrophilic granules appear in the cytoplasm. The maturation pool is sometimes called the **marrow granulocyte reserve**, as it is believed to be the main source of extra neutrophils which enter the bloodstream in acute infections and other pathological states. The mature neutrophils, once released into the bloodstream, stay there for about 7–10 hours before they migrate to the tissues, where they function as mobile phagocytes.

Haemopoietic growth factors

The formation of all blood cells is sustained throughout life by a group of glycoprotein growth factors, the *haemopoietic growth factors* (collectively called *colony-stimulating factors*, **CSF**). The first to be discovered was erythropoietin. Others which control the production of white blood cells include: multipotential CSF, granulocyte–macrophage CSF and granulocyte CSF. Recently, these growth factors have found important clinical uses by stimulating the bone marrow activity in disease conditions such as bone marrow failure, haematological malignancies and infectious diseases.

Neutrophils in the bloodstream

Mature neutrophils leave the bone marrow to enter the blood. Some of them join the blood circulation—the so-called **circulating granulocyte pool**. These are the cells available for blood sampling and counting. Others are deposited along the walls of the small vessels (**marginal granulocyte pool**), where they are in a state of rapid and continuous exchange with the circulating cells, and from this site they can be mobilized by exercise or by an adrenaline (epinephrine) injection. The entry of these cells into the circulating pool accounts for the increased white cell count (leucocytosis) that accompanies exercise and other stressful situations.

Functions of leucocytes

The general function of leucocytes is defence against infection. However, the different types of leucocytes contribute to a different extent towards this general function.

Functions of neutrophils

The neutrophils are also called **polymorphonuclear leucocytes** because the nucleus is formed of two to five lobes. This cell is the most important cell in the cellular defences of the body against infection. To achieve this goal, neutrophils execute several integrated functions: (i) the neutrophils must reach the site of infection (**chemotaxis**); (ii) they must ingest the foreign organism (**phagocytosis**); and (iii) they must kill or inhibit the multiplication of the microorganism (**microbial killing**).

Chemotaxis

The neutrophils are actively motile cells; they can move more rapidly than any other cell in the body. Their movement is directed towards bacteria in a purposeful manner, being attracted to bacteria or the site of infection or inflammation by a variety of chemotactic substances, e.g. products of certain bacteria, damaged leucocytes or other tissue components. The property of directed movement of the neutrophils is named **chemotaxis**. It accounts for the accumulation of neutrophils at sites where they are needed, e.g. infected wounds. Impaired chemotaxis can lead to increased susceptibility to infectious diseases, especially in children.

When neutrophils approach the infected site, they lie along the walls of the closest capillaries—a process called **margination**. Then individual neutrophils squeeze themselves between endothelial cells and gradually move out from the capillary—a process called **diapedesis**. Since neutrophils are motile cells, they move towards the bacteria.

Phagocytosis

Phagocytosis is the process whereby a cell eats particulate matter (Fig. 2.6).

Fig. 2.6 Schematic diagram of the process of phagocytosis by a neutrophil. An opsonized microbe (M) after being recognized by the neutrophil is contained in an invagination of the neutrophil membrane. Thereafter, the particle is enclosed in a phagocytic vacuole. Some of the neutrophil granules (G) stick to the wall of the vacuole and then release their bactericidal substances, which induce killing and ultimate digestion of the microbe.

One of the remarkable features of neutrophils is their fine capacity to distinguish foreign cells like bacteria from homologous body cells and aged or damaged cells from fresh ones. This is due to the presence in plasma of certain substances (**opsonins**), such as **γ-globulins** (especially immunoglobulin G (IgG)) and **complement C4**, which coat bacteria and ageing cells, thereby making them 'palatable' to neutrophils. To opsonize means to prepare for eating. An opsonin is an agent in plasma which acts on foreign particles to increase their palatability to phagocytes.

Recognition is followed by close adhesion between the outer membrane of the neutrophil and the bacterium. This is followed by invasion of the neutrophil membrane and complete encirclement of the bacterium by pseudopodia. The pseudopodia fuse to enclose the bacterium in a phagocytic vacuole.

Microbial killing

Following the ingestion (phagocytosis) of the bacterium, the following sequence of events take place:

1 The fusion of the neutrophilic granules with the phagocytic vacuole.

2 Discharge of antimicrobial agents from the granules into the vacuole. These agents include lysozymes, myeloperoxidase and lactoferrin, which are capable of destroying a wide range of bacteria.

3 Killing and digestion of the ingested organism.

Functions of eosinophils (acidophils)

The eosinophils are characterized by the presence of coarse, bright red granules in their cytoplasm. These granules contain an arginine-rich basic protein which attracts red acidic dyes like eosin. The eosinophil nucleus is often seen as two large lobes. Eosinophil functions are not very different from those of the neutrophil.

Chemotaxis

Unlike neutrophils, eosinophils are attracted more towards areas of chronic inflammation rather than acute inflammation. **Chemotactic substances** for eosinophils include histamine, antigen–antibody complexes, 5-hydroxytryptamine (5-HT), bradykinin and a specific 'eosinophil chemotactic factor'.

Eosinophils tend to accumulate at the sites of histamine release, as is seen in allergic diseases of the skin or lungs.

Phagocytosis

Eosinophils are capable of ingesting a variety of particles, ranging from bacteria and destroyed cells to antigen–antibody complexes. Phagocytosis involves the same sequence of events as already described for neutrophils. However, antimicrobial activity is considerably less than that of the neutrophil. Eosinophils also release **major basic protein** (MBP) which is highly toxic to larvae of parasites.

Eosinophils and inflammation

In inflamed tissues, eosinophils have been shown to be capable of antagonizing and inactivating histamine and other chemical mediators of inflammation, such as 5-HT and bradykinin. Through this function, the eosinophil helps to limit and circumscribe the inflammatory process.

The eosinophilic response to an inflammatory stimulus is characterized by accumulation of eosinophils in the inflamed tissues, with a simultaneous increase both in the production of eosinophils by the bone marrow and in the number of circulating eosinophils (eosinophilia), on their way from the bone marrow to the inflammatory sites. Chronic eosinophilia occurs in response to complex antigens, as in helminthic (worm) infestations (e.g. hookworm, ascaris and bilharzia) and in response to allografts (e.g. skin grafts).

The accumulation of eosinophils in inflammatory sites may be inhibited by high doses of corticosteroids, which also depress the chemotactic attraction of eosinophils.

Eosinophilia

From the foregoing account we may deduce that eosinophilia occurs in pathological states as a result of an antigen—antibody reaction.

Common causes of eosinophilia include:

1 Parasitic disease, e.g. worm infestations of the gut.
2 Allergic conditions:
   (a) Bronchial asthma.
   (b) Allergic rhinitis (hay fever).
   (c) Drug reactions, e.g. penicillin sensitivity.
3 Tropical eosinophilia, which represents a reaction to the filaria parasite.
4 Dermatological diseases.

Functions of basophils

The distinguishing morphological feature of the basophil is the large blue-black granules which appear to fill the cytoplasm, overlie the nucleus and tend to obscure nuclear configuration. Basophil granules contain abundant acid mucopolysaccharide, which accounts for their strong affinity for basic dyes such as methylene blue. Heparin is one of the important acid mucopolysaccharide constituents; other constituents include histamine, 5-HT and ribonucleic acid (RNA). The basophil is the carrier of **histamine** in the blood and, due to its being rich in both heparin and histamine, it bears a strong resemblance to **tissue mast cells**. The function of basophils is not known with certainty but they may have a role related to their content of the physiologically active substances, such as heparin, histamine and 5-HT. Mast cells and basophils have surface Igt receptors which bind IgE coated antigens, degranulate and release histamine leading to allergic reactions e.g. urticaria.

Monocytes (blood macrophages)

This macrophage has its origin in the bone marrow monoblast and promonocyte. The mature monocyte reaches the bloodstream, where it stays for a variable period of time, ranging from a few hours to 6 days. Then it leaves the circulation for the tissues, where it undergoes transformation to the larger and more effective phagocyte—**tissue macrophage (histiocyte)**.

Functions

The macrophage contributes directly to the body defence systems by phagocytosis and killing of invading bacteria and, indirectly, by interacting and cooperating with lymphoid cells in both the afferent (or recognition of foreign material) and efferent (effector) limbs of the **immune response**. In the afferent limb, macrophages process the antigen and present it to lymphocytes.

Macrophages phagocytose damaged or altered host cells and microscopic debris, which justifies the descriptive name '**tissue scavengers**'.

Lymphocytes

Much of our knowledge about the cellular elements of the blood has been based on the concept that cells may be recognized and classified by morphological criteria. This concept, however, does not hold in relation to recognizing and classifying cells of the lymphoid series. The blood lymphocytes constitute a family of cells of different origins, migration patterns, sizes, staining characteristics, ultrastructure, lifespan and function.

Formation (lymphopoiesis)

Lymphocytes originate from the primitive unipotent stem cell (lymphoid-committed precursor) in the **thymus, lymphoid tissues** and **bone marrow** and then proceed along a known maturation line via the 'lymphocyte production pathway', which includes the following cellular stages:

1 *Lymphoblasts*. Normally these are only seen in lymphopoietic organs and almost never observed in peripheral blood.
2 *Intermediate (transitional) forms* (large blast cells).
3 *Small and large lymphocytes* (blood lymphocytes).

These stages are not unidirectional. The process can, under certain circumstances, go in the reverse direction and small lymphocytes can grow into large lymphocytes and lymphoblasts. Such blastic transformation can be demonstrated *in vitro* by growing small lymphocytes in a suitable culture medium containing a non-specific mitogen, such as *phytohaemagglutinin (PHA)*, or a specific antigen, e.g. *tuberculin*.

Lymphocytes in the bloodstream

Lymphocytes enter the peripheral blood either directly, by passing through the walls of blood-vessels in the various lymphopoietic organs, or indirectly, by entering the lymph stream and eventually reaching the bloodstream through the thoracic duct and other lymph ducts in the neck.

Classification

When seen under an ordinary light microscope, blood lymphocytes can be divided into **small** (5–8 μm diameter) and **large lymphocytes** (8–15 μm diameter). The majority of blood lymphocytes are of the small type.

Functions

Lymphocytes are the central cells in immunity. On the

basis of this function, lymphocytes are divided into two types:

1 *Thymus-dependent lymphocytes (T cells)* are so called because they originate in the thymus or bone marrow and migrate to the thymus where they mature and are reprogrammed to recognize foreign antigens. They have a lifespan of 100–300 days or even more (hence the name long-lived lymphocytes). This long lifespan is closely related to their property of constant movement from blood to tissues to lymph to blood again (*recirculation of lymphocytes*).

T lymphocytes are the principal mediators of **cellular immune responses,** such as rejection of tissue graft, e.g. kidney transplant, and delayed hypersensitivity reactions. They also play a minor role in the synthesis of immunoglobulins (antibodies).

2 *Thymus-independent lymphocytes (B cells).* In humans, the B cells develop in the bone marrow, the germinal centres of lymph nodes and the red pulp of the spleen. Their lifespan is 2–7 days (hence the name short-lived lymphocytes). They have been called B cells because they are known as bursa cells. When the B cells are properly stimulated by an antigen, they develop successively into large lymphocytes and, lastly, plasma cells. The plasma cells are lymphoid cells which are capable of producing **antibodies.** Thus, the B lymphocytes are the principal mediators of the **humoral immune response.**

Total leucocyte count

Although it is usually quoted in textbooks that the total leucocyte count is 4000 to 10 000 cells per cubic millimetre of blood, it should be emphasized that this range applies more to Europeans than to residents of hot tropical countries. It is not uncommon to find a total leucocyte count among healthy students and blood donors in these geographical locations of between 2000 and 4000 cells/mm³. Because there is a relatively low count of neutrophils, this is called *neutropenia.*

Differential white cell counts

The normal proportions of white blood cells are as follows:

Neutrophils	60–70%
Lymphocytes	20–30%
Monocytes	2–8%
Eosinophils	2–4%
Basophils	0–2%

Leucocytosis and leucopenia

An increase in the total leucocyte count above the normal is called leucocytosis. This may occur in health (physiological leucocytosis) or disease.

Physiological leucocytosis may occur under several conditions:

1 Diurnal variation: leucocyte counts are lowest in the morning and increase to a maximum in the afternoon.

2 After a protein meal.

3 Following physical exercise.

4 Stimulation by stress or an injection of adrenaline (epinephrine).

Disease states which commonly cause leucocytosis are bacterial infections (pyogenic infections), e.g. tonsillitis, infected wounds or inflamed appendix. In these conditions, measurement of the total leucocyte count is essential for diagnosing the existence of the infection. The differential white cell count is also useful. In general, acute bacterial infections cause an increase in the neutrophil count, while chronic and viral infections are associated with an increased lymphocyte count.

Leucopenia is a decrease in the total leucocyte count below the normal. It is often seen in conditions of malnutrition and is also an important feature of typhoid fever. Some drugs may depress the bone marrow and therefore result in leucopenia and, in particular, a decrease in the granulocyte count (agranulocytosis). Leucopenia can also be caused by a deficiency of vitamin B_{12} or folic acid.

Leukaemia

Neoplastic growth of the stem cells in the bone marrow or lymphoid tissue leads to myeloid or lymphocytic leukaemia, respectively. Leukaemia can be acute or chronic, depending on the time course of the disease. The total white cell count is usually very high (> 50 000 mm³). The leucocyte precursors in the bone marrow proliferate extensively and occupy more and more bone marrow space, resulting in a concomitant depression in the production of red cells, leading to anaemia, and of platelets, leading to thrombocytopenia and the risk of bleeding. The causes of the leukaemias are not fully understood, but among the known factors are chromosomal abnormalities, radiation and chemical agents, including drugs and some viruses.

The reticuloendothelial system (macrophage system)

The term macrophage was first used by Metchnikoff to refer to large mononuclear phagocytes to distinguish them from the smaller neutrophil polymorphs—microphages. He established the concept of phagocytosis and intracellular digestion as the essential primary mechanism of defence against bacterial agents. Afterwards, the term reticuloendothelial system was introduced by Aschoff and Landon in 1924 to refer to cells which take the vital stain trypan blue when injected into experimental animals. These cells included certain endothelial cells and reticular cells in addition to some macrophages. Thus, the concept was established that there is a system of cells within the body whose function is to collect, by a process of active phagocytosis, finely particulate material such as dyes or colloidal particles.

Cellular components

1 Macrophages lining lymph sinuses in lymph nodes and blood sinuses in the liver (Kupffer cells), spleen, bone marrow, adrenal cortex and anterior lobe of the pituitary gland. It is important to realize that ordinary vascular endothelium (blood or lymph) is not phagocytic. This highly specialized function is reserved for the endothelium lining the sites mentioned above.
2 Reticular cells of lymph nodes, spleen and bone marrow.
3 Tissue macrophages (histioytes): distributed widely throughout solid tissues.
4 Blood macrophages (monocytes).
Monocytes and histiocytes are sometimes referred to as mobile reticuloendothelial cells, i.e. the reticular and endothelial macrophages.

The reticuloendothelial system is, therefore, not a sharply defined system, either anatomically or physiologically, and its component cells have great powers of proliferation and regeneration. Furthermore, because of their wide distribution, reticuloendothelial cells have ready access to foreign particles that circulate in the bloodstream, as well as to materials which originate interstitially and find their way into lymphatics.

Functions

1 Phagocytosis of bacteria and any foreign particles, the remains of dead tissue cells, erythrocytes, leucocytes, etc.
2 Breakdown of haemoglobin and the formation of bile pigments.
3 Assisting the immune system by the processing of antigens and their presentation to lymphocytes (see the immune response below).
4 Storage of iron.

The basis of immunity

the human body is in constant threat from foreign organisms that have a great potential to cause disease. To meet these threats there exists in the body a special defensive (homoeostatic) mechanism of immense potentiality which is mobilized when the body is invaded by foreign organisms and which is especially adapted to respond to the effects of the particular invader in question. This special mechanism is immunity. Its study (immunology) is of great importance in the understanding of disease processes and their prevention.

The immune system

The immune system consists of a series of specialized cells localized in tissues and organs throughout the body, e.g. the thymus, lymph nodes, spleen, bone marrow and the wall of the gastrointestinal tract. This system enables the human body to respond by means of cellular or humoral factors to the harmful effects of foreign macromolecules, e.g. bacteria, that get access to the internal environment and tend to alter its basic characteristics (the constancy of the internal environment), as is seen in disease conditions. The immune system is, therefore, one of the important *homoeostatic* mechanisms that maintain normal health and prevent disease.

In addition, the immunological defences operate against transplanted tissues and organs as well as malignant tumours or cancerous growth in the body. On all these fronts, the immune system specifically recognizes and selectively eliminates the foreign invader and neutralizes its harmful toxic products.

Immunocompetent cells

Immunocompetent cells are cells capable of responding to contact with an antigen by manifesting or developing a specific cellular or humoral immunological capacity. These cells are equipped with cell surface receptors which are specific to given antigens. They also possess the mechanisms to respond to antigenic stimulation. Immunocompetent cells are lymphocytes, sometimes called virgin lymphocytes, of which there are two functionally distinct types: B lymphocytes, responsible for humoral immune responses, and T lymphocytes, which mediate the cellular immune responses.

The immune response

An antigen is a substance capable of invoking a specific immunological response. It may be part of a virus, a bacterium or a transplanted or foreign tissue cell. Chemically, antigens may be proteins, polysaccharides, nucleic acids or a combination of these. It is now known that for any antigen there exists one or more genetically predetermined immunocompetent cells that can be stimulated to elicit an immune response. The antigen is recognized by the immunocompetent cells, either directly or after being processed by macrophages (Fig. 2.7).

Fig. 2.7 Schematic representation of the interaction of an antigen (AG) with: (i) B lymphocyte (B cell), which is activated to proliferate to a large pyroninophilic (pyron.) cell, which ultimately gives rise to an antibody-producing cell, i.e. humoral immune response; and (ii) T lymphocyte (T cell), which is stimulated to proliferate to become an activated T cell (effector cell or sensitized lymphocyte), the mediator of the cellular immune response. MAC, macrophage: helps in the processing of the antigen in the early stage of the immune response.

Antibody (immunoglobulin) is a γ-globulin produced by special immunocompetent cells (plasma cells). Immunoglobulins have the property of interacting specifically with and binding the antigen in response to which they have been produced.

When an organism is first exposed to an antigen, a **primary immune response** is elicited, after a latent period due to division, proliferation and maturation of immunocompetent cells. It reaches a maximum in 1–2 weeks after exposure to the antigen. A good example is vaccinations, e.g. against smallpox or yellow fever. Usually the vaccination will be taken as effective only after the latent period has passed.

Upon re-exposure to the same antigen that provokes the primary response, the **secondary immune response** is obtained, which is more brisk. Its latent period is shorter and the antibody level rises faster and higher than in the primary response. This is because a large number of responsive cells become available to react with the antigen. The secondary immune response has given rise to the idea that the body has acquired some sort of immunological memory of the antigen due to the production of memory cells (Fig. 2.7). These memory cells have the capacity to produce both effector and memory cells upon subsequent stimulation by the original antigen.

Humoral immune response (Fig. 2.7)
B lymphocytes have surface receptors for the interaction with the antigen. When the cell binds with the antigen,

it is stimulated to proliferate and develop into large pyroninophilic cells, which may divide and ultimately give rise to the mature plasma cell. Plasma cells are individually capable of secreting one specific **antibody** or **immunoglobulin**. The antibody initiates the destruction of the antigen and promotes its removal by the phagocytic cells of the reticuloendothelial system. Antibody production is the manifestation of the **humoral immune response**.

The antigen–antibody reaction is designed to oppose the antigen as a threat to the human body. The reaction takes many forms, including neutralization, precipitation, agglutination and lysis.

Antibodies are responsible for this desirable reaction, which participates in the killing of the microbe and the neutralization of its harmful effects. However, they also have several forms of heightened reactivity to antigens collectively, named immediate-type hypersensitivity (or allergy). This is commonly seen in individuals allergic to dust, pollen of flowers or certain drugs, such as penicillin.

While executing these functions, antibodies do not work on their own but get the help of the reticuloendothelial system and other phagocytic cells in the blood. The complement system is a complex group of enzymes in normal blood that work together with antibodies and play an important role as mediators of both immune and allergic reactions.

The cellular immune response
On contact with the antigen, T lymphocytes proliferate and

give rise to several types of effector cells with heightened reactivity towards the antigen. This reactivity is expressed in a variety of properties of these effector cells, among which are the following:

1 They are directly cytotoxic (cytotoxic T cells) and are capable of the destruction of foreign cells, which are eventually phagocytosed by macrophages, monocytes and neutrophils.

2 They help B lymphocytes and cytotoxic T cells to differentiate and proliferate—hence the name helper T cells.

3 They secrete a variety of polypeptides called **cytokines**, which are capable of: (i) attracting macrophages and other phagocytic cells to the site of antigen–antibody reactions; (ii) stimulating further division and proliferation of lymphocytes, especially B lymphocytes; (iii) inflicting damage on all cells except lymphocytes; and (iv) attacking a variety of viruses, thus preventing viral replication. The cytokines with the latter ability, called interferon, have received much attention in view of their potential therapeutic use as an antiviral and also anticancer agent.

Cellular immunity is actively involved in the following:

1 Rejection of tissue or organ grafts, e.g. kidney transplant.

2 Delayed hypersensitivity reactions, e.g. tuberculin reaction.

3 Antitumour immunity, which involves the cellular immune mechanism in the defence against mutant or cancer cells.

4 Cooperation with B cells in humoral immune responses.

The acquired immune deficiency syndrome (AIDS)

In a healthy person the cellular immune responses are performed with a predominance of circulating T-helper lymphocytes (T4 or CD4 cells) over T-suppressor lymphocytes (T8 or CD8 cells); the normal ratio is 2 : 1. The AIDS virus selectively destroys and therefore causes a decrease in the number of **T-helper cells** and a reversal in the T-helper/T-suppressor cell ratio, with T-suppressor cells predominating. This results in generalized inhibition of the immune system and the affected person therefore loses resistance against infective agents, e.g. bacteria, viruses, etc.

Plasma proteins

Blood plasma contains 91% water and 9% solids, of which 7% are proteins and the rest are inorganic salts (mainly sodium and bicarbonate), in addition to substances being transported from one part of the body to another.

Types of plasma proteins

Plasma proteins are divided into three types with average concentrations (in g/100 ml) as follows:

Albumin	4.8
Globulins	2.3
Fibrinogen	0.3
Total	7.4

Albumin (molecular weight = 69 000)

Albumin is synthesized by the liver. Ten to 12 grams are produced each day and it has a half-life of 20 days. Because albumin is a relatively small molecule, plasma albumin accounts for 80–90% of the plasma colloid osmotic pressure (25 mmHg) although it makes up about 60% of the total plasma protein mass. Therefore, albumin is important in the formation and absorption of tissue fluids and in preserving a fluid balance between blood and tissues. When the concentration of plasma albumin falls to low levels, less than 2 g/100 ml (**hypoalbuminaemia**), fluids leave the circulation readily and accumulate in excessive amounts in the interstitial compartment, leading to oedema. The commonest cause of hypoalbuminaemia in tropical countries is decreased intake of protein, as seen in children with malnutrition. Liver disease, with gross damage to liver cells, results in decreased synthesis of albumin. Kidney disease (nephrotic syndrome) results in excessive losses of albumin in the urine.

Albumin plays a role in the transportation of calcium, bilirubin and sulphonamides in the blood.

Globulins (molecular weight = 90 000–1 300 000)

On the basis of electrophoretic mobility, globulins are subdivided into α_1-, α_2-, β- and γ-globulins. Alpha- and β-globulins are synthesized in the liver and γ-globulins in the reticuloendothelial system by plasma cells.

Transport function of α- and β-globulins. Alpha-globulins transport lipoproteins, lipids, hormones (cortisol-binding globulin, CBG; thyrozine-binding globulin, TBG) and bilirubin in plasma.

Beta-globulins transport lipoproteins, lipids, cholesterol, iron (transferrin) and copper (ceruloplasmin).

The binding of vitamins A, D and K and some hormones by plasma proteins prevents them from being filtered in the kidney and lost in urine and also provides a stable blood reservoir of hormones on which tissues can draw.

Gamma-globulins (immunoglobulins). All the known antibodies are **γ-globulins**. The newborn child is protected by globulins which cross the placenta from the maternal to the fetal circulation. Local immunity is conferred to the gastrointestinal tract via colostrum (first breast milk), which contains a special type of immunoglobulin

Table 2.1 Cell antigens, plasma agglutinins and genotypes of the ABO blood groups.

Blood group	Antigen or agglutinogen in the red cells	Antibodies or agglutinins in plasma	Genotype
A	A	Anti-B (B)	AA, AO
B	B	Anti-A (A)	BB, BO
AB	A and B	—	AB
O	None	Anti-A and anti-B	OO

(IgA). By 6–9 months the infant is able to produce his/her own immunoglobulins (IgG, IgM, IgD, IgE), which give **active** immunity against a variety of diseases. Solutions of γ-globulins are used therapeutically to give **passive** immunity.

A number of proteins with specific physiological functions have been isolated from the globulin fraction, e.g. prothrombin, transferrin, plasminogen, haptoglobins and many others. Haptoglobins are a group of globulins which have the distinctive property of binding free haemoglobin in the plasma. When there is excessive destruction of erythrocytes, free haemoglobin is picked up by haptoglobin, which can bind up to 150 mg Hb/100 ml blood and pass it to the reticuloendothelial system. When free haemoglobin levels exceed haptoglobin binding capacity, free haemoglobin appears in the urine (haemoglobinuria).

Summary of the functions of plasma proteins

1 Transport functions (α- and β-globulins).
2 Defensive (immunoglobulins).
3 Reserve of body proteins.
4 Osmotic function (albumin) through control of the exchange of fluid between blood and tissues.
5 Viscosity of plasma is due mainly to fibrinogen and globulins.
6 Fibrinogen is the precursor of fibrin in the blood clot. Prothrombin is an α_2-globulin and most of the remaining clotting factors are β-globulins.

The blood groups

On the surface of human red blood cells are found a series of genetically determined glycoproteins and glycolipids that act as blood group antigens. They appear in early fetal life and remain unchanged throughout life. More than 100 blood antigens have been described, out of which at least 15 well-defined red blood cell group systems exist in most racial groups. Of these, only two are of major importance in clinical medicine—the ABO and rhesus (Rh) systems.

The ABO system

The ABO system depends on whether the *red cells* of an individual contain one, both or neither of the two blood group antigens A and B. Therefore, there are four main ABO groups: A, B, AB and O (Table 2.1).

These blood antigens are also called agglutinogens since, in the presence of the respective antibody (agglutinin), agglutination of red blood cells occurs.

The plasma may contain antibodies (agglutinins) against the A and B antigens: anti-A or alpha, anti-B or beta. These agglutinins are not present at birth but they appear between the 2nd and 8th month of life, most probably in response to A and/or B antigens taken in food of animal origin, especially meat, and in some bacteria. The anti-A and anti-B antibodies are described as **naturally occurring antibodies**. In the blood of any individual, the antibody present is the reciprocal of the antigen. Therefore, the ABO system can be defined with respect to both the characteristic antigen present on the red cells and the characteristic antibody present in the plasma or serum.

Inheritance of blood groups (Table 2.1)

The inheritance of the A and B antigens is dictated by the A and B genes. The O gene does not produce any demonstrable red cell antigen. This is the reason why group A genotype can be AA (homozygous) or AO (heterozygous). Similarly, for group B the possible genotype is BB or BO, while for blood group O the only possible genotype is OO. Group AB has both A and B genes and the only possible genotype is AB. Knowledge of these genotypes is useful in working out the probable blood group of an offspring on the basis of the knowledge of the blood genotypes of the father and mother. It is also helpful in sorting out disputed parentage of the child.

Frequency distribution of blood groups

The frequency of the different blood groups in the ABO system varies widely in different ethnic groups, as is shown in Table 2.2.

Table 2.2 Distribution of the ABO blood groups in different ethnic populations (%).

	A	B	AB	O
Europeans	40	8	2	50
Arabs	27	20	4	49
Asians	21	28	7	44
West Africans	26	19	4	51

Table 2.3 Possible combinations that may occur in blood transfusion.

	Donor red cell			
Recipient	AB	A	B	O
AB	–	–	–	–
A	+	–	+	–
B	+	+	–	–
O	+	+	+	–

+, reaction; –, no reaction.

The rhesus (Rh) blood group system

The Rh system is described on the basis of the presence or absence of the rhesus antigen (D) on the surface of red blood cells. If present, the individual is said to be D-positive or Rh-positive; 85% of Europeans, 90–95% of Arabs and Africans and 98% of Asians are Rh- or D-positive. If absent, the individual is described as D- or Rh-negative.

Rhesus antigens

There are at least three sets of alternative antigens in the Rh system: D or d, C or c, E or e. However, D is a strong antigen and therefore clinically more important than the others. In blood banks, Rh grouping is performed with anti-D serum.

Rhesus antibodies

Rhesus antibodies are not naturally occurring antibodies but are described as **immune antibodies**, i.e. developed in response to a known antigenic stimulus. Anti-D antibody may be acquired as a result of immunization resulting from:

1 Transfusion of a Rh-negative individual with Rh-positive blood. This mishap usually occurs if the technician typing the blood in a blood bank makes a clerical error when determining the Rh blood group of either the donor or recipient or when issuing blood to a patient.

2 Presence of a Rh-positive fetus in a Rh-negative mother. Although fetal and maternal circulations are separate, entry of fetal Rh-positive cells into the maternal circulation may occur in the later weeks of pregnancy but mostly at the time of placental separation and delivery of the child. These Rh- or D-positive cells may provoke the production of anti-D.

Importance of blood groups in clinical medicine

Blood transfusion

The importance of blood groups becomes apparent when one considers the necessity of transfusing blood from one individual to another. For a safe blood transfusion, the following steps are followed:

1 The ABO and Rh blood grouping of both donor and recipient should be carried out.

2 When a suitable donor's blood for the recipient is found, a cross-matching test is done. The donor cells are mixed with the recipient's serum to find out whether the recipient's plasma contains an antibody which may react with the donor cells.

Table 2.3 summarizes the possible combinations that may arise in blood transfusion practice. It is clear that group AB recipients, because their plasma contains neither anti-A nor anti-B antibodies, can safely receive blood from donors of all ABO groups—thus the name **universal recipient**. Similarly, group O donors are referred to as **universal donors**, since their cells lack both antigens A and B and therefore their blood can be given safely to recipients of all ABO groups. In the case of the universal recipients, the antibodies anti-A and anti-B in the plasma of group O, A or B donated blood are diluted in group AB recipients' plasma so that the antibodies are unlikely to react with the recipients' cells. For the universal group O donors, the anti-A and anti-B present in the donors' plasma are diluted in the recipients' plasma and therefore will not react with the recipients' cells. However, in recent years haemolytic reactions have arisen due to the use of universal donor blood containing anti-A or anti-B at a high titre. When used for transfusion of patients other than group O, these antibodies react with the recipient cells and cause a haemolytic reaction. The cardinal rule in blood banks nowadays is to transfuse patients with blood of the same ABO group; low-titre group O donors are used as universal donors only in emergency situations.

Similarly, when the universal recipients are transfused with group A, group B or group O blood with a high titre of anti-A or anti-B, a transfusion reaction may occur. Therefore, group AB recipients should always be transfused with group AB blood.

Complications of blood transfusion

Transfusing blood and blood products (fresh frozen plasma, platelet concentrate, etc.) into patients is common hospital practice in accidents and other emergency situations or during surgical operations. Strict precautions are followed before giving blood or any of its products to avoid certain reactions that may accompany their transfusion.

Most of the complications of blood transfusion result from antigen–antibody reactions between donor and recipient (incompatible blood transfusion). The outcome may be haemolytic, allergic or febrile reactions, which may occur at the time of giving blood or may be delayed for days or weeks. Other complications include transmission of disease from the donor to the recipient, e.g. malaria, syphilis, viral hepatitis and the AIDS virus. Nowadays in blood banks, donated blood is routinely screened for the presence of the infective agents that transmit syphilis, viral hepatitis and AIDS.

Rhesus incompatibility between mother and fetus (haemolytic disease of the newborn)

Rhesus incompatibility arises when a Rh-negative woman gets pregnant and the fetus is Rh-positive, having inherited the D gene from the father. As mentioned earlier, the mother may develop anti-D antibody as a result of such an incompatible pregnancy or if she has received incompatible (D+) blood before pregnancy. The first baby usually escapes the effects. Such immune antibodies, usually of the IgG type, may cross the placenta in future pregnancies. If the second fetus is Rh-positive, the immune anti-D may react with and destroy fetal red cells, resulting in the disease called haemolytic disease of the newborn. The fetus may be born with haemolytic anaemia, which, if severe, may necessitate exchange blood transfusion. Blood group O Rh-negative is infused in the newborn at one point while the haemolysed blood is gradually withdrawn from the infant at another point. Haemolytic disease of the newborn has an overall reported incidence of one in 200 of all pregnancies. This figure has decreased further with the use of prophylactic anti-D antibody, which is injected into Rh-negative mothers immediately after delivery of their first Rh-positive child. The injected antibody will react with and get rid of fetal Rh-positive cells before they immunize the mother.

Haemostasis

Haemostatic mechanisms prevent blood loss from intact vessels and stop excessive bleeding from severed vessels. Normal haemostasis is dependent upon a complex series of interactions between several components, which include: (i) local vascular factors; (ii) platelets; (iii) coagulation (fibrin formation); and (iv) fibrinolysis.

Bleeding seen in clinical practice often results from a defect in more than one of these components. Understanding of the integrated concept of the physiology of haemostasis is best achieved by considering the role of each of the above components.

Vascular factors

Localized vasoconstriction is the immediate response of the vessel wall to injury. It is transient and lasts for less than 1 minute. The mechanism of vascular constriction is uncertain, but systemic or localized humoral and neural factors are believed to be important, particularly for the initial intense local constriction. The humoral factors involved include the localized release of the vasoconstrictor serotonin 5-HT from platelets and the systemic release of catecholamines from the adrenal medulla. However, the ability of the injured vessel to respond to these factors may be influenced by the general metabolic state of the patient. Acute hypoxia and metabolic acidosis diminish this important response.

Platelets

Platelets originate in the bone marrow, where the most recognizable primitive precursor, the megakaryoblast, matures through the stages of promegakaryocyte and megakaryocyte. This last cell has a diameter of 24–30 μm. Platelets of diameter 2–3 μm are formed by the breaking off of pieces of the cytoplasm of the megakaryocyte. Formation of platelets (thrombocytes) is under the effect of the hormone *thrombopoietin*, which increases markedly in conditions of low platelet count (thrombocytopenia). Once released from the bone marrow, the platelets pass through the spleen before reaching the bloodstream, where they survive for 3–5 days. The normal platelet count in peripheral blood is 100 000–400 000 platelets/mm^3 (average 250 000).

The functions of platelets can be summarized in the following processes:

1 The interaction of platelets with the vessel wall. Platelets in the circulation are in a quiescent state and are discoid in shape. A few seconds after injury to a blood-vessel, platelets rapidly adhere to the damaged area. Collagen exposed in the vessel wall attracts platelets to adhere to it and is also responsible for triggering the release of endogenous platelet adenosine diphosphate (ADP), which increases the stickiness of platelets, and is therefore a potent platelet aggregation substance.

2 The interaction of platelets with one another (platelet aggregation). In the presence of released ADP, platelets aggregate with one another to form a fragile and reversible **primary haemostatic plug**, which is not capable of satisfactory haemostasis.

3 Soon after aggregation, platelets start releasing the following substances:

(a) 5-HT, a potent vasoconstrictor.

(b) Platelet phospholipid or platelet factor 3 (PF_3), which is essential in the process of blood coagulation.

(c) Proteins, e.g. platelet β-thromboglobulin (β-TG) and platelet factor 4 (PF_4, heparin-neutralizing factor).

(d) Thromboxane A_2 (TXA_2), a prostaglandin formed from arachidonic acid. It is a potent vasoconstrictor and aggregating agent. Aspirin ingestion inhibits TXA_2 formation and prevents platelet aggregation. This is the basis of the use of aspirin in the prevention of thrombotic disorders, e.g. coronary heart disease.

The further stability of the platelet plug requires the availability of thrombin, which is generated as a result of the simultaneous activation of the coagulation system. Thrombin induces structural changes in platelets. The platelets swell and interlock with each other. The simultaneous formation of fibrin, which infiltrates the platelet plug, results in a reinforced (concrete-like) structure. This final step is described as **irreversible aggregation**.

Platelets contribute in several ways to blood clotting. They contribute **platelet phospholipid**, without which coagulation fails. Platelet phospholipid (PF_3) is an integral part of the platelet membrane. Once the platelet is activated, the membrane phospholipid undergoes certain physical changes whereby it becomes exposed to the plasma. This phospholipid is essential for the process of blood coagulation. **Clot retraction** to about 10% of the original clot size is due to platelets. Platelet pseudopodia attached to fibrin contract, pulling the fibrin fibrils tightly together. This is due to the presence in platelets of large quantities of contractile proteins, actin, myosin, tropomyosin and troposin. Moreover, there exists within the platelet a calcium ion-regulating mechanism resembling the sarcoplasmic reticulum of muscle cells. When internal contraction occurs in platelets, it facilitates the following:

1 Extrusion of the platelet release products.

2 Contraction of the aggregates.

3 Retraction of the blood clot.

4 Sealing of the porous haemostatic plug.

Blood coagulation

The coagulation mechanism is a complete set of bio-chemical reactions which terminate in the production of the enzyme thrombin, which, in turn, changes the soluble plasma protein fibrinogen into insoluble fibrin. A large number of factors participate in this process; however, only 12 clotting factors have been identified and given numerical designations in the order of their discovery. A simplified schematic representation of the interactions of these clotting factors is shown in Fig. 2.8. This is based on the McFarlane cascade or waterfall hypothesis.

Mechanism of blood coagulation

The clotting factors circulate in the bloodstream in the form of inactive precursors. Their activation may occur along the two following pathways.

Intrinsic pathway

The intrinsic pathway is dependent on certain clotting factors, all of which are present in the blood—hence the name intrinsic pathway. The trigger to this pathway is the activation of factor XII by contact with a foreign surface, i.e. any surface other than the smooth natural endothelial surface. Therefore, activation of factor XII may occur when blood comes in contact with exposed collagen when the vessel wall is injured. Activation also occurs when blood comes in contact with glass when coagulation is tested for in the laboratory. Once factor XII is converted into active factor XII (XIIa), it activates factor XI to form active factor XI (XIa), which, in turn, activates factor IX to form active factor IX (IXa). Active factor IX, in the presence of factor VIII (antihaemophilic globulin), platelet phospholipid and calcium ions, activates factor X to activate factor X (Xa). Beyond this point the blood coagulation mechanism continues along a pathway common to both intrinsic and extrinsic mechanisms of the clotting system.

Extrinsic pathway

The extrinsic pathway is triggered by a material (tissue factor or tissue thromboplastin) from damaged tissues, which forms a complex with factor VII and this complex, in the presence of calcium ions, activates factor X to Xa. Thus, the extrinsic pathway takes a shorter time than the intrinsic pathway.

The common pathway for both the intrinsic and extrinsic mechanism of activation of the clotting system proceeds as follows (Fig. 2.8). Active factor X (Xa), in association with factor V, platelet phospholipid (platelet factor 3, PF_3) and calcium ions, forms what is known as the thrombokinase complex, which converts prothrombin to thrombin. Thrombin is a proteolytic enzyme which splits two short peptide chains, fibrinopeptides A and B,

Fig. 2.8 A diagrammatic representation of the interaction of the various clotting factors in the intrinsic and extrinsic pathways of the activation of the coagulation mechanism. PF_3, platelet factor 3.

from both ends of the fibrinogen molecule. The resulting residues, called fibrin monomers, join end to end to form long strands of fibrin polymer, which aggregate to form a three-dimensional network of fibrin. As such, this aggregate is soft and friable and is therefore not strong enough to give a satisfactory haemostatic plug. Final bonding and polymerization of these fibrin monomer strands to form a more stable fibrin gel requires the presence of factor XIII (fibrin-stabilizing factor) and calcium ions.

Additional points on the clotting system

1 Both intrinsic and extrinsic pathways are necessary for normal haemostasis.

2 Both pathways are activated when blood leaves the blood-vessels for the tissues.

3 Thrombin is a key factor in both the intrinsic and extrinsic systems, in addition to its action on fibrinogen.

4 The activation of the clotting mechanism along the shorter extrinsic pathway results in the rapid formation of thrombin, which feeds back to activate the intrinsic pathway through factors VII and V. Factor VII can activate factor X to active factor X, and this forms an activation connection between both pathways.

5 Thrombin stimulates platelets to release ADP and TXA_2 and therefore enhances further aggregation of platelets.

6 Thrombin is essential for platelet morphological changes during haemostasis, which lead to the formation of the primary haemostatic plug.

Fibrinolysis

Fibrinolysis is the enzymatic breakdown of fibrin. Fibrinolysis is a normal function of the blood and it makes a major contribution to the maintenance of the patency of blood-vessels in health and disease. It can be considered as a counterbalance to the equally important clotting process,

Fig. 2.9 The fibrinolytic enzyme system. FDP, fibrin degradation product.

the former laying down fibrin and the latter removing it. If either side of the balance is tipped, the end result will be either a bleeding tendency, due to excessive digestion of fibrin, or thrombosis and blocking of blood-vessels, due to excessive clotting. Fibrinolysis, in the physiological sense, is produced by the enzyme plasmin, which is derived from a stable plasma protein precursor, plasminogen (a β-globulin) (Fig. 2.9). The conversion of plasminogen into plasmin requires activators which are present in the blood, tissues and urine. Plasmin digests unwanted intra- or extravascular deposits of fibrin, which is the desired physiological effect. However, it is a non-specific proteolytic enzyme, which can digest certain clotting factors, including fibrinogen, factor V and factor VIII. Under normal circumstances the fibrinolytic enzyme system is kept in check by inhibitors of plasminogen activators and also by inhibitors of plasmin (antiplasmins), which are produced by the liver. The liver also inactivates circulating plasminogen activators. Human tissue plasminogen activator (tPA) is now produced by recombinant DNA techniques and is currently used with some success in dissolving coronary clots (thrombi) in patients who suffer acute coronary thrombosis.

Anticoagulants

Anticoagulants are substances which inhibit the process of blood coagulation. The following anticoagulants are in common use in clinical practice:

1 *Substances which remove calcium ions from the blood*:
  (a) Citrate, used in collection of blood in blood banks.
  (b) Oxalate and ethylenediamine tetra-acetate (EDTA), used for blood collection in clinical laboratories.
2 *Heparin* is a mucopolysaccharide found in many tissues, with the highest concentration in the liver, lungs, granules of mast cells and basophil leucocytes. Heparin is

a very potent anticoagulant. It interferes with the clotting process in two ways: first, it acts as a direct antithrombin and, second, it prevents the conversion of prothrombin to thrombin.

Heparin is commonly used for keeping blood in the fluid state during open-heart surgery and to prevent the occurrence of venous thrombosis in the postoperative period. It is also used for blood collection in laboratories. .
3 *Warfarin and phenindione*. These substances suppress the synthesis of vitamin K-dependent factors (II, VII, IX and X) by the liver. Warfarin and phenindione are widely used in clinical practice. Their advantage over heparin is that they are given by mouth, while heparin can only be given by injection. Their effect continues for up to 48 hours, while the action of heparin lasts for 6–8 hours.

Naturally occurring anticoagulants

Naturally occurring anticoagulants are present in small concentrations in normal plasma, where their main function is to keep the clotting mechanism in check. The best known of the naturally occurring anticoagulants are antithrombin III and protein C, which inactivate clotting factors VIII and V.

Haemorrhagic (or bleeding) disorders

Haemorrhagic disorders are disease conditions characterized by an excessive bleeding tendency due to a defect in the haemostatic system. Bleeding disorders may be caused by:
1 Vascular defects: either congenital or acquired.
2 Platelet defects: either a decrease in the number of circulating platelets (thrombocytopenia) or a defect in platelet function.
3 Coagulation defects: either congenital or acquired.

Congenital coagulation defects

The commonest congenital bleeding disorders are haemophilia A, due to factor VIII deficiency, and haemophilia B, or Christmas disease, due to deficiency of factor IX. Haemophilia is characterized by excessive bleeding, which may occur spontaneously in the skin, mucous membranes and joints, or after minor trauma or surgery, e.g. tooth extraction. Bleeding in these situations can only be stopped by replacing the missing clotting factor in the form of fresh frozen plasma or clotting factor concentrate.

Acquired coagulation defects

Acquired defects may be due to diminished production of a clotting factor, as in liver disease and vitamin K deficiency, or to consumption of platelet and clotting factors, as in the serious condition disseminated intravascular coagulation (DIC), in which extensive activation of the clotting system occurs *in vivo*. This may end in fatal bleeding.

Further reading

1 Babior, B.M. & Stossel, T.P. (1994) *Haematology: A Pathophysiological Approach*. Churchill Livingstone, London.

3 / Excitable Tissues

Introduction

Receptors in the skin and other sense organs act as transducers which change various stimuli, such as heat, cold, light or sound, into electrical signals. Nerve fibres are responsible for conduction of these signals, which are known as nerve impulses, to the central nervous system (CNS) and also from the various parts of the CNS to effector organs such as muscles and glands. Nerves and muscles are called excitable tissues because they respond to chemical, mech-anical or electrical stimuli. Muscle cells demonstrate this excitation by producing mechanical contractions, which take place in skeletal muscle, heart muscle and smooth muscle cells. However, in a general sense, all living cells are excitable because they respond to external stimuli and possess special properties which reside in the cell membrane. The most important properties of cell membranes necessary for excitation are:

1 They can maintain different concentrations of positively charged cations and negatively charged anions outside and inside their membranes (see Chapter 1).

Objectives
On completion of the study of this section, the student should be able to:
1 Understand the basic properties of cell membranes which underlie the process of excitation.
2 Comprehend the ionic basis of the resting and action potentials of the cell membrane, particularly that of nerve and muscle, so as to make appropriate use of diagnostic techniques such as electrocardiography, electromyography and electroencephalography.
3 Explain the basis of the process of transmission at synaptic junctions.
4 Describe the molecular basis of contraction and relaxation of muscle fibres in order to explain the links between the electrical and mechanical events.

2 Their permeability changes when they are appropriately stimulated.

3 When the permeability changes, only specific types of ions can pass in a certain direction.

A stimulus on the cell membrane first produces a **change in permeability** (or **conductance**). This is followed by movement of ions across the cell membrane. As the ions have different electrical charges, their movement from one side of the cell membrane to the other produces a difference in **electrical potential** between the outside and inside of the cell membrane. The difference in voltage across the cell membrane at rest (i.e. not being stimulated) is called the **resting membrane potential** (RMP). When the cell membrane is stimulated, the resting membrane potential is temporarily reversed and an **action potential** is produced. The action potential is transmitted along nerves and causes muscles to contract and glands to release secretions.

This chapter will explain the main mechanisms concerned with maintenance of the resting membrane potential and the production of the action potential. Furthermore, the mechanisms whereby the action potential causes muscle to respond will be described.

Ionic distribution across the cell membrane

The composition of the interstitial fluid (the internal environment) must be kept constant (as explained in Chapter 1). It is essential that the difference in ionic gradients between the inside of the cell and the outside is maintained for the RMP and action potential to develop. If no action potential can be produced by a maximal stimulus, then the cell is considered unexcitable.

Origins of the resting cell membrane potential

A number of forces act on cell membranes at rest. These forces are responsible for: (i) the maintenance of the resting membrane potential; (ii) the development of the action potential; and (iii) bringing the cell back to its resting state after the action potential is over. These forces are: **diffusion, electrical gradients** and **active transport**.

Diffusion

Diffusion is the movement of molecules from a region of higher concentration to a region of lower concentration. The rate of diffusion is proportional to the difference in concentration of the molecules in the two places. This is called the **concentration gradient** or **chemical gradient**. Ions are electrically charged (Na^+, K^+, Cl^-) and therefore positive ions move to the negative area and negative ions move to the positive area. This is called the **electrical gradient**.

Electrical gradient

In Chapter 1, we have learned that there is a high concentration of non-diffusible protein anions in the intracellular fluid. The presence of such ions on one side of the membrane produces a form of equilibrium known as the **Donnan effect**. The negative charge of protein molecules hinders entry of diffusible anions and favours entry of cations (Fig. 3.1). The Donnan effect predicts that the distribution of diffusible ions in this case will be such that their *concentration ratios* inside (i) and outside (o) the membrane will be equal, as follows:

$$\frac{[K^+]_i}{[K^+]_o} = \frac{[Cl^-]_o}{[Cl^-]_i}$$

Also, the product of the concentrations of diffusible ions of the same valence on each side will be equal, i.e.:

$$[K^+]_i \times [Cl^-]_i = [K^+]_o \times [Cl^-]_o$$

Equilibrium potentials and the Nernst equation

If the cell membrane is permeable to only one ion, an equilibrium is reached when there is no net movement of that ion. This is called the **equilibrium potential** (E) for that ion. If a cell is placed in a medium similar to the extracellular fluid (ECF) but containing K^+ only, K^+ will diffuse out

Fig. 3.1 Forces acting across the cell membrane and the resting membrane potential. ECF, extracellular fluid; ICF, intracellular fluid.

of the cell (efflux). This occurs because K^+ concentration (chemical gradient) inside the cell is much higher (concentration gradient). As this outward movement continues, there is a gradual build-up of an opposing force acting in the opposite direction. This force, which tends to keep K^+ inside the cell, is the electrical gradient due to the attraction between the positively charged K^+ and the negatively charged intracellular protein and other intracellular anions. As more and more K^+ diffuses out, this electrical gradient will progressively increase until it ultimately reaches a value which balances the force of the chemical gradient and prevents further net K^+ efflux. At this potential, where the electrical gradient becomes equal to the chemical gradient, K^+ is said to be at **electrochemical equilibrium** and the potential is referred to as the K^+ **equilibrium potential** (E_{K^+}). The **Nernst equation** is used to calculate the *equilibrium potential* of individual ions.

In the case of positively charged ions such as K^+, the Nernst equation at 37°C is:

$$E_{K^+} = 61 \log \frac{[K^+]_o}{[K^+]_i} = 61 \log \frac{5 \text{ mmol/l}}{150 \text{ mmol/l}} = -90 \text{ mV}$$

and in the case of negatively charged ions such as Cl^-:

$$E_{X^-} = 61 \log \frac{[X^-]_i}{[X^-]_o} \text{ (in mV)}$$

where E_{X^-} is the equilibrium potential of the ion X^-, $[X^-]_i$ is the concentration of X^- inside the cell, and $[X^-]_o$ is the concentration of X^- in the extracellular medium. The Nernst equation depends on two assumptions:

1 The membrane is freely permeable to the ion being examined.

2 There is no other ion exerting an opposing influence in the medium.

The equilibrium potential for Na^+ or Cl^- can be calculated as follows:

$$E_{Na^+} = 61 \log 150/15 = +61 \text{ mV}$$
$$E_{Cl^-} = 61 \log 9/125 = -70 \text{ mV}$$

The sign of the potential refers to the polarity of the inside of the membrane.

Equilibrium potentials are never reached in normal cells because, when one ion is moving in one direction, other ions are moving in the opposite direction and this tends to prevent the development of the equilibrium potential. The equilibrium potential can be measured for a particular ion only *under experimental conditions*.

Active transport

Active transport requires energy because it transports ions against their concentration gradients. The most important active transport system is the **sodium–potassium pump**, which is responsible for transport of Na^+ to the outside and K^+ to the inside against their concentration gradients. There is an enzyme called Na^+–K^+ adenosine triphosphatase (ATPase) present on the cell membrane. This enzyme is activated by intracellular Na^+ to hydrolyse adenosine triphosphate (ATP) and release the energy needed to pump Na^+ to the outside of the cell and K^+ to the interior. The Na^+–K^+ pump is responsible for keeping the different concentrations of Na^+ and K^+ in resting cells.

The resting membrane potential (RMP)

If a microelectrode is inserted into a cell, another electrode is placed into the interstitial fluid surrounding the cell and the two electrodes are connected to a voltmeter, the inside of the cell will show a negative deflection of about −70 mV (−50 to −90) with respect to the outside (Fig. 3.1). This potential is called the resting membrane potential and its value depends on the type of tissue. It is negative inside the cell with respect to the outside because of the following:

1 The resting cell membrane is 10–100 times more permeable to K^+ than to Na^+. K^+ tends to leak out of the cell down its concentration gradient, carrying positive charge with it, and is unable to carry Cl^- with it because Cl^- has a higher concentration outside. This tends to make the cell interior *more negative*.

2 The non-diffusible anions (protein, sulphate and phosphate ions) cannot leave the cell. According to the Donnan effect, there is a slight excess of cations outside the cells and a slight excess of anions inside. This leaves the *inside negative* with respect to the outside.

3 A very small amount of sodium also diffuses into the cell down its concentration gradient because the cell membrane is only slightly permeable to Na^+. If K^+ continued to leak to the outside and Na^+ to the inside, a state of equilibrium would be reached and there would be no potential difference between the two sides of the membrane. This does not happen because of the Na^+–K^+ pump.

The main function of the Na^+–K^+ pump is to maintain the concentration gradients between the inside and outside of the membrane. Leaking K^+ and Na^+ ions are returned. The pump returns two K^+ ions to the inside of the cell while it removes three Na^+ ions from the inside. In this way the Na^+–K^+ pump maintains the electronegativity of the cell membrane. Inhibition of the Na^+–K^+ pump, e.g. by metabolic inhibitors, leads to a decrease in the RMP.

The resting membrane remains **polarized** because the movements of ions at rest do not favour either an inward or an outward flux. A state of equilibrium is maintained.

The Nernst equation, though useful for the determination of the equilibrium potential of individual ions, is not accurate for the calculation of the RMP. For this purpose, the **Goldman equation** is more suited. It takes into account the equilibrium potential of the three important ions (K^+, Na^+ and Cl^-) which exist together in the body fluids. It also takes into consideration the differential membrane permeability to these ions:

$$\text{RMP (mV)} = 61 \log \frac{P_{K^+}[K^+]_o + P_{Na^+}[Na^+]_o + P_{Cl^-}[Cl^-]_i}{P_{K^+}[K^+]_i + P_{Na^+}[Na^+]_i + P_{Cl^-}[Cl^-]_o}$$

where P_{K^+}, P_{Na^+} and P_{Cl^-} are membrane permeabilities to K^+, Na^+ and Cl^-, respectively; $[K^+]_o$, $[Na^+]_o$ and $[Cl^-]_o$ are extracellular concentrations of K^+, Na^+ and Cl^-; and $[K^+]_i$, $[Na^+]_i$ and $[Cl^-]_i$ are intracellular concentrations of K^+, Na^+ and Cl^-.

Certain facts need to be pointed out:

1 Since RMP = E_{Cl^-} (–70 mV), it becomes evident that Cl^- distribution across the membrane depends exclusively on physiochemical forces and needs no active transport to maintain this distribution (unlike K^+ and Na^+, which need the Na^+–K^+ pump). There is evidence that Cl^- does not contribute to the value of the RMP and changing the extracellular Cl^- concentration does not affect the RMP. Hence, Cl^- can be omitted from the above equation, which becomes:

$$\text{RMP (mV)} = 61 \log \frac{P_{K^+}[K^+]_o + P_{Na^+}[Na^+]_o}{P_{K^+}[K^+]_i + P_{Na^+}[Na^+]_i}$$

2 Because P_{K^+} is almost 100 times P_{Na^+}, the RMP depends primarily on K^+ with very little contribution from Na^+. Increasing the extracellular potassium concentration causes a marked reduction in the RMP, whereas changing the extracellular sodium concentration does not significantly affect the RMP.

The action potential (AP)

The action potential is a sudden reversal of membrane polarity produced by a stimulus. Action potentials occur in living organisms to produce physiological effects such as:

1 Transmission of impulses along nerve fibres.
2 Release of neurosecretions or chemical transmitters in synapses.
3 Contraction of muscle.
4 Activation or inhibition of glandular secretion.

Many cellular functions in animals and plants are induced by action potentials. During stimulation of muscle or nerve, an action potential can be recorded by inserting a microelectrode inside a cell with a reference electrode in the extracellular fluid (Fig. 3.2). By this method a **monophasic potential** is recorded. Action potentials recorded from the surface of nerves or muscles using two surface electrodes are called **biphasic** because they have two waves, one negative and the other positive (Fig. 3.3). The different action potentials can be recorded by a cathode ray oscilloscope, which transforms changes in voltage into the graphic records shown in Figs 3.2 and 3.3.

Development of the AP

When a cell membrane is stimulated by a physical or a chemical stimulus, the cell membrane permeability to Na^+ is dramatically increased. **Sodium channels** open and the sodium ions rush through the channels to the inside of the cell, causing the inside of the membrane to become positive with respect to the outside. This is called **depolarization**, because it changes the membrane polarity from its polarized negative state. The membrane potential actually becomes reversed and reaches +35 mV.

Towards the end of depolarization, sodium permeability decreases and potassium permeability increases abruptly and K^+ ions leave the cell down their concentration gradient, causing the inside of the membrane to return quickly to its original potential. This is called **repolarization** and the membrane potential is brought back to –70 mV. The duration of the action potential in skeletal muscle and nerves (depolarization and repolarization) is about **1–5 ms (1/1000 s)**.

The Na^+–K^+ pump moves sodium out of the cell and potassium to the inside against their concentration gradients and the membrane regains its resting membrane potential and is ready for another action potential. Figure 3.4 gives a graphic representation of the changes in permeability of the cell membrane which take place during the action potential.

A stimulus which is just strong enough to move the RMP from a resting value (–70 mV) to the level (–55 mV) that

Fig. 3.2 Monophasic action potential recorded with one of the recording electrodes inside the cell.

leads to the production of an action potential is called a **threshold stimulus** (Fig. 3.5). **Subthreshold** stimuli result only in **transient local responses**, which are proportional in amplitude (height) to the strengths of the corresponding subthreshold stimuli. In each of these instances, the stimulus leads to the opening of some sodium channels, resulting in Na$^+$ influx and membrane depolarization. This, however, is short-lived because it is promptly counteracted by local repolarizing processes, which overcome it and return the membrane potential (MP) to −70 mV. These **local potentials**, which tend to resist any change in the membrane potential, comprise potassium efflux and chloride entry into the cell.

The threshold stimulus, on the other hand, succeeds in taking the MP to the critical value of −55 mV, at which the local repolarizing processes can no longer overcome and stop depolarization. From here onward, opening of Na$^+$ channels leads to opening of more and more Na$^+$ channels. This progressive increase in Na$^+$ conductance (permeability) is, of course, accompanied by Na$^+$ influx, which causes depolarization and moves the MP toward E_{Na^+} (+60 mV). This value, however, is never reached because depolar-

ization gets switched off at an MP value around +30 to +40 mV by two factors:

1 Inactivation and closure of Na$^+$ channels, which occur soon and automatically after their opening. Inactivated Na$^+$ channels cannot be reactivated (opened) until the MP has returned to a value close to the RMP.

2 Delayed opening of K$^+$ channels takes place and leads to K$^+$ efflux, which is responsible for repolarization of the membrane. Sometimes a third component of the AP is observed: this is a **hyperpolarization** coming after repolarization. It is an inconsistent finding and is of variable duration. The Na$^+$–K$^+$ pump takes Na$^+$ out of the cell and K$^+$ into it and maintains the RMP.

Recording of APs

Action potentials are recorded by oscillographs and oscilloscopes. When the recording is obtained between an intracellular active (or recording) electrode and an extracellular (or reference) electrode, the potential is called a monophasic potential, because one positive or one negative deflection is recorded. When both the recording and reference electrodes are placed on the surface of a muscle or

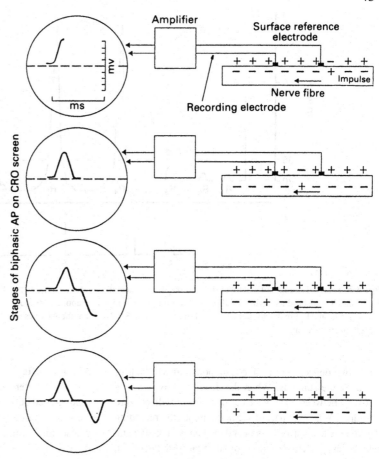

Fig. 3.3 Biphasic action potential recorded with both the reference and the recording electrodes outside the cell. CRO, cathode ray oscilloscope.

Fig. 3.4 Graphic representation of the changes in Na$^+$ and K$^+$ permeability (conductance) of the cell membrane during the action potential. (Reproduced with permission from Hodgkin, A.L. (1958) *Proc. R. Soc. Lond (Biol).*, **148**, 1, based on Hodgkin, A.L. & Huxley, A.P. (1952) *J. Physiol.* **117**, 500–44.)

Fig. 3.5 Effect of strength of electrical stimulation. A, point of entry of microelectrode into the cell. Local graded responses (R_1, R_2 and R_3) are produced when subthreshold stimuli (S_1, S_2 and S_3) are applied. Response R_4 is due to a threshold stimulus. Responses R_5 and R_6 are due to suprathreshold stimuli (S_5 and S_6). Note that the AP does not increase in amplitude with increased strength of stimulation.

nerve, two deflections or a biphasic potential will be produced by the stimulus. When the depolarization wave is half-way between the two electrodes there will be zero recording. When the part of the nerve under the recording electrode is depolarized, its outside becomes negative and the recording electrode will record a negative deflection in relation to the reference electrode. When the depolarization wave reaches the reference electrode, the recording electrode will record a positive deflection in relation to the reference electrode (Fig. 3.3).

Changes in cell excitability during AP
During depolarization and for a short period following it, the nerve or muscle cannot be excited by even the strongest stimulus. This is called the **absolute refractory period** (ARP). A second stimulus given in the early part of the ARP cannot produce a second AP over the first one because Na^+ channels are already maximally open and cannot be opened further. Similarly, if given in the latter part of ARP, a second stimulus cannot produce a second AP because Na^+ channels are now in the inactivation phase and cannot be opened. The ARP is followed by the **relative refractory period** (RRP), which covers repolarization and hyperpolarization. During the RRP, an action potential of a lower amplitude than normal can be elicited, but only by a stimulus stronger than the threshold stimulus (i.e. by a **suprathreshold stimulus**).

All-or-none law
The action potential, unlike the local response (see below), is not graded but obeys the all-or-none law. This means that a given stimulus either elicits no AP or produces a full AP whose amplitude (height) cannot be increased by further increase in the stimulus intensity. As shown in Fig. 3.5, subthreshold stimuli fail to elicit the AP and suprathreshold stimuli fail to make it bigger. Although normally the AP of a given cell has a fixed amplitude, it can become smaller if elicited in the relative refractory period of the cell or if the extracellular Na^+ concentration is low.

Graded potentials
Graded potentials are local, non-propagated responses whose amplitude varies with the strength of the stimulus applied. A depolarizing local response leads to a reduction in the membrane potential, taking it closer to the threshold level at which the action potential develops and thereby making the cell more excitable. **Excitability** refers to the ability of the cell to produce action potentials. Such a **local depolarizing potential** can arise from movement of positive ions (e.g. Na^+) into the cell or exit of negative ions from the cell. It can also be produced by cathodal stimulation, which deposits negative charges on the outer side of the cell membrane, thereby reducing the membrane potential.

A **hyperpolarizing local potential**, on the other hand, makes the membrane more negative inside and thereby

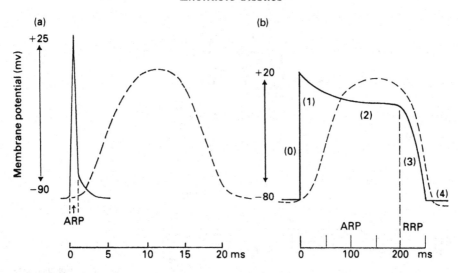

Fig. 3.6 (a) Action potential of skeletal muscle compared with (b) AP of cardiac muscle (note the time-scale). The broken line indicates the muscle contraction in each case. For cardiac muscle, (0) indicates depolarization due to Na^+ influx; (1) is due to initial rapid repolarization due to closure of sodium channels; (2) is the plateau to slow prolonged opening of Ca^{2+} channels; and (3) is due to closure of Ca^{2+} channels and opening of K^+ channels causing final repolarization and the resting state (4).

reduces excitability of the cell. It can result from entry of negative ions (e.g. Cl^-) into the cell, exit of positive ions (e.g. K^+) from the cell, or anodal stimulation. Graded potentials die out within 1–2 mm from their point of origin. They cannot transmit sensory or motor information for long distances. They are, however, very useful as **receptor potentials**, serving for the initial recognition of a stimulus at the sensory receptor. They are also of utmost importance for integration of information at synapses. Furthermore, they can summate (add up) to reach the threshold level necessary for generation of the action potential (Fig. 3.5). There are two ways for this **summation** to occur:

1 *Spatial summation* occurs when several subthreshold stimuli arrive simultaneously at the neuron, add up and become strong enough to depolarize the neuron to the threshold level.

2 *Temporal summation* occurs when several subthreshold stimuli are delivered rapidly and successively so that each is added on top of the preceding one before that one dies out, until the threshold level is reached and an action potential is generated.

Examples of graded potentials that will be discussed later include **excitatory postsynaptic potential** (EPSP), **inhibitory postsynaptic potential** (IPSP) and muscle **end-plate potential** (EPP).

Action potential of cardiac muscle

Depolarization of heart muscle is similar to that of skeletal

muscle, i.e. it is due to increased membrane permeability to sodium ions. At the end of depolarization, the membrane potential does not return to the resting level but stays positive (above zero) for about **200–250 ms** (Fig. 3.6). This is called the plateau (flat top). The plateau phase is due to opening calcium channels with consequent Ca^{2+} influx.

Towards the end of the plateau K^+ leaves the cells, producing repolarization. Due to the delay in repolarization, the **absolute refractory period** (ARP) of heart muscle lasts for nearly the entire duration of the contraction. The RRP is short and lasts from the end of the absolute refractory period until shortly after repolarization. A second AP, triggered during the RRP, gives a weak contraction superimposed on the semirelaxed phase of the first contraction. It is weak because the shorter duration of the second AP results in less than normal Ca^{2+} entering the cell. Therefore, unlike skeletal muscle, ventricular muscle cannot develop summation and **tetanus** during high-frequency stimulation. The prolonged refractory period protects the ventricles from too rapid re-excitation and allows them to relax long enough to be filled with blood. It also allows AP conduction through the muscular network to be completed before a second excitation can occur. This prevents recycling of excitation in the heart.

Electrical properties of smooth muscle

There are three types of smooth muscle:

(a)

Propagation

Depolarization

Refractory

(b)

Depolarization

ECF

ICF

Myelin sheath

Fig. 3.7 (a) Continuous conduction in unmyelinated nerve. (b) Saltatory conduction in myelinated nerve. AP, action potential; ECF, extracellular fluid; ICF, intracellular fluid; RMP, resting membrane potential.

1 *Spontaneously active smooth muscle.* These muscles can contract spontaneously in the absence of external innervation. They generate electrical activity, which spreads by gap junctions and produces contractions. Two types of electrical activity can be seen:

(a) *Pacemaker potentials*: a focal **pacemaker** area depolarizes adjacent regions to produce action potentials. The pacemaker potential is due to slow influx of Ca^{2+}. The pacemaker region is not fixed and can shift from one location to another. This can be observed in the uterus and taeniae coli. Note that the AP in smooth muscle is brought about by influx of Ca^{2+} rather than Na^+.

(b) *Slow wave depolarizations*: examples of these can be seen in the stomach and intestine. They are made up of slow, plateau-like waves, which last 2–8 s. Their frequency is determined by the cells whose rate is fastest. On reaching the threshold, they initiate action potentials. External innervation serves merely to regulate these spontaneous activities by stimulating them (parasympathetic, acetylcholine) or by inhibiting them (sympathetic, noradrenaline).

2 *Electrically unexcitable smooth muscle.* These do not generate electrical activity and depend upon external stimulation to contract. Examples are bronchial and tracheal smooth muscles.

3 *Intermediate smooth muscle.* This type shows spike-like electrical activity on stimulation. The force of contraction is proportional to the frequency of action potentials. Examples of these are found in the piloerector muscles, blood-vessels, vas deferens, seminal vesicles and iris.

Propagation of the AP (impulse transmission)

Nerve fibres can be classified as myelinated and unmyelinated. An action potential developing at one point also stimulates adjacent parts of the membrane, causing new action potentials to spread in both directions. This process enables one stimulus to depolarize a whole cell and enables nerves to carry impulses from one part of the body to the other. The process of transmission is illustrated in Fig. 3.7.

Propagation of the action potential in unmyelinated (C) fibres occurs by continuous conduction. The depolarized area of the membrane depolarizes the area immediately next to it and itself becomes refractory for a brief period. This prevents propagation in the reverse direction and ensures unidirectional transmission (Fig. 3.7). In myelinated nerves, however, there is **saltatory conduction**, whereby the impulse jumps from one **node of Ranvier** to the next. This is a much quicker way of impulse transmission. When the myelin sheath is lost in some diseases, e.g. diabetes mellitus, conduction in fast nerves becomes slow and sensations like fast pain are lost.

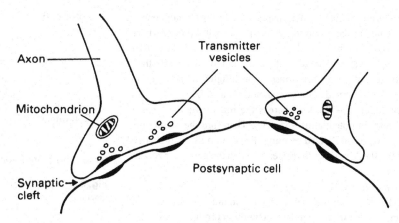

Fig. 3.8 A typical synapse.

Synaptic transmission

A **synapse** is the junction between two neurons where the electrical activity of one neuron is transmitted to the other. Most synapses occur between the axon terminals of one neuron (presynaptic neuron) and the cell body or soma and dendrites of another, **postsynaptic**, neuron (Fig. 3.8). The presynaptic endings enlarge slightly to make the **synaptic knob**. The synaptic knob is separated from the postsynaptic membrane by the **synaptic cleft**. The synaptic knob contains **vesicles** which contain a **transmitter** substance. When the action potential arrives from the axon, it causes the calcium channels to open, i.e. increases the membrane permeability to Ca^{2+}. The intracellular Ca^{2+} attracts the vesicles to fuse with the membrane and release their contents by exocytosis. The released transmitter diffuses into the synaptic cleft and combines with specific receptors for that transmitter on the postsynaptic membrane. This changes the permeability of the postsynaptic membrane to specific ions and results in a postsynaptic potential. If this potential is depolarizing and is summated with others to reach the membrane threshold level, an AP results. The postsynaptic membrane usually contains no transmitter; this is why nerve conduction occurs in only one direction.

Mechanism of AP generation in a postsynaptic cell

Postsynaptic potentials (PSPs)

Postsynaptic potentials are local potentials produced in the postsynaptic membrane by the release of a transmitter. Depending on the type of synapse or transmitter, these potentials can be **excitatory** or **inhibitory**. Single PSPs do not usually cause any excitation or inhibition in the postsynaptic neuron because the change in membrane potentials does not reach the threshold to produce a response, but they may produce partial depolarization or hyperdepolarization. Threshold is reached by spatial or temporal summation and can be excitatory or inhibitory, as explained below.

Spatial summation. A number of synaptic knobs release their transmitter at the same time on a single postsynaptic membrane and each produces a local depolarization of a fraction of a millivolt. When small depolarization currents from transmitters released by the other knobs are added together, they depolarize the membrane by about 11 mV. This will cause an action potential to be generated in the postsynaptic cell, which is transmitted down the postsynaptic axon. If they do not reach threshold, these potentials decay and die away. This type of summation of EPSPs to reach threshold is called **spatial summation**, i.e. summation due to stimulation of a number of synaptic knobs releasing transmitter on one postsynaptic neuron.

Temporal summation. If one synaptic knob is repetitively stimulated, its postsynaptic local potential may add up and reach threshold to fire an action potential. This is called **temporal summation**.

Excitatory and inhibitory postsynaptic potential. If the transmitter released at the synapse opens Na^+ channels and thereby *depolarizes* the small area immediately under the synaptic knob, the result will be an **excitatory postsynaptic potential** (EPSP).

If the transmitter opens Cl^- channels and thereby *hyperpolarizes* the postsynaptic membrane an **inhibitory postsynaptic potential** (IPSP) will result. EPSPs make the postsynaptic cell easier to excite. Conversely, IPSPs make the postsynaptic cell more difficult to excite.

Summation of several EPSPs causes the **generator zone** of the postsynaptic neuron to reach the threshold and an

AP is elicited in the postsynaptic cell. The generator zone is situated at the origin of the axon (the axon hillock) where it arises from the cell body. It is the region where APs are generated. The generator zone is more excitable than the rest of the axon because it has a lighter concentration of voltage-gated sodium channels. It also has a threshold potential of -59 mV (whereas the rest of the axon has a threshold potential of -55 mV). Therefore the membrane has to be depolarized by only 11 mV from its resting value of -70 mV in order to trigger an AP in the generator zone.

Synaptic delay

After maximal stimulation, the minimum time required for an impulse from a presynaptic knob to produce a response in the postsynaptic neuron is 0.5 ms. This is called the synaptic delay. This is the time taken for the transmitter to be released from vesicles and to produce an action potential in the postsynaptic membrane. A monosynaptic neuron pathway will have a delay of about 0.5 ms, while a polysynaptic pathway will have a delay corresponding to the number of synapses.

Electrical transmission

Some synapses transmit signals electrically or without transmitters. In such synapses the synaptic cleft is replaced by a low-resistance bridge, which allows the passage of the electrical impulse with ease. This type of transmission has a short synaptic delay and occurs only in the brain.

Neuromuscular transmission

Transmission of impulses from nerves to muscles occurs at **neuromuscular junctions**, which are a special type of synapse. Each nerve fibre loses its myelin sheath, branches several times and supplies from three to several hundred muscle fibres. The motor nerve and all the muscle fibres it supplies is called the **motor unit**. Each muscle fibre, however, receives innervation from only one neuron. The nerve endings enlarge slightly to make the synaptic knob, which fits into an invagination of the muscle cell membrane called the motor end-plate. At the **motor end-plate** the muscle postjunctional membrane makes numerous folds called the **subneural** or **junctional folds**. These, like villi, greatly increase the membrane surface area of the motor end-plate (Fig. 3.9).

Acetylcholine is the only transmitter at the synaptic knobs that is synthesized in the neural cytoplasm, from choline and acetylcoenzyme A. The subneural clefts contain the enzyme **acetylcholinesterase (AChE)**, which is capable of rapidly hydrolysing acetylcholine (ACh) to prevent its accumulation: Choline is released as a result

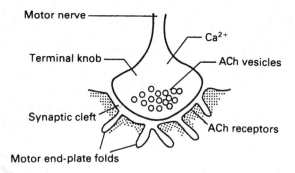

Fig. 3.9 Diagrammatic representation of the neuromuscular junction.

of ACh breakdown and is taken up by the nerve and reutilized.

The events of **neuromuscular transmission** are similar to those occurring at synapses. The incoming action potentials increase the permeability of the nerve ending to calcium ions. Ca^{2+} enters the nerve endings, causing attraction and rupture of the acetylcholine vesicles. The acetylcholine diffuses in the synaptic cleft and therefore the subneural folds and combines with acetylcholine receptors on the motor end-plate. This opens the sodium channels on the end-plate and produces a depolarization called the end-plate potential. Therefore, neuromuscular junctions are excitatory only. The amount of acetylcholine released by an impulse is enough to activate 10 times the receptors needed to produce a full end-plate potential. This is not waste but a safety factor to ensure that the message gets across. The end-plate potential is a local, graded, non-propagated response which is present only in the end-plate region. It serves to depolarize the adjacent muscle membrane to its threshold level. Action potentials are generated on both sides of the end-plate and are conducted by the local current mechanism to both ends of the muscle fibre. As we shall see later in this chapter, the muscle action potentials will eventually produce muscular contraction.

Myasthenia gravis

Myasthenia gravis is a serious disease caused by a failure of transmission at the neuromuscular junction. It is characterized by tiredness and progressive paralysis of muscles; death commonly occurs due to failure of respiratory muscles. It is an autoimmune disease in which some of the acetylcholine receptors are destroyed by circulating antibodies. Acetylcholine released by the impulses cannot produce an immediate effect and is destroyed by AChE. Drugs such as neostigmine inhibit the action of AChE and allow accumulation of adequate amounts of acetylcholine to stimulate the remaining receptors. Such drugs are used for the management of this disease.

Some drugs that modify neuromuscular transmission

1 *Muscle relaxants* are drugs widely used during general anaesthesia and in some other medical conditions to produce muscle relaxation. **Curare** is an example of non-depolarizing blockers, which occupy ACh receptors reversibly without producing depolarization. **Succinylcholine**, on the other hand, is an example of depolarizing blockers. It produces an initial depolarization of the sarcolemmal membrane, which prevents ACh from producing a response in the depolarized membrane. A few minutes later, as the membrane becomes repolarized, a second phase of decreased receptor sensitivity to ACh takes place.

2 *Alpha-bungarotoxin* is a chemical extracted from snake venom. It binds irreversibly to ACh receptors. The victim becomes totally paralysed. When labelled with radioactive iodine, it is used in a histochemical technique to estimate the number of ACh receptors at the neuromuscular junction.

3 *Anticholinesterase drugs*, such as **neostigmine**, reversibly combine with AChE and thus allow ACh to accumulate in the cleft, giving it a more favourable opportunity to act on the receptors. They are used in the management of myasthenia gravis, as mentioned above.

4 *Organophosphate compounds* combine irreversibly with AChE, leading to long-term increases in neuromuscular transmission. They are used as insecticides and, regrettably, as a chemical weapon. They produce muscle fasciculations, abdominal cramps, respiratory distress, sweating and convulsions. They are a frequent cause of poisoning in agricultural areas when they are accidentally ingested.

Neurotransmitters

Transmission of impulses in synapses and in neuromuscular junctions requires chemical transmitters. Transmitters are found in the presynaptic knob and each transmitter has a specific receptor in the postsynaptic membrane. A transmitter can be excitatory or inhibitory depending on the ionic permeability that it will produce. **Acetylcholine** and **catecholamines** are usually excitatory transmitters because they increase sodium permeability, while **gamma-aminobutyric acid** (GABA) and **glycine** are inhibitory transmitters because they increase chloride permeability and therefore produce hyperpolarization. After producing their action, transmitters either are degraded by specific enzymes, are taken up into the synaptic knob or diffuse into the tissue fluid.

Contraction of muscle

Contraction is defined as the active process of generating a mechanical force in muscle. The force exerted by a contracting muscle on an object is known as **muscle tension** and the force exerted on a muscle by a weight is known as the **load**. To lift a load, muscle tension must be greater than the muscle load. To lift a load the muscle must shorten and this type of contraction is called an **isotonic** (constant tension) contraction because the load remains constant throughout the period of shortening. When muscle shortening is prevented by a load that is greater than the force of contraction, the development of tension occurs at constant muscle length and this is called **isometric** (constant length) contraction. Body movements involve mainly isotonic contractions, which involve movement. Supporting a weight in a fixed position or maintaining the erect posture (e.g. standing) involves isometric contractions. Both types of contractions are involved together in most muscular activities.

Mechanics of skeletal muscle contraction

Simple muscle twitch

The mechanical response (contraction) to a single action potential is called a simple muscle twitch (Fig. 3.10a). Following the stimulus, there is an interval of a few milliseconds, known as the **latent period**, before contraction begins. This is the time taken for the action potential to develop. If the muscle is stimulated through its nerve, the latent period is longer because of the time taken in transmission at the neuromuscular junction. Figure 3.10(b–d) shows the effect of two successive stimuli.

Summation of contraction

A single twitch is of no mechanical value because its duration is very short. To produce sustained and coordinated muscle movements, single twitches summate in two different ways:

1 *Spatial summation*. The muscle fibres, together with the motor neuron which innervates them, constitute a **motor unit**. In spatial summation, stimulation of numerous nerve fibres causes an increasing number of motor units to be excited. The responses of single motor units are therefore added together to produce a strong contraction by the muscle.

2 *Temporal summation*. Separate muscle contractions are caused by single action potentials when their frequency is low. When frequency of stimulation rises above 10/s the second stimulus causes a contraction to develop before

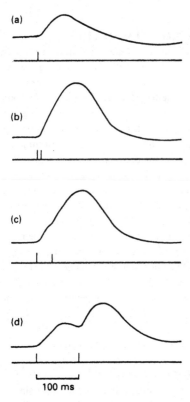

Fig. 3.10 (a) A single muscle twitch (contraction) due to a single short-lived stimulus; (b) complete summation of two contractions; (c) and (d) show incomplete summation as the interval between the two stimuli widens.

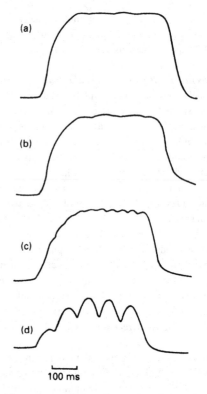

Fig. 3.11 Responses of a muscle to various frequencies of stimulation. Note that at (d) 20/s stimulation produces summation, at (c) 40/s incomplete fusion or clonus, and at (a & b) 80/s and 100/s, respectively, there is complete fusion or tetanus, which is a smooth maintained contraction.

the first one is over. As frequency increases, the degree of summation becomes greater, producing stronger contractions every time in a stepwise fashion (Fig. 3.11). When muscle is stimulated at a progressively greater rate, a frequency is reached at which contractions fuse together and cannot be distinguished. This is called tetanization and the contraction is a **tetanic contraction**, which is smooth and maintained. Most contractions of muscles in everyday life are of this nature. They allow useful work to be done.

Types of muscle contractions

Isometric contractions
When the muscle is not allowed to shorten (isometric), the tension developed during contraction increases to reach a maximum (as shown in Fig. 3.12). The relationship shown in the diagram is known as a length–tension relationship. It is seen from Fig. 3.12 that there is an optimum length of the

Fig. 3.12 Isometric contraction (length–tension curve). At point 100 mm, the length represents the resting length of the muscle, which gives the maximum strength of contraction.

muscle at which it develops maximum tension when it is stimulated. This depends on the effect of stretch or relaxation of the muscle on the degree of overlap of the actin and myosin filaments in the sarcomere. Isometric contractions do not result in external work being performed. However, they are useful for maintenance of posture and supporting activities.

Isotonic contractions

When a muscle is allowed to shorten, it will exert mechanical work (e.g. lifting a load). In this case the tension developed is constant (isotonic) and is equal to the load. Figure 3.13 shows the force–velocity curve during isotonic contractions. It is seen from this relationship that the **velocity** decreases as the load increases. The initial length of the muscle also affects the velocity of contraction. The **power** of contraction equals the force times velocity. Muscle power is usually maximum when only one-third of the maximum tension develops, i.e. isotonic contraction lifting one-third of the maximum load.

Molecular basis of muscle contraction

Both skeletal and cardiac muscles show striations (alternating dark and light bands) under the light microscope and are therefore called striated muscles. The striated muscle fibre (cell) has a diameter ranging between 50 and 200 μm and can be as long as 15 cm. Each contains several hundred

Fig. 3.13 Isotonic contraction (force–velocity curve). The velocity of contraction is inversely related to the load.

myofibrils in the cytoplasm. The myofibril is made up of contractile units called **sarcomeres**, whose length lies between 1.5 and 3 μm depending upon how much the muscle is stretched (Fig. 3.14).

The sarcomere consists of thick **myosin** filaments, thin **actin** filaments and two regulatory proteins called

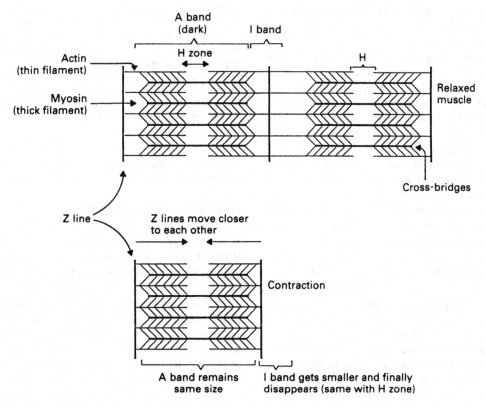

Fig. 3.14 Molecular structure of sarcomeres.

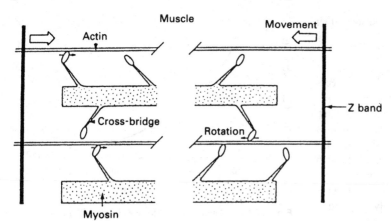

Fig. 3.15 Movement of actin and
myosin filaments showing rotation of
the cross-bridge head of the myosin
molecule. (Reproduced from Bray, J.J.,
Cragg, P.A., Macknight, A.D.C., Mills,
R.G. and Taylor, D.W. (eds) (1989)
Lecture Notes in Physiology, 2nd edn.
Blackwell Scientific Publications,
Oxford.)

troponin and tropomyosin. It is bound on either side by
a plate-like protein structure called the **Z line**, to which
actin filaments are attached. The dark **A band** lies in the
middle of the sarcomere and is formed of overlapping
myosin and actin (Fig. 3.14). The light **I band** is made
of actin. The **H zone** is made of myosin only. During contraction actin and myosin slide upon each other, increasing
the extent of their overlap and bringing the Z lines closer
together. This leads to the narrowing and finally disappearance of the I band and H zones, but the A band remains
unaffected.

The **myosin molecule** has a cross-bridge head and a
rod-like tail (Fig. 3.15). The joint-like or neck region
between the head and tail allows the head to swivel through
an angle of 45–50° during contraction. The head has a site
for binding ATP and it also contains an ATPase enzyme.
This enzyme, however, gets activated only when the myosin
head binds to actin. Each myosin filament (Fig. 3.16b) is
made up of 150–360 **myosin molecules** arranged so that
the heads project from the sides of the filament.

The **actin molecule** is a globular protein, 400 of which
form a chain called **F-actin**. Two F-actin chains intertwine
to form one actin filament (Fig. 3.16a). The actin molecules
contain binding sites for the heads of myosin.

Tropomyosin is a relaxing or inhibitory protein which
has a long thread-like molecule lying between the two
F-actin chains, a bit to the side of the groove between
them, and covering the binding sites on actin molecules.
It thereby prevents the myosin head from combining with
actin in the relaxed state of the muscle.

Troponin molecules have calcium-binding sites and are
attached to the **tropomyosin molecule** at 40 nm intervals.
When Ca^{2+} binds to troponin, this moves the tropomyosin
threads sideways into the groove between the two F-actin
chains, thereby uncovering the binding sites on actin. The

Fig. 3.16 Actin filament, formed of a spiral of two chains of
actin molecules. The thread-like tropomyosin molecules lie
between the two chains of actin molecules, slightly to one side of
the groove between them, covering the binding sites for myosin.
Troponin molecules are spaced at 40 nm intervals. (b) Myosin
filament (made up of 150–360 myosin molecules). (Reproduced
from Bray, J.J., Cragg, P.A., Macknight, A.D.C., Mills, R.G. and
Taylor, D.W. (eds) (1989) *Lecture Notes in Physiology*, 2nd edn.
Blackwell Scientific Publications, Oxford.)

myosin heads immediately get attached to these sites, forming cross-bridges.

The events in muscle contraction

As mentioned earlier, acetylcholine released by the motor
nerve at the neuromuscular junction leads to formation
of the EPP. This, in turn, depolarizes the **sarcolemma**
(muscle cell membrane), leading to formation of the muscle action potential. The muscle action potential spreads
to the inside of the cell via a system of transverse tubules
(**T tubules**), which are invaginations in the muscle cell
membrane. Arrival of the AP at the **sarcoplasmic reticulum**, which serves as a Ca^{2+} store and contains a high concentration of Ca^{2+}, leads to opening of Ca^{2+} **channels** on its
membrane. Consequently, Ca^{2+} diffuses out into the cell
cytoplasm and combines with **troponin**. This makes troponin pull tropomyosin sideways into the groove between

the two F-actin chains, thereby exposing the active sites on actin. Myosin heads, with ATP on them, get attached to actin, resulting in the formation of a high-energy actin–myosin complex. This binding of actin to myosin activates the **ATPase enzyme** present in the myosin head, leading to hydrolysis of ATP:

$$ATP \xrightarrow{ATPase} ADP \xrightarrow{ATPase} AMP$$
$$P_i + E \qquad P_i + E$$

where E represents energy and P_i represents inorganic phosphate.

This hydrolysis of ATP needs magnesium (3 µmol/litre). The energy thus liberated is used for movement of cross-bridges between actin and myosin so that these filaments slide upon each other, bringing the Z lines closer together and making the sarcomere shorter. Summing up of all increments of shortening occurring in all sarcomeres results in the overall shortening of the muscle. When ATP is hydrolysed and lost, what remains is called a **rigor complex** or a low-energy actin–myosin complex. When a new ATP molecule comes and occupies the vacant site on the myosin head, this triggers detachment of myosin from actin. The free myosin head now swings back to its original position and then gets attached to another actin molecule and the cycle gets repeated (i.e. hydrolysis of ATP, swivelling of cross-bridges over 45–50°, sliding of filaments, detachment of myosin from actin, and so on). The rigor complex is very stable and, unless an ATP molecule becomes available to occupy the vacant site on myosin and trigger the release of myosin from actin, the actin remains permanently attached to myosin. In this circumstance the muscle becomes extremely rigid, a situation referred to as **rigor mortis**. It occurs following death due to cessation of metabolism and lack of ATP.

Relaxation of muscle is an active process. ATP is used to pump Ca^{2+} back into the sarcoplasmic reticulum, calcium is detached from troponin, tropinin ceases pulling on tropomyosin, and this returns to its original position and covers the active sites on actin, preventing formation of cross-bridges, and the muscle relaxes. Therefore, ATP is needed for both contraction and relaxation:

1 ATP hydrolysis provides energy for movement of cross-bridges during contraction.

2 ATP is needed for breakdown of the rigor complex and disengagement between actin and myosin.

3 ATP is used for pumping Ca^{2+} back into its stores and thereby promoting muscle relaxation.

Further reading

1 Ganong, W.F. (1999) Excitable tissues: nerve. In: *Review of Medical Physiology*, 19th edn, pp. 43–56. Appleton & Lange, San Mateo, California.

2 Ganong, W.F. (1999) Synaptic and junctional transmission. In: *Review of Medical Physiology*, 19th edn, pp. 80–112. Appleton & Lange, San Mateo, California.

3 Keynes, R.D. & Aidley, D.J. (1981) *Nerve and Muscle*. Cambridge University Press, Cambridge.

4 / The Autonomic Nervous System

Introduction

The whole nervous system can be *anatomically* divided into *central* and *peripheral*. The central is encased within the bones of the cranium and the vertebral column. Thus, the central nervous system (CNS) consists of the brain and the spinal cord. The peripheral nervous system consists of nerve connections between the CNS and the various organs and tissues. These connections include nerve trunks, plexuses and all the smaller nerve fibres which distribute themselves to muscles, skin and other organs.

On the other hand, there are *physiological* divisions of the nervous system. The *somatic* part of the nervous system mainly deals with the voluntary and conscious aspects of neurological control such as skeletal muscle movement and the various somatic sensory functions. The other division, which is the subject of this section, is the **autonomic nervous system**, which deals with involuntary control mechanisms, such as regulation of the heart, the circulation and digestive functions, i.e. *visceral functions*. It is important to note that, anatomically, each of the somatic and autonomic divisions has a central and peripheral component.

The control of visceral functions

The division of the nervous system into autonomic and somatic is not to say that they function independently. There is a great deal of integration between the two. In fact, overlap occurs in the part dealing with emotions and the psyche. This is of particular importance in the manifestations of psychosomatic disorders, when emotional or

Objectives
On completion of the study of this section, the student should be able to:
1 Understand the functional relationships between the somatic and autonomic nervous systems in order to differentiate between somatic and autonomic disorders.
2 Understand the anatomical and functional aspects of the sympathetic and parasympathetic divisions of the autonomic nervous system so as to appreciate the integration of the control of visceral functions.
3 Understand the nature of chemical transmission and the types of autonomic receptors in order to explain the mechanism and site of action of drugs which modify the functions of organ systems.
4 Understand the roles of visceral sensation so as to explain visceral control mechanisms and the physiology of visceral pain.
5 Describe the higher control of the autonomic nervous system so as to appreciate the relationships between psychological factors and visceral disorders.

psychological factors manifest themselves as visceral or somatic symptoms and signs.

Since the autonomic nervous system is directly concerned with regulating visceral or involuntary functions, it is responsible for many mechanisms which control the internal environment. Autonomic nerves also enable the body to react automatically to external environmental inputs such as heat or light. The main integrating station for autonomic functions is the part of the brain known as the **hypothalamus**. From the hypothalamus impulses pass down to the various autonomic nerve cells which supply the internal organs and tissues.

Divisions of the autonomic nervous system

The motor fibres (efferents) of the autonomic nervous system can be divided, from a functional point of view, into two types: the **sympathetic** and the **parasympathetic**. Anatomically they also have different origins in the central nervous system. Sympathetic fibres leave the central nervous system in the thoracic and upper two or three lumbar spinal nerves; hence the name *thoracolumbar outflow*. These nerves distribute themselves widely to supply blood-vessels, the heart, lungs and abdominal viscera.

Parasympathetic fibres leave the central nervous system in some of the cranial nerves, namely the 3rd, 7th, 9th and 10th **cranial nerves** (oculomotor, facial, glossopharyngeal and vagus nerves, respectively). The first three of these nerves supply structures in the head and neck while the vagus nerve is distributed mainly to the thoracic and abdominal organs. Other parasympathetic fibres leave the central nervous system in the **sacral spinal nerves**; hence the other name of the parasympathetic division, the *craniosacral outflow*.

The **sympathetic** division enables the body to mobilize and spend energy and to prepare organ systems to face emergency situations. The **parasympathetic** division functions in the state of relaxation and therefore contributes to the regulation of visceral functions to enable the body to perform restorative and vegetative functions.

Organization of the autonomic nerves

In general, the autonomic nerves, whether sympathetic or parasympathetic, consist of two neurons. The first neuron has its cell body in the central nervous system (the brain nuclei or the grey matter of the spinal cord). The second neuron has its cell body in a **ganglion** which lies outside the CNS. Thus, the two neurons are called **preganglionic** and **postganglionic** respectively. In this respect the autonomic nerves are different from somatic nerves. Somatic nerve cell bodies are never found outside the CNS.

It is noteworthy that a single preganglionic neuron synapses with several postganglionic neurons, thus spreading the effect over a larger area. The sympathetic and parasympathetic parts have some differences and some similarities in their structure and function. Although they generally have opposite effects, there is often a degree of integration in their functions.

The sympathetic division

Anatomical considerations
The **preganglionic** fibres of the sympathetic nerves originate in the lateral horn cells in the spinal grey matter. These lateral horns constitute a column of cells which characterizes the grey matter of all the thoracic and the upper two lumbar segments. The preganglionic fibres leave the spinal cord in the ventral roots. Outside the vertebral column these fibres leave the spinal nerves in the **white rami communicantes** (WRC) and synapse with the postganglionic neurons in the *paravertebral ganglion* (Fig. 4.1). These ganglion neurons have connections between them and therefore they form the **sympathetic chain** which lies on

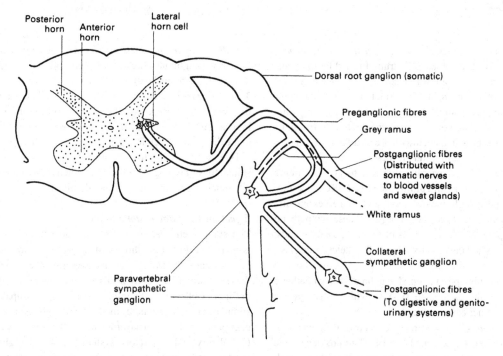

Fig. 4.1 The organization of pre- and postganglionic fibres of the sympathetic nervous system. Preganglionic fibres are shown as solid lines and postganglionic fibres as broken lines.

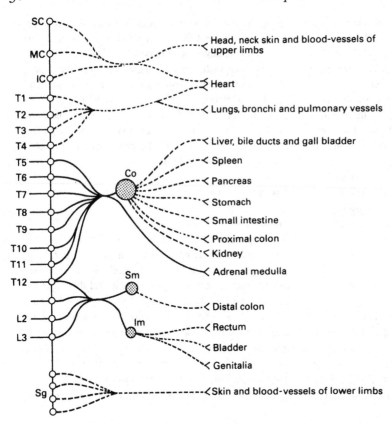

SC
MC
IC
T1
T2
T3
T4
T5
T6
T7
T8
T9
T10
T11
T12
L2
L3
Sg

Co

Sm

Im

Head, neck skin and blood-vessels of upper limbs
Heart
Lungs, bronchi and pulmonary vessels
Liver, bile ducts and gall bladder
Spleen
Pancreas
Stomach
Small intestine
Proximal colon
Kidney
Adrenal medulla
Distal colon
Rectum
Bladder
Genitalia
Skin and blood-vessels of lower limbs

Fig. 4.2 Diagrammatic representation showing the origins and distribution of sympathetic nerves. The solid lines are preganglionic fibres and the broken lines are postganglionic fibres. SC, MC and IC are the superior, middle and inferior cervical ganglia, respectively. Co, Sm, Im and Sg are the coeliac, superior mesenteric, inferior mesenteric and sacral ganglia, respectively.

both sides of the vertebral bodies on the posterior wall of the thorax. The sympathetic trunk formed by interganglionic connections allows synapses to be made several segments above or below the point of exit of the preganglionic fibre from the spinal cord. Some preganglionic fibres, however, do not synapse in the **paravertebral ganglia** but pass through them to synapse in **collateral ganglia**, e.g. the coeliac ganglion and the mesenteric ganglia.

The paravertebral ganglia give rise to postganglionic fibres in the **grey rami communicantes** (GRC) (see Fig. 4.1). The postganglionic fibres join somatic nerves and distribute themselves to the target organs. These sympathetic fibres supply the blood-vessels of the skin, sweat glands, hair follicles and the blood-vessels in the skeletal muscles.

Sympathetic fibres which do not synapse in the thoracic and upper lumbar paravertebral ganglia of the sympathetic chain leave the ganglia to synapse with postganglionic neurons in other ganglia (Fig. 4.2):

1 *Cervical ganglia*. These receive an upward extension of the sympathetic trunk from T1 to T4. Their postganglionic fibres distribute themselves to structures in the head, neck and upper limbs.

2 *Collateral ganglia*. These are found in the abdomen and their postganglionic fibres supply the abdominal viscera down to the proximal part of the colon.

3 *Sacral ganglia*. These receive a caudal extension of the sympathetic trunk from the lower thoracic and upper lumbar segments. They distribute their postganglionic fibres to the distal colon, pelvic organs and lower limbs.

Due to the proximity of paravertebral ganglia to the spinal cord, the preganglionic sympathetic fibres are usually much shorter than the postganglionic ones.

Effects of sympathetic stimulation

The sympathetic part of the autonomic nervous system is activated during conditions of stress and emergencies (e.g. fear, anxiety, hypoglycaemia, severe pain, etc.). Under these conditions the body needs to be prepared for 'fight or flight'. Collectively, therefore, the effects of sympathetic stimulation will promote mechanisms which increase energy metabolism and the efficiency of the supply systems (circulatory and respiratory systems). Table 4.1 gives a summary of the various effects brought about by sympathetic and parasympathetic stimulation.

Table 4.1 Effects of sympathetic and parasympathetic stimulation.

Organ	Sympathetic effects	Parasympathetic effects
The eye		
Iris	Dilatation of pupil	Constriction of pupil
Ciliary muscle	Relaxation (far vision)	Contraction (near vision)
Lacrimal glands	None	Lacrimation
The brain	Increased alertness	None
	Increased blood flow	None
The heart		
SA node	Increased heart rate	Decreased heart rate
Myocardium	Increased strength of contraction	No effect?
Coronary blood-vessels	Dilatation	Dilatation
Blood-vessels to skeletal muscles	Dilatation (cholinergic)	None
Skin	Vasoconstriction	None
	Sweating	
Bronchial muscle	Relaxation (increased blood O_2 content)	Constriction
Gastrointestinal tract		
Salivary glands	Decreased secretion	Increased secretion
Pancreas	Decreased secretion	Increased secretion
Stomach	Decreased secretions and motility	Increased HCl secretions and motility
	Decreased	Increased
Intestinal secretions and motility	Constriction	Relaxation
Sphincters		
Ureters and urinary bladder	Relaxation	Contraction
Detrusor muscle	Contraction	Relaxation
Internal sphincter	Ejaculation	Erection
Male sex organs	Secretion of adrenaline and	None
Adrenal medulla	noradrenaline	

SA, sino-atrial; HCL, hydrochloric acid.

The parasympathetic division

Anatomical considerations

The parasympathetic fibres originate in the nuclei of the cranial nerves mentioned above and in the sacral segments of the spinal cord. The ganglia of parasympathetic fibres are usually situated near or within the tissues or organs supplied. Thus, the postganglionic fibres are very short compared with the preganglionic fibres. The distribution of parasympathetic fibres is given in Fig. 4.3.

Effects of parasympathetic stimulation

The physiological effects of parasympathetic stimulation are related to those activities associated with relaxed states connected with vegetative functions, such as feeding, resting and sexual stimulation. The responses of the digestive system to food intake are due to parasympathetic stimulation, e.g. salivary secretion, secretions of the stomach, pancreas and intestine. Parasympathetic stimulation also increases the motility of the gastrointestinal system and the urinary tract (see Table 4.1).

Chemical transmitters

The effects of sympathetic and parasympathetic stimulation are produced by the release of chemical substances or transmitters which serve two functions: (i) to transmit the nerve impulse from the preganglionic fibre to the postganglionic neuron in the autonomic ganglia; and (ii) to combine with receptors in the target cells so as to produce the desired physiological effect.

In all the ganglia, whether sympathetic or parasympathetic, the transmitter substance is *acetylcholine*. Therefore, all the preganglionic fibres release acetylcholine at the synapse between the pre- and postganglionic neurons. The adrenal medulla is homologous with a sympathetic ganglion. The fibres reaching it come from preganglionic neurons and therefore release acetylcholine (see Fig. 4.3). In the sympathetic ganglia there are interneurons which

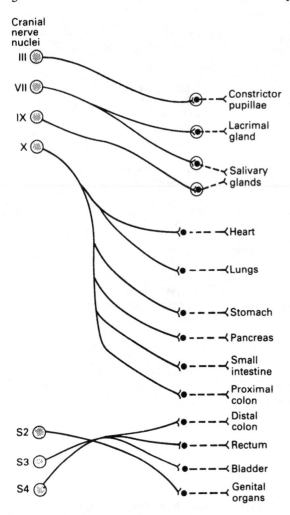

Cranial
nerve
nuclei

III

VII

IX

X

Constrictor
pupillae

Lacrimal
gland

Salivary
glands

Heart

Lungs

Stomach

Pancreas

Small
intestine

Proximal
colon

Distal
colon

Rectum

Bladder

Genital
organs

S2

S3

S4

Fig. 4.3 The origins and distribution of parasympathetic
nerves. III, VII, IX and X are the cranial nerves which contain
parasympathetic fibres. S2, 3 and 4 indicate the 2nd, 3rd and
4th sacral segments. Note the long preganglionic fibres;
postganglionic fibres are usually within the target organ.
However, some of the cranial nerves have separate ganglia,
denoted by the open circles.

at this stage). Some postganglionic cholinergic neurons
also release vasoactive intestinal peptide (VIP). On the
other hand, most of the **sympathetic** postganglionic fibres
release **noradrenaline** (norepinephrine). The postganglionic sympathetic fibres which supply the sweat glands
and the blood-vessels in skeletal muscles are an exception;
they release acetylcholine. Figure 4.4 gives a summary of
autonomic transmitter substances and their sites of release.

In addition to the above well-known transmitters, there
are some *non-adrenergic non-cholinergic (NANC)* autonomic neurons which release other transmitters, mainly
peptides. NANC neurons are also found in the intrinsic
nerves of the gut or *enteric nervous system (ENS)*. In the
gut these transmitters regulate gastrointestinal motility and
the release of hormones. Table 4.2 gives examples of some
well-known transmitters of NANC neurons.

The chemical transmitters act locally either at the
synapse or at the target cell receptors. Their effect lasts only
for a few seconds because they are either destroyed or
removed from the site of their release. Acetylcholine is
broken down by the enzyme *cholinesterase*, which is
found in the terminal endings of all cholinergic nerves.
Noradrenaline, on the other hand, is rapidly taken up by the
nerve endings by active transport. This process accounts
for the removal of most of the noradrenaline released. The
remainder diffuses out with the surrounding extracellular
fluid and is removed by the circulation, where it is quickly
destroyed by enzymes.

Adrenergic receptors

A quick review of the effects of sympathetic stimulation
reveals that in some organs contraction of smooth muscle
is produced, e.g. constriction of blood-vessels. In other
organs, sympathetic stimulation produces relaxation of
smooth muscle, e.g. coronary vessels, intestine and urinary
bladder. The explanation of this is the presence of different
receptors on the target cells. Two main types of adrenergic
receptors, known as **alpha- (α-)** and **beta- (β-) receptors**,
have been described. In general, alpha receptors are stimulatory and beta receptors are inhibitory, although this is not
always the case (Table 4.3).

Certain drugs have been found to block or inhibit some
of the effects of alpha or beta receptor stimulation. On the
basis of this observation, such drugs have been classified as
α-blockers and β-blockers.

The distribution of adrenergic receptors in the various
tissues can be deduced from the effects of drugs. Table 4.3
gives examples of α- and β-receptor effects of sympathetic
stimulation. Within one organ more than one type of receptor may be found. The alpha and beta receptors have been

are also acted upon by preganglionic fibres and they themselves synapse on the postganglionic neuron. These interneurons secrete **dopamine** as an inhibitory transmitter.
Their functional significance is to damp transmission at the
ganglia and therefore to limit preganglionic stimulation.

Acetylcholine and noradrenaline (norepinephrine) are
the two main transmitters released by the postganglionic
fibres. In general, all postganglionic fibres of the **parasympathetic** release *acetylcholine* as the main transmitter (with a few exceptions which will not be mentioned

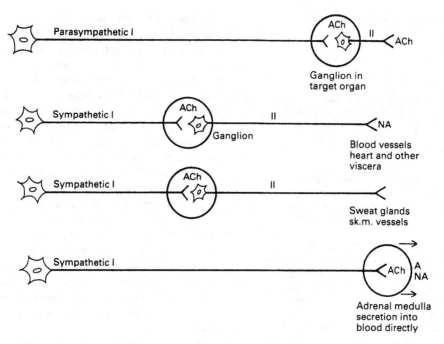

Fig. 4.4 Schematic representation of the various sites of release of autonomic transmitters. I and II refer to preganglionic and postganglionic fibres, respectively. A, adrenaline (epinephrine); ACh, acetylcholine; NA, noradrenaline (norepinephrine); sk.m., skeletal muscle.

Table 4.2 Examples of the transmitters of NANC neurons.

Transmitter	Site(s)	Possible effects
Dopamine	ANS ganglia	Modulates effects of ACh
	Some sympathetic postganglionic neurons	Renal sympathetic blood-vessels
	ENS	
Encephalin	ENS	Secretomotor and interneuronal activity inhibits peristalsis
		May stimulate secretion
GABA (gamma-aminobutyric acid)	ENS	Relaxant effect on the gut
GRP (gastrin-releasing peptide)	ENS	Excitatory stimulus to G cells, which release gastrin
NO (nitric oxide)	ANS	Cotransmitter with ACh in some cholinergic neurons
	ENS	Inhibitory cotransmitter at gut neuromuscular junctions
VIP (vasoactive intestinal peptide)	ANS	Cotransmitter with many cholinergic neurons
	ENS	A vasodilator
		Secretomotor in ENS

ACh, acetylcholine. ANS, autonomic nervous system.

Table 4.3 The effects of α- and β-adrenergic receptors.

Sympathetic effects due to α-receptors	Sympathetic effects due to β-receptors
Dilatation of iris (mydriasis)	*Beta$_1$-receptors*
Constriction of blood-vessels in gut, skin, salivary glands, lungs and cerebral circulation	Cardioacceleration
	Increased myocardial contractility
	Lipolysis
Constriction of sphincters in GI tract	Renin secretion
Increased motility of ureters	*Beta$_2$-receptors*
Contraction of trigone and internal sphincter of urinary bladder	Coronary vasodilatation
	Skeletal muscle vasodilatation
Ejaculation	Skeletal muscle tremor
Sweating, slight and localized	Bronchodilatation
Pilomotor muscle contraction	Relaxation of uterus
Decreased secretion of salivary glands	Intestinal relaxation
	Bladder relaxation
Decreased secretion of pancreatic juice	Calorigenic effect
	Glycogenolysis
Decreased insulin and glucagon secretion	Amylase secretion

Table 4.4 Some examples of adrenergic receptor blockers.

Alpha-receptor blockers	Beta-receptor blockers
Phenoxybenzamine (Dibenyline)	*Non-selective*
	Propranolol (Inderal) (β$_1$ and β$_2$)
Phentolamine (Rogitine)	Oxprenolol (β$_1$ and β$_2$)
Dihydroergotamine	
Prazosin (α$_1$)	*Selective*
Yohimbine (α$_2$)	Atenolol (Tenormin) (β$_1$)
	Metoprolol (β$_1$)
	Practolol (β$_1$)
	Butoxamine (β$_2$)

subdivided into α$_1$-, α$_2$-, β$_1$- and β$_2$-receptors. New drugs are now available with more selective action on specific receptors. Table 4.4 gives examples of adrenergic receptor blockers. These drugs are becoming more and more important in therapeutics, e.g. in the treatment of hypertension and coronary heart disease.

Cholinergic receptors

Acetylcholine is released in all preganglionic nerve endings, i.e. in the sympathetic and parasympathetic ganglia. On the basis of the effects of drugs which have similar actions to acetylcholine, it has been found that the receptors in the ganglia are different from those in peripheral tissues supplied by postganglionic fibres. Thus, *nicotine* produces effects similar to those of preganglionic stimulation (nicotinic actions of acetylcholine). On the other hand, the drug *muscarine* produces effects similar to postganglionic parasympathetic fibres (muscarinic effects of acetylcholine). Cholinergic receptors in the autonomic ganglia can be blocked by drugs such as *hexamethonium*. On the other hand, the muscarinic actions of acetylcholine at the postganglionic endings are blocked by *atropine*. In fact, atropine blocks all the autonomic cholinergic effects except those at the autonomic ganglia.

Apart from the autonomic nerves, acetylcholine is also the transmitter at the neuromuscular junction of skeletal muscle. The cholinergic receptors in skeletal muscle can also be stimulated by nicotine but they are not identical with those found in autonomic ganglia. At the neuromuscular junction, the action of acetylcholine is blocked by the drugs *curare* and *tubocurarine*. Furthermore, acetylcholine is an important neurotransmitter in the central nervous system.

Myasthenia gravis is a disease caused by autoimmune destruction of acetylcholine receptors at the neuromuscular junction of skeletal muscle (see Chapter 3).

Visceral afferent fibres

Visceral functions are continuously monitored by various sensory receptors situated in the organs or in the central nervous system. Examples of peripheral receptors are the **chemoreceptors** and **baroreceptors** which are concerned with the regulation of cardiovascular and respiratory functions. Examples of central receptors are the **thermoreceptors** and **osmoreceptors** in the hypothalamus which are concerned with the regulation of body temperature and water balance, respectively. There are also receptors for pain and stretch in the viscera.

Afferent fibres from the viscera travel in the fibres of the autonomic nervous system (see Fig. 4.1). These afferent fibres are essential for the regulation of the various organ systems. The visceral afferent fibres have their cell bodies in the *cranial nerve ganglia* and in the *dorsal root ganglia* of the spinal cord. Thus, we find visceral nerves in the facial nerve, glossopharyngeal nerve and vagus. Visceral afferent fibres are also found in the thoracic and upper two or three lumbar nerves and the sacral nerves, i.e. all the spinal nerves which have sympathetic or parasympathetic components. Therefore, visceral pain goes to these segments of the spinal cord and is sometimes felt on the part of the body or skin supplied by somatic nerves of the same segment. This is called **referred pain**. A good example of this is shoulder pain due to diaphragmatic irritation or gall-bladder disease.

In the spinal cord, visceral afferent fibres travel in the spinothalamic tracts. In the brain they are found in the fibres of the thalamic radiation. Cortical representation is in the postcentral gyrus and is found to be intermixed with somatic representation.

Special features of autonomic functions

The following special features characterize the mechanisms responsible for autonomic functions. They are highlighted here for the sake of contrast with somatic functions.

1 The viscera have their own intrinsic functions and therefore autonomic denervation does not result in complete loss of function or paralysis. Autonomic nerves seem to control the *level of activity* and its modulation according to requirements.

2 Autonomic nerves have a basal level of discharge or tone, which can be increased or decreased according to physiological requirements. *Sympathetic tone* is the term given to the continuous basal discharge to blood-vessels which keeps them in a state of partial or tonic contraction at rest. Vasoconstriction is produced by increasing the sympathetic tone and vasodilatation is produced by decreasing it.

The parasympathetic or *vagal tone* to the heart at rest keeps the heart rate at the right level for maintenance of the resting cardiac output. An increase in the heart rate can be produced by reducing the vagal tone. Increasing the tone results in slowing of heart rate.

Similarly, abolition of vagal tone to the gastrointestinal tract results in temporarily decreased motility and slow passage of food, recovery occurring within 24 hours. However, gastric acid secretion is permanently decreased, which allows a peptic ulcer to heal, thereby providing a rationale for surgical section of the vagus nerve in the surgical management of peptic ulcers.

3 One of the characteristics of sympathetic functions is the *mass discharge*. This means that sympathetic discharge can occur simultaneously to many parts of the body. Thus, in the 'fight or flight' response there are numerous effects occurring at the same time, e.g. increased cardiac output, increased blood flow in the skeletal muscle, decreased blood flow in the skin and splanchnic area, increased rate of metabolism, increased blood glucose, mental alertness, etc.

This is not the case with parasympathetic reactions, which tend to be localized specific responses, e.g. the heart rate decreases in response to a rise in blood pressure by increasing vagal tone; salivary secretion in response to the smell and taste of food; secretion of gastric juice; emptying of the rectum and urinary bladder, penile erection, etc.

Higher control of autonomic functions

There are several areas of the brain which are concerned with autonomic regulation. Neurons in the *posterior* part of the *hypothalamus* regulate sympathetic functions, such as blood pressure and heart rate, while those in the *anterior hypothalamus* regulate some parasympathetic effects, such as contraction of the urinary bladder. There is, however, considerable overlap in this distribution of hypothalamic nuclei. Other areas, such as the reticular formation of the medulla and pons, exert influences on autonomic functions such as heart rate, blood pressure and gastrointestinal secretions and motility.

Autonomic functions are initiated by reflexes which have their centres in the spinal cord or the cranial nerve nuclei in the brain stem. These reflexes are influenced by the higher centres mentioned above. Some of the reflexes, like the voiding of urine and defecation, are also controlled by higher voluntary centres.

The hypothalamus is situated at the base of the brain. It is closely related to the **limbic system**, of which it is considered by some as an integral part. There are numerous nuclei and areas in the hypothalamus. These have been given various names, the most well known of which are the supraoptic and paraventricular nuclei (see Chapter 16). These nuclei are not anatomically as well defined as they might appear in diagrams. The hypothalamus receives information from various parts of the CNS and gives outputs both to the cerebrum above and to the brain stem below (Fig. 4.5). It sends outputs to the anterior thalamus and the limbic cortex in the cerebrum. It also sends outputs to the reticular formation of the brain stem and the vital centres of the medulla.

The hypothalamus is largely concerned with vegetative or visceral functions (see Table 4.5). It mediates some of the effects of the autonomic nervous system. For this reason it is sometimes called the *head ganglion of the autonomic nervous system*. Section of the brain stem above the medulla, however, does not affect most basal functions of the autonomic nervous system. This emphasizes the importance of spinal and medullary centres in autonomic responses.

The *limbic system* consists of those parts of the brain which are responsible for instinctive behaviour and emotions. In lower animals this part of the brain represents the

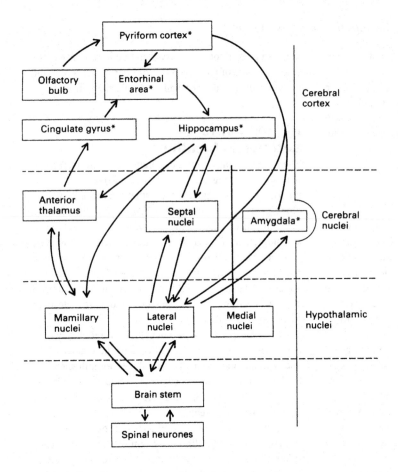

Fig. 4.5 Diagrammatic representation of the major connections of the hypothalamus. Parts of the cerebral cortex and cerebral nuclei are marked (*) to indicate that they are part of the limbic system.

Table 4.5 Functions of various nuclei of the hypothalamus.

Anterior hypothalamus*	Posterior hypothalamus*
Preoptic nucleus Bladder contraction Decreased heart rate Decreased blood pressure	*Posterior hypothalamic nucleus* Dilatation of pupil Increased blood pressure Shivering
Supraoptic nucleus Antidiuretic hormone release	*Perifornical nucleus* Hunger Increased blood pressure
Paraventricular nucleus Oxytocin release	Rage
	Ventromedial nucleus Satiety
Anterior hypothalamic area Temperature regulation, sweating	
	Dorsomedial nucleus Stimulation of GI tract
Lateral hypothalamic nuclei Thirst centre Feeding centre	
	Mammillary bodies Feeding reflexes

* The lateral hypothalamic nuclei overlap both the anterior and posterior nuclei on both sides. One of the main functions of the lateral nuclei is to provide connections with the cerebral nuclei, e.g. the thalamus and the limbic nuclei. GI, gastrointestinal.

largest portion of the cerebral hemispheres. In humans it is restricted mainly to parts around the hilum of the cerebral hemisphere (see Chapter 16). The close connections of the hypothalamus with the limbic system help to explain the causation of abnormal autonomic reactions. Such conditions have been collectively known as **psychosomatic disorders**, characterized by hyper- or hypoactivity of autonomic functions. Peptic ulcer, hypertension, ulcerative colitis and migraine are frequently encountered examples of these conditions. Almost all diseases have a psychological element in them. The patient's reaction to his/her complaints are influenced by his/her psyche and by social factors in the environment. The doctor is well advised to take account of these factors in communication with patients as well as in diagnosis and management.

Further reading

1 Ganong, W.F. (1999) The autonomic nervous system. In: *Review of Medical Physiology*, 19th edn, pp. 214–220. Appleton & Lange, San Mateo, California.
2 Guyton, A.C. & Hall, J.E. (1997) The limbic system. In: *Textbook of Medical Physiology*, 9th edn, pp. 769–781. Saunders, Philadelphia.

5 / The Cardiovascular System

Objectives

On completion of the study of this section, the student should be able to:

1 Acquire basic information on the properties of cardiac muscle and the electrical events taking place in the heart, so as to use the electrocardiogram (ECG) in order to identify conduction defects, arrhythmias, ischaemic heart disease, etc.

2 Describe the events of the cardiac cycle and correlate the electrical events with the contraction and relaxation phases and the heart sounds so as to explain the pathophysiology of valvular and congenital heart disease.

3 Comprehend the factors which influence and regulate the cardiac output so as to use this information in the diagnosis and management of heart failure.

4 Understand the relationships between pressure, flow and resistance in the circulatory system so as to explain the pathophysiology of blood-pressure abnormalities, heart failure and oedema.

5 Understand the circulation in various special regions (pulmonary, coronary, cerebral) so as to explain abnormalities of blood flow such as myocardial and cerebral ischaemia.

Introduction

The heart provides two pumps in series which drive the circulation of blood through the systemic and pulmonary vessels. The circulation of blood serves many functions, e.g.: (i) transport of substances absorbed from the gastrointestinal tract (GIT) and O_2 to the tissues; (ii) return of CO_2 to the lungs; (iii) transport of waste products of metabolism for excretion; (iv) thermoregulation; and (v) transport of hormones and other agents that regulate cell function. The heart and blood-vessels respond to physical and chemical changes in the internal and external environments and therefore play a major role in homoeostasis. Adjustments in the pumping action of the heart and the distribution of blood flow help to bring the altered parameters back to normal. For example, changes in blood O_2, CO_2 or pH give rise to important cardiovascular responses which correct these changes. A rise or fall of the skin or deep body temperatures also produces cardiovascular responses which help in the regulation of body temperature. For these reasons, the cardiovascular system can be regarded as a homoeostatic system.

Fig. 5.1 The chambers and valves of the heart. The arrows indicate the direction of flow. (Reproduced from Bray, J.J., Cragg, P.A., Macknight; A.D.C., Mills, R.G. & Taylor, D.W. (eds), (1989) *Lecture Notes in Physiology*, 2nd edn. Blackwell Scientific Publications, Oxford.)

Labels on figure: Aorta; Pulmonary artery; Pulmonary vein; Left atrium; Bicuspid atrioventricular valve; Aortic semilunar valve; Chordae tendineae; Papillary muscle; Left ventricle; Myocardium; Superior vena cava; Right atrium; Pulmonary semilunar valve; Tricuspid atrioventricular valve; Inferior vena cava; Right ventricle

Anatomical considerations of the heart

Atria

The atria are thin-walled chambers which receive blood either from the systemic circulation or from the pulmonary circulation. The atria open into the ventricles via the atrioventricular valves (Fig. 5.1).

The ventricles

The ventricles are thick-walled chambers which pump blood into the pulmonary trunk and the aorta. The wall of the left ventricle is three to four times thicker than the right ventricle, because of the greater work it has to do against aortic impedance due to the arterial blood pressure. The right ventricle works against much less pressure in the pulmonary arteries. However, each ventricle has the same capacity and pumps the same volume of blood in a given period of time. Even minor differences over long periods of time result in heart failure. This leads to congestion of the systemic veins in the case of **right ventricular failure**, and congestion of the pulmonary circulation in the case of **left ventricular failure**.

There is a fibrous tissue ring separating the atria from the ventricles. It separates the myocardium of the atria from that of the ventricles. Therefore, electrical activity in the atria cannot go directly to the ventricles. The fibrous tissue also gives attachment to the muscle cells of the heart and the atrioventricular valves.

The valves of the heart

There are no valves where the great veins enter the atria. However, the heart itself has four sets of valves which ensure that the blood flows in one direction and that no regurgitation occurs between the chambers of the heart. The right atrioventricular opening is guarded by the **tricuspid** valve (three cusps). At the left atrioventricular opening, there is the **mitral valve** or bicuspid valve (two cusps). The openings of the aorta and the pulmonary trunk are guarded by the **semilunar valves**.

The atrioventricular cusps are held by **chordae tendineae** to papillary muscles. These muscles contract as part of the ventricular myocardium. Therefore, during ventricular contraction the cusps are held down so that they do not flap into the atria causing back flow of blood (see Fig. 5.1).

The conducting tissues

The conducting tissues of the heart consist of specialized myocardial cells. The pacemaker cells are found in the **sinoatrial (SA) node** in the right atrium near the junction with the superior vena cava. The **atrioventricular (AV) node** lies above the fibrous ring and represents the only myocardial connection between the atria and ventricles. The **bundle of His** starts in the AV node and gives rise to two branches (right and left), which descend into the interventricular septum. The terminal branches of the conducting tissue end in the subendocardial muscle of the ventricles.

Cardiac innervation

The heart receives extrinsic nerve supply from both **sympathetic** and **parasympathetic** divisions of the autonomic nervous system. The preganglionic neurons of the cardiac sympathetic nerves originate from the lateral horn cells of the upper thoracic segments. They relay in the sympathetic chain. The postganglionic nerves run in the cardiac sympathetic nerve and innervate the SA node, the atrial myocardium, the AV node and the ventricular myocardium. The parasympathetic supply to the heart originates in the neurons of the **nucleus ambiguus** of the medulla oblongata, also known as the **cardioinhibitory area**. The nerve fibres reach the heart in the vagus nerves. Preganglionic fibres synapse in parasympathetic ganglia near the heart. The postganglionic fibres are short and supply the SA node in the atrial muscle and the AV node.

Properties of cardiac muscle

To understand the properties of cardiac muscle, we must first take into account some basic anatomical considerations.

When seen under the light microscope, cardiac muscle appears striated but it differs in several ways from striated skeletal muscle. It consists of branching and interdigitating fibres which are closely attached to one another by structures known as **intercalated discs** (Fig. 5.2). Intercalated discs provide a strong union between fibres, maintaining cell-to-cell cohesion. They provide low-resistance bridges for the spread of excitation from one fibre to another. Therefore they permit cardiac muscle to function as a syncytium because of the presence of **gap junctions**. Cardiac muscle cells contain a large number of elongated mitochondria in close contact with the myofibrils.

Cardiac muscle has four characteristic properties, which will be considered below: **contractility, rhythmicity, excitability** and **conductivity**.

Contractility

Contractility is the ability of the cardiac muscle to convert chemical energy into mechanical work. The heart acts as a muscular pump and the strength of its contractility determines its pumping power.

The mechanism of contraction depends on the contractile units, the myofibrils, which contain the protein molecules

Fig. 5.2 Microstructure of cardiac muscle showing intercalated discs between muscle cells. (Reproduced from Bray, J.J., Cragg, P.A., Macknight, A.D.C., Mills, R.G. & Taylor, D.W. (eds) (1989) *Lecture Notes in Physiology*, 2nd edn. Blackwell Scientific Publications, Oxford.)

actin and myocin. The shortening of the myofibrils (see Chapter 3) takes place with energy derived from adenosine triphosphate (ATP). Almost all the energy needed for contraction is derived from **aerobic metabolism**, so an adequate oxygen supply is essential for cardiac contractility.

Factors affecting myocardial contractility

Factors which affect myocardial contractility are said to have an inotropic effect. Those which increase contractility are called positive **inotropic factors** and those which decrease contractility are called negative inotropic factors. The factors which affect myocardial contractility are as follows:

1 *Starling's law of the heart*. The contractility of cardiac muscle depends on the initial length of its fibres. If the **venous return** is increased, this will stretch the cardiac muscle so that the initial length of the muscle fibres will increase. As a result of this increase in diastolic volume, the strength of contraction will increase, provided that the fibres are not stretched above their elastic limits. Starling's law explains how cardiac muscle accommodates itself to the changes in venous return.

2 *Cardiac innervation*. Cardiac muscle is supplied by both divisions of the autonomic nervous system. In the heart, cholinergic and noradrenergic nerve fibres end on the sinoatrial node, AV node and bundle of His. Noradrenergic fibres also innervate the ventricular muscle. Sympathetic stimulation produces an increase in contractility and vagal stimulation produces a decrease in contractility.

3 *Hormonal and chemical factors or drugs*. Adrenaline (epinephrine), noradrenaline (norepinephrine), alkalis, digitalis and calcium ions are all positively inotropic. Acetylcholine, acids, ether, chloroform, some bacterial toxins (e.g. diphtheria toxin) and K^+ ions are all negatively inotropic.

4 *Physical factors*. Warming increases contractility while cooling decreases it.

5 *Oxygen supply*. This depends on the condition of the coronary vessels. Hypoxia (low oxygen content in the blood) depresses contractility.

6 *Mechanical factors*:

(a) Because cardiac muscle behaves as a syncytium, it obeys the 'all-or-none law', i.e. minimal or threshold stimuli lead to maximal cardiac contraction.

(b) Cardiac muscle shows the **treppe** or **staircase phenomenon**, i.e. if an isolated heart is stimulated by successive equal and effective stimuli, the first few contractions show a gradual increase in the magnitude of contraction.

(c) Cardiac muscle cannot be excited while it is contracting. This is due to the **long absolute refractory** period of cardiac muscle (see Chapter 3). Therefore, the muscle must relax before it can be restimulated. The length of the refractory period is vital to the functions of the heart as a pump. It prevents cardiac muscle from being tetanized like skeletal muscle. If it were possible to tetanize cardiac muscle, the heart would be thrown into a state of continuous contraction, i.e. it would stop and the subject would die of circulatory failure.

(d) Cardiac muscle can perform both **isometric** and **isotonic** types of contractions as will be explained later.

Rhythmicity (automaticity)

Rhythmicity is the ability of cardiac muscle to contract in a regularly constant manner. The rhythmicity is **myogenic** in origin, i.e. its origination has nothing to do with the nerves of the heart. It is not neurogenic. This is proved by: (i) the finding that, if the apex of the frog heart is cut off and placed in Ringer's solution, it will continue to contract in a rhythmic manner although it is devoid of any nervous tissue; (ii) the fact that the heart of the human or the chick embryo shows rhythmic contraction before the development of any nervous connections to it.

The pacemaker of the heart

The frog's heart is different from the human heart in that it has five chambers instead of four. The extra chamber is the sinus venosus (SV), which is similar to the sinoatrial (SA) node in the human heart. Experiments with frogs' hearts have proved that rhythmicity is not the same in the different chambers of the heart. In the human heart there are specialized pacemaker tissues which are characterized by an unstable membrane potential. A slow decrease in K^+ permeability causes a progressive decline in K^+ efflux and towards the end of this phase influx of Ca^{2+}. The membrane potential declines steadily until the firing level is reached and another action potential is triggered. This **pacemaker potential** is also known as a **prepotential** (Fig. 5.3). It is evident in the SA node and the AV node. The depolarization phase is due to Ca^{2+} influx and opening of some Na^+ channels as well. The repolarization phase is due to K^+ influx. There are 'latent pacemakers' in other parts of the conduction system, which are called upon when the SA and AV nodes are not functioning. Atrial and ventricular muscles do not have the prepotential characteristic. Evidence for the pacemaker of the heart has been derived from the following observations:

1 If heat or cold is applied to the different chambers of the frog's heart, the rhythm is found to change only when the heat or cold is applied to the SV. No change is noted when the temperature stimulus is applied to the atria or ventricles.

Fig. 5.3 Pacemaker potential and K^+ conductance in sinoatrial node. Note the prepotential indicating instability of the resting membrane potential (RMP). (Reproduced from Bray, J.J., Cragg, P.A., Macknight, A.D.C., Mills, R.G. & Taylor, D.W. (eds) (1989) *Lecture Notes in Physiology*, 2nd edn. Blackwell Scientific Publications, Oxford.)

2 If the SV is separated from the atria of the frog's heart, the atria and ventricles will stop immediately, while the SV will continue to beat in its normal rhythm. After some time the ventricles will start contracting again but at a slower rhythm. This is called the **idioventricular rhythm**.

3 Measurement of the electrical potential changes over the different chambers of the heart has shown that the SA node is the first part of the heart to show electrical negativity.

Factors affecting rhythmicity

Nervous, physical and chemical factors affect rhythmicity as follows:

1 *Neural factors*. Vagal stimulation (or application of acetylcholine) increases the permeability of SA nodal tissue to K^+ ions and decreases the opening of Ca^{2+} channels. This decreases the slope of the prepotential and the rate of firing of the SA node and results in slowing of the heartbeat (**bradycardia**). Strong stimulation of the vagus nerve may lead to complete stoppage of SA nodal activity. Sympathetic stimulation (or application of noradrenaline [norepinephrine]) decreases the permeability of the nodal tissue to K^+ ions and decreases the resting membrane potential. This increases the slope of the prepotential and the rate of firing, resulting in acceleration of the heart (**tachycardia**).

2 *Physical factors*. Moderate warming of the SA node increases rhythmicity, while cooling decreases it.

Fig. 5.4 Time relationship between the action potential and the contraction of ventricular muscle. ARP, absolute refractory period; ECG, electrocardiogram; RRP, relative refractory period. Note that summation of contraction is not possible.

3 *Effects of ions.* Application of Na$^+$ ions can initiate rhythmicity but cannot maintain it. A decrease in extracellular K$^+$ ions increases the slope of diastolic depolarization and therefore increases the rhythmicity. An increase in extracellular K$^+$ ions decreases the rhythmicity and may stop the heart in **diastole** (relaxed phase) by decreasing the slope of diastolic depolarization.

4 *Chemical factors.* Thyroid hormones and catecholamines increase the rhythmicity of the heart while acetylcholine, digitalis, some metabolites and oxygen lack decrease the heart rate.

Excitability (irritability)

Excitability is the ability of the cardiac muscle to respond to adequate stimuli by generating an action potential followed by a mechanical contraction (Fig. 5.4).

Changes in the extracellular K$^+$ concentration affect the resting membrane potential of cardiac muscle, while changes in extracellular Na$^+$ concentration affect the magnitude of the action potential. The initial depolarization is due to an increase in Na$^+$ permeability. The plateau in the slope of the action potential is due to a slower increase in Ca^{2+} permeability. Repolarization is due to a delayed increase in K$^+$ permeability.

Excitability passes through two phases:

1 *Absolute refractory period (ARP).* In cardiac muscle the ARP is very long compared with that in nerve or skeletal muscle cells. The ARP occupies the whole period of systole

(contraction phase of cardiac muscle). The ARP corresponds to the period of **depolarization**, during which the excitability of the heart muscle becomes zero, i.e. no stimulus, however strong, can excite the muscle or produce any response. The difference between cardiac muscle and skeletal muscle in this phase is very important from a functional point of view. Skeletal muscle can be tetanized while cardiac muscle cannot, because the ARP occupies the whole contraction phase (systole).

2 *Relative refractory period.* This occupies the time of diastole of cardiac muscle and corresponds to **repolarization**. A strong enough stimulus can give rise to contraction during the relative refractory period. The refractory period can be affected by the heart rate, temperature, bacterial toxins, vagal stimulation, sympathetic stimulation and drugs.

Responses of the cardiac muscle are all or none in character, i.e. the muscle fibres contract fully if they respond at all. Due to the presence of the ARP property, the cardiac muscle cannot be tetanized, which in itself is a safety measure. Tetanization of cardiac muscle (if it could be induced) would be fatal.

Conductivity

Conductivity is the ability of cardiac muscle fibres to conduct the cardiac impulses that are initiated in the SA node, which is the pacemaker of the heart.

The cardiac conduction system is composed of the:
1 Sinoatrial (SA) node.
2 Internodal pathways.
3 Atrioventricular (AV) node.
4 Bundle of His and its branches.
5 Purkinje system.

The conduction system is richer in glycogen and has more sarcoplasm than the rest of the cardiac muscle fibres. The **SA node** develops from the right side of the embryo and the **AV node** develops from the left side. The right vagus, therefore, supplies the SA node, while the left vagus supplies the AV node. Both nodes receive noradrenergic nerves from the cervical sympathetic ganglia via the cardiac nerves.

The SA node is the normal cardiac **pacemaker** because it discharges most rapidly and dictates the rate at which the heart beats. From the SA node the impulses are conducted to the AV node through atrial musculature and internodal pathways, which are three in number. They connect the SA node to the AV node. From the AV node the impulses pass to the AV bundle (bundle of His), which divides into two branches, right and left, and transmit the impulses to the ventricles. From the apex of the heart the impulses are conducted to the base of the heart through the Purkinje fibres.

Conduction velocity in the bundle of His is 1 m/s and in the Purkinje fibres 4 m/s (fastest); it is about 0.4 m/s in ventricular muscle and 0.05 m/s in the SA node. It is slowest (0.01 m/s) in the AV node. The AV nodal delay gives time for the ventricles to be filled with blood before they contract (ventricular systole).

The electrocardiogram (ECG)

Introduction

Definitions
• 'A **graphic recording** of electrical activity generated by the heart.'
• 'The **techniques** of recording electrical activity from the heart.'
• '**Tracing** of the **surface cardiac potentials** recorded **against time**.'
• 'A record of the changing potentials of the **electrical field** imparted by the heart.'
In essence, it is a clinical test used as an indicator of cardiac function. It is most useful in detecting *cardiac arrhythmias* and the *assessment of the myocardium*.

Historical background
Kolliker and Muller in 1856 demonstrated the presence of an action current associated with the heart beat. The correlation between a measurable amount of current in the human body and cardiac contraction was discovered by Walter and Ludwig in 1887. These basic concepts were registered and translated into a quantitative form by Willem Einthoven in 1901, who is considered to be the father of the ECG.

Apparatus and patient preparation
Initially a string galvanometer was introduced by Einthoven to record the heart beat; it was replaced by the oscilloscope later. Today immediate and direct recordings of ECGs are possible by using vacuum-tube amplification equipment. A good-quality, effective contact between the electrodes and skin is important. Jelly is used as a conductor. The patient should be warm to avoid shivering so as to minimize baseline interference.

The leads
The routine ECG includes 12 leads. A pair of electrodes applied to the appropriate parts of the body is called a lead.
1 The limb leads. These are six leads—three bipolar and three unipolar (Fig. 5.5). The standard limb leads are named leads I, II and III. Lead I connects the arms, lead II

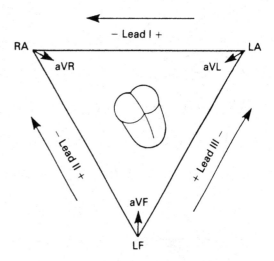

Fig. 5.5 Einthoven's triangle and the limb leads. RA, LA and LF are right arm, left arm and left leg, respectively; aVR, aVL and aVF are augmented limb leads. The arrows indicate the direction in which each lead detects the electrical activity of the heart. (Reproduced from Bray, J.J., Cragg, P.A., Macknight, A.D.C., Mills, R.G. & Taylor, D.W. (eds) (1989) *Lecture Notes in Physiology*, 2nd edn. Blackwell Scientific Publications, Oxford.)

connects the right arm with the left leg and lead III connects the left arm with the left leg. These are known as **bipolar** leads since two electrodes are used for recording each standard lead. The **unipolar** limb leads include aVR, aVL and aVF, which are labelled according to the limb to which the positive terminal of the ECG machine is connected. The letter 'a' signifies the augmentation (increase in the magnitude of recording by 1.5 times). By combining the six limb leads, the Einthoven triangle (Fig. 5.5) can be constructed.
2 The chest (precordial) leads. These are also **unipolar** leads and include leads V1–V6, as shown in Fig. 5.6:
• V1: in the 4th intercostal space (ICS) just to the right of the sternum.
• V2: in the 4th ICS just to the left of sternum.
• V4: at the midclavicular line in the 5th ICS.
• V3: halfway between V2 and V4.
• V5: in the anterior axillary line at the same level as V4.
• V6: in the midaxillary line at the same level as V4 and V5.

The 12 leads record the algebraic sum of the **vectors** generated as a result of the cardiac muscle action potentials. The vector is a term which describes the direction and magnitude of the depolarization wave, usually represented by an arrow pointing in the positive direction. The leads facing the resultant vector record an upright deflection (positive deflection), while those recording a vector travelling away

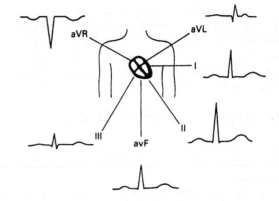

Fig. 5.8 ECG records from bipolar limb leads and unipolar augmented limb leads. (Reproduced from Bray, J.J., Cragg, P.A., Macknight, A.D.C., Mills, R.G. & Taylor, D.W. (eds) (1989) *Lecture Notes in Physiology*, 2nd edn. Blackwell Scientific Publications, Oxford.)

Fig. 5.6 Diagram showing the position of the unipolar chest leads. (Reproduced from Bray, J.J., Cragg, P.A., Macknight, A.D.C., Mills, R.G. & Taylor, D.W. (eds) (1989) *Lecture Notes in Physiology*, 2nd edn. Blackwell Scientific Publications, Oxford.)

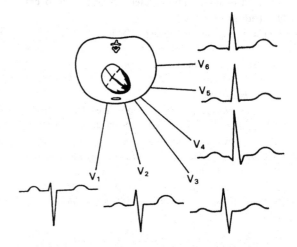

Fig. 5.9 ECG records from chest leads. (Reproduced from Bray, J.J., Cragg, P.A., Macknight, A.D.C., Mills, R.G. & Taylor, D.W. (eds) (1989) *Lecture Notes in Physiology*, 2nd edn. Blackwell Scientific Publications, Oxford.)

Fig. 5.7 General appearance of ECG record at rest. (Reproduced from Bray, J.J., Cragg, P.A., Macknight, A.D.C., Mills, R.G. & Taylor, D.W. (eds) (1989) *Lecture Notes in Physiology*, 2nd edn. Blackwell Scientific Publications, Oxford.)

from the lead will show a negative deflection as compared with the **isoelectric line** (Figs 5.7, 5.8 & 5.9). The ECG tracings are made at a standard recording speed of 25 mm/s and an amplification (amplitude) of 1 mV = 1 cm deflection. On standard ECG paper, each small horizontal division represents 0.04 s and each large division is 0.2 s, while each small vertical division represents 0.1 mV (Fig. 5.7). This information will help us later in interpreting the different ECG wave durations and the magnitude of their voltage, as well as the duration of the different ECG intervals.

The normal ECG

ECG waves and intervals

ECG waves. The wave-forms observed in the ECG are labelled as P, QRS, T and U waves (Fig. 5.7).
• **P wave**. This is the first positive deflection (as compared with the isoelectric line). It is produced by atrial activation. Electrically it represents the depolarization of the atria. It is rounded in shape, with 0.2 mV amplitude and 0.12 s duration (Fig. 5.7).
• **QRS complex**. This is the second mainly positive deflection. It is generated by ventricular depolarization secondary to the spread of the excitation wave down the interventricular septum and across the ventricles. The duration of the QRS complex is 0.12 s. This information is useful when we consider conduction delay abnormalities. Also note that the amplitude of the QRS complex can give a clue to the state of ventricular hypertrophy.
• **T wave**. This is the third positive deflection in a normal ECG tracing. It represents ventricular repolarization. Its amplitude ranges from 0.1 to 0.7 mV.
• **U wave**. This is a small, rounded, positive deflection (< 0.1 mV) which sometimes follows the T wave. Like the T wave, it is also due to ventricular repolarization. Its amplitude is increased as a result of drugs (e.g. quinidine) or hypokalaemia. An inverted U wave is sometimes seen in association with myocardial ischaemia.

The P–R interval. This interval is measured from the onset of the P wave to the onset of the QRS complex (0.12–0.22 s). It includes the time for intra-atrial, AV nodal and His–Purkinje conduction. Its prolongation beyond the normal range usually indicates a conduction delay in the AV system.

Q–T interval. This is measured from the onset of the QRS complex to the end of the T wave. It gives an approximation of the refractory period of the ventricles. Since it varies with the heart rate, the *Bazett formula* may be used to measure the Q–T interval corrected to the heart rate:

$$Q\text{--}Tc \text{ interval} = \frac{Q\text{--}T}{\sqrt{R\text{--}R}}$$

where Q–Tc is the corrected Q–T interval in ms., Q–T is the measured interval from the onset of QRS to the end of the T wave and R–R is the measure between two successive QRS complexes for the heart rate. The upper limit of the normal Q–Tc interval is 0.39 s for men and 0.44 s for women. The significance of this interval is that, if it

is prolonged, the patient becomes vulnerable to serious arrhythmias.

Electrical axis
The axis refers to the vector of impulses generated by the heart. The hexaxial reference system is used for the determination of the mean electrical axis. Although there is no uniform agreement regarding the definition of normal and abnormal axes, the following criteria are generally accepted:
• The normal axis falls between 0° and +90°.
• The left axis deviation (LAD) lies between 0° and −90°.
• The right axis deviation (RAD) falls between +90° and 270°.
For further information on axis deviation, a textbook on the ECG should be consulted.

Major conditions causing LAD are *hypertension, aortic stenosis* and *ischaemic heart disease*. RAD is caused by *chronic obstructive lung disease, pulmonary emboli* and *congenital heart disease*.

Interpretation of the ECG
The ECG should be interpreted in the context of the patient's age, gender and clinical status. A systematic approach cannot be overemphasized. One scheme of ECG interpretation is as follows:
1 Check the patient's particulars and ECG standardization.
2 Heart rate and rhythm assessment.
3 Screen the ECG intervals and durations of waves and complexes.
4 Measure QRS voltage.
5 R-wave progression.
6 Look for abnormal waves.
7 Calculate the mean electrical axis.
8 Important clinical correlates or inferences should be mentioned. One should not forget to compare the recent ECG with previous ECGs (if available).

The abnormal ECG
This subject will be discussed under the following headings:
• Rate and rhythm abnormalities.
• Conduction disturbances.
• Chamber hypertrophy.
• Myocardial ischaemia and infarction.
• Effects of metabolic factors and drugs.

Rate and rhythm abnormalities
The normal resting heart beats at a rate of 60–100 beats per minute (bpm). **Tachycardia** is defined as a heart rate of > 100 bpm, while **bradycardia** is < 60 bpm. Sinus

Fig. 5.10 Atrial flutter. The ECG shows regular abnormal P waves (F flutter waves giving the characteristic saw-toothed appearance). The ECG also shows a 4 : 1 atrioventricular block.

Fig. 5.11 Atrial fibrillation. Note the absence of P waves with irregular QRS complexes. The baseline shows irregular oscillations.

arrhythmia denotes the normal variation in the heart rate with respiration. The heart rate increases during inspiration and decreases during expiration. This phenomenon is common in children.

Atrial arrhythmias

1 *Paroxysmal atrial tachycardia* (PAT). The rate is fast (140–220 bpm). Onset is sudden and usually precipitated by caffeine, alcohol or anxiety. It lasts for seconds or minutes.

2 *Atrial premature contractions* (APCs). Also known as atrial extrasystoles, these are diagnosed by the presence of a premature P wave followed by a normal QRS. It is a benign condition and no treatment is usually required.

3 *Atrial flutter.* This is due to either an ectopic focus or a re-entry phenomenon. The wave conducted through the AV system recircles instead of going in one direction. The heart beats at a rate of 220–350 bpm. The P wave has a saw-toothed appearance on the ECG. The rhythm of rapid, identical, undulating waves is known as flutter or **F waves** (Fig. 5.10). Some degree of AV block is usually present at a 2 : 1, 3 : 1 or 4 : 1 ratio, i.e. the ventricular rate is decreased by the given ratio compared with that of the atria. Common causes of atrial flutter are *rheumatic mitral valve disease* and *ischaemic heart disease (IHD)*.

4 *Atrial fibrillation.* Fibrillation results from random chaotic depolarization of the atria. There is no organized electrical activity, which results in failure of effective pumping activity. The ECG will demonstrate a fine or coarse irregular baseline, with or without F waves. Atrial fibrillation is inferred from the *complete irregularity of QRS* complexes with *absent P waves*. The atrial rate in atrial fibrillation is usually impossible to count but is generally between 450 and 650 bpm. Common causes of atrial fibrillation include *mitral valve disease, thyrotoxicosis, ischaemic heart disease (IHD)* and *hypertension* (Fig. 5.11).

Ventricular arrhythmias

1 *Ventricular premature contractions (VPCs).* These are bizarre and wide QRS complexes (> 0.12 s) appearing

Fig. 5.12 Ventricular premature contractions (VPCs) are seen following the T wave of a normal complex. The abnormal route of these ventricular extrasystoles causes a wide, abnormally shaped QRST complex.

prematurely without a preceding ectopic P wave. They are also known as **ventricular extrasystoles**. They may originate from a single focus or multiple foci anywhere in the ventricles. Although VPCs are commonly found in healthy adults, frequent and multifocal VPCs always indicate organic heart disease and/or *digoxin toxicity* (Fig. 5.12).

2 *Ventricular tachycardia.* This is diagnosed by the presence of rapid, broad and often bizarre QRS complexes, with T waves which are usually opposite in direction to the main QRS complex deflection. The heart rate is usually above 140 bpm. The common causes of ventricular tachycardia include IHD (particularly during acute *myocardial infarction*) *digoxin toxicity, rheumatic heart disease, hypertension* and *cardiomyopathies*.

3 *Ventricular flutter and fibrillation.* These are usually lethal arrhythmias precipitated by chaotic depolarization in the ventricles, which causes loss of organized ventricular contractions. They are the cause of most sudden cardiac arrest secondary to circulatory arrest. Regular and consecutive undulations occur in ventricular flutter and a grossly irregular undulation of varying amplitude is present in ventricular fibrillation, but no true QRS complexes are seen. These arrhythmias nearly always occur in serious organic heart disease. Unless urgently treated by direct current (DC) shock, patients die within minutes.

(a)

(b)

(c)

Fig. 5.13 (a) and (b) Incomplete heart block. (c) Complete heart block. See explanation in the text. (Reproduced from Emslie-Smith, D., Paterson, C.R., Scratcherol, T. & Read, N.W. (eds) (1988) *BDS Textbook of Physiology*, 11th edn. With permission from Churchill Livingstone, Edinburgh.)

Conduction disturbances

The electrical activity starts at the SA node and spreads, through the intra-atrial pathways, to the AV node. From there the activity is transmitted to the ventricles through the His–Purkinje system after some delay at the AV node. Interruption of the conduction at any level in this pathway will result in conduction delays. Such effects can be detected in the ECG as follows.

AV nodal block

1 *First-degree heart block (1° HB).* This occurs when the P–R interval is prolonged (> 0.21 s) with normal conduction to the ventricles and without failure of transmission. It is a benign condition; mostly idiopathic, but can be caused by drugs or infection; usually no treatment is required.

2 *Second-degree heart block (2° HB).* Two types are described. In **Mobitz type I** (*Wenckebach*), there is progressive prolongation of the P–R interval until one impulse fails to be transmitted (Fig. 5.13a). In **Mobitz type II**, P waves are blocked periodically without a preceding prolongation of the P–R interval. It is much less common than

Mobitz type I. However, in practice, the presence of a 2 : 1 AV block in association with **bundle-branch block (BBB)** indicates that the diagnosis of Mobitz type II is almost certain (Fig. 5.13b). The clinical significance of Mobitz type I and type II is quite different. While Mobitz type I produces few or no symptoms, Mobitz type II is associated with congestive heart failure (CHF) or *Adams–Stokes syncopal attacks*. The prognosis in type I is generally good, whereas type II has a serious outcome.

3 *Third-degree heart block (3° HB), or complete heart block (CHB).* When atrial impulses fail to conduct to the ventricles due to complete AV block, both atria and ventricles beat independently. In the ECG, there will be no association between the P wave and the QRS complex known as marshing P (Fig. 5.13c). The commonest cause of CHB is degenerative, which could be primary or secondary to ischaemic heart disease (IHD). It may occasionally be congenital. If transient, it may be reversible; otherwise a **permanent pacemaker** is the treatment of choice.

4 *Intraventricular block.* An abnormal sequence of ventricular excitation occurs when the electrical impulse passing through the right or left bundles of His are blocked.

    Left bundle-branch block (LBBB) can be diagnosed when:

- The QRS complex is prolonged > 0.12 s.
- There is an 'M' pattern of QRS in I, aVL and V4–V6.
- There are secondary ST and T changes in I, aVL and V4.

The presence of LBBB almost always indicates organic heart disease, e.g. ischaemic heart disease, hypertension, aortic stenosis, congenital heart disease and cardiomyopathy.

    In **right bundle-branch block (RBBB)**, the diagnostic criteria include:

- Prolonged QRS complex (> 0.12 s).
- 'M' (rSR) pattern of QRS (i.e. a small R wave followed by an S wave and an abnormal R due to slow propagation) in V1–V3.
- Deep and slurred S waves in I, aVL and V4–V6.
- Secondary ST and T changes in V1–V3.

RBBB can occur in normal individuals, but it is also associated with ischaemic heart disease, hypertension or myocarditis.

Chamber hypertrophy

Atrial hypertrophy

1 *Left atrial hypertrophy* (LAH) is characterized by a wide P wave (≥ 0.11 s) and a notched, double-humped P wave (P-mitrale). Causes of LAH include *mitral valve disease*, *hypertension* and *hypertrophic cardiomyopathy*.

2 *Right atrial hypertrophy* (RAH) is characterized by a tall, peaked P wave in II, III and aVF (P-pulmonale). The amplitude of the P wave is 2.5 mm or more. RAH is always associated with *pulmonary hypertension*, which may be precipitated by chronic obstructive pulmonary disease (COPD), *pulmonary embolism* or *mitral valve disease*.

Ventricular hypertrophy

1 *Left ventricular hypertrophy* (LVH). Several ECG criteria have been suggested for the diagnosis of LVH, of which the following are commonly accepted:

    (a) Increased QRS voltage; R wave in lead I plus S wave in lead III of 25 mm or more.

    (b) S wave in V1 plus R wave in V5 or V6 of 35 mm or more.

    (c) R wave in a VL of 13 mm or greater.

    (d) Secondary ST and T-wave abnormalities.

    (e) Left axis deviation is seen in < 50% of cases of LVH.

Common causes of LVH include *hypertension, aortic stenosis* and *coarctation of the aorta*.

2 *Right ventricular hypertrophy* (RVH). Diagnostic criteria for RVH include:

    (a) Tall R wave in V1.

    (b) 'M' (rSR) pattern in V1.

    (c) T-wave changes in V1.

Causes of RVH are characterized by high pressure in the right ventricle or pulmonary arteries, such as *chronic cor pulmonale, pulmonary stenosis, mitral valve stenosis, tetralogy of Fallot, atrial septal defect* and *tricuspid insufficiency*.

Myocardial ischaemia and infarction

Myocardial ischaemia. *Anginal pain* is of diagnostic importance, since the ECG can be normal in IHD. Myocardial ischaemia results in ST-segment and T-wave changes. There is ST-segment elevation in the leads overlying the ischaemic area and ST-segment depression in leads on the opposite side of the heart (Fig. 5.14).

Myocardial infarction. A transmural infarct results in a wide, deep Q wave from the leads overlying the infarcted area. These leads also demonstrate ST-segment elevation. Due to the advent of **thrombolytic therapy** in saving human lives when used in treating acute myocardial infarction, the ECG is becoming indispensable in early diagnosis of patients with this condition. It must be remembered that the ECG plays a supportive role to the clinical diagnosis and assessment of serial cardiac enzymes in the management of acute myocardial infarction.

Effects of metabolic factors and drugs

Several electrolytes and drugs alter the ECG. The most

Fig. 5.14 Inferior myocardial infarction. The ECG shows depression of the ST segment in lead I and elevation of the ST segment and peaked T waves in leads II and III. Note also the dissociation of the P wave and the QRS complex in this record.

important of these will be discussed below, e.g. **hyper-** and **hypokalaemia, hypocalcaemia, digitalis** and some **antiarrhythmic drugs**.

Usually the effect of electrolytes or drugs is a complex process. Several other variables may modify this effect, such as the patient's age and sex, as well as the nature and seriousness of the underlying heart disease and any associated metabolic abnormalities.

Potassium. This is the electrolyte that most commonly produces ECG alterations and cardiac arrhythmias. In **hyperkalaemia**, the ECG changes correlate reasonably well with the serum level of potassium, as shown in Table 5.1. **Hypokalaemia** prolongs ventricular depolarization with prominent U waves. The heart is more prone to digitalis toxicity if hypokalaemia coexists.

Calcium. **Hypocalcaemia** prolongs phase 2 of the action potential, as reflected by prolongation of the ST segment and Q–T interval. Prolongation of the Q–T interval predisposes the patient to a serious type of arrhythmia (*torsade de pointes*), which can be fatal.

Digitalis (e.g. digoxin). Although this is a potent antiarrhythmic agent, digoxin toxicity can produce all types

Table 5.1 Correlation between level of hyperkalaemia and ECG changes.

K+ serum level (mmol/l)	ECG changes
5.5	Peaked, tall (tent-shaped) T waves
	Slight QRS-complex widening
7.5–8.5	Marked intraventricular blocks and VPCs
> 8.5	Wide QRS
	Complete AV block
	Ventricular arrhythmias and death

of cardiac arrhythmias. Advanced age, acute myocardial infarction, renal insufficiency and hypokalaemia reduce the patient's tolerance to digitalis and precipitate toxicity. Examples of digitalis-induced cardiac arrhythmias include atrial fibrillation or flutter, AV block, ventricular arrhythmias and standstill.

Other antiarrhythmic drugs (e.g. quinidine and amiodarone). These can produce prolongation of the Q–T interval. This may precipitate lethal ventricular arrhythmias (e.g. *torsade de pointes*).

Hypothermia

A drop in core body temperature below 32°C (95°F) prolongs repolarization, with a distinctive convex elevation of the J point (which is the junction point on the ECG following the QRS complex) and marked bradycardia. These changes may culminate in atrial fibrillation or flutter.

The cardiac cycle

The heart, as a pump, goes through phases of contraction (**systole**) and relaxation (**diastole**). During these phases there are associated changes in pressure and volume, which take place in the different chambers of the heart and in the great vessels. There are also vibrations, mainly generated by the closure of the valves. These vibrations result in the heart sounds. The correlation of these events with each other and their time sequence during the **cardiac cycle** help us to understand dynamic cardiovascular functions.

Of special interest is the correlation of the mechanical changes with the electrical events (the ECG). The ECG demonstrates that the cardiac muscle of the atria acts as one unit and that of the ventricles as another. The timing of the electrical waves is seen to precede the mechanical contraction and relaxation phases.

The wave of contraction which occurs first in the atria

and then in the ventricles is triggered off by depolarization of the pacemaker (SA node). The electrical signal results in depolarization followed by contraction of the atria. The signal is transmitted to the ventricles through the AV node. It cannot be transmitted through other sites because of the presence of fibrous tissue separating the cardiac muscles of the atria from those of the ventricles. There is a *delay in conduction* at the AV node and this allows time for the ventricles to fill with blood before their own contraction begins. The terms diastole and systole, if not qualified, usually refer to the phases of relaxation and contraction of the *ventricles*. But we can also speak of atrial diastole and atrial systole.

The cardiac cycle can be divided into three main parts for the sake of conveniently describing the various events:
1 Atrial systole.
2 Ventricular systole.
3 Diastole of both atria and ventricles.

Throughout the following description of the cardiac cycle, refer to Fig. 5.15.

Atrial systole

The contraction of the atria starts towards the end of ventricular diastole and helps to complete the filling of the ventricles. About 70% of ventricular filling takes place *passively* through the AV valves, due to the pressure gradient brought about by relaxation of the ventricles. Thus, the atrial systole only adds 30% of ventricular filling.

During atrial systole, there is slight regurgitation of blood into the venae cavae, which results in the generation of pressure waves in the veins near the heart (**jugular venous pulse**).

Ventricular systole

The contraction of the ventricles follows immediately upon completion of atrial systole. The rise in ventricular pressure results in immediate *closure of the AV valves*. This causes the *first heart sound*, which marks the beginning of systole. The semilunar valves, however, do not open until ventricular contraction has raised the pressure in the ventricles enough to oppose the aortic and pulmonary artery pressure levels. This takes about 0.5 s. During this time the ventricles are closed chambers, because both the AV and the semilunar valves are closed, and therefore there is no change in the volume of the ventricles. This period is called the **isovolumetric contraction phase**. When the pressure reaches about 80 mmHg in the left ventricle, the aortic valve opens, and, when it reaches 10 mmHg in the right ventricle, the pulmonary valve opens. When both of these valves open, there follows the *rapid ejection phase* of systole. This soon slows down and causes the systolic pressure

Fig. 5.15 Events of one cardiac cycle in the left side of the heart at rest. (Reproduced from Bray, J.J., Cragg, P.A., Macknight, A.D.C., Mills, R.G. & Taylor, D.W. (eds) (1989) *Lecture Notes in Physiology*, 2nd edn. Blackwell Scientific Publications, Oxford.)

peak of about 120 mmHg in the aorta and 25 mmHg in the pulmonary artery.

At rest, during ventricular systole, each ventricle ejects about 70–90 ml of blood, which is known as the **stroke volume**. This is about 65% of the ventricular volume at the end of diastole. A residual reserve volume of about 50 ml is left in each ventricle at the end of systole (end-systolic volume). The term *protodiastole* refers to the last 0.04 s of systole. During protodiastole, the pressure in the ventricles falls, due to the flow of blood from the aorta into the systemic circulation.

Diastole

Atrial relaxation precedes ventricular relaxation and continues through the greater part of ventricular diastole. At the beginning of ventricular diastole, the *aortic* and *pulmonary valves close*. This causes the *second heart sound*, which marks the beginning of diastole. The drop in pressure in the ventricles relative to that in the aorta and the pulmonary artery causes these valves to close immediately. The aortic valve closes when the pressure in the left ven-

tricle falls to about 80 mmHg and the pulmonary valve closes when the pressure in the right ventricle falls to about 12 mmHg. Normally, the two valves close synchronously (at the same time).

In early diastole and after the closure of the semilunar valves, the AV valves do not open immediately. This is because the pressure in the ventricles is still higher than that in the atria. It takes about 0.04 s for ventricular pressure to fall to a level below that in the atria and only then do the AV valves open. This period between the closure of the semilunar valves and the opening of the AV valves is called the **isovolumetric relaxation phase**. The ventricle during this period is a closed chamber and there is no change in volume; there is only a fall in pressure.

When the AV valves open, blood rapidly flows into the relaxed ventricles. This is the **rapid filling phase of diastole**. Towards the end of diastole, the atria contract and complete the filling of the ventricles, as previously described. Thus, one cardiac cycle is completed.

Variation in the duration of systole and diastole

It is found that cardiac muscle can depolarize faster when the heart rate is rapid. The duration of the action potential can be decreased from 0.25 s to 0.15 s. At rest, systole lasts for 0.3 s but it can be shortened to 0.16 s when the heart rate is 190–200/min. Similarly, diastole is decreased from 0.53 to 0.14 s.

The refractory period is also affected by an increased heart rate. The absolute refractory period is shortened from 0.2 to 0.13 s and the relative refractory period from 0.05 to 0.02 s.

Pressure changes during the cardiac cycle

Aortic pressure

At the beginning of ventricular systole, there is no change in aortic pressure because the aortic (Ao) valve is still closed (isovolumetric phase of systole). When the Ao valve opens, there is a quick rise of pressure during the *rapid ejection* phase, which soon flattens at a peak of about 120 mmHg at rest (systolic pressure). The aortic pressure rises to a value slightly above that in the ventricles, due to the momentum of blood flow, i.e. kinetic energy becomes converted into pressure.

The last quarter of systole (**protodiastole**) is characterized by a fall in aortic pressure. This is due to *slow ejection* and the flow of blood from the aorta into the systemic circulation. At the beginning of diastole, the pressure is about 80 mmHg (diastolic pressure). During diastole there is a slow and slight decrease in aortic pressure due to the

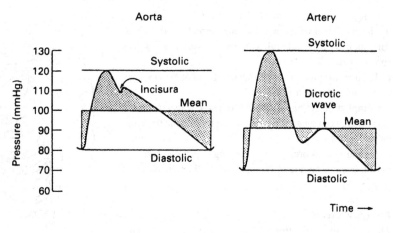

Fig. 5.16 Pressure waves in the aorta and a large artery. The shaded areas above and below the mean pressure are equal. (Reproduced from Bray, J.J., Cragg, P.A., Macknight, A.D.C., Mills, R.G. & Taylor, D.W. (eds) (1989) *Lecture Notes in Physiology*, 2nd edn. Blackwell Scientific Publications, Oxford.)

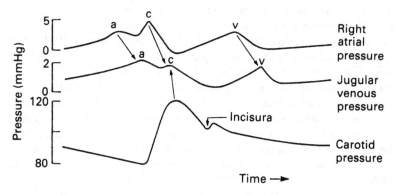

Fig. 5.17 The jugular venous pressure wave shown against the atrial and carotid pressure waves. (Reproduced from Bray, J.J., Cragg, P.A., Macknight, A.D.C., Mills, R.G. & Taylor, D.W. (eds) (1989) *Lecture Notes in Physiology*, 2nd edn. Blackwell Scientific Publications, Oxford.)

continued flow of blood from the aorta into the systemic circulation.

Arterial pressure waves

The arterial pressure wave reflects the systolic peak and diastolic trough. However, these waves are sharper than those seen in the aorta (Fig. 5.16). There is an irregularity in the descending limb, called the dicrotic notch. This has been attributed to a rebound of the aortic valves upon closure and to oscillations in the aorta. Figure 5.16 also shows the calculation of the mean pressure from the arterial pressure wave.

Pressure changes in the pulmonary artery

Pressure waves in the pulmonary artery are similar to those in the aorta. The difference is only in magnitude. The systolic pressure is about 21–25 mmHg and the diastolic is about 5–10 mmHg.

Atrial pressure

The atrial pressure changes result in three waves (Fig. 5.17).

The 'a' wave is due to **atrial systole** and is 4–6 mmHg in the right atrium and 7–8 mmHg in the left atrium. The 'c' wave is due to the rise in ventricular pressure causing the AV valves to bulge into the atria during the isometric contraction phase. It is also partly due to pulling of the atrial muscle during ventricular contraction. The 'v' wave is due to a build-up of pressure in the atria while the AV valves are closed. This wave falls once the AV valves open.

Jugular venous pulse and pressure (JVP)

The jugular pulse represents venous pulsations, seen at the neck, which are transmitted from the right atrium and great veins. When recorded, this pulse wave is composed of:
1 An **a** wave, due to atrial systole.
2 A **c** wave, due to bulging of the tricuspid valve into the atria during isometric ventricular contraction.
3 A **v** wave, which occurs when the atrial pressure rises before the tricuspid valve opens during diastole (Fig. 5.17).

The clinical significance of the jugular venous pressure wave lies in the fact that it can help in the diagnosis of cardiac disease, e.g.:

1 Congestive heart failure (CHF): the JVP rises beyond the normal level of 4 cm above the sternal angle (which corresponds to a **central venous pressure (CVP)** of approximately 9 cm H_2O).

2 Tricuspid regurgitation: produces **giant c waves** with each ventricular systole.

3 Complete heart block (CHB): cannon waves (**giant a waves**) are seen when the atria contract while the tricuspid valve is closed.

Jugular venous pressure rises during expiration and falls during inspiration due to changes in intrathoracic pressure (Fig. 5.17)

Electrical events
The waves of the electrocardiogram are changes in voltage detected on the surface of the body. They are conducted potential differences from cardiac muscle. Each wave is the sum of millions of action potentials occurring in individual cardiac muscle fibres. The characteristic pattern of the ECG shows waves named P, QRS complex and T. The details of the electrocardiogram and its clinical uses have been discussed earlier in this chapter.

During the cardiac cycle it is seen that the P wave precedes atrial systole and the QRS complex precedes ventricular systole, i.e. electrical depolarization comes before the mechanical event. Also note that the T wave (repolarization of the ventricles) corresponds to the later part of the ventricular systole and the beginning of diastole.

The heart sounds
The heart sounds can be detected over the anterior chest wall by means of a **stethoscope** (auscultation) or by the use of a sound recording device (**phonocardiography**). There are certain areas where the heart sounds can be heard best (Fig. 5.18). Usually, two sounds can be heard with ease and are known as the **first** and **second heart sounds**. Sometimes a third and fourth sound can be detected.

The first heart sound is due to the vibrations produced by closure of the mitral and tricuspid valves. It occurs at the beginning of systole. In fact, it is a good clinical indicator of the onset of ventricular systole. It is of a low pitch and is slightly longer in duration (0.15 s). The second heart sound is shorter (0.11 s) and higher in pitch. The two sounds can be simulated by the words '*lub dup*'. The second heart sound is caused by the closure of the aortic and pulmonary valves and it marks the beginning of ventricular diastole. The second heart sound may become split into two sounds during inspiration. This is called physiological splitting, brought about by the delay in closure of the pulmonary valve. The *third heart sound* is probably caused by the rush

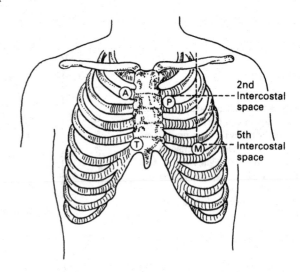

Fig. 5.18 Precordial auscultation areas for heart sounds. A, aortic area; M, mitral area; P, pulmonary area; T, tricuspid area.

of blood during rapid ventricular filling in diastole. The *fourth heart sound*, which is rarely heard, occurs just before the onset of systole, i.e. just before the first heart sound, and has also been attributed to ventricular filling.

Auscultation of the heart is useful in clinical diagnosis of valve disease. Students of medicine are advised to familiarize themselves with the normal pattern and characteristics of the normal heart sounds so that they may be able to detect abnormal heart sounds (**murmurs**) or additional vibrations, which are called **bruits** and **thrills**. Murmurs are heard when there is abnormal flow, causing turbulence to occur. Abnormal vibrations can be caused by valve disease, e.g. narrowing (**stenosis**) or incompetence (**regurgitation**). Bruits can be heard over a highly vascular organ, e.g. a highly vascular, enlarged and active thyroid gland, or over an arteriovenous fistula or shunt. Thrills are vibrations which can be felt by the hand when placed over the chest wall and they accompany a murmur caused by valve disease.

Murmurs are described as *systolic* or *diastolic* according to their timing in the cardiac cycle. Thus, a murmur heard after the first heart sound and before the second is a systolic murmur, and one which comes after the second and before the first is a diastolic murmur. The valve source of the murmur can be discovered according to the location of the murmur in the areas of auscultation, as shown in Fig. 5.18. Thus, a murmur due to mitral stenosis occurs during diastole (because blood flows through this valve in diastole) and is best heard at the apex of the heart. Similarly, aortic stenosis will cause a systolic murmur, heard best at the base of the heart. A systolic murmur at the mitral area indicates abnormal back flow through the mitral valve (mitral incompetence), which should be closed during systole. A murmur due to aortic regurgitation is heard in diastole (because blood should not be flowing through this valve in diastole), but this time it is heard best at the base of the heart over the aortic area.

Cardiac murmurs are also produced by congenital malformations of the heart, such as *interventricular septal defect*, *pulmonary atresia* and *patent ductus arteriosus*.

The cardiac output

The cardiac output is defined as the volume of blood pumped by *each ventricle* per unit time. In healthy adults it is about 5 litres/min. The cardiac output (COP) depends on the heart rate and on the stroke volume. In fact, it is equal to the product of these two parameters.

$$COP = \text{Stroke volume} \times \text{heart rate}$$

Example

$$COP = 70 \text{ ml} \times 72/\text{min}$$
$$= 5040 \text{ ml/min (approximately 5 litres)}$$

This volume will vary with the size of the individual. Women have smaller cardiac outputs than men, and children have smaller outputs than adolescents or adults. Because of this variation, it is preferable to use the **cardiac index (CI)**. Cardiac index equals $COP/\text{min}/\text{m}^2$ of body surface area. The normal range of CI is 2.6–4.2. During moderate muscular exercise the cardiac output may increase by two- or threefold. In athletes the cardiac output may reach 30 litres/min or more.

Measurement of cardiac output

From the definition stated above, it is clear that the COP is equal to the volume of blood that flows in the pulmonary artery or the aorta per min. **Fick's principle** states that the amount of a substance taken up by an organ in a given time equals the difference in concentration of that substance between arterial and venous blood, multiplied by the volume of blood flowing through the organ during the same period of time, i.e.:

$$\begin{array}{c}\text{Amount of substance} \\ \text{taken up by organ}\end{array} = \begin{array}{c}\text{Arteriovenous} \\ \text{difference}\end{array} \times \begin{array}{c}\text{Blood} \\ \text{flow}\end{array}$$

If we take O_2 uptake in the lungs as an example, we can use Fick's principle to calculate the cardiac output. Each minute the blood flow in the lungs is equal to the output of the right ventricle. We therefore need to measure the O_2 uptake per minute and the arteriovenous (a-v) O_2 difference.

Example

O_2 uptake in the lungs	$= 250 \text{ ml/min}$
a-v oxygen difference	$= 20/100 - 15/100 \text{ ml}$
	$= 5 \text{ ml/100 ml}$

COP (pulmonary blood flow) = O_2 uptake $\div$ a-v O_2 difference

By substitution in the above formula:

$$COP = \frac{250}{5} \times 100 = 5000 \text{ ml/min}$$

Another method used for measurement of cardiac output is known as the indicator or **dye dilution method**. This method depends on the observation that a dose of isotope or a dye injected into the right atrium will flow as a bolus in the pulmonary circulation and through the left side of the heart and then into the arterial system before it recirculates and completely mixes with the blood. This makes it possible to calculate the blood flow per unit time. Figure 5.19 shows the curve obtained by plotting the dye concentration in arterial blood against time during the first circulation of the dye bolus. This curve is used to obtain the time taken by the dye to circulate once through the heart.

The dye concentration is plotted on a logarithmic scale and time on a linear scale. The log-linear plot makes the descending limb of the curve a straight line, which is extrapolated to zero concentration. The point of intersection gives the theoretical time taken by the dye bolus to circulate through the lungs and to leave the heart.

The average concentration of the dye is calculated by integration of the area under the curve. Dividing the amount of dye (Q) by the average arterial concentration (C) gives the volume of blood (V) required to carry the dye, i.e.:

$$Q/C = V$$

This volume is the cardiac output during the time given by the curve for one circulation of the dye.

Example

Five milligrams of dye was injected and the average arterial concentration was found to be 1.5 mg/litre. A single circulation time, as shown in Fig. 5.19, is 40 s.

$$\text{Cardiac output in 40 s} = \frac{5 \text{ mg}}{1.5 \text{ mg/litre}}$$
$$= 3.33 \text{ litres}$$

$$\text{Cardiac output/min} = 3.33 \times \frac{60}{40} = 4.995 \text{ litres}$$

There are other techniques for measuring cardiac output, such as thermodilution methods and echocardiography, which are outside the scope of this text.

Fig. 5.19 The indicator or dye dilution method for determination of cardiac output. The broken line is the extrapolation drawn to find the circulation time.

Control of cardiac output

The control of cardiac output is essential for adjustments of the blood-pressure and blood-flow requirements under different physiological and pathological states. For example, muscular exercise increases the demand for O_2 carriage and this, in turn, requires more blood flow to carry O_2 from the lungs and to deliver it at a higher rate to working muscles. In cases of fever or exposure to heat, there is dilatation of the vascular bed with consequent lowering of arterial blood pressure. This requires a higher cardiac output so as to maintain the blood pressure. Cardiac output is simply controlled by means of adjustments to the **heart rate** and the **stroke volume**. The regulation of these two important parameters will now be discussed in detail.

Regulation of the heart rate

The mechanisms which influence the heart rate are either **neural** or **humoral**. The neural mechanisms depend on cardiac innervation. The sympathetic and the parasympathetic (vagus) nerves exert their influence on the SA node and therefore modify the heart rate by their effect on the pacemaker. The inherent rhythm of the SA node in the denervated heart is higher than the heart rate at rest (about 70/min). This is because the vagus exerts a continuous flow of impulses, known as **vagal tone**, which tends to slow the heart rate. Inhibition of vagal tone causes the heart to beat faster. On the other hand, inhibition of the sympathetic

nerves will cause a slight decrease in the heart rate, but their stimulation results in a great increase in sinus rhythm.

The neural regulation of the heart rate by means of autonomic nerves is achieved by means of **cardiac centres**, mainly in the medulla oblongata. Figure 5.20 shows a diagrammatic representation of the cardiac centres. The **cardioinhibitory** centre (depressor area) and the **vasomotor centre** (pressor area) receive inputs from various sensory receptors in the body. The most important of these are the **baroreceptors** and the **chemoreceptors**.

The **baroreceptors** are stretch receptors located in the arterial system, the most well known of which are in the carotid sinus at the bifurcation of the common carotid artery and in the arch of the aorta. The chemoreceptors are special cells (known as *glomus bodies*) situated in the carotid and aortic bodies in close proximity to the location of the baroreceptors and they send their afferent impulses through the buffer nerves (Fig. 5.21). The receptor cells are sensitive to changes in Po_2, H^+ concentration and Pco_2. The following is a description of some of the more important reflexes which regulate the heart rate.

The baroreceptor reflex. Stimulation of the baroreceptors takes place when the blood pressure rises. In fact, there is a direct relationship between the rate of firing of the baroreceptors and the blood pressure, i.e. the higher the blood pressure, the higher the frequency of impulses generated in

Fig. 5.20 Diagrammatic representation of the medulla and pons showing the location of cardiovascular centres. (Reproduced from Bray, J.J., Cragg, P.A., Macknight, A.D.C., Mills, R.G. & Taylor, D.W. (eds) (1989) *Lecture Notes in Physiology*, 2nd edn. Blackwell Scientific Publications, Oxford.)

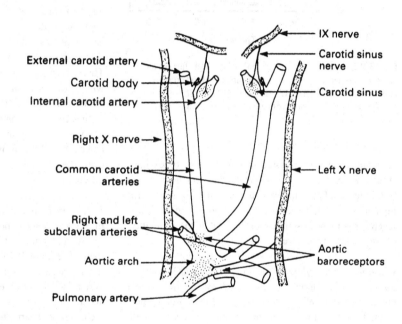

Fig. 5.21 Afferent nerves of the baroreceptors and chemoreceptors and the cranial nerves which connect them to the cardiovascular centres in the medulla. For simplicity, the aortic bodies have been omitted. (Reproduced from Bray, J.J., Cragg, P.A., Macknight, A.D.C., Mills, R.G. & Taylor, D.W. (eds) (1989) *Lecture Notes in Physiology*, 2nd edn. Blackwell Scientific Publications, Oxford.)

the baroreceptors (Fig. 5.22). There are very few impulses in the nerves coming from the baroreceptors when the pressure is low, but this increases when the mean pressure rises. The baroreceptor reflex is found to be more sensitive to changes in pressure within the physiological range and less so when the pressure is too low or too high.

Stimulation of the baroreceptors by a rise in blood pressure produces reflex slowing of the heart by excitation of the *cardioinhibitory centre*. This works through the vagus, which causes slowing of the SA node, and results in decreasing the cardiac output. On the other hand, there is also reflex *inhibition* of the vasomotor centre. This causes a decrease in the sympathetic vasoconstrictor tone

to blood-vessels, leading to *vasodilatation* in the peripheral circulation. Two effects result: a decrease in the *peripheral resistance* and an increase in the capacity of the peripheral circulation. In this way, the baroreceptor reflex causes not only a decreased cardiac output but also a decreased peripheral resistance, both of which contribute to decreasing the blood pressure and bringing it back to normal.

Conversely, when the blood pressure falls, the baroreceptor impulses rapidly decrease in frequency. This initiates an immediate *sympathetic response* through the *vasomotor centre*. There is an increase in the *heart rate*, an increase in the *strength of myocardial contraction* and peripheral *vasoconstriction*. All of these result in rapidly

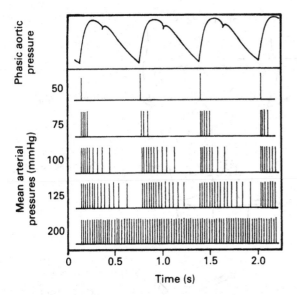

Fig. 5.22 Frequency of impulse traffic in a single fibre of the carotid sinus nerve in relation to mean arterial blood pressure. (Reproduced from Berne, R.M. & Levy, M.N. (1986) *Cardiovascular Physiology*, 5th edn. By permission of C.V. Mosby Co., St Louis.)

elevating the blood pressure to normal. The reflex constitutes an important life-saving mechanism in response to falling blood pressure, which is valuable for short-term regulation of blood pressure. The responses of the baroreceptors will be discussed further when the regulation of arterial blood pressure is considered.

Chemoreceptor reflexes. The Po_2, H^+ and CO_2 concentrations in the blood are monitored by the **peripheral chemoreceptor** cells in the carotid and the aortic bodies. It has been found that these bodies have a very high rate of blood flow in relation to their size. This characteristic makes the glomus cells most suitable for monitoring the chemical composition of the blood. Oxygen, being one of the vital components, stimulates the peripheral chemoreceptors if its partial pressure falls (**hypoxia**). Also, if the **pH** falls, as in acidosis, stimulation of the chemoreceptors takes place. High Pco_2 can affect the peripheral chemoreceptors, but only to a minor extent. As will be discussed in the chemical control of respiration (Chapter 6), Pco_2 is more effective on central chemoreceptors. The chemoreceptors are also stimulated when the blood pressure falls. Their rich blood supply also makes them sensitive to a decrease in blood pressure because it leads to a diminished O_2 supply (hypoxia).

Hypoxia also leads to anaerobic glycolysis, with excessive production of lactic acid. Lactic acidosis causes a drop in the blood pH, which stimulates the chemoreceptors. When the carotid and aortic chemoreceptors are stimulated by the above changes, they send impulses to the cardiac centres in the medulla. The result is a reflex *increase in the heart rate* due to stimulation of cardiac acceleratory neurons, which work through *sympathetic* stimulation. These responses increase the cardiac output and therefore the blood pressure and improve the O_2 delivery and CO_2 uptake by the circulation.

The Bainbridge reflex. It has been found that stretch of the right atrium by an increased venous return results in a reflex increase in the heart rate (tachycardia). However, when the heart rate is already high, the reflex produces a decrease in the heart rate or may be absent. The sensory nerves of this reflex are in **vagal afferent** fibres from the right atrium. The reflex is abolished when the vagus is cut. The efferents are in both the vagus and the sympathetic, which produce an increase in the heart rate and possibly the stroke volume. The Bainbridge reflex acts as a safeguard against accumulation of blood in the right side of the heart and the venous system. The heart responds to an increase in venous return by increasing the cardiac output. However, the physiological significance of this reflex is still unsettled.

Receptors in joints and tendons. Movement of skeletal muscles increases the heart rate. There are receptors in joints and tendons which detect the skeletal muscle movement. These are called **proprioceptors**. Impulses originating in these receptors will travel to the central nervous system, where they are relayed to hypothalamic and cardioacceleratory neurons. This reflex is partly responsible for the increased heart rate during muscular exercise.

Higher centres. It is well known that emotional factors, working through the senses of hearing or vision or even initiated by thought or dreams, can affect the heart rate. These effects seem to work through the **limbic system** and the **hypothalamus**. There are neurons in the anterior part of the hypothalamus which cause the sympathetic nerves to accelerate the heart.

Regulation of the stroke volume

The stroke volume mainly depends on the amount of blood coming back to the heart (**venous return**), but it also depends on the **condition of the myocardium** and several factors which affect **myocardial contractility**.

The effect of Na⁺, K⁺ and Ca²⁺ ions on myocardial contractility. Excess **K⁺** ions (hyperkalaemia) cause the myocardium to become hyperpolarized. The cardiac muscle fibres become relaxed and extremely weak. This is due to a decrease in the resting membrane potential and the action potential. As the action potential becomes smaller, the myocardial contraction becomes weaker. Excess K^+ can block conductions at the AV node. The heart comes to a standstill with the myocardium relaxed.

The effect of **excess Ca²⁺** is the opposite of that of excess K^+. Excess Ca^{2+} causes the myocardium to contract more strongly and the heart may go into spasm (Ca^{2+} rigor). This is probably due to a direct effect of Ca^{2+} on the contractile process. On the other hand, low Ca^{2+} causes relaxation of cardiac muscle. Under physiological conditions, however, serum Ca^{2+} is not allowed to vary widely. A decrease in serum Ca^{2+} will cause death due to skeletal muscle and nerve excitation resulting in tetany before the heart is affected. Similarly, high levels of Ca^{2+} usually result in deposition of Ca^{2+} in tissues rather than hypercalcaemia which affects the heart.

Slow *calcium channel-blockers*, such as *nifedipine* and *verapamil*, suppress Ca^{2+} entry into the cardiac muscle cell and the conducting tissues. These drugs can also inhibit the contraction of vascular smooth muscle. They therefore cause vasodilatation and decrease arterial blood pressure and thus help the myocardium by decreasing the **afterload** on the left ventricle (see below).

Excess Na⁺ ions depress myocardial contractility. This is because the Na^+ ion competes with Ca^{2+} receptors in the contractile process. Low Na^+, on the other hand, may result in cardiac fibrillation.

Mechanical factors. These are related to the state of stretch of the cardiac muscle at the beginning of contraction and also to the resistance offered to the muscle during contraction. The stretch of the ventricular muscle is related to cardiac filling, which depends on the venous return. This is often referred to as **preloading** of the cardiac muscle. On the other hand, the resistance to myocardial contraction is proportional to the pressure in the aorta and pulmonary arteries. This is referred to as impedance to flow and also as afterloading of the cardiac muscle. This impedance does not affect the cardiac output within the normal range of blood pressure.

1 *The length-tension relationship (preloading).* The stretch of the myocardium by blood causes the muscle to contract more strongly. The famous physiologist, Starling, stated that the strength of myocardial contraction is proportional to the initial length of the muscle fibres. This

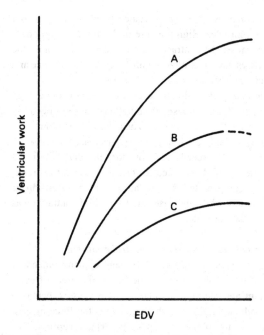

Fig. 5.23 Relationship between myocardial stretch (end-diastolic volume (EDV)) and tension (ventricular work). Curve A shows the effect of sympathetic stimulation, B shows the relationship at rest, and C the effect of myocardial depressants (e.g. parasympathetic stimulation, hypoxia, hypercapnia and acidosis).

statement became known as *Starling's law of the heart*. Thus, the myocardial strength increases as the filling of the heart increases. Therefore, it can be regarded as an intrinsic **autoregulation** of the myocardium, which enables the heart to cope with increased venous return. This autoregulatory mechanism also ensures that the output of the right and left ventricles are matched for each beat. It safeguards against blood accumulating in the venous system or in the pulmonary circulation.

The curves shown in Fig. 5.23 illustrate the relationships between the stretch of cardiac muscle and the *strength* of contraction (length–tension curve). The degree of stretch is given by the **end-diastolic volume (EDV)**. The strength of contraction (tension) is given by **myocardial work** (myocardial performance). The curves have become known as the *Frank-Starling curves*. It should be noted, however, that the degree of stretch works positively up to a certain limit or optimum. If this limit is exceeded, then further stretching produces a negative effect on contractility.

2 *Aortic and pulmonary impedance (afterloading).* The pressure in these great arteries affects the force of

contraction by offering resistance to blood flowing out of the ventricles. High pressure in the aorta or pulmonary artery causes the contractile force to decrease because the ventricles have to contract against increased resistance and therefore the stroke volume is decreased.

3 *The heart rate* indirectly affects the force of contraction. As the heart rate increases, the duration of diastole becomes shorter and the EDV smaller. Thus, the stroke volume, according to Starling's law, should be decreased. Only when the heart rate exceeds 120/min does the diastolic filling become significantly affected. During muscular exercise, this is compensated for by an increased **sympathetic** stimulation, which increases the strength of contraction as well as the heart rate.

Effects of neural regulation on stroke volume

1 *Sympathetic stimulation.* The main regulatory mechanism of the stroke volume is the **inotropic** effect of **catecholamines**. During muscular exercise there is increased sympathetic discharge, which increases the force of ventricular contraction through β_1-**adrenergic receptors**. This increases the stroke volume by decreasing the residual or end-systolic volume of the ventricles. Similarly, during stimulation of the *baroreceptor reflex* by *hypovolaemia*, sympathetic discharge is responsible for increasing the stroke volume.

2 *Effects of parasympathetic stimulation.* There is little negative inotropic effect on the ventricle, while the atrial contraction is decreased. The effects of sympathetic and parasympathetic stimulation can be seen in Fig. 5.23 superimposed on the length–tension relationship as shown by the Frank–Starling curves.

The venous return

Several mechanisms help to return the blood through the venous system to the heart:

1 The most important of these is the venous pressure gradient, due to the pumping action of the heart, which is usually less than 10 mmHg. The pressure in the right atrium is zero or negative. This **pressure gradient** is enough to ensure a venous return equal to the cardiac output at rest. The blood volume and the state of constriction or dilatation of the systemic veins determine the pressure gradient and, in particular, the central venous pressure (i.e. pressure in the great veins and the right atrium). In the case of haemorrhage, **venoconstriction** ensures adequate venous pressure and venous return.

2 During walking or other forms of muscular work, contracting muscles squeeze the capillaries and veins within them. The deep veins lying between muscles are also squeezed. Due to the presence of valves in the veins, the blood flows towards the heart. This mechanism is known as the **muscle pump**. Standing for long periods of time without movement can result in pooling of blood in the lower extremities, decreasing the venous return and the cardiac output. **Fainting** can occur if the blood flow to the brain is decreased.

3 During inspiration the intrathoracic pressure becomes negative relative to atmospheric pressure. The thin walls of the atria and great veins allow the central venous pressure to become negative as well. Therefore, a suction force, known as the **respiratory pump**, draws blood into the venae cavae and the right atrium. This is assisted by the descent of the diaphragm, which increases the pressure in the abdominal cavity. The opposite of the respiratory pump occurs during the *Valsalva manoeuvre*, i.e. forced expiratory effort against a closed glottis, as during coughing or straining. The venous return decreases and so does the cardiac output and blood pressure. As a result, an increase in the heart rate is brought about by the baroreceptor reflex.

4 Gravity also plays a role in the venous return from the head and neck. Conversely, if the body is erect, pooling may result in the lower limbs. On lying down, venous return is improved. This is why the head should be kept down and the legs raised as a first-aid procedure in cases of hypotension, e.g. after severe blood loss. In cases of congestive heart failure, lying flat on the back causes dyspnoea due to more venous return to the heart and therefore pooling of blood in the lungs, causing breathlessness.

The effect of gravity may become exaggerated in patients receiving drugs which block the sympathetic ganglia. **Postural hypotension** may occur on standing up from the lying position due to vasodilatation and pooling of blood in the lower extremities, together with failure of the sympathetic response.

Summary of nervous regulation of the heart

Sympathetic stimulation

Sympathetic stimulation causes an increase in the **heart rate** through β_1-adrenergic receptors in the SA node. There is also a shortening of the **conduction time** in the AV node and a **positive inotropic effect** on the atrial and ventricular muscle. These effects cause an increase in the cardiac output and the arterial blood pressure.

Parasympathetic stimulation

Parasympathetic stimulation releases acetylcholine and slows the heart rate by suppressing the pacemaker potential. Conversely, suppression of vagal tone or blocking acetylcholine by atropine causes an increase in the **heart rate** up to 150–180/min. Acetylcholine causes slowing or blocking of conduction in the junctional myocardium of the AV node. There is also a **negative inotropic effect** on the atria but little or no such action on the ventricles. This effect is brought about by hyperpolarization of the resting membrane potential and shortening the duration of the action potential.

Indirect effects on the ventricles include a decrease in the **stroke volume** due to poor atrial contraction, which leads to a decrease in ventricular filling and therefore a negative effect on Starling's law. Together with a decreased heart rate, this effect leads to a decrease in cardiac output and arterial blood pressure.

Cardiac centres

The cardioinhibitory area consists mainly of the **nucleus ambiguus of the vagus** nerve in the medulla oblongata. Cardioinhibitory neurons are also found in the **nucleus of the tractus solitarius** (NTS). A rise in blood pressure stimulates arterial baroreceptors and produces bradycardia through excitation of the cardioinhibitory area. Conversely, a fall in blood pressure will produce tachycardia by inhibiting vagal tone and increasing sympathetic discharge. Emergency situations produce tachycardia by sympathetic stimulation, but there is no '**cardioacceleratory centre**' as such.

The **vasomotor centre** (VMC) or pressor area is situated in the ventrolateral part of the medulla oblongata, including the cardioinhibitory area. It sends fibres to the preganglionic sympathetic nerves of the lateral horn cells of the spinal cord. Both excitatory and inhibitory neurons from the medulla converge on the sympathetic preganglionic neurons. Excitation will bring about an increase in the heart rate, vasoconstriction and a rise in blood pressure. Inhibition of **sympathetic vasomotor tone** causes vasodilatation and a decrease in arterial blood pressure.

Reflexogenic areas

Numerous receptors and reflexes have been described in the cardiovascular system. Only well-studied receptors and reflexes will be described here. Arterial blood pressure is monitored by the systemic **baroreceptors**. Those in the carotid sinus send impulses via the sinus nerve, which is a branch of the glossopharyngeal nerve, and those in the aortic arch send impulses in the afferent fibres of the vagus nerve. Fibres from the baroreceptors synapse in the vicinity of the NTS, from which interneurons make connections with the nucleus ambiguus and the vasomotor centre. The latter controls vasomotor tone via the lateral horn cells of the spinal cord. An increase in blood pressure sends excitatory impulses to the cardioinhibitory centre and inhibitory impulses to the vasomotor centre. The total response will therefore be slowing of the heart rate and vasodilatation (i.e. a fall in the peripheral resistance). Both effects will decrease the blood pressure.

Systemic **arterial chemoreceptors** are situated in the carotid bodies near the bifurcation of the common carotid artery and in aortic bodies near the aortic arch. The cells of these bodies receive a rich blood supply. They are stimulated by a decrease in Po_2 and pH and an increase in Pco_2. A decrease in the perfusion of the chemoreceptor bodies (e.g. after a fall in arterial blood pressure) will also result in local hypoxia and stimulation of the chemoreceptors. Afferent nerve fibres from the chemoreceptors reach the NTS in the same nerves as those from the arterial baroreceptors. In the medulla these afferent fibres converge on the VMC and produce reflex tachycardia and a positive inotropic effect.

Chemoreceptor stimulation by hypoxia also results in secretion of **adrenaline** (epinephrine) by the adrenal medulla, which causes tachycardia and an increase in cardiac output.

Low-pressure stretch receptors are found in the right atrium. Stimulation of the **atrial receptors type B**, which respond to an increase in venous return, results in tachycardia mediated by sympathetic nerves. These receptors may be responsible for the *Bainbridge reflex*. Other atrial receptors, when stimulated, result in vasodilatation. Both the above responses can be considered as safety mechanisms against excessive increases in venous return or central venous pressure.

Pulmonary receptors. In the pulmonary circulation (with uncertain location), there are receptors stimulated by vascular distension which mediate reflex bradycardia and a fall in systemic arterial blood pressure. Their physiological significance and that of possible pulmonary chemoreceptors are still uncertain.

Metabolism of cardiac muscle

Under basal conditions, 35% of the energy needs of the human heart are provided by carbohydrates, 60% by fat and 5% by ketones and amino acids. However, the nutritional status of the individual affects these ratios. One per cent of the total energy is provided by anaerobic metabolism, but this figure increases to as much as 10% during hypoxic states. As cardiac muscle has a high protein turnover, amino acid uptake is mainly used for protein synthesis and maintenance of cardiac muscle.

The immediate source of energy for myocardial contraction is high-energy phosphate from ATP. Stores of ATP are resynthesized from creatine phosphate. This indicates that an adequate supply of O_2 is essential for myocardial contractions. In fact, myocardial oxygen consumption (MVO_2) is closely related to the work of the heart. In hypoxia (as in severe muscular exercise), the heart reverts to anaerobic glycolysis, supplying limited energy and resulting in formation of lactate, which cannot be utilized as a main source of energy. In severe myocardial ischaemia, ATP is soon depleted resulting in the formation of adenose monophosphate (AMP) and adenosine. The latter leaks out of the cell. This curtails resynthesis of ATP. If the ischaemia persists, myocardial cellular death begins in about 30 min. Medications used to dissolve coronary clots are best used as early as possible, preferably within the first half-hour of the attack.

The work of the heart

The work of the heart as a pump is converted into: (i) pressure (pressure work); and (ii) flow (kinetic work). By far the greater part goes to the building up of blood pressure in the arterial system. The energy used for this pressure work by the left ventricle is about seven times that of the right ventricle. This is due to the higher impedance in the aorta and the thickness of the left ventricle wall. As a result the oxygen consumption of the left ventricle is far greater than that of the right. The kinetic work of each ventricle is only about 1–2% of the total work done at rest, but increases significantly during exercise because of the increase in the velocity of flow due to increased cardiac output.

Cardiac reserve

In healthy persons at rest, the heart uses only a fraction of its maximum output. This margin of difference is called the **cardiac reserve**. In a sedentary adult the cardiac reserve is five times the resting cardiac output, while in athletes it can be sevenfold. The cardiac reserve is called upon during stress, such as muscular exercise, or disease conditions which require cardiovascular adjustments, such as heart failure, valvular disease and blood loss. Many disease conditions result in decreased cardiac reserve. In such cases the patient fatigues quickly, e.g. feels *breathless*, the heart rate becomes too fast or the muscles become painful due to inadequate oxygen supply.

The physiological mechanisms activated to achieve the cardiac reserve are *cardiac acceleration* and the increase in *stroke volume*. These are discussed in detail in the appropriate parts of this chapter. In chronic disease, such as

hypertension and aortic stenosis, *myocardial hypertrophy* contributes to the cardiac reserve.

In clinical practice, measurement of the cardiac reserve is a useful assessment of the condition of the heart. However, the cardiac output may be difficult to measure in most hospitals. Indirect methods, such as *exercise tolerance* tests (the so-called stress test), are carried out instead (see Chapter 13).

Applied physiology

Heart failure

The condition of heart failure is not a disease entity. It can be defined as failure of the heart to pump adequate amounts of blood to maintain the various functions of the body. It can be due to a variety of disease processes, which can be grouped into three categories: (i) those due to **myocardial failure**, such as myocardial infarction, chronic overload, or toxins and poisons; (ii) **mechanical abnormalities**, such as valvular disease, congenital cardiac anomalies and increased impedance to forward flow (e.g. hypertension and aortic stenosis); and (iii) **cardiac arrhythmias**, such as fibrillation and flutter.

The pathophysiology of heart failure varies with the underlying pathology. In all cases there is a decreased cardiac output for a given EDV, i.e. depression of the Frank-Starling curve.

Congestive heart failure (CHF)

As a result of decreased cardiac output, left atrial pressure increases, leading to back pressure and pulmonary congestion. This is the cause of shortness of breath or **dyspnoea**, which increases when the patient lies down (orthopnoea).

After myocardial infarction the immediate adjustments that take place in heart failure are due to decreased cardiac output and systemic venous congestion. Activation of cardiovascular reflexes takes place mainly due to the baroreceptors, chemoreceptors and cerebral ischaemia. There is an increase in the heart rate and strength of myocardial contraction, due to sympathetic activation. This results in *partial compensation* for the damaged myocardium and an almost normal cardiac output is maintained.

In chronic states in which both ventricles are involved, there is activation of the *renal mechanisms* that result in fluid retention. These lead to: (i) decreased glomerular filtration, brought about by decreased renal blood flow; (ii) secretion of **renin** and activation of the **renin-angiotensin** system; and (iii) secretion of **aldosterone**. These effects cause Na^+ and water retention. The increased blood volume increases the venous return and right atrial pressure, leading to an improvement of the cardiac output. At rest the patient may have no symptoms but becomes breathless on effort because of the decreased cardiac reserve.

When the cardiac output cannot maintain adequate renal function, more fluid is retained. This leads to a progressive rise in the **right atrial** pressure, venous congestion and increased capillary pressure, leading to **oedema** of the lower limbs or of the lower back in recumbent patients. Venous congestion also leads to **liver enlargement**, congestion of the abdominal viscera and **ascites**. These are the classical signs of CHF.

Further retention of fluid leads to stretch of the myocardium and oedema of the cardiac muscles and eventually leads to death from **decompensated heart failure**. In the terminal stages oedema of the lung takes place with extreme shortness of breath. This state calls for immediate therapy; otherwise the patient soon dies.

Left ventricular failure

This can occur in acute myocardial infarction, in mitral or aortic valve disease or as a result of severe hypertension. In such cases, the left ventricle fails without involvement of the right ventricle. The result is severe **pulmonary congestion** brought about by the normal right ventricular output and severe rise of pressure in the left atrium. **Pulmonary oedema** occurs and the patient coughs up frothy sputum, often bloodstained. Left ventricular failure can be fatal in less than half an hour unless appropriate measures are taken.

Right ventricular failure

This rarely occurs due to pulmonary hypertension or mitral stenosis without involvement of the left ventricle. In such cases systemic venous congestion is a prominent feature. The liver becomes enlarged and systemic oedema and ascites occur (i.e. **CHF**). In this case **dyspnoea** is due to low pulmonary perfusion leading to hypoxia and respiratory stimulation by the **chemoreceptors**.

High cardiac output failure

This is a term given to describe conditions where the cardiac output is higher than normal but still inadequate to meet demands of oxygen consumption or haemodynamic adjustments, e.g. **thyrotoxicosis**, vitamin B_1 deficiency (**beriberi**) and cases of large **arteriovenous shunts**.

The systemic circulation

Oxygenated blood is pumped by the left ventricle into the aorta, from which systemic arteries supply the various

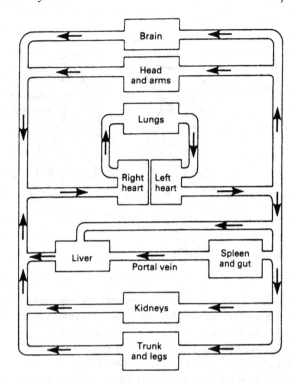

Fig. 5.24 Schematic diagram of the circulatory system showing the main vascular beds. (Reproduced from Bray, J.J., Cragg, P.A., Macknight, A.D.C., Mills, R.G. & Taylor, D.W. (eds) (1989) *Lecture Notes in Physiology*, 2nd edn. Blackwell Scientific Publications, Oxford.)

organs and limbs. Figure 5.24 shows that each main artery supplies a defined vascular bed, which is drained by a main vein. The veins join the **venae cavae**. Organ or regional blood supply is arranged *in parallel*. This makes it possible to regulate parts of the systemic circulation independently to meet local needs, without affecting the general circulation.

The **arteries** are large-diameter vessels. The thick walls are composed mainly of circular smooth muscle with a good proportion of elastic tissue. This permits stretching during systole and recoil during diastole and gives the *damping effect*, which converts pulsatile blood flow into a more steady stream. From small arteries the blood flows into the **arterioles**, whose walls contain a thick layer of smooth muscle and much less elastic tissue than arteries. This permits control of the diameter of the arterioles and therefore the *peripheral resistance* to blood flow. For this reason the arterioles have been called the **resistance vessels**. An arteriole has a diameter of about 20 μm. The total cross-sectional area of the arterioles in the whole body is about 400 cm^2.

Venule

Arteriole

Metarteriole

Thoroughfare
channel

Ateriovenous
anastomosis

Precapillary
sphincter

Capillary

Venule

Fig. 5.25 Diagrammatic representation
of microcirculation. (Reproduced from
Bray, J.J., Cragg, P.A., Macknight,
A.D.C., Mills, R.G. & Taylor, D.W. (eds)
(1989) *Lecture Notes in Physiology*, 2nd
edn. Blackwell Scientific Publications,
Oxford.)

Blood flows from the arterioles into the **capillaries** which have thin walls made of one layer of flat **endothelial cells**. There are **precapillary** smooth-muscle **sphincters**, which are not innervated but which respond to chemical substances in the blood or interstitial fluid. The final part of an arteriole (**metarteriole**) appears to be connected to a venule by a **main capillary channel** (throughfare channel). True capillaries form a network around this main vessel (Fig. 5.25). The diameter of a true capillary is about 5 μm at the arteriolar end and about 9 μm at the venular end. Therefore, the red cells have to squeeze through the capillaries and become convex discs, with their convexity towards the direction of flow and their edges closely applied to the capillary wall. This favours exchange of O_2 taking place between the interstitial fluid and the haemoglobin in the red blood cells. The capillaries are called **exchange vessels**.

At any one time, only 5% of the **blood volume** is in the systemic capillaries, but this proportion is the most vital part of circulating blood because it is across the capillary membrane that gas and nutrient exchange takes place. The transit time from the arteriolar end to the venular end of the capillary is 1–2 s. In an adult the total **cross-sectional area** of the capillaries is about 4500 cm^2 and their **surface area**, which is available for exchange, is about 6300 m^2. The **pressure** in the capillaries varies considerably. Typical values in human nail-bed capillaries are 32 and 15 mmHg at the arteriolar and venular ends, respectively. There is a small pulse pressure of about 5 mmHg in capillaries.

The structure of the capillary wall, the barrier between the plasma and the interstitial fluid, varies from one vascular bed to another. It behaves like a membrane that is impermeable to colloids, which exert an osmotic pressure of about 25 mmHg (called oncotic pressure). The exchange of fluid across the capillary membrane and the formation of oedema is described in Chapter 1.

Capillary **pores** at the junctions between endothelial cells allow molecules of up to 10 nm in diameter to pass through the capillary wall. These gaps are much smaller in brain capillaries and thus contribute to the **blood–brain barrier**. Larger gaps (20–100 nm) or **fenestrae** are found in the intestinal villi and some of the kidney capillaries.

The **veins** and venules are thin-walled vessels with much less muscle in them than in the arteries. However, they are still capable of a certain degree of contraction. The total **cross-sectional area** of the venules is 4000 cm^2, while that of the **veins** is about 40 cm^2. However, the venules and veins together hold more than 60% of the blood volume. This is why they are called the **capacity vessels**. Changes in blood volume can be compensated for by venoconstriction or dilatation and provide important vascular responses to **changes in blood pressure**. The veins have **valves**, which are made of crescent-shaped folds of **intima**. These valves play an important role in **venous return**, as already described.

Normally, the fluid leaving the capillaries is more than that returning to them. The extra fluid does not accumulate because it is drained by the **lymphatics**. Lymph flows back through the thoracic duct into the great veins in the thorax. The lymph is propelled by rhythmic contractions in the walls of the right **lymphatic duct** and the **thoracic duct**. The flow of lymph is helped by the **respiratory pump** and by the muscle pump, in the same way as they help the venous return. The lymph vessels and the large ducts also have valves, which prevent back flow.

Fig. 5.26 The upper drawing shows laminar and turbulent flow. The lower (graph) gives the relationship between pressure and velocity of flow. Laminar flow becomes turbulent when a certain critical velocicy is reached. (Reproduced from Bray, J.J., Cragg, P.A., Macknight, A.D.C., Mills, R.G. & Taylor, D.W. (eds) (1989) *Lecture Notes in Physiology*, 2nd edn. Blackwell Scientific Publications, Oxford.)

The arterial blood pressure

To ensure a steady blood flow or perfusion to the tissues, the **mean arterial blood pressure** is maintained at about 100 mmHg. This is achieved by control of the **cardiac output** and by variations in the **diameter of the arterioles**, which are responsible for regulation of the **peripheral resistance**. Local and central mechanisms help to regulate the blood flow through specific parts of the circulation. This section deals with the relationships between **pressure, flow** and **resistance** (i.e. **haemodynamics**) and the regulation of arterial blood pressure under physiological conditions. The above terms will be explained and defined. The applied physiology of arterial blood pressure will also be considered.

Basic concepts of haemodynamics

The perfusion of tissues depends on the pressure generated by the pumping action of the heart. The difference in mean blood pressure between the aorta and the right atrium (i.e. **effective perfusion pressure**) determines the blood flow in the systemic circulation. **Flow** is defined as the volume of blood which passes a given point in the circulation per unit time in ml/s. Flow should not be confused with **velocity**, which is defined as displacement of blood from one point in the circulation to another in cm/s.

Resistance (R)

Resistance to flow in tubes is generally determined by the diameter (radius, r) of the tube, the viscosity (η) of the fluid and the length (L) of the tube, as given by the following formula (**Poiseuille–Hagen formula**):

$$R = \frac{8\eta L}{\pi r^4}$$

This relationship is accurate for rigid tubes (e.g. glass or steel). In blood-vessels (which are not rigid) this mathematical relationship is applicable within limits. However, it is important to note that the main influence on variation of resistance is the **diameter of the blood-vessels** (expressed as r^4). Adjustment of the diameter of the arterioles is the primary mechanism for the regulation of the peripheral resistance.

In summary, the relationship between pressure, flow and resistance is similar to that in **Ohm's law**, which applies to electricity:

Ohm's law:

$$I \text{ (current)} = \frac{V \text{ (voltage)}}{R \text{ (resistance)}}$$

Similarly:

$$F \text{ (flow)} = \frac{P \text{ (pressure difference)}}{R \text{ (resistance)}}$$

and:

$$P = F \times R$$

Blood flow

Blood flow can be **laminar** or **turbulent** (Fig. 5.26). **Turbulence** is associated with the generation of sounds in the cardiovascular system (e.g. heart sounds and murmurs).

The degree of turbulence depends on the density of the fluid, the diameter of the vessel, the velocity of flow and

Fig. 5.27 Measurement of systolic and diastolic blood pressure using the sphygmomanometer.

the viscosity of the fluid. Turbulence is given by **Reynold's number** (*Re*):

$$Re = \frac{\text{Density} \times \text{diameter} \times \text{velocity}}{\text{viscosity}}$$

The greater the Reynolds number, the greater the turbulence. Murmurs are heard over the heart if there is narrowing (**stenosis**) or insufficiency of the valves, which affects the diameter of cardiac orifices between the heart chambers. Viscosity may be greatly decreased in anaemia, which is also associated with tachycardia and therefore greater velocity. This may explain the systolic murmurs commonly heard in anaemic patients.

Measurement of arterial blood pressure

If a glass tube is connected with an artery, blood will rise into the tube to a height of about 2.5 m. The top of the blood column will be seen to move up and down with each contraction and relaxation of the left ventricle. These were the basic observations made in AD 1732 by Stephen Hales in an experiment on a horse.

We can now measure the blood pressure indirectly but conveniently by using a **sphygmomanometer** (Fig. 5.27). A rubber bag is wrapped around the upper arm and inflated by a hand-pump. The cuff is connected to the mercury manometer. When the cuff is inflated to a pressure above

that in the brachial artery, blood flow to the forearm stops and the radial pulse cannot be felt by **palpation** of the radial artery at the wrist. The cuff is now deflated slowly until the pulse is felt again. The pressure reading at this point is the **systolic pressure**. This is called the **palpation method**. When a stethoscope is placed on to the antecubital fossa and the cuff inflated to a pressure higher than the systolic pressure, there is no flow and no sounds can be heard (Fig. 5.28). On slow deflation, sounds are heard

Fig. 5.28 Using the auscultatory method, systolic arterial blood pressure is taken at the point when the sounds start and the diastolic is read when the sounds either start to fade or disappear completely.

when the pressure falls to the systolic pressure. These are known as **Korotkov sounds**. They are due to turbulent blood flow, because the artery opens for a limited period of time only when the blood pressure exceeds that inside the cuff. On further deflation the sounds become louder and sharper. Suddenly they fade or stop. In adults at rest, the point at which the sounds disappear is taken as the **diastolic pressure**. In children and in adults after exercise, the point at which the sounds fade is more accurate. Thus, by using the **auscultation method**, we can obtain readings of both the systolic and the diastolic arterial blood pressure.

Normal blood pressure is often quoted as 120 mmHg systolic and 80 mmHg diastolic. However, it is difficult to define normal values because of the errors of sphygmomanometric measurement, age variation and the state of relaxation (**basal state**) or otherwise of the individual.

Regulation of arterial blood pressure

The **neural regulation** of arterial blood pressure is closely linked with that of the heart. Normal arterial pressure depends on the **cardiac output**, the **peripheral resistance** and the **blood volume**. It is the regulation of these three variables which determines the arterial blood pressure. Variation in cardiac output mainly determines the systolic blood pressure. The regulation of cardiac output, namely the heart rate and stroke volume, has been described. The following will deal with the other two parameters.

Regulation of peripheral resistance

Variations in the **peripheral resistance** determine the **diastolic blood pressure**. The diameter of the arterioles is regulated by varying the **sympathetic vasomotor tone**. There are several reflex mechanisms which regulate the vasomotor tone, the most important of which are the baroreceptor and chemoreceptor reflexes:

1 The **baroreceptors** send a continuous flow of signals to the **vasomotor centre** and the vagal centre. The frequency of these signals is directly proportional to the arterial blood pressure. When blood pressure falls, there is a *decrease* in the signals reaching the vasomotor centre, resulting in a reflex increase in sympathetic vasomotor tone (**vasoconstriction**) and consequently an increase in the peripheral resistance. As mentioned before, there is also an increase in the heart rate and therefore in COP. Conversely, an increase in blood pressure leads to *inhibition* of *vasomotor tone*, *vasodilatation* and reflex vagal slowing of the heart.

2 The **chemoreceptors** are stimulated by low Po_2, high Pco_2 and low plasma pH. Although the main function of the chemoreceptors is in respiratory control, they also exert important effects on the **vasomotor centre**. They can be stimulated during **hypotension** (e.g. after haemorrhage), which causes **hypoxia** due to decreased blood flow to the chemoreceptor cells. The result is reflex **vasoconstriction** and therefore an increase in the blood pressure. There is also an increased output of **catecholamines** from the **adrenal medulla**, leading to tachycardia. Increased Pco_2 has a direct effect on the vasomotor centre, producing reflex **vasoconstriction**. In the tissues, however, hypoxia and hypercapnia produce *local vasodilatation*. Therefore, the central and local effects oppose each other and there is little or no general effect on arterial blood pressure.

Cerebral ischaemia or local hypercapnia, produced by increased intracranial pressure or diminished cerebral blood flow, has a direct effect on the vasomotor centre, which tends to increase the blood pressure. A reflex bradycardia usually results, due to baroreceptor stimulation.

The reflex vasomotor effects mentioned above are most active in the **skin splanchnic area** and **muscle**. These tissues can tolerate decreased O_2 supply without damage to the cells. The brain and heart tissue cannot function without a constant blood supply and therefore their blood-vessels are only partly under neural control.

3 Other vasomotor reflexes can be initiated by receptors in various organs. **Atrial stretch receptor** stimulation (e.g. by increased venous return) produces reflex vasodilatation and a fall in blood pressure. **Thermoreceptors** in the skin or hypothalamus produce skin vasodilatation on exposure to heat and vasoconstriction on cooling. These responses help to maintain body temperature. **Pulmonary receptors** have been described which produce vasoconstriction as a result of lung inflation.

4 **Hormonal agents** also play an important role in the regulation of peripheral resistance. However, both resistance and capacity vessels can be involved.

Adrenaline (epinephrine) and noradrenaline (norepinephrine) are secreted from the adrenal medulla on sympathetic stimulation (e.g. in emergency or stressful situations, asphyxia and hypoglycaemia). **Noradrenaline** (norepinephrine) is vasoconstrictor, while adrenaline (epinephrine) is vasoconstrictor in most parts of the circulation but vasodilator in skeletal muscle. Therefore, noradrenaline increases the peripheral resistance, while adrenaline has no marked effect on **total peripheral resistance**, which may even decrease if the skeletal muscle vasodilatation is great.

Other hormonal agents include angiotensin, kinins, prostaglandins and histamine. Angiotensin II has a powerful vasoconstrictor effect but the others have, so far as is known, no role in the normal regulation of blood pressure.

Regulation of blood volume

The mechanisms which regulate blood volume are mainly renal. There are low-pressure **volume receptors** in the walls of the right atrium, which send impulses to the brain via the vagus. Some of these receptors may also be responsible for secretion of the hormone known as **atrial natriuretic peptide (ANP)**. The volume receptors and ANP have an important role in regulation of **aldosterone** and **sodium excretion**. Retention of sodium is one of the main mechanisms for maintaining blood volume. The **macula densa** cells of the juxtaglomerular apparatus in the kidney may also be considered as volume receptors, because they are stimulated by decreased blood flow in the kidney. They secrete renin in response to decreased renal blood flow and therefore trigger off the **renin–angiotensin system**, the most important mechanism for aldosterone regulation (see Chapter 9). **Angiotensin II** has a powerful vasoconstrictor effect, which contributes to the hormonal control of peripheral resistance.

Antidiuretic hormone (ADH), or **vasopressin**, of the posterior pituitary is released when volume receptors are stimulated, e.g. by hypovolaemia. This hormone is also released in response to osmoreceptor stimulation and therefore helps in the regulation of body water and the thirst mechanism (see 'Regulation of ADH', Chapter 9).

Large blood losses affect the **cardiac output** and therefore the arterial blood pressure and the baroreceptors. This leads to vasomotor stimulation, which results in an increase of **cardiac output** and **peripheral resistance**. There is also **venoconstriction**, which compensates for the volume loss by decreasing the capacity of the venous system.

Summary

The mean arterial pressure is determined by the cardiac output and the total peripheral resistance. The **systolic pressure** is a function of the stroke volume and therefore is determined mainly by the **cardiac output**. The **diastolic pressure** depends more on the **peripheral resistance**. Regulatory mechanisms depend on fast-acting reflexes which control the **heart rate**, **stroke volume** and **peripheral resistance**. Long-term mechanisms are mainly concerned with regulation of the body fluids and blood volume (Fig. 5.29).

Fast-acting reflex mechanisms

1 The baroreceptor reflex regulates the heart rate and peripheral resistance through vasomotor tone.
2 Chemoreceptor reflex regulates the heart rate and vasomotor tone.
3 Central nervous system ischaemic reflex.

4 Adrenal medullary hormones.
5 Vasopressin vasoconstrictor effect.

Long-term regulatory mechanisms.

These work through renal water and electrolyte regulation:
1 Renin–angiotensin system.
2 Aldosterone secretion.
3 Vasopressin antidiuretic effect.
4 ANP secretion.

Local regulation of blood flow

As the main goal of the circulation is to maintain adequate perfusion of the tissues, the **blood flow** (volume per unit tissue mass per unit time) determines the supply of O_2 and nutrients. It has been explained that regulation of the cardiac output and the peripheral resistance maintains a pressure gradient for adequate blood flow in the various organs. However, the activities and demands of different organs may vary from time to time. For this reason, *local regulation* of the blood flow in a particular organ or region of the body can take place without affecting the entire circulation. The following mechanisms are responsible for local circulatory adjustments of blood flow in organs or tissues:

1 There are **intrinsic mechanisms** which enable bloodvessels to react to local conditions. An increase in perfusion pressure stretches the arteriolar wall, which reacts by contraction of its smooth muscle and therefore decreases the diameter. Thus, an increase in **perfusion pressure** results in a **myogenic response**, which tends to keep the flow constant. This mechanism is particularly well developed in the kidney and the brain and is referred to as **autoregulation**. It enables these organs to keep their blood flow constant, despite wide variations of the perfusion pressure. However, this is not true of very low or very high perfusion pressures. At a certain low pressure, called the critical closing pressure, the arterioles collapse and blood flow stops (Fig. 5.30).

In addition to the myogenic response described above, another theory of autoregulation holds that an increase in perfusion pressure causes an increase in **tissue fluid formation** and therefore a rise of extramural pressure, causing the vessels to be compressed. This may partly explain autoregulation in an encapsulated organ like the kidney.

2 A second intrinsic mechanism depends on **metabolites**. Accumulation of products of metabolism in active tissues causes vasodilatation. This explains the increased blood flow, or **reactive hyperaemia**, in a limb after brief ischaemia. The factors known to produce vasodilatation are CO_2, hydrogen ions, potassium excess and oxygen lack. This is called **metabolic autoregulation**; it enables tissues to regulate their blood flow according to their activity and

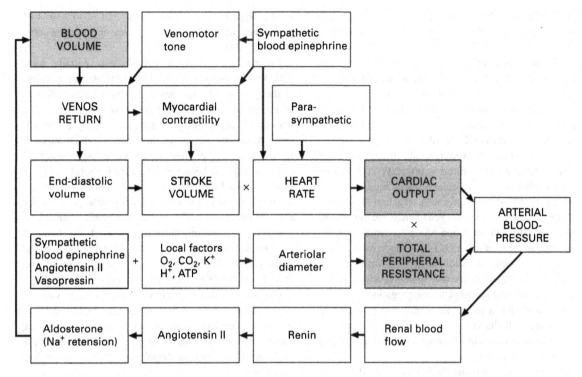

Fig. 5.29 Summary diagram of the determinants of arterial blood pressure. See text for the mechanisms responsible for the regulation of the various parameters. Shaded boxes indicate the main variables which directly affect the arterial blood pressure.

Fig. 5.30 The graph shows the relationship between blood flow and the pressure in blood-vessels. Note the critical closing pressure.

metabolic rate. It is particularly effective in the regulation of blood flow in cardiac and skeletal muscle. An increase in other metabolites, such as ATP, adenosine diphosphate (ADP), adenosine, pyruvate and lactate, has also been found to cause vasodilatation.

3 A third local regulatory mechanism depends on **humoral agents** released in the tissues. The release of the enzyme **kallikrein** by active salivary and sweat glands and by other exocrine glands converts plasma kininogens into active vasodilator substances or **kinins**, such as **bradykinin** and **kallidin**. Kinins are also formed in inflammation and in response to allergic reactions, and they contribute to the vasodilatation seen in these conditions. Other humoral vasodilators include **histamine**, which is produced by mast cells and granulocytes in allergy and inflammation. Some **prostaglandins** are vasodilators, while others are vasoconstrictors. These are produced in inflamed tissues and their synthesis can be suppressed by anti-inflammatory agents such as aspirin.

4 A fourth local mechanism is the effect of **temperature**. Warming of an organ produces local vasodilatation, while cooling results in vasoconstriction. This is an essentially local effect, which can occur in denervated limbs. The effect may be explained partly by a direct effect on vascular smooth muscle and partly by local changes in tissue metabolite production.

5 Finally, it has now been recognized that the **endothelium** is probably the largest and most active paracrine organ in the body. It produces several substances which influence local blood flow and intravascular coagulation, e.g.:

(a) **Prostacyclin (PGI$_2$)**, a potent relaxant of vascular smooth muscle, is also an inhibitor of platelet aggregation. Its release is stimulated by *hypoxia, shear stress* and *low-density lipoprotein (LDL)*. The mechanism of action of PGI$_2$ is mediated by elevation of the intracellular concentration of cyclic AMP.

(b) **Endothelium-derived relaxing factor (EDRF)**. This is believed to be **nitric oxide (NO)**. It has a relaxing effect on the vascular smooth muscle and an inhibitory role on adhesion and aggregation of platelets. The effect is mediated via cyclic guanosine monophosphate (GMP) and inhibition of Ca^{2+} release from the endoplasmic reticulum. EDRF sets the resting arterial tone and in stress conditions it controls vascular tone. Both EDRF and PGI$_2$ interact synergistically to dilate blood-vessels and inhibit platelet aggregation.

(c) **Endothelin**, a potent vasoconstrictor produced by vascular endothelial cells.

(d) **Thrombomodulin**. This serves as an endothelial receptor for thrombin.

(e) **Plasminogen activator** and many other substances.

Endothelial dysfunction is initiated by oxidized LDL, which influences monocyte adhesion and migration. Endothelial dysfunction is also associated with impaired endothelium-dependent vasodilatation, reduced release of nitric oxide and elevated levels of endothelin, which cause abnormal vasoconstriction. Decreased vasodilatation can directly contribute to coronary ischaemia; it is considered to be a factor in the pathogenesis of coronary heart disease. Other causes of defective release of EDRF include hypertension and hyperlipidaemia.

Applied physiology

Hypertension and hypotension

Hypertension
Elevated arterial blood pressure (hypertension) is diagnosed when the **diastolic pressure** is higher than 90 mmHg. Usually, both systolic and diastolic pressures are raised. It is a disease with no known cause in about 90% of cases. These are diagnosed as having **essential** or **benign hypertension**, which means we do not know the primary cause. The remaining cases can be secondary to **renal disease**, hypersecretion of aldosterone (**Conn's syndrome**), excess glucocorticoids (**Cushing's syndrome**) or a catecholamine-secreting tumour of the adrenal medulla (**phaeochromocy-**

toma). Hypertension is also a symptom of **toxaemia of pregnancy**, which may be due to a pressor peptide released by the placenta.

Patients with essential hypertension initially have periodic elevations of blood pressure which are exaggerated physiological responses to physiological stimuli such as exercise, cold or excitement. These responses can be managed by sympatholytic drugs. Eventually the blood-pressure elevation becomes continuous, which suggests failure of the baroreceptors to respond or that their normal range of response becomes readjusted (or set) at a higher level. Increased arterial blood pressure is due to an increase in either cardiac output or peripheral resistance. Since the cardiac output is usually normal in chronic, established, essential hypertension, the main cause of the sustained increase in blood pressure is the peripheral resistance. The underlying mechanism is excessive arteriolar constriction and/or structural abnormalities in the resistance vessels.

Chronic hypertension may continue for many years as uncomplicated hypertension, but it may rapidly develop into **malignant hypertension**, due to unknown triggering factors, more in men than in women. This causes swelling of the optic disc (**papilloedema**), renal failure and cerebral symptoms.

Hypotension
Hypotension may occur in normal subjects as a result of the effect of gravity on venous return. On prolonged standing, pooling of up to 500 ml of blood occurs in the lower limbs. Interstitial fluid also accumulates in the lower extremities, due to increased hydrostatic pressure. These effects may cause a decrease in **venous return** and **cardiac output**. If the blood flow to the brain decreases to a critically low level, **fainting** occurs. However, compensatory mechanisms involving the baroreceptors and volume receptors lead to an increase in the heart rate and activation of the renin–angiotensin system. These help to maintain normal cardiac output and the state of constriction of blood-vessels. Local autoregulation in the cerebral circulation also helps to maintain normal cerebral blood flow.

Attacks of fainting or **syncope** may be precipitated by hypotension due to a *reflex vasomotor inhibition*, usually when the patient is standing. Consciousness is recovered quickly on lying down. Severe emotions can cause syncope due to fall of blood pressure mediated by the limbic system and the hypothalamus. A possible mechanism is *skeletal muscle vasodilatation*, brought about by release of adrenaline and activation of the sympathetic **cholinergic vasodilator system** to skeletal-muscle vessels.

Orthostatic or **postural hypotension** may occur in some subjects on standing up from a lying-down position. It causes transient dimness of vision and dizziness or a fainting attack. The mechanism seems to involve failure of the sympathetic compensatory mechanisms which readjust vascular tone on standing. There is also failure of adrenal medullary secretion of noradrenaline in response to baroreceptor stimulation. Patients with hypovolaemia due to a variety of causes are more likely to develop postural hypotension.

Hypotension may be due to **heart failure**, when the heart is unable to maintain a systolic pressure of 100 mmHg. This occurs in coronary artery disease due to myocardial damage and in mitral stenosis and aortic stenosis. Attacks of fainting are common in such patients. Peripheral vasodilatation, as caused by exposure to heat or vasodilator drugs, may precipitate such attacks. If a fainting attack is prolonged (coma), cerebral ischaemia and brain damage may occur.

Haemorrhage

Acute blood loss is serious because it leads to a sudden drop in **venous return**, a decrease in end-diastolic volume and therefore a reduction in **cardiac output** and **arterial blood pressure**. If the blood loss is less than 20% of the blood volume, rapid compensatory mechanisms are usually adequate, and spontaneous readjustment of the blood pressure takes place. However, if the blood loss is more than 20%, the compensatory mechanisms are not enough and blood transfusion must be given as early as possible.

The rapid **compensatory mechanisms** increase the peripheral resistance and the cardiac output to restore the arterial blood pressure as follows:

1 Responses initiated by the **arterial baroreceptors**. Their rate of discharge falls and this releases the pressor area of the vasomotor centre to increase its discharge. The result is generalized **vasoconstriction** due to increased sympathetic vasomotor tone. This is accompanied by increased **venoconstriction**, especially in the splanchnic area. Therefore, both the peripheral resistance and the **central venous pressure** are increased. The baroreceptor reflex also causes **tachycardia** by means of increased sympathetic discharge as well as inhibition of vagal centres (cardioinhibitory neurons).

2 The above mechanisms are augmented by stimulation of the **peripheral chemoreceptors**. These are stimulated by lack of O_2 due to diminished blood flow (stagnant hypoxia) and decreased O_2 carrying capacity of the blood. H^+ concentration also rises due to increased anaerobic glycolysis and lactic acid formation.

Cerebral blood-vessels are not constricted because they have little vasomotor control. The coronary vessels are dilated due to increased myocardial metabolism. However, renal blood flow may be compromised due to constriction of afferent and efferent arterioles. This causes decreased urine formation (**oliguria**), sodium retention and increased blood urea.

3 Responses due to the **adrenal medulla**. Sympathetic stimulation due to the baro- and chemoreceptor reflexes stimulates the adrenal medulla to release catecholamines into the bloodstream. Noradrenaline also reaches the circulation from sympathetic postganglionic fibres. The catecholamines augment the vasomotor tone and also increase the stroke volume and dilate the coronary vessels. Other effects of catecholamines after haemorrhage include an increase in secretion of adrenocorticotrophic hormone (ACTH) and cortisol and enhancement of blood coagulation by releasing fibrinogen and prothrombin from the liver and by activation of factor V.

The rapid compensatory mechanisms described above explain the signs of hypovolaemia: pale, cool skin and tachycardia with low-volume (thready) pulse. There is also an increase in the respiratory rate, mediated by O_2 lack and acidosis. Tachypnoea helps increase the venous return and the efficiency of oxygenation of blood. Restlessness (increased skeletal muscle movement), in some cases, is probably due to stimulation of the reticular formation. Muscle movements increase the venous return through the 'muscle pump'.

Thirst is also a prominent symptom of hypovolaemia. It is due to cellular dehydration. This is explained as follows. When the arterioles constrict, the capillary pressure falls. This leads to net movement of interstitial fluid into the bloodstream. The decreased interstitial fluid volume causes net movement of fluid out of the intracellular compartment, leading to thirst.

4 Angiotensin II is a powerful vasoconstrictor. Its formation in response to hypovolaemia is due to activation of the **renin–angiotensin system**. Angiotensin II exerts a generalized vasoconstrictor effect, which contributes to the increase in peripheral resistance. It also contributes to the thirst mechanism by acting centrally. Angiotensin II is an important stimulus for **aldosterone** secretion and therefore it helps to retain Na^+ and increase the extracellular fluid (ECF).

The **long-term** or delayed mechanisms are mainly concerned with the restoration of blood volume and red blood cell (RBC) formation, as follows:

1 Restoration of plasma volume. The movement of ECF into the circulation leads to haemodilution and a fall

Type of shock   Causes   Effects

Hypovolaemic:

Cardiogenic:

Distributive:

Fig. 5.31 Flow diagram showing the types of shock, their causes and effects. Note vicious circles which lead to worsening of the condition of the patient, e.g. decreased arterial pressure causing decreased myocardial function and low organ perfusion leading to multiorgan failure.

of plasma protein concentration. Preformed albumin is released from the liver and is eventually followed by increased plasma protein synthesis. The plasma proteins are restored in 3–4 days.

As long as hypovolaemia exists, stimulation of aldosterone and ADH (vasopressin) secretion continues to play an important role in the restoration of ECF volume (see Chapter 9).

2 Red blood cell formation is stimulated by the renal hormone **erythropoietin**, which is released in response to hypoxia (see Chapter 2). Anaemia following haemorrhage is associated with an increase in the concentration of **2,3-diphosphoglycerate (2,3-DPG)**. This is also stimulated by hypoxia and favours the delivery of O_2 from haemoglobin to the tissues, causing a shift of the O_2 dissociation curve to the right.

Shock

Shock can be defined as a state of the circulation in which decreased blood flow disturbs the functions of organ systems. It is usually the result of **heart failure**. The patient presents with a **pale**, **cold** and **sweaty skin** due to sympathetic stimulation. There is also **tachycardia**, **restlessness**, **thirst**, decreased formation of urine and metabolic acidosis. If not treated adequately it may become refractory, with brain damage, multiorgan failure and death.

When the main problem lies with the cardiac output, as in coronary artery occlusion, this is called **cardiogenic shock** or central circulatory failure. When the fault is

in the blood volume or peripheral resistance, it is known as **peripheral circulatory failure**. The systolic blood pressure is usually less than 80 mmHg. The main disturbance is either blood loss or dehydration or massive serum loss due to extensive skin burns. (**hypovolaemic shock**), together with a large vascular bed. Other causes of shock are due to maldistribution of blood or body fluids (**distributive**). The causes of this group include **septicaemia**, anaphylaxis (severe allergy) and **neurogenic shock** (due to damage to the central nervous system) and **adrenal cortical failure**. In this group there is failure of vasoconstrictor compensatory mechanisms (study Fig. 5.31).

Circulation in special regions

This section deals with the adjustments of the blood flow in special vital regions of the body. Aspects of blood flow in other organs will be found in the various chapters dealing with organ systems.

Pulmonary circulation

The pulmonary arterial system has low resistance (about one-tenth that in systemic circulation). The pulmonary vessels are thinner-walled, shorter and more compliant. The blood pressure in the pulmonary arteries is about 25 mmHg systolic and 10 mmHg diastolic (mean 15 mmHg). In the pulmonary capillaries it is 10 mmHg and in the left atrium it is about 8 mmHg during diastole. However, the total blood flow, the cross-sectional area and the velocity of flow in the pulmonary circulation are similar to those in the systemic circulation. At rest, a red blood cell takes about 0.75 s to pass through a pulmonary capillary and much less than that during exercise. The amount of blood in the lungs during standing is about 450 ml; on lying down it may increase to nearly double this amount. This causes a decrease in the vital capacity and explains **dyspnoea** (breathlessness) on lying flat (**orthopnoea**) in patients with cardiac failure or pulmonary disease.

The regulation of pulmonary blood flow is mainly passive, due to the high **distensibility** of the pulmonary vessels. When the cardiac output increases, as in muscular exercise, the blood flow in the lungs increases, pulmonary arterial pressure increases and parts of the lungs normally with little perfusion receive increased blood flow. There are, however, important vascular responses to alveolar O_2. **Hypoxia** causes **vasoconstriction**. Note that this is the opposite effect to that in the systemic circulation. Therefore, hypoxic alveoli tend to have less blood flow. This helps to divert blood flow to well-ventilated alveoli and thus gaseous exchange is enhanced. However, during exposure to hypoxia of *high altitude* or in lung disorders causing decreased ventilation, pulmonary vasoconstriction has obvious disadvantages, such as increased vascular resistance. This causes an increase in pulmonary blood pressure and increases ventricular workload. Accumulation of CO_2 in underventilated areas leads to a rise in **hydrogen ion** concentration, which also causes vasoconstriction.

The pulmonary blood-vessels are supplied by sympathetic nerves, which produce *vasoconstriction*, and parasympathetic nerves, which are *vasodilators*. Adrenaline administration or sympathetic stimulation can decrease the pulmonary blood flow by about one-third.

Fig. 5.32 A diagram showing phasic blood flow in the coronary arteries. (Reproduced from Berne, R.M. & Levy, M.N. (1988) *Physiology*, 2nd edn. By permission of C.V. Mosby Co., St Louis.)

Coronary circulation

The coronary arteries are the first branches arising from the aorta, just above the aortic valves. The **left coronary artery** supplies most of the left ventricle and part of the anterior surface of the right ventricle, as well as the interventricular septum. The **right coronary artery** supplies most of the right ventricle and the posterior wall of the left ventricle. The sinoatrial node is supplied by both arteries. The atrioventricular node and bundle are supplied by the right coronary artery. The right bundle branch is supplied by the right coronary artery while the left terminal bundle branch is supplied by both arteries.

The coronary arteries supply the myocardium with blood mainly *during diastole* (Fig. 5.32). About 80% of coronary blood flow takes place during diastole. *During systole* the blood flow is still maintained because the aortic

cusps are kept away from the coronary orifices by **eddy currents**. When the myocardium is in a state of contraction, the blood-vessels are compressed and flow is decreased. Subendocardial myocardial tissue in the left ventricle is further compressed by the high pressure inside the ventricle. This part of the heart muscle is most affected by ischaemic damage (myocardial infarction). In the right ventricle and both atria, coronary flow is better due to the greater pressure gradient between these chambers and the aorta.

The **venous drainage** of the left ventricle is mainly through venules which run with the small arteries and converge to form the coronary sinus and the anterior cardiac veins. This is known as the **superficial drainage system**. There is a **deep system** which drains the remaining parts of the heart. It is made up of arteriosinusoidal vessels which open directly into the heart chambers.

Regulation of coronary blood flow

Coronary blood flow is mainly regulated by **metabolic autoregulation**. The degree of coronary dilatation is proportional to myocardial O_2 **consumption**. **Hypoxia** is a potent vasodilator. Cardiac muscle has a high oxygen consumption relative to its mass. At rest it receives 250 ml of blood/min and extracts about 30 ml of O_2/min (i.e. 60%). Other tissues extract about 25% of arterial O_2 supply. Therefore, during exercise there is little further O_2 extraction and the increased O_2 uptake has to come from an increased coronary blood flow. Hypoxia is thought to release a vasodilator substance, probably **adenosine** released from ATP during myocardial metabolism. Low Po_2 can increase the coronary blood flow fivefold. Reactive hyperaemia occurs when blood flow is temporarily obstructed. This increases blood flow in capillaries rather than in arteriovenous shunts. Other chemical factors involved in autoregulation include Pco_2, H^+, K^+ and **prostaglandins**.

Adrenaline (epinephrine) from the adrenal medulla causes vasodilatation in the coronary arteries by acting on β_2 **receptors**. Therefore, in conditions where adrenaline (epinephrine) is released, the coronary blood flow is increased.

Neural regulation depends on sympathetic and parasympathetic nerves, which play a smaller role in regulation of coronary blood flow than autoregulation. **Parasympathetic cholinergic** nerves produce vasodilatation. Noradrenaline (norepinephrine) produces mild vasoconstriction by acting on α-adrenergic receptors. However, after sympathetic stimulation of the cardiac nerves, the increase in the heart rate and myocardial contractility increases the O_2 uptake and the net result is vasodilatation (by *metabolic autoregulation*) rather than vasoconstriction. Similarly, during exercise the coronary blood flow is maintained by autoregulation despite the increase in the heart rate and the shorter duration of diastole. When there is narrowing of the coronary arteries (**atherosclerosis**), the myocardial blood flow on exertion may not be sufficient, and myocardial ischaemia gives rise to chest pain (**angina pectoris**).

The pressure in the aorta, compared with that in the coronary arteries, significantly affects the coronary blood flow, especially during late systole, when both pressures fall simultaneously. Also, the mean and systolic aortic pressure affects the coronary blood flow indirectly when there is a change in aortic impedance, which, in turn, affects the work of the heart and its O_2 consumption.

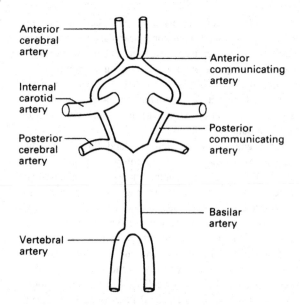

Fig. 5.33 The circle of Willis. (Reproduced with permission from Emslie-Smith, D., Paterson, C.R., Scratcherol, T. & Read, N.W. (eds) (1988) *BDS Textbook of Physiology*, 11th edn. Churchill Livingstone, Edinburgh.)

Cerebral circulation

The brain receives its blood supply from the two **internal carotid arteries** and the **vertebral arteries**. These two sources communicate through the **circle of Willis** (Fig. 5.33), ensuring adequate circulation even when a major artery is occluded. The cerebral arteries have less developed muscle layers. The veins drain into the venous sinuses, which are kept patent by the attachments of the dura mater. This ensures venous drainage even when there is an increase in intracranial pressure. The blood flow to the brain is about 50 ml/100 g, i.e. if the brain is about 1400 g, then it receives 700 ml, which amounts to 15% of the cardiac output.

The capillaries in the brain have special endothelial tight junctions and lack the fenestrae commonly found in other capillaries. This is believed to be the structural basis of the **blood–brain barrier**, one of the protective mechanisms of the brain and the spinal cord.

The cerebral blood flow is kept constant mainly by **myogenic autoregulation**. Thus, the arteries dilate when the blood pressure decreases and constrict when the blood pressure is high. This is effective over a wide range of mean arterial blood pressure (50–150 mmHg). Significant hydrostatic pressure changes occur on changing the position of the head in relation to the heart, e.g. performing a handstand. The camel and the giraffe have to lower the head by about 2–4 m when drinking water. Autoregulatory mechanisms maintain a constant blood flow to the brain despite the effect of gravity. Venous congestion and oedema are prevented by ECF passing to the cerebrospinal fluid, which is reabsorbed in the cerebral ventricles.

Metabolic autoregulation also plays an important role. The cerebral arterioles are particularly sensitive to P_{CO_2} changes and a low blood pH. Marked vasodilatation can cause up to a twofold increase in cerebral blood flow when the P_{CO_2} rises from 40 to 100 mmHg. Conversely, a marked vasoconstriction occurs when the P_{CO_2} falls below 40 mmHg. There is a decrease in cerebral blood flow, which may cause dizziness, when the P_{CO_2} decreases, e.g. due to hyperventilation (as in high altitudes) or due to excessive laughter or crying (as in hysterical attacks). The P_{O_2} plays a smaller role than P_{CO_2}. Hypoxia produces little vasodilatation when P_{O_2} decreases from 100 to 50 mmHg.

The cerebral blood-vessels have both sympathetic and parasympathetic supply but they seem to play a minor role in blood-flow regulation.

Cerebral blood flow can be affected by change of the intracranial pressure. An increase in the **intracranial pressure** occurs in cases of hydrocephalus, brain tumours or meningitis. The cerebral blood flow is decreased due to compression of the intracranial blood-vessels. This causes hypoxia and hypercapnia in the cerebral circulation and directly stimulates the **vasomotor centres**, leading to an increase in the blood pressure. There is also local metabolic vasodilatation. The increase in perfusion pressure and the vasodilatation helps to keep the blood flow constant. The increase in arterial blood pressure is responsible for reflex **bradycardia**, usually observed in cases of increased intracranial pressure. It is mediated by the baroreceptors and is known as *Cushing's reflex*.

Further reading

1 Guyton, A.C. & Hall, J.E. (1996) Cardiac output, venous return, and their regulation. In: *Textbook of Medical Physiology*, 9th edn, pp. 239–252. Saunders, Philadelphia.

2 Guyton, A.C. & Hall, J.E. (1996) Dominant role of the kidneys in long-term regulation of arterial pressure and in hypertension; the integrated system for pressure control. In: *Textbook of Medical Physiology*, 9th edn, pp. 221–238. Saunders, Philadelphia.

3 Guyton, A.C. & Hall, J.E. (1996) Muscle blood flow and cardiac output during exercise; the coronary circulation: and ischemic heart disease. In: *Textbook of Medical Physiology*, 9th edn, pp. 253–264. Saunders, Philadelphia.

4 Guyton, A.C. & Hall, J.E. (1996) Muscular distensibility and functions of the arterial and venous systems. In: *Textbook of Medical Physiology*, 9th edn, pp. 171–181. Saunders, Philadelphia.

5 Guyton, A.C. & Hall, J.E. (1996) Nervous regulation of the circulation, and rapid control of arterial pressure. In: *Textbook of Medical Physiology*, 9th edn, pp. 209–219. Saunders, Philadelphia.

6 Guyton, A.C. & Hall, J.E. (1996) Overview of the circulation and medical physics of pressure, flow, and resistance. In: *Textbook of Medical Physiology*, 9th edn, pp. 161–170. Saunders, Philadelphia.

7 Ganong, F.G. (1999) *Review of Medical Physiology*, 19th edn. Appleton & Lange, Stamford, Connecticut.

8 Wilson, J.D. (1998) *Harrison's Principles of Internal Medicine*, 14th edn. McGraw-Hill, New York.

6 / The Respiratory System

Objectives

On completion of the study of this chapter, the student should be able to:

1 Understand the mechanics of breathing leading to normal ventilation.

2 Understand the relationship between volume and pressure in the lungs so as to explain abnormalities of lung compliance.

3 Describe the processes of gas exchange in the pulmonary alveoli and tissues so as to explain defects of these mechanisms leading to hypoxia or hypercapnia.

4 Understand the neural and chemical control of **ventilation** so as to explain the variations that occur in physiological and pathological states.

5 Describe the role of the respiratory system in the regulation of blood pH so as to explain the mechanisms of respiratory acidosis and respiratory alkalosis.

6 Become aware of the pulmonary function tests used in the diagnosis and management of respiratory disorders.

Introduction

The respiratory system serves two major functions in the human body: (i) it provides mechanisms for **exchange of oxygen and carbon dioxide** between the environment and tissues; and (ii) it plays a main role in the **regulation of pH** of the extracellular fluid. To achieve these two functions, the respiratory system provides the mechanical movements which result in **ventilation**, i.e. movement of the air in and out of the lungs during breathing. The lung alveoli provide mechanisms for the exchange of gases between the blood and the alveolar air. The regulation of breathing is closely linked with this exchange of gases and the breathing is stimulated or depressed according to the need to get more oxygen and to remove excess carbon dioxide. The removal of CO_2 provides a mechanism for getting rid of carbonic acid, which is a major factor in the regulation of blood pH.

The respiratory system has other subsidiary functions, which will be mentioned in the discussion of other body functions.

Ventilation

Ventilation is the process dealing with the air movement between the lung and atmospheric air.

Lung volumes and capacities

For convenience, definitions of certain volumetric parameters commonly used in respiration are presented before the description of the mechanics of breathing. It should be explained at this stage that, when a volumetric parameter comprises more than one volume, it is referred to as a **capacity**.

1 *Tidal volume* is the volume of air inspired or expired at each breath. At rest (quiet breathing) the tidal volume is about 500 ml in a normal adult male. Its volume varies with body size, sex, age and activity. It is measured by a spirometer or gas meter. The tidal volume is increased with depth of breathing, as in exercise.

2 *Respiratory minute volume or pulmonary ventilation* is the volume of air breathed in or out of the lungs each minute. In other words, it represents the volume of air which ventilates the lung every minute. If the resting tidal volume is 500 ml and if the resting respiratory rate is 12/min, then the pulmonary ventilation rate or lung minute volume is $500 \times 12 = 6000$ ml/min.

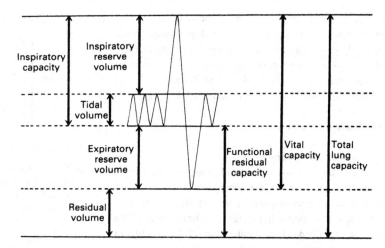

Fig. 6.1 Graphic representation of lung volumes and capacities during normal breathing, maximum inspiration and maximum expiration.

3 *Inspiratory reserve volume* is the extra volume of air which can be inspired by a maximal inspiratory effort over and above the tidal inspiration. It is defined as the volume of air inspired by a maximal inspiratory effort after normal inspiration. It is also measured by a spirometer or gas meter.

4 *Inspiratory capacity.* Since inspiration starts after the end of expiration, the amount of air that can be inspired is equal to the tidal volume plus the inspiratory reserve volume. This is referred to as the inspiratory capacity (it is called capacity because it is formed of more than one volume, i.e. tidal volume plus inspiratory reserve volume). It is defined as the volume of air inspired by a maximal inspiratory effort after normal expiration.

5 *Expiratory reserve volume* is the extra volume of air which can be expired by a maximal expiratory effort over and above the tidal expiratory volume. It is defined as the volume of air expired by a maximal expiratory effort after normal expiration. It is measured by a spirometer or gas meter.

6 *Vital capacity* is the total volume of air that can be exchanged between the lungs and the environment in one respiratory cycle. It is defined as the volume expired by a maximal expiratory effort after maximal inspiration. It comprises tidal volume plus inspiratory reserve volume plus expiratory reserve volume. The vital capacity also depends on the size, age and sex of the individual. It is a good test for assessment of lung function and can be measured by a spirometer or gas meter.

7 *Residual volume* is the volume of air that remains in the lung after maximal expiration. Since it is the volume of air that cannot be expired, it is not available for measurement by a spirometer or gas meter; other methods have to be used (see 'Lung function tests'). Assessment of the residual volume is a good index of the state of the lung. It is usually

Table 6.1 Normal lung volumes and capacities in litres for adult males and females.

	Volume (litres)	
	Male	Female
Tidal volume (TV)	0.5	0.5
Inspiratory reserve volume (IRV)	3.3	1.9
Expiratory reserve volume (ERV)	1.0	0.7
Residual volume (RV)	1.2	1.1
Inspiratory capacity (IC)	3.8	2.4
Functional residual capacity (FRC)	2.2	1.8
Vital capacity (VC)	4.8	3.1
Total lung capacity (TLC)	6.0	4.2

All pulmonary volumes and capacities are 20–25% less in females than in males.

increased by age and lung disease when the lung elasticity or bronchial diameter is affected.

8 *Functional residual capacity (FRC)* is the volume of air remaining in the lung after normal expiration. It includes the expiratory reserve volume and the residual volume. Like the residual volume, it cannot be measured by a spirometer or by a gas meter. As the FRC is large (2.2 litres) and the part of inspired tidal air which reaches the alveoli is small (0.35 litre), the composition of alveolar air remains relatively constant during the inspiration–expiration cycle.

9 *Total lung capacity* is the maximal volume of air that can be accommodated in the lungs. It comprises tidal volume, inspiratory reserve volume, expiratory reserve volume and residual volume.

The various volumes and capacities are shown graphically in Fig. 6.1 and their normal values are shown in Table 6.1.

Age, sex and body size have a significant effect on some of the lung volumes and capacities. For example, both residual volume and functional residual capacity increase with age while vital capacity decreases with age. Similar changes are usually observed in lung diseases affecting elasticity and expansibility (compliance) of the lungs.

Mechanics of breathing

Anatomical considerations

The lungs are enclosed in an airtight compartment formed of the thoracic cage and the diaphragm. Their only connection with the atmosphere is through the mouth, nose and respiratory conducting system of tubes—airways. The lungs are surrounded by a minute space filled with a film of fluid, the **pleural space**, lying between the visceral pleura, attached to the lung surface, and the parietal pleura, which lines the inner surface of the thoracic cage and the thoracic surface of the diaphragm. The thin film of fluid in the pleural space lubricates the movements of the two surfaces during breathing. The chest wall is formed of muscles, ribs and vertebrae. On the outside it is covered by skin, subcutaneous tissue and muscle. The **diaphragm** is a muscle attached to the lower portion of the thoracic cage. It separates the thorax from the abdominal cavity. The oesophagus passes through the diaphragm to the stomach. The diaphragm, when relaxed, assumes a dome shape with its convexity towards the thoracic cavity. When it contracts during inspiration, it descends and becomes less convex.

The ribs are connected by two layers of muscles: **external** and **internal** groups of intercostal muscles. The two groups of muscles differ in the direction of their muscle fibres from their origin to their insertion. The external intercostal muscles pass downwards and forwards from their origin to their insertion, while the internal intercostal muscles pass downwards and backwards from their origin to their insertion (Fig. 6.2). The ribs are articulated posteriorly to the vertebral column by socket joints and anteriorly to the mobile manubrium and sternum by cartilage joints. From their attachment posteriorly to the vertebral column the ribs curve downwards and laterally, forwards and then medially.

Chest movements

The arrangement of the ribs and intercostal muscles is such that movements of the ribs cause alterations in the dimensions of the chest. When the **external intercostal muscles** contract they raise the upper ribs and sternum. This movement will displace the sternum and ribs forward, increasing the **anteroposterior diameter** of the thoracic cavity. More-

Fig. 6.2 Diagrammatic representation showing the arrangement of fibres of external and internal intercostal muscles and position of ribs during expiration. The dashed line indicates the position during inspiration.

Fig. 6.3 Movements of the ribs and sternum during inspiration to increase the anteroposterior diameter of the thoracic cavity. Compare with their position in expiration.

over, as the arched ribs are raised, they rotate outward in a '*bucket handle*' movement, increasing the transverse diameter of the chest slightly. Contraction of the **internal intercostal muscles** tends to lower the ribs and sternum, reducing the anteroposterior diameter of the thoracic cavity (Fig. 6.3).

When the **diaphragm** contracts, it becomes less convex and pushes the abdominal viscera downwards. This increases the vertical diameter of the thoracic cavity (Fig. 6.4).

During normal resting inspiration, the increase in the vertical diameter of the chest, brought about by the descent of the diaphragm, contributes about 70% of the increase in the volume of the thoracic cavity. The increase in the anteroposterior diameter, brought about by upward movement of the sternum and ribs, contributes about 25–30% of the volume change, while the increase in the transverse diameter, brought about by the rotation of the ribs, contributes about 1–2%.

Intrapleural pressure

A manometer connected to a needle inserted into the pleural space will record subatmospheric pressure (**negative pressure**) throughout the respiratory cycle during normal

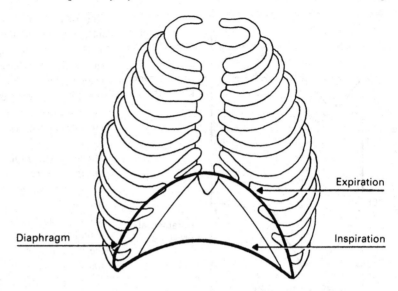

Fig. 6.4 Movement of the diaphragm during inspiration to increase the vertical diameter of the thoracic cavity.

Fig. 6.5 The effect of introducing air into the pleural cavity through the chest wall. The lung will recoil inward (collapse) and the chest wall will recoil outward.

quiet breathing. The pressure will vary between −4 mmHg at the end of normal expiration to about −6 mmHg during inspiration (Fig. 6.5). During forcible inspiration, it may fall to −70 mmHg. During forcible expiration against a closed glottis (**Valsalva manoeuvre**), the intrapleural pressure becomes positive, rising to 50 mmHg or more above atmospheric pressure.

The changes in oesophageal pressure detected by a balloon inserted into the oesophagus reflect the changes in intrapleural pressure fairly accurately.

Causes of subatmospheric (negative) intrapleural pressure. Several factors contribute to the creation of a negative intrapleural pressure:

1 *The lungs.* The walls of the lungs are rich in elastic tissue, which tends to collapse the lungs because the elastic recoil of the lung acts in an inward direction. Thus, with advancing age due to loss of elastic tissue, intrapleural pressure rises towards the atmospheric pressure. The lung recoil is also potentiated by the surface tension of the fluid lining the alveoli and alveolar sacs. However, the surface tension forces are normally reduced by **surfactant**, a lipoprotein secreted by type II cells of the alveolar epithelium. Congenital deficiency of surfactant (*hyaline membrane disease of the newborn*) may be one of the causes of the failure of the lungs to expand at birth.

2 *The chest wall.* Formed of ribs, cartilage and muscle, the chest wall has a tendency to recoil outward, i.e. in an opposite direction to the elastic recoil of the lungs. At equilibrium, these two opposing forces lead to a negative pressure in the pleural cavity. If air is introduced into the pleural cavity by opening the chest wall, the lungs will collapse (recoil inward) while the chest wall will recoil outward and the intrapleural pressure becomes atmospheric (Fig. 6.5).

3 *Pleural capillaries and lymphatics.* The intrapleural space is rich in blood capillaries and lymphatics, which tend to absorb fluid from the pleural cavity. This adds to the negativity of the intrapleural pressure.

Fig. 6.6 Graphic representation of intrapleural and intra-alveolar pressures during a full respiratory cycle. For full explanation see text. EXP, expiration; INS, inspiration.

Intra-alveolar (intrapulmonary) pressure

Pressure within the alveoli of the lungs varies with the different stages of the respiratory cycle. When recorded at the end of expiration with the glottis open, it is atmospheric. During inspiration, because the lungs are expanding with the increasing size of the thoracic cage, the pressure tends to fall below atmospheric. If the glottis is open, air will be drawn into the lungs. During quiet inspiration, the pressure falls to about −1 mmHg but with forcible inspiration it may fall much lower, to about −70 mmHg. During expiration, as the lungs recoil, the intra-alveolar pressure rises above atmospheric and forces the air out of the lungs if the airway is open. With normal quiet expiration intra-alveolar pressure usually rises to 1 mmHg. The changes of the intra-alveolar pressure are related directly to those in the intra-pleural space. Figure 6.6 illustrates the following.

1 During inspiration, the intra-alveolar pressure drops below the atmospheric pressure.

2 During expiration, the intra-alveolar pressure rises above the atmospheric pressure.

3 At the end of both inspiration and expiration, the alveolar pressure becomes equal to atmospheric pressure.

At these points there is no air flow because the pressure in the lungs is at equilibrium with the outside.

4 Throughout the respiratory cycle the intrapleural pressure stays lower than the intra-alveolar pressure. This keeps the lungs inflated at all times.

During forceful expiration with the glottis closed (Valsalva manoeuvre) the intra-alveolar pressure may rise up to 100 mmHg above atmospheric.

Mechanism of air flow between the lung and the atmosphere

The external intercostal muscles and the diaphragm are innervated by somatic nerves, the intercostal and the phrenic nerves, respectively. Stimulation of the nerves leads to contraction of the external intercostal muscles, increasing the anteroposterior diameter and, to a lesser extent, the transverse diameter of the chest, while contraction of the diaphragm increases the vertical diameter. The resulting increase in the volume of the chest tends to lower the intrapleural pressure. Consequently, because of their expansile properties, the lungs expand. The expansion of the lung lowers the intra-alveolar pressure below atmospheric so that, if the glottis is open, air will be drawn into the lungs.

When inspiration comes to an end by cessation of impulses to the inspiratory muscles, the muscles relax. The diaphragm ascends to assume a more convex shape, reducing the vertical diameter of the chest. On relaxation of the external intercostal muscles, the sternum and ribs descend and the thoracic wall recoils. Consequently, the intrapleural pressure rises (becomes less negative). The elastic lung then recoils and compresses the air in the alveoli, leading to the rise of the intra-alveolar pressure above atmospheric. If the airways are open, air is forced out of the lungs.

It is evident from the above description of the mechanisms of inspiration and expiration that during quiet breathing inspiration is an *active* process, involving muscular contraction, while expiration is a *passive* process, brought about by the relaxation of muscles of inspiration, recoil of the chest wall and elastic recoil of the lungs.

Accessory muscles of respiration

A distinction should be made between an increase in inspiration and an increase in pulmonary ventilation (minute volume).

During quiet breathing, only about one-tenth of the muscle fibres of the external intercostal muscles and the diaphragm are active at any one time. With more powerful inspiration, more muscle fibres are recruited into activity until all fibres become active during maximal inspiration.

This alone can increase pulmonary ventilation 10-fold, up to about 60 litres/min. However, there are other muscles involved in increasing pulmonary ventilation. These groups of muscles are designated accessory muscles of respiration; some are inspiratory and others are expiratory. They act by increasing the depth of inspiration even further, and by decreasing the airway resistance to air flow to allow quick and easy flow of air between the lungs and the atmosphere.

A group of muscles attached to the thoracic cage can be brought into action during maximal ventilation or whenever there is difficulty in breathing from any cause. When these muscles contract, they lift the entire thoracic cage upwards. This chest movement tends to facilitate inspiration by a further increase in the anteroposterior diameter of the chest, but a more important effect is that it straightens the airways, decreasing their resistance to air flow. The most important accessory muscles of inspiration are the **sternocleidomastoids**, the **anterior serrati** and the **scaleni**.

Normally, expiration is a passive process that does not involve active muscular contraction. However, during maximal expiratory efforts, as in severe exercise or when there is difficulty in breathing, e.g. bronchial obstruction in bronchial asthma, expiration becomes an active process with active muscular contraction. Other muscles can also be identified as having an accessory role during expiration. The **internal intercostal** muscles, by depressing the sternum and ribs, decrease the anteroposterior diameter of the chest. When the **abdominal recti** contract, they depress the thoracic cage, while also reducing the anteroposterior diameter of the chest. At the same time, they compress the abdominal viscera, pushing them upwards against the diaphragm, which will rise further and reduce the vertical diameter of the chest. The internal intercostal muscles and the abdominal recti are the main accessory muscles of expiration.

Fatigue of the respiratory muscles

Breathing continues throughout life. It involves voluntary muscular contraction. One of the properties of voluntary muscles is fatigability. The question may be asked whether the diaphragm and external intercostal muscles get fatigued since they are voluntary muscles. In fact they do, but, because during quiet breathing only *one-tenth* of the fibres are actively contracting, their activity is taken up by other fibres when they get fatigued. This will ensure that quiet breathing will continue indefinitely.

Work of breathing

During quiet breathing, inspiration is an active process requiring energy. This amounts to about 2–3% of the total energy expenditure of the body under resting conditions. During severe exercise both the total energy expenditure of the body and that required for the work of breathing increase. Although the absolute total energy expenditure of the work of breathing increases significantly during activity, in the region of 15–20-fold, its percentage of the total body energy expenditure may not change significantly.

There are several components of breathing that require energy:

1 Energy is required by the contracting muscles of breathing, by the diaphragm and external intercostal muscles during quiet breathing and by accessory muscles of respiration during maximal or laboured breathing.

2 Energy is required to overcome the viscosity of the expanding lung tissue and of the tissues of the thoracic cage. This is designated as the non-elastic tissue resistance. When the lungs become diseased, e.g. consolidated or fibrotic, the non-elastic resistance increases.

3 Energy is required to stretch the thoracic and lung elastic tissues (elastic tissue resistance) and to overcome the surface tension in the alveoli and alveolar sacs during inspiration. This energy requirement will increase when the surfactant is deficient.

4 Energy is required to overcome airway resistance to air flow. The narrower the airways, the greater is the resistance to air flow and the more will be the energy requirement, as in the case of *bronchial asthma* or *obstructive emphysema*.

Compliance

Compliance means the ability to expand or stretch. It is the reciprocal of elasticity. The compliance of the lung is a useful measurement for the diagnosis of respiratory disease.

Definitions

Elastance

Elastance can be defined as the stretching force which must be applied to a certain body to produce a unit change in length.

Compliance

Compliance is the **change in length or volume per unit change in the stretching force**. Lung compliance refers to the change in lung volume caused by the pressure gradient.

It has already been stated that, when the intra-alveolar pressure falls below atmospheric, air is drawn into the lungs. Conversely, when the intra-alveolar pressure rises above atmospheric, air is forced out of the lungs. The changes in intra-alveolar pressure are determined by changes in intrapleural pressure, which closely correspond to changes in oesophageal pressure.

Normally, when the lungs are *in situ* within the chest, the combined compliance of the lungs and thorax is measured; it is about 0.11 litre/cm H_2O pressure (i.e. when the intra-alveolar pressure increases by 1 cm H_2O, the thorax and lung expand by a volume of 0.1 litre). When measurement is made on the lungs alone after being removed from the chest, its compliance is found to be greater than the combined compliance of the lungs and thorax. The compliance of the lungs alone is around 0.2 litre/cm H_2O pressure. Because the lungs and chest wall act in series, their combined compliance add as reciprocals, i.e.:

$$\frac{1}{\text{Combined compliance}} = \frac{1}{\dfrac{1}{\text{Lung compliance}} + \dfrac{1}{\text{Chest wall compliance}}}$$

Measurement of compliance of the lungs and thorax combined

Combined compliance can be measured using a mouthpiece fitted with a flowmeter and a valve. A balloon is introduced into the oesophagus to record the oesophageal pressure (intrapleural pressure). The nose is closed by a nose clip. The subject inspires in increments of approximately 100 ml at a time. At the end of each increment of inspiration, the valve is shut and the subject relaxes his inspiratory muscles while the oesophageal pressure is recorded. The process is repeated until the inspired increments of air equal the normal tidal volume. The same procedure is repeated again during a tidal expiration. Now the subject expires in increments of about 100 ml of air at a time till the end of tidal expiration. The oesophageal pressure is noted each time. The volume change is then plotted against the oesophageal pressure change for inspiration and expiration.

Figure 6.7 shows a normal compliance curve. From this curve the work of breathing can be calculated. The total work of breathing is indicated by the area OAECFO. Of this, area OADCFO represents work done to overcome elastic resistance (compliance work). The shaded area AECDA represents work to overcome airway and tissue resistance (viscous resistance). Area ADCBA represents the work done against airway and tissue resistance during expiration. This is normally part of the work done to overcome elastic resistance during inspiration. On expiration, the work is passively done by the elastic recoil of the tissues expanded during inspiration.

Fig. 6.7 The lung compliance curve. See text for explanation. FRC, functional residual capacity.

Usually a high compliance indicates that a given change in pressure moves a large volume of air into the lungs. Lung compliance is decreased when there is fibrosis, congestion, oedema or bronchial obstruction or when the surface tension of fluid lining the alveoli is increased. The compliance is usually small in the newborn but it increases gradually with age. In adults it decreases with old age. Therefore, the main factors which affect compliance are lung congestion, lung size and surface tension, which is mainly related to surfactant.

Lung congestion leads to decreased compliance and is well documented clinically. Lung size is directly proportional to compliance. For this reason, the term *specific compliance* was introduced. It is the compliance per unit volume of lung.

Surfactant is a substance which lowers the surface tension of the alveoli. Surfactant contains phospholipids (dipalmitoyl-phosphatidyl-choline) neutral lipids, protein and carbohydrates. It is produced by type II alveolar epithelial cells. The importance of surfactant lies in the fact that it prevents the collapse of alveoli during expiration when their volume is small (law of Laplace). Another important function is that surfactant increases the compliance of the lungs and therefore decreases the work of breathing. By decreasing the surface tension around lung capillaries, surfactant also decreases the formation of tissue fluids in the lungs. In the absence of surfactant, the lungs become rigid, oedema is formed and the alveoli collapse. These features are characteristically seen in *respiratory distress syndrome* (RDS) of the newborn.

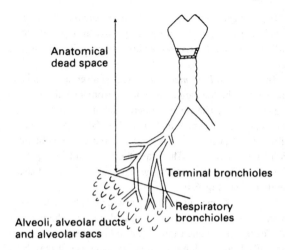

Anatomical dead space

Terminal bronchioles

Respiratory bronchioles

Alveoli, alveolar ducts and alveolar sacs

Fig. 6.8 Diagram to show the anatomical dead space, where no gas exchange takes place, and the parts of the lungs where gas exchange does take place.

Distribution of pulmonary ventilation

Pulmonary ventilation is the volume of air breathed in or out per minute. Inspired air is distributed to distinct spaces in the lungs:

1 Part of it occupies the air-conducting system of tubes which extends from the mouth and nose down to the terminal bronchioles. In this specific anatomical space there is no gas exchange with blood. It is therefore referred to as the **anatomical dead space**.

2 The rest of the inspired air occupies the space distal to the terminal bronchioles (the respiratory bronchioles), the alveolar ducts, alveoli and alveolar sacs, where gas exchange takes place (Fig. 6.8).

The volume of air that actually undergoes exchange with the blood will be equal to:

$$\text{(Tidal volume − anatomical dead space)} \times \text{respiratory rate}$$

This volume is referred to as the **alveolar ventilation rate**, as distinct from the total respiratory minute volume or pulmonary ventilation rate. In a normal subject, the anatomical dead space is approximately one-third of the normal resting tidal volume.

If, in a normal subject, the resting volume is 500 ml and the respiration rate is 12/min, then:

1 Minute volume (pulmonary ventilation rate) is equal to:

$$500 \times 12 = 6000 \text{ ml/min}$$

2 Alveolar ventilation rate is equal to:

$$\tfrac{2}{3} \times 500 \times 12 = 4000 \text{ ml/min}$$

3 Dead-space ventilation is equal to:

$$\tfrac{1}{3} \times 500 \times 12 = 2000 \text{ ml/min}$$

If the tidal volume is significantly decreased, it can lead to a marked decrease in alveolar ventilation. This occurs even if the pulmonary ventilation is maintained at normal levels by an increase in the respiratory rate. The following example illustrates this fact.

In an adult male the following results were obtained:

Tidal volume = 300 ml
Respiratory rate = 20/min
Pulmonary ventilation = 300 × 20
= 6000 ml/min
Alveolar ventilation = $[300 − (\tfrac{1}{3} \times 500)] \times 20$
= (300 − 167) × 20
= 133 × 20
= 2660 ml/min
Dead-space ventilation = $\tfrac{1}{3} \times 500 \times 20$
= 3340 ml/min

It is evident that, although the minute volume is normal, alveolar ventilation is significantly decreased. This is because the dead space is a constant volume and its share of pulmonary ventilation has increased (from 2000 ml/min in a normal person to 3340 ml/min) as the respiratory rate increased. A small reduction in tidal volume may therefore lead to a considerable decrease in gas exchange.

Measurement of anatomical dead space

Expired air is a mixture of air coming from the alveoli (alveolar air) and air in the anatomical dead space, which is atmospheric. Alveolar air normally contains about 6% CO_2, while expired air contains around 4% CO_2. If we assume that atmospheric air (which normally contains 0.04% CO_2) has 0%, we can calculate the dead-space volume as follows:

Tidal volume × 4%
= Alveolar air × 6%
= (Tidal volume − anatomical dead space) × 6%

Therefore:

Anatomical dead space
$$= \text{Tidal volume} \times \frac{6 − 4}{6}$$

Or, in other words:

Anatomical dead space

$$= \frac{\text{Tidal volume} \times (\text{alveolar } CO_2 - \text{expired air } CO_2)}{\text{Alveolar } CO_2}$$

This is Bohr's equation.

The above method of measuring the anatomical dead space assumes normal perfusion of the lung. In certain lung diseases this assumption is not valid. When some alveoli do not receive adequate perfusion with blood, they become non-functional. The volume or anatomical dead space plus that of unperfused alveoli is known as the **physiological dead space**. In normal persons the anatomical and physiological dead spaces are nearly equal. In diseases of the lungs which decrease gas exchange, the physiological dead space may be 10 times the anatomical dead space or more, i.e. 1000–2000 ml.

Uneven ventilation

In the upright subject the bases of the lungs are found to be better ventilated than the apices. This can be demonstrated by breathing radioactive xenon. The uneven ventilation is due to the effect of gravity. Similarly, a subject in the supine position will have better ventilation of the posterior parts of the lungs than the anterior parts. Uneven ventilation can significantly affect gas exchange in the lungs.

Gas exchange in the lungs

Oxygen is continuously taken up from the lungs by the blood, and carbon dioxide is likewise continuously removed from the blood. At the end of expiration, the air remaining in the alveoli has higher levels of CO_2 and lower levels of O_2. Air reaching the alveoli during inspiration mixes with air already in the alveoli. Consequently, alveolar air contains less oxygen and more carbon dioxide than inspired air. Air expired will constitute a mixture of alveolar air and the dead-space air, which is atmospheric. Table 6.2 gives approximate normal values of atmospheric air, expired air and alveolar air.

The exchange of oxygen and carbon dioxide between the alveoli and blood is a purely passive process of gas diffusion. However, several factors influence the diffusion of gases:

1 *Alveolar–capillary membrane*. This is a semipermeable membrane which separates alveolar air from the pulmonary capillary blood. The electron micrograph in Fig. 6.9 shows alveoli, capillaries and red blood cells (RBCs) in a section of rat lung. Several layers separate the red-cell membrane from the alveolar air. These are the fluid film lining the alveoli, the alveolar membrane, interstitial fluid and the capillary wall (Fig. 6.10).

Naturally, change in thickness of the alveolar–capillary membrane will affect the rate of gas diffusion. The thickness of the membrane cannot be diminished significantly, but with deep breathing, as in severe exercise, it may be decreased. In disease it can become much thicker, e.g. by fibrosis or accumulation of fluid in the alveoli, as in pulmonary oedema. This may lead to alveolar–capillary block.

2 *Partial pressure gradient of gases across the alveolar–capillary membrane*. In a gas mixture like air, the **partial pressure** of a gas is the pressure exerted by that gas in relation to the total pressure of the gas mixture. The **partial pressure** of a gas is the product of the total pressure of the mixture and the fractional concentration of the gas under consideration. Table 6.2 gives the composition and partial pressures of inspired air (atmospheric air), alveolar air and expired air. The partial pressure of oxygen (Po_2) in the mixed venous blood reaching the alveoli is about 40 mmHg, while the partial pressure of oxygen in the alveolar air is around 100 mmHg. Oxygen therefore diffuses from the alveolar space to the capillary blood along a partial pressure gradient of about 60 mmHg.

The partial pressure of carbon dioxide (Pco_2) in the mixed venous blood reaching the alveoli is about 46 mmHg, while in the alveolar air it is about 40 mmHg. Thus carbon dioxide diffuses from the capillary blood to the alveolar space along a partial pressure gradient of about 6 mmHg.

	Atmospheric air		Alveolar air		Expired air	
	%	PP (mmHg)	%	PP (mmHg)	%	PP (mmHg)
O_2	20.84	159	13.6	104	15.7	120
CO_2	0.04	0.3	5.3	40	3.6	27
N_2	78.62	597	74.9	569	74.5	566
H_2O	0.50	3.7	6.2	47	6.2	47
	100	760	100	760	100	760

Table 6.2 Composition of respiratory gases.

PP, partial pressure.

Fig. 6.9 Electron micrograph showing the alveoli, capillaries and red blood cells in a section of rat lung. (Courtesy of Dr Michael Scott, King Fahad Medical Research Centre, King Abdulaziz University, Jedda, Saudi Arabia.)

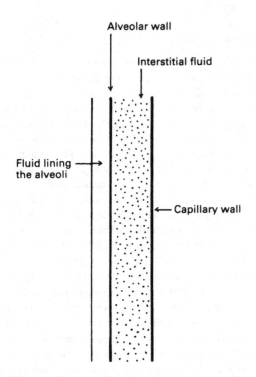

Fig. 6.10 Components of the alveolar–capillary membrane.

3 *The physical properties of gases*. The solubility and molecular weight of gases are a factor in the rate of diffusion. The more soluble the gas, the faster it will diffuse through the alveolar–capillary membrane, which is a fluid membrane. The higher the molecular weight of the gas, the slower it will diffuse through. Carbon dioxide is 23-fold more soluble than oxygen.

The solubility of a gas and its molecular weight determine its **diffusion coefficient**. This is defined as the rate of diffusion through a unit area of a given membrane per unit pressure difference:

$$\text{Diffusion coefficient} = \frac{\text{Solubility}}{\sqrt{\text{Molecular weight}}}$$

If we take the diffusion coefficient of oxygen to be 1.0, that of carbon dioxide is approximately 20.0. Carbon dioxide can therefore diffuse through the alveolar capillary membrane 20 times faster than oxygen. Consequently, diffusion failure will affect oxygen long before carbon dioxide diffusion is impaired.

4 *Surface area*. As the surface area of the alveolar–capillary membrane increases, the total volume of a gas exchanged will be proportionately increased. The **alveolar–capillary membrane** surface, in adult males, is approximately 70 m^2. During severe exercise, the depth of breathing is significantly increased, which increases the alveolar ventilation. The cardiac output is likewise increased severalfold. This normally leads to the opening up of small pulmonary capillaries, which results in an increase of the capillary surface area. What is important for diffusion purposes is not an increase of the alveolar surface alone or of the capillary surface alone; what is important is the effective surface area, i.e. the functioning alveoli in contact with functioning capillaries. It is reasonable, therefore, to expect an increase in the effective surface area during severe exercise. In diseases which decrease alveolar ventilation, e.g. *emphysema* and *obstructive lung diseases*, and in diseases which interfere with normal alveolar perfusion, e.g. *pulmonary embolism* and *restrictive lung diseases*, the effective surface area is decreased.

5 *Ventilation/blood flow ratio*. As mentioned above, the rate of diffusion of gases is determined by the effective surface area, i.e. the functional alveoli in contact with functioning capillaries, where the alveolar air comes in contact with capillary blood.

$$\frac{\text{Ventilation/}}{\text{blood flow ratio}} = \frac{\text{Alveolar ventilation}}{\text{Blood flow}}$$

In a normal adult male at rest:

Alveolar ventilation = 4 litres/min
Pulmonary blood flow (cardiac output) = 5 litres/min
Ventilation/blood flow ratio = $\frac{4}{5}$ = 0.8

As an extreme example of disturbed ventilation/blood flow ratio, no exchange of gases is expected to take place in functioning alveoli not perfused with capillary blood (**wasted ventilation**); nor does any gas exchange take place if blood is perfusing non-functioning alveoli (**wasted perfusion**).

Perfusion of the lungs is also uneven. The bases of the lungs receive more blood than the apices. The **ventilation/perfusion ratios** are 3.3 at the apices and 0.63 at the bases. This shows that perfusion is more uneven than ventilation. During exercise, however, lung perfusion becomes more uniform.

In normal individuals, an average ventilation/perfusion ratio of 0.8 is ideal for effective exchange of gases because each lung will have the same ratio as the overall ratio for both lungs together.

Example 1. Even ventilation with even blood flow:

	Alveolar ventilation (litres/min)	Blood flow (litres/min)	Ventilation/ perfusion ratio
Right lung	2	2.5	2/2.5 = 0.8
Left lung	2	2.5	2/2.5 = 0.8
Both lungs	4	5.0	4/5.0 = 0.8

However, if there is uneven ventilation or perfusion, the overall ventilation/perfusion ratio (of both lungs combined) may be normal but the ratio is abnormal for individual lungs, leading to wasted ventilation or wasted perfusion.

Example 2. Uneven ventilation with even blood flow:

	Alveolar ventilation (litres/min)	Blood flow (litres/min)	Ventilation/ perfusion ratio
Right lung	1	2.5	1/2.5 = 0.4
Left lung	3	2.5	3/2.5 = 1.2
Both lungs	4	5.0	4/5.0 = 0.8

In the right lung there is wasted blood flow, leading to a low ventilation/perfusion ratio in that lung, while in the left lung there is wasted ventilation, resulting in a high ventilation/perfusion ratio. It is clear that, although the overall ventilation/perfusion ratio is normal, the ratio is significantly disturbed in the individual lungs, leading to ineffective exchange of gases.

Example 3. Even ventilation with uneven blood flow:

	Alveolar ventilation (litres/min)	Blood flow (litres/min)	Ventilation/ perfusion ratio
Right lung	2	1	2/1 = 2.0
Left lung	2	4	2/4 = 0.5
Both lungs	4	5	4/5 = 0.8

In the right lung there is wasted ventilation whereas in the left lung there is wasted perfusion. Although the overall ventilation/perfusion ratio is normal, it is significantly disturbed in the two lungs separately, leading inevitably to reduced gas exchange between the blood and alveolar air.

6 *Chemical reactions*. Haemoglobin readily combines reversibly with oxygen and carbon dioxide. If blood contains the normal value of 150 g of haemoglobin per litre of blood, and if haemoglobin is fully saturated with oxygen, i.e. at partial pressure of O_2 of 100 mmHg, blood will carry $150 \times 1.34 = 200$ ml O_2/litre of blood (since 1 g of haemoglobin, when fully saturated, combines with 1.34 ml O_2 at standard temperature and pressure, dry (STPD)). The O_2 dissolved in 100 ml of blood at an oxygen partial pressure of 100 mmHg is only $0.003 \times 100 = 0.3$ ml, since 100 ml of blood carries only 0.003 ml O_2/1 mmHg partial pressure.

About 98.5% of the total oxygen transported in arterial blood is combined with haemoglobin. If there were no haemoglobin, the blood volume would need to increase about 70 times to transport the same volume of oxygen. Conversely, a partial pressure of O_2 of about 7600 mmHg (7 atmospheres) would be needed for 100 ml plasma to hold 20 ml O_2 in the dissolved form.

The situation is not so critical with carbon dioxide, as it is about 20 times more soluble than oxygen. Haemoglobin binds about 20% of the total carbon dioxide transported in blood.

Table 6.3 Diffusion capacity for O_2 and CO_2 at rest and during severe exercise.

	Diffusion capacity	
	At rest	During severe exercise
O_2	20 ml/min/mmHg Po_2	65 ml/min/mmHg Po_2
CO_2	400 ml/min/mmHg Pco_2	1300 ml/min/mmHg Pco_2

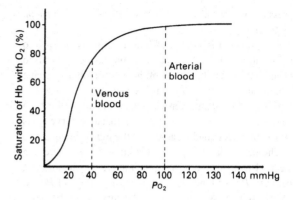

Fig. 6.11 The oxygen–haemoglobin dissociation curve.

7 *Temperature*. The rate of diffusion of gases is normally dependent on temperature, but, since body temperature is normally maintained within narrow limits, it has no influence on the rate of exchange of gases across the alveolar–capillary membrane.

The **diffusion capacity** of a gas is defined as the total volume of the gas that diffuses across the alveolar–capillary membrane per unit time per unit partial pressure (ml/min/mmHg). All the above factors affect the diffusion capacity of any particular gas. One would therefore expect that, all other factors being the same, carbon dioxide, because of its greater solubility, would have a higher diffusion capacity than oxygen—about 20 times more.

During exercise, both alveolar ventilation and blood flow increase. The alveolar membrane is stretched, leading to increased surface area and decreased thickness. Previously unperfused pulmonary capillaries open up and existing capillaries dilate, leading to increased surface area of the capillary membrane. Consequently, the effective surface area for gas exchange increases, leading to increased diffusion capacity for both oxygen and carbon dioxide (Table 6.3).

Diseases that affect any of the factors concerned with diffusion across the alveolar–capillary membrane lower the diffusion capacity of oxygen more than that of carbon dioxide. Impaired diffusion of oxygen reaches fatal levels long before the diffusion capacity of carbon dioxide is significantly decreased.

Gas transport

Transport of oxygen

Oxygen is transported in the blood in two forms:

1 The main mode of transport is in the form of **oxyhaemoglobin**. Over 98% of the total oxygen carried in arterial blood is in this form. Under normal resting conditions, the pulmonary capillary blood is fully equilibrated with alveolar air, i.e. the Po_2 in the capillary blood is nearly

100 mmHg. However, the Po_2 in systemic arterial blood is usually below 100 mmHg (about 95 mmHg) even though it may be 100 mmHg in pulmonary capillary blood. The reason for this is that some venous blood mixes with arterial blood. There are two main sites for this **physiological shunt**:

(a) Some of the bronchial venous blood drains into the pulmonary veins. The deep bronchial veins eventually end in a main pulmonary vein or the left atrium. The superficial bronchial veins also communicate with the pulmonary veins.

(b) Some of the venous blood from the coronary circulation drains directly into the left side of the heart via venae cordis minimae, which drain into all four chambers of the heart.

2 Less than 2% of oxygen in arterial blood is in **dissolved form**. At Po_2 of 100 mmHg, about 0.3 ml O_2 dissolves in 100 ml of blood. In venous blood (Po_2 of 40 mmHg) about 0.12 ml O_2/100 ml of blood is in dissolved form.

Oxyhaemoglobin

Haemoglobin has great affinity for oxygen. It combines loosely and reversibly with oxygen by a process of oxygenation (not oxidation). The reaction is very fast, requiring less than 10 ms. The combination of oxygen with haemoglobin is a function of the **partial pressure** of oxygen, in a relationship outlined by the oxygen–haemoglobin dissociation curve (Fig. 6.11). This relationship forms the basis of oxygen uptake in the lungs and its release to the tissues. At zero partial pressure of oxygen the percentage saturation of haemoglobin with oxygen is zero, while at Po_2 of 100 mmHg the saturation is about 97.5%.

The oxygen dissociation curve (plotting percentage saturation of haemoglobin with oxygen against partial

Chapter 6

pressure of oxygen) is characteristically *sigmoid in shape* (S-shaped).

Haemoglobin is formed of four haem units attached to polypeptide chains. Oxygenation of one haem unit leads to changes in the configuration of the haemoglobin molecule which increase the *affinity* of the second unit, and oxygenation of the second unit increases the affinity of the third and so on. This is the reason why the dissociation curve starts slowly but gains quickly, assuming the sigmoid shape.

The other characteristic of the curve is that there is a steep rise in the percentage saturation of haemoglobin between Po_2 of 0 mmHg and 75 mmHg. Beyond Po_2 of 75 mmHg there is a slow rise in the curve and it becomes more or less flat at Po_2 of 80 mmHg or above.

The partial pressure of oxygen in arterial blood is about 95 mmHg, while in the tissues it drops to about 40 mmHg.

At Po_2 of 40 mmHg, haemoglobin is 75% saturated; at Po_2 of 95 mmHg, haemoglobin is 97% saturated. When 1 g of haemoglobin is fully saturated with oxygen, it binds up to 1.34 ml of oxygen at standard temperature and pressure (STP). Therefore, if haemoglobin concentration is 150 g/litre of blood and arterial blood is 97% saturated, then the oxygen content of arterial blood will be about:

$$1.34 \times 150 \times \frac{97}{100} = 195 \text{ ml/litre of blood}$$

In venous blood, saturation of haemoglobin with oxygen is 75%. Therefore, the oxygen content of venous blood will be approximately:

$$1.34 \times 150 \times \frac{75}{100} = 150 \text{ ml/litre of blood}$$

This means that the **arteriovenous oxygen difference** is approximately 45 ml/litre of blood. Indeed, under resting conditions in a normal person, oxygen uptake by the tissues is about 40–50 ml/litre of blood.

During exercise, however, oxygen expenditure by the active muscles is considerably increased. The Po_2 in the tissues may drop to 15 mmHg (or even lower), corresponding to a percentage saturation of haemoglobin of about 20%, or oxygen content of about:

$$1.34 \times 150 \times \frac{20}{100} = 40 \text{ ml/litre of blood}$$

The arteriovenous oxygen difference may then rise to about 150 ml/litre of blood during severe exercise.

It is evident that the **quantity** of oxygen carried in a volume of blood is dependent on the Po_2 as well as the haemoglobin concentration. The percentage saturation of

Fig. 6.12 Effect of anaemia on oxygen content of the blood at different Po_2 values.

haemoglobin with oxygen is dependent on Po_2 and totally independent of **haemoglobin concentration**. If oxygen content (instead of percentage saturation of haemoglobin with oxygen) is plotted against Po_2, the level of the curve will be dependent on the haemoglobin concentration of the sample of blood (Fig. 6.12). But when plotting **percentage saturation** against Po_2, as is usually done, the curve will always be the same, whatever the haemoglobin concentration is, if other factors remain the same.

Factors which affect the oxygen–haemoglobin dissociation curve. There are several factors that may affect the oxygen–haemoglobin dissociation curve. They may shift the curve to the right, indicating **lowered affinity** of haemoglobin for oxygen, or shift it to the left, indicating **increased affinity** for oxygen.

1 *Partial pressure of carbon dioxide.* A rise in Pco_2 decreases the affinity of haemoglobin for oxygen and hence shifts the oxygen dissociation curve to the right (Fig. 6.13). This is called the **Bohr effect**. In the tissues, Pco_2 is high, and the more active the tissues are, the higher it will be. Therefore, more oxygen will be available for the tissues to meet this extra activity. In the lung, Pco_2 is lower than in the tissues—about 40 mmHg. The affinity of haemoglobin for oxygen in the lungs will be increased, leading to easier uptake of oxygen by haemoglobin in the lungs.

2 *Blood pH.* Fall of pH (rise in hydrogen ion concentration) shifts the curve to the right, indicating a lowered affinity of haemoglobin for oxygen. During activity, pH of

Fig. 6.13 The effect of P_{CO_2} on the oxygen–haemoglobin dissociation curve (Bohr effect).

Fig. 6.15 The effect of temperature on the oxygen–haemoglobin dissociation curve.

Fig. 6.14 The effect of pH on the oxygen–haemoglobin dissociation curve.

Fig. 6.16 The oxygen dissociation curves for: (a) adult haemoglobin (AHb); (b) fetal haemoglobin (FHb); and (c) myoglobin (Mb).

the tissues drops, due to the production of greater amounts of CO_2 and organic acids, such as lactic acid. This facilitates the release of oxygen to the active tissues (Fig. 6.14).

3 *Temperature.* A rise of core body temperature also shifts the dissociation curve to the right. In active tissues, mainly due to oxidative processes, heat is generated and more oxygen is released from haemoglobin to provide the extra requirements of the tissues (Fig. 6.15).

4 *2,3-Diphosphoglycerate (2,3-DPG).* 2,3-DPG is found in red blood cells bound to haemoglobin. It tends to decrease the affinity of haemoglobin for oxygen and therefore shifts the dissociation curve to the right. It helps the release of oxygen to the tissues. Its concentration in the red blood cells tends to increase in hypoxia, e.g. at high altitude.

Fetal haemoglobin has a greater affinity for oxygen than that of adult haemoglobin, probably because it binds less effectively with 2,3-DPG. Its oxygen dissociation curve is more to the left than that of adult haemoglobin, but,

because it is formed of four haem units, it still posseses the sigmoid shape (Fig. 6.16).

Myoglobin is an iron pigment found in red muscle. Because it is formed of one haem unit, its oxygen dissociation curve does not exhibit a sigmoid shape; it is a rectangular hyperbola. Myoglobin has greater affinity for oxygen than adult or fetal haemoglobin. Its oxygen dissociation curve is further to the left than that of fetal haemoglobin (Fig. 6.16). Myoglobin releases its oxygen at a much lower P_{O_2} than haemoglobin. It is therefore very useful in muscles that are subjected to sustained contractions, during which blood supply is usually markedly decreased. Myoglobin will then provide the necessary oxygen supply for these muscles, where P_{O_2} may drop nearly to zero.

P_{O_2} in tissues during severe exercise drops considerably, to about 10 mmHg or less. This results in greater release of oxygen from blood in tissues (Fig. 6.17).

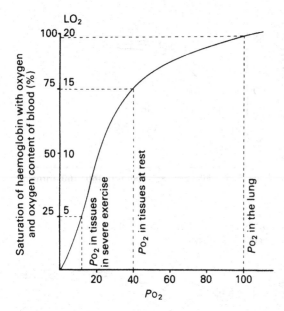

Fig. 6.17 Effect of severe exercise on Po_2 in tissues. Note the corresponding saturation of blood (25–75%), which indicates greatly enhanced oxygen release.

Fig. 6.18 The relationship between Po_2 and dissolved oxygen in plasma.

Dissolved oxygen

There is a direct relationship between Po_2 and dissolved oxygen (Fig. 6.18). As oxygen is poorly soluble, within the normal values of Po_2 in blood, only a minute fraction of oxygen is transported in the dissolved form. In 100 ml of blood at body temperature, 0.003 ml of O_2 dissolves 1.0 mmHg Po_2. Therefore, in arterial blood, dissolved oxygen does not normally exceed 0.3 ml/100 ml, and in venous blood it is about 0.12 ml/100 ml. The dissolved

O_2 is in equilibrium with the O_2 combined with haemoglobin. It is the dissolved O_2 which gets transferred to the tissue fluid and becomes replaced from O_2 carried by haemoglobin.

Dissolved oxygen, although it constitutes less than 2% of the total oxygen transport in blood, is essential for tissues that do not have a blood supply, like the **cornea** and **cartilage**, which depend on oxygen dissolved in the tissue fluids. Dissolved oxygen can be considerably increased by breathing pure or *hyperbaric oxygen*. This is part of the rationale for oxygen therapy.

Carbon dioxide transport

Carbon dioxide is transported from the tissues, where it is produced by metabolism, to the lungs, where it is unloaded to be removed to the atmosphere. It is transported by the plasma and by the red blood cells.

Transport of carbon dioxide by the plasma

Carbon dioxide produced by active cells diffuses by concentration gradient into the tissue fluid and the blood capillaries to reach plasma, where it is carried in several forms:

1 Some of it is transported in **dissolved** form.

2 A small amount reacts with water to form **carbonic acid**:

$$CO_2 + H_2O \rightarrow H_2CO_3$$

The reaction proceeds very slowly because in the plasma there is no **carbonic anhydrase**, which catalyses the reversible reaction. The carbonic acid then dissociates into hydrogen ions and bicarbonate:

$$H_2CO_3 \rightleftharpoons H^+ + HCO_3^-$$

3 Carbon dioxide in the plasma reacts with the amino group of plasma proteins to form **carbamino proteins**.

Transport of carbon dioxide in the red blood cells

1 Most of the carbon dioxide that diffuses from the tissues into plasma enters the red blood cells and dissolves in the intracellular fluid.

2 Some of the dissolved CO_2 reacts with water to form carbonic acid. The reaction is a fast one due to the presence of **carbonic anhydrase** in red cells.

In active tissues, due to the *high concentration of carbon dioxide*, the reaction proceeds to the right, i.e. formation of carbonic acid. The acid formed dissociates into:

$$H_2CO_3 \rightleftharpoons H^+ + HCO_3^-$$

The bicarbonate ions accumulating in the red blood cell diffuse into the plasma due to a **concentration gradient**.

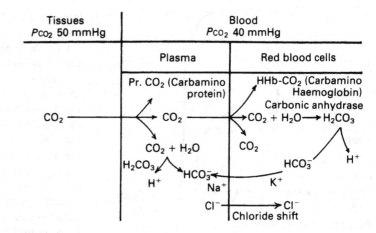

Fig. 6.19 The diagram illustrates the mechanism of carbon dioxide transport in blood, namely, as bicarbonate (70%), as carbamino compounds (20–25%) and as dissolved CO_2 (5–10%). It also shows the movement across the red cell membrane, which explains the chloride shift.

Since the main cation within the cell is potassium, which cannot freely diffuse out of the cell, **electrical equilibrium** is maintained by diffusion of chloride ions, the main extra-cellular anion, into the cell. This is called the **chloride shift**.

The hydrogen ions produced are buffered by haemoglobin which has unloaded its oxygen. The plasma bicarbonate is mainly the bicarbonate that diffuses out of the cell (Fig. 6.19).

3 A portion of the dissolved CO_2 in the intracellular water reacts with the amino group of the reduced haemoglobin to form **carbaminohaemoglobin**.

In summary, carbon dioxide is transported in the blood in three forms: in the dissolved form, as bicarbonate and as carbamino compounds. Under resting conditions about 4 ml of CO_2 is taken up by 100 ml of blood draining the tissues and is consequently released in the lungs. Of this amount, approximately 2.8 ml (70%) is transported as bicarbonate, 0.8 ml (20%) as carbamino compounds and 0.4 ml (10%) in dissolved form.

Plasma transports more than 60% of the carbon dioxide which diffuses in the blood from tissues. The chemical reaction taking place in the red blood cells, due to the presence of the enzyme carbonic anhydrase, provides practically all of the bicarbonate ions transported in plasma.

Carbon dioxide dissociation curve

The volume of carbon dioxide carried in the blood is determined by the partial pressure of carbon dioxide (Pco_2). The dissolved form is directly proportionate to Pco_2 (0.06 ml dissolved in 100 ml of blood/litre mmHg Pco_2).

Figure 6.20 shows the relationship of the carbon dioxide content of blood to Pco_2 (carbon dioxide dissociation curve). The curve is affected by the saturation of haemoglobin with oxygen (**Haldane effect**). Oxyhaemoglobin shifts the curve to the right, i.e. in the lungs carbon dioxide is released from the blood. Reduced haemoglobin shifts the curve to the left, i.e. more carbon dioxide is taken up by the blood in the tissues. Thus, Pco_2 influences oxygen saturation of haemoglobin (Bohr effect) and Po_2 influences the CO_2 dissociation curve (Haldane effect). However, the Bohr effect is much more potent and more important than the Haldane effect.

Control of ventilation

Since the main functions of respiration are to supply oxygen to the tissues, to remove CO_2 from the tissues and to play a major role in the regulation of blood pH, it has to be capable of readjustment in states of *hypoxia* or *hypercapnia* or during metabolic disturbance of the *acid–base balance*.

Fig. 6.20 The carbon dioxide dissociation curve with oxygenated and reduced haemoglobin (Haldane effect).

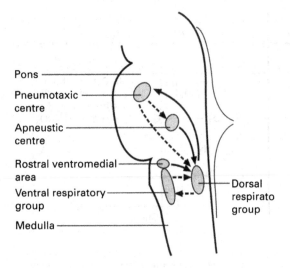

Pons

Pneumotaxic centre

Apneustic centre

Rostral ventromedial area

Ventral respiratory group

Medulla

Dorsal respirato group

Fig. 6.21 Diagrammatic representation of the medulla and pons showing areas with respiratory neurons. The solid arrows indicate stimulation and the dashed ones indicate inhibition. The two dashed arrows between the inspiratory (dorsal) neurons and the ventral group indicate reciprocal inhibition.

The readjustment is achieved by several mechanisms involved in the regulation of ventilation. These mechanisms can be grouped into two main categories, referred to as **nervous** and **chemical** control mechanisms, which are closely integrated.

The respiratory centre

There are three groups of respiratory neurons located bilaterally in the medulla and pons which are collectively known as the respiratory centre.

1 The dorsal respiratory group (DRG). The main inspiratory drive comes from the **dorsal respiratory group (inspiratory group)** located along the dorsal aspect of the medulla oblongata. The neurons of this group are mainly found in the *nucleus of the tractus solitarius (NTS)* and in the reticular formation. The NTS also plays an important role as a relay station for sensory neurons in the vagus and glossopharyngeal nerves. These nerves convey signals from the chemoreceptors, the baroreceptors and a variety of receptors in the lungs.

The DRG has no rhythmicity of its own. Recently it has been found that spontaneous rhythm arises in the **rostral ventromedial medulla (RVM)** located at the rostral end of the ventral respiratory group (Fig. 6.21). The rate of the inspiratory drive from DRG seems to be determined by the rhythmicity of the RVM and other inputs. The exact neural interaction between these centres is not fully understood.

However, the following description is a generally accepted scenario.

From the **inspiratory group** a volley of impulses arises which increases gradually for 2 s (ramp signal) and then they stop for 3 s. This produces the inspiratory and expiratory periods of the respiratory cycle. When the inspiratory signals are subjected to regulatory inputs, this may lead to: (i) the ramp signal being cut short, allowing a more rapid *rate of breathing*; or (ii) the ramp becoming steeper, i.e. the signals increase rapidly, allowing a *deeper inspiration*.

The inspiratory group signals to the spinal motor neurons of the diaphragm and external intercostal muscles, causing inspiration, while passive elastic recoil of the lungs and the chest wall causes expiration.

2 The ventral respiratory groups (VRG). These neurons function during inspiration and expiration and lie mainly in the *nucleus ambiguus* and *nucleus retroambiguus* of the medulla oblongata. They remain silent during quiet breathing.

The ventral group do not seem to have a spontaneous rhythm. However, when the dorsal inspiratory drive increases as in exercise, there is activation of the ventral group and they augment the inspiratory drive. Other neurons in the ventral group are expiratory and they send expiratory signals to the abdominal muscles during deep expiration.

3 The pneumotaxic centre. This group of respiratory neurons is located in the upper pons. It transmits inhibitory signals to the inspiratory group, which cut short the ramp signal and therefore limit inspiration. When the pneumotaxic centre is inhibited, inspiration becomes prolonged and deep, and the rate of breathing is slow. Conversely, a strong signal from the pneumotaxic centre can cause rapid, shallow breathing.

A fourth group of respiratory neurons has been described in the lower pons, the 'apneustic centre'. Its effects have been demonstrated in experimental animals. When the vagi are cut and a section in the mid-pontine region separates the pneumotaxic centre from the other respiratory neurons, the apneustic centre causes prolongation of the ramp signal. This causes deep inspiration with short gasping expirations. It is suggested that the apneustic centre acts as an 'overdrive' and, together with the pneumotaxic centre, regulates the depth of breathing.

The respiratory centre receives several inputs. For convenience they have been divided into two groups: **nervous** and **chemical**. The chemical regulation of respiration is all-important because the main function is to remove excess CO_2 and provide O_2 so that blood leaving the pulmonary circulation has the correct amounts of these gases.

Respiratory control provides adequate ventilation for this function to be achieved. Nervous regulation, on the other hand, is concerned with inputs other than chemical ones, e.g. central nervous system (CNS) inputs and mechano-receptors in the lungs and other parts of the body.

Chemical control of ventilation

As the final purpose of ventilation is to maintain arterial Po_2 and Pco_2, these gases play an important role in the regulation of the respiratory centre. This effect is achieved through a chemosensitive area in the medulla (**central chemoreceptors**) or through **peripheral chemoreceptors** situated in the aortic and carotid bodies.

1 Central chemoreceptors. Pco_2 is responsible for the minute-to-minute regulation of the respiratory centre. There is a chemosensitive area located close to the ventral surface of the upper part of the medulla. This area lies in close proximity to the various parts of the respiratory centre. The central chemoreceptors are excited by increased Pco_2 and hydrogen ions. In fact, the receptors are sensitive mainly to hydrogen ions. However, H^+ do not enter the **blood–brain barrier** but CO_2 easily diffuses from the capillaries and penetrates this barrier into the tissue fluids of the brain. CO_2 then reacts with water in the interstitial fluid to form carbonic acid, which dissociates to give H^+ + bicarbonate. The H^+ excite the central chemoreceptors. For this reason, blood CO_2 has a strong stimulatory effect on the central chemoreceptors, while blood H^+ concentration has no effect. It is worthy of note that it is the rise in H^+ due to increased Pco_2 in the brain extracellular fluid (ECF) that puts a stop to voluntary breath-holding.

In the same way, CO_2 enters the cerebrospinal fluid (CSF) very quickly through the arachnoid plexuses of vessels. The H^+ concentration rises rapidly in the CSF because it has little in the way of protein buffers. This excites the chemosensitive area within seconds, in contrast to CO_2 passing directly through the blood–brain barrier, where H^+ concentration is buffered by interstitial fluid protein. The effect of a rise in Pco_2 in the latter case takes 1 or more minutes to appear.

The central chemoreceptors are not stimulated by O_2 lack. In fact they can be depressed if Po_2 reaches a critical level. O_2 supply to the brain and other tissues can be maintained at normal levels when alveolar ventilation fluctuates between 3 litres and 20 litres per minute. Therefore Po_2 does not play any role in central chemoreceptor regulation of ventilation. However, Po_2 does have an important and life-saving effect on peripheral chemoreceptors when it falls to dangerous levels.

2 Peripheral chemoreceptors. Unlike the central chemo-receptors, the peripheral chemoreceptors are sensitive to low Po_2 as well as to high Pco_2 and H^+ concentration. Most of the peripheral chemoreceptors are located in the *carotid bodies* and some are found in *aortic bodies*, as well as other places. Nerve fibres from the carotid body receptors travel in the IX cranial nerve (glossopharyngeal). Fibres from aortic bodies travel in the vagi. These inputs relay in the NTS and influence the dorsal inspiratory group.

The cells of the chemoreceptor bodies 'receive direct blood supply from the large arteries they are attached to and have an extremely high blood flow rate. This characteristic makes them well situated to detect blood gas changes in the arterial system. A fall in arterial Po_2 (hypoxaemia) below 60 mmHg has a strong effect on the peripheral chemoreceptors. A progressive increase in the frequency of impulses from the chemoreceptors arises when the Po_2 starts to fall below normal. The sensitivity of the receptors is greatest between Po_2 60 and 90 mmHg. This is the same range within which the oxygen saturation of haemoglobin shows the fastest drop. A decrease in the blood flow to the carotid and aortic bodies caused by low arterial blood pressure (e.g. hypovolaemia or heart failure) produces a similar effect to hypoxaemia. The Po_2 may be normal due to normal dissolved O_2 although the total amount of O_2 carried in the blood may be dangerously low, as in severe anaemia and carbon monoxide (CO) poisoning. The patient dies of tissue deprivation of O_2.

Table 6.4 gives a summary of the chemical regulation of ventilation.

The combined effects of blood gases

The effect of breathing air with low O_2 partial pressure at rest results in lowering the Po_2, which stimulates the peripheral chemoreceptors and increases ventilation. This leads to increased removal of CO_2 from the blood and lowering the Pco_2, consequently depriving the central chemoreceptors of the H^+ which drives the respiratory centre. The net result is a slight increase in ventilation. This is not so when arterial Po_2 falls but Pco_2 is maintained at the normal level. The effect of falling Po_2 in this case is very strong. Ventilation starts to increase at Po_2 levels below 100 mmHg, triples at Po_2 40 mmHg and becomes sixfold at Po_2 20 mmHg. An example of this situation is encountered in patients with pulmonary disease which interferes with gas exchange. We get low Po_2 with normal or increased Pco_2 and H^+ concentration, which leads to increased ventilation, seen as breathlessness at rest (**dyspnoea**), which improves through O_2 therapy. This may lead to decreased ventilation (**hypoventilation**) due to abolishing the effect of low Po_2 on peripheral

Table 6.4 Summary of the site of action and the effects of chemical factors on the regulation of ventilation. Note that CO_2 can also penetrate the blood–brain barrier (BBB) and dissolve in the cerebrospinal fluid (CSF), giving H^+ which can rapidly act on central chemoreceptors.

| Chemoreceptors | Effects of Pco_2, Po_2 and H^+ in blood | | |
	Pco_2	Po_2	H^+
Central	Strong stimulation. Main control of ventilation. Hypercapnia depresses respiratory centre when $Pco_2 > 70$ mmHg	Depresses respiratory centre when < 60 mmHg	H^+ does not enter BBB but CO_2 diffuses from brain capillaries into ECF $H_2CO_3 \leftrightharpoons H^+ + HCO_3^-$ H^+ stimulates respiratory centre
Peripheral	Weak stimulation. Minor effect compared with above	Stimulation when < 60 mmHg. Life-saving in hypoxia	Stimulation important in non-H_2CO_3 acidosis

Fig. 6.22 The effect of Pco_2 on alveolar ventilation: The number against each curve indicates the Po_2 in mmHg. The solid curves show the effect of Pco_2 when alveolar Po_2 is kept constant at normal pH. Note that at lower Po_2 the same change in Pco_2 produces a greater effect on ventilation. The dashed curves show the effect of decreased pH. Note that the curves for the same Po_2 are parallel, i.e. a shift in threshold of the response without an increase in sensitivity to Pco_2.

chemoreceptors. When this happens, serious **respiratory acidosis** may result, due to accumulation of CO_2 in the blood.

The above effects of Po_2 on ventilation show that there are differences between the effect of Po_2 alone and when combined with increased Pco_2. Figure 6.22 shows that, when alveolar Po_2 is held constant, the increase in Pco_2

results in increased sensitivity of the respiratory centre response, as shown by the slope of the curves, i.e. the change in Pco_2 is seen to give a greater effect when the Po_2 is lower. There is no change in the threshold, as shown by the intercepts of the curves on the Pco_2 axis. However, when the pH drops, as in metabolic acidosis, the whole family of curves is shifted to the left.

Nervous control of ventilation
The inspiratory neurons send excitatory impulses via the intercostal and phrenic nerves to the external intercostal muscles and the diaphragm, respectively. The respiratory centre is influenced by higher brain centres, by other centres in the brain stem and by signals from special receptors which give rise to respiratory reflexes.

The role of the respiratory centre
1 **Dorsal respiratory group (DRG)**. This contains mainly neurons which are active during inspiration. They are driven by rhythm generated in the **rostral ventromedial medulla (RVM)**.
2 **Ventral respiratory group (VRG)**. These consist of both inspiratory and expiratory neurons. They become active during active expiration or inspiration.
3 The **pneumotaxic centre** acts by means of a negative feedback loop, with the inspiratory neurons putting an end to normal quiet inspiration giving rise to the respiratory cycle.
4 The **apneustic centre** gives an extra boost to the inspiratory neurons, which prevents total inhibition of the inspiratory neurons. Presumably this balance between the apneustic and the pneumotaxic centres provides smooth inspiration and expiration.

Fig. 6.23 Diagrammatic representation of the various central and peripheral nervous inputs to the medullary respiratory centre.

Higher brain centres

1 Impulses from the **cerebral cortex** bring about voluntary modification of breathing. This is indicated by the ability to hyperventilate voluntarily and by temporary cessation of breathing (voluntary apnoea). One can only modify breathing voluntarily but cannot completely control it.

2 Impulses from the **cerebellum** coordinate breathing with other activities such as swallowing, talking and coughing.

3 Impulses from the **hypothalamus** and the centres for emotion and temperature regulation, modify breathing. Breathing is modified during emotional stress, such as fear, excitement or anger, and by change in body temperature. Panting in dogs (shallow hyperventilation) is a mechanism for dissipation of heat from the body, controlled by hypothalamic centres.

Figure 6.23 is a schematic diagram illustrating the arrangement of the various inputs controlling respiration.

Special receptors

The respiratory centre also receives nervous impulses from peripheral parts of the body which control ventilation reflexes. The following are the main examples of receptors associated with modification of breathing:

1 Sensory vagal fibres arising from *stretch receptors* in the smooth muscles of bronchi and bronchioles send inhibitory impulses to the **inspiratory neurons** during hyperinflation as in exercise. They put a stop to inspiration and protect against overinflation. This is known as the **Hering–Breuer inflation** reflex, which acts as a feedback mechanism in a way similar to the pneumotaxic centre. It can increase the rate of breathing in the same way. Cutting vagal fibres arising from the lungs prolongs inspiration. The breathing becomes deep and slow. It has also been demonstrated that there are vagal fibres arising from the lungs which are stimulated by deflation. They tend to bring expiration to an end, and allow inspiration to start. This reflex is referred to as the **Hering–Breuer deflation** reflex. It is a much weaker reflex than the inflation reflex.

2 It has also been found that active or passive movement of **muscles and joints** will stimulate breathing, even when their blood supply is cut off, while their nerve supply is left intact. These are *proprioceptive* impulses arising from muscle and joint receptors all over the body, including the diaphragm, which is rich in muscle spindles. Proprioceptive stimulation of breathing may be the main stimulus for ventilation at the onset of muscular exercise.

3 Stimulation of the **skin receptors** by noxious stimuli may also stimulate ventilation. Stimulation of baroreceptors in the aortic arch and carotic sinuses may give rise to reflex modification of breathing.

Hypoxia

Hypoxia refers to conditions in which there is deficient oxygen supply to the tissues. Disturbances which interfere with oxygen availability or uptake in the lungs, its transport in blood and its delivery to the tissues may lead to hypoxia. Accordingly, hypoxia can be divided into four main categories:

1 *Hypoxic hypoxia* results from any disturbance which interferes with normal oxygenation of the arterial blood, leading to low arterial Po_2. It can therefore be due to: (i) factors in the atmosphere, such as **high altitude**; (ii) factors interfering with normal O_2 **diffusion** in the lung; or (iii) mixing of arterial blood with venous blood, as in **venoarterial shunts** and congenital heart disease. In hypoxic hypoxia, arterial Po_2 is low and the percentage saturation of haemoglobin with oxygen in arterial blood is also low. Consequently, the oxygen content per unit volume of blood is low.

Clinical causes of hypoxic hypoxia include ventilation defects, e.g. paralysis of respiratory muscles, airway obstruction and poisoning with drugs that inhibit the respiratory centre, e.g. morphine and barbiturates. Hypoxia due to hypoventilation is always associated with high arterial Pco_2.

Shunting of venous blood can also occur when there is wasted perfusion, i.e. when a larger number of alveoli do not get adequate ventilation. This leads to a large amount of venous blood passing through the lungs without being oxygenated.

Diffusion defects can occur in conditions which cause thickening of the pulmonary membrane, e.g. lung fibrosis, oedema and consolidation, as in pneumonia. In this case, there would be wasted ventilation.

Therefore, the concept of the *ventilation/perfusion ratio* ($\dot{V}/\dot{Q}$, where $\dot{V}$ = alveolar ventilation and $\dot{Q}$ = cardiac output, both in litres/min) is most important in the causation of hypoxic hypoxia due to pulmonary or cardiac disease. In a situation where there is *wasted ventilation*, $\dot{V}/\dot{Q}$ will be more than 1.0. In this case, the **physiological dead space** is increased because some ventilated alveoli have inadequate perfusion. In conditions where there is *wasted perfusion*,

certain alveoli, although well perfused, do not get adequate ventilation. In this case oxygen therapy does not give the desired effect.

2 *Anaemic hypoxia.* This is due to lowering of the oxygen-carrying capacity of the blood. It may therefore be caused by anaemia, by abnormal haemoglobins or by rendering haemoglobin unavailable for oxygen uptake, as in **carbon monoxide poisoning**.

In this type of anaemia the arterial Po_2 is normal; the percentage saturation of haemoglobin with oxygen is also normal, except in carbon monoxide poisoning. However, the oxygen content of arterial and venous blood per unit volume of blood is lowered, because there is insufficient haemoglobin to carry it.

3 *Stagnant hypoxia.* In this type of hypoxia there is slow or no circulation to the tissues. It may be a localized disturbance of circulation to a certain part of the body, e.g. the limbs, or it may be generalized or central, as in heart failure.

In this type of hypoxia, arterial Po_2 is normal, percentage saturation of haemoglobin in arterial blood is normal and O_2 content per unit volume of arterial blood is normal. The only disturbance can be seen in the venous blood, where Po_2, percentage saturation of haemoglobin and oxygen content are all lowered significantly.

4 *Histotoxic hypoxia.* The disturbance is in the uptake of oxygen by the tissues, either due to poisoning of cellular enzymes or due to a long diffusion distance between the capillaries and cells, as may occur in tissue oedema. In this type of hypoxia, all parameters in the arterial blood are normal. As there is little or no utilization of O_2 by the tissues, the Po_2, percentage saturation of haemoglobin and oxygen content of venous blood will all be higher than normal.

Table 6.5 shows blood gas findings in the various types of hypoxia.

Hypoxia is best treated with oxygen therapy and by correcting the underlying cause.

Cyanosis

Cyanosis is a blue coloration of the skin and mucous membranes. It starts to show when the level of **reduced haemoglobin** in capillary blood is more than 5 g/100 ml of blood. Reduced haemoglobin is dark in colour and, when its concentration exceeds 5 g/100 ml, its colour can overshadow the colour of oxygenated haemoglobin, no matter what the total haemoglobin concentration is.

Cyanosis can be localized (*peripheral*) or it can be generalized (*central*).

The peripheral type is most commonly seen at the tips of the fingers when the person is exposed to severe cold. Cold

Table 6.5 Comparison of blood gas findings in the various types of hypoxia.

Type of hypoxia	Arterial blood			Venous blood		
	Po_2	% Sat	% O_2	Po_2	% Sat	% O_2
Hypoxic	Low	Low	Low	Low	Low	Low
Anaemic	Normal	Normal (except CO poisoning)	Low	Low	Low	Low
Stagnant	Normal	Normal	Normal	Low	Low	Low
Histotoxic	Normal	Normal	Normal	High	High	High

% Sat, % saturation of haemoglobin; % O_2, O_2 content in ml/dl blood.

leads to vasoconstriction, which will decrease the blood flow through peripheral parts. This allows more time for extraction of oxygen from the blood, which results in a higher level of reduced haemoglobin.

The generalized type of cyanosis is due to a central cause, such as **venoarterial shunts**, or severe hypoxia, as may occur in the newborn or in persons exposed to atmospheric air at very high latitudes.

Since cyanosis occurs when the capillary blood contains more than 5 g/100 ml of reduced haemoglobin, it is more commonly seen with **polycythaemia** and very rarely with anaemia, especially severe anaemia. It is therefore more evident in conditions associated with polycythaemia, e.g. polycythaemia vera, high altitudes or congenital heart diseases with right-to-left shunts, and in the newborn.

The role of the respiratory system in the acid–base balance

Definitions and normal values
The normal range of arterial pH is 7.35–7.45, with an average of 7.4. **Acidosis** is defined as any condition in which arterial pH is less than 7.35, while **alkalosis** is defined as any condition in which arterial pH is more than 7.45. Values of pH below 7.0 or above 7.8 are incompatible with life.

The pH of the blood is mainly determined by the ratio of concentration of **bicarbonate** to **carbonic acid**, i.e. the ratio of salt to acid as given by the **Henderson–Hasselbalch equation**:

$$pH = pK + \log \frac{salt}{acid}$$
pK for carbonic acid = 6.1

In normal persons, the concentration of bicarbonate is about 24 mmol/litre, while that of carbonic acid is approximately 1.2 mmol/litre, giving a ratio of 20 : 1:

$$\log 20 = 1.3$$
$$pH = 6.1 + 1.3 = 7.4$$

The concentration of carbon dioxide (CO_2) in the body fluids is determined by the rate of CO_2 production in the tissues and the rate of its removal by the lungs. There is a time-lag between its production and removal, leading to its accumulation in the body fluids to a concentration of about 1.2 mmol/litre under resting conditions. If the rate of production in the tissues exceeds the rate of removal by the lungs, as in very severe exercise, its concentration in the body fluids will increase.

It is evident that, if the ratio of salt to acid (in this case bicarbonate to carbonic acid) increases, either by increase of the salt or decrease of the acid, pH will rise, and vice versa. For example:

1 In the case of hyperventilation, CO_2 is washed out, leading to lowered carbonic acid concentration in the blood. The ratio of bicarbonate to carbonic acid will therefore increase and pH will rise. This is referred to as **respiratory alkalosis**.

2 Conversely, if CO_2 is retained in the body, as in respiratory failure or impaired removal of CO_2 for any reason, the ratio of bicarbonate to carbonic acid will decrease and pH will consequently fall. This is referred to as **respiratory acidosis**.

In the case of respiratory acidosis, the kidney excretes more acid urine in the form of non-carbonic acids, e.g. acid phosphate, and retains more bicarbonate, thus raising the level of bicarbonate in the blood. This approximates the bicarbonate/carbonic acid ratio towards the normal ratio. The reverse happens in respiratory alkalosis, i.e. the kidney retains and secretes fewer hydrogen ions and less bicarbonate.

When the acidosis is not due to carbonic acid, it is referred to as **metabolic acidosis**, as in diabetes mellitus, where acidosis is due to excess keto acids, or in cases of severe diarrhoea, where there is excessive loss of bicarbonate and potassium coming from pancreatic and intestinal secretions.

When there is excess bicarbonate in the blood as a result of excessive ingestion, or if there is excessive loss of hydrochloric acid in persistent vomiting, **metabolic alkalosis** will result.

In conclusion, the role of the lung in pH regulation depends on the sensitivity of the respiratory centre to CO_2 and of the peripheral chemoreceptors to H^+. Metabolic acidosis stimulates respiration and consequently more CO_2 is washed out of the blood and the pH rises. On the other hand, alkalosis of metabolic origin depresses respiration and therefore accumulation of CO_2 brings the pH back to normal. These responses represent the *respiratory compensatory mechanisms* in the regulation of the acid–base balance (see also Chapter 11).

Investigation of pulmonary disease

When investigating lung disease, a certain protocol is usually followed:

1 History-taking and clinical examination.
2 Radiological examination.
3 Laboratory tests of lung function.
4 Other laboratory tests and procedures, e.g. bacteriological examination of blood, sputum or pleural fluid.

These tests help to locate and identify the pathology of the lesion. However, in this text only the tests for lung function will be considered. The question arises: 'Why do we perform lung function tests?'

1 They help in the diagnosis and management of patients with lung disease.
2 They are useful in preoperative assessment of fitness for general anaesthesia and surgery.
3 They assist in the follow-up of the progress of disease and therapy.
4 They are utilized in epidemiological surveys, e.g. industrial hazards and occupational lung diseases.
5 They are used for insurance purposes and when assessing compensation for disability.

Lung function tests

The lung function tests basically assess the following:

1 Ventilatory functions.
2 Gas diffusion (across the pulmonary membrane).
3 Elastic properties of the lungs.
4 Airways resistance.
5 Ventilation/perfusion relationship.

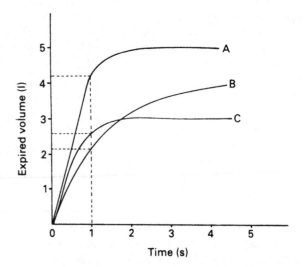

Fig. 6.24 Spirograms recorded by a 'vitalograph' for three patients. The maximum volume expired is the FVC for each patient. A: FVC = 5 litres; FEV_1 = 4.2 litres; FEV_1 = 84%—normal; B: FVC = 4 litres; FEV_1 = 2.2 litres; FEV_1 = 55%—obstructive lung disease; C: FVC = 3 litres; FEV_1 = 2.7 litres; FEV_1 = 90%—restrictive lung disease.

Ventilatory functions

1 *Measurement of lung volumes and capacities* (see Fig. 6.1) Using a bell-type spirometer, the subject breathes normally and records tidal volume. Following a normal inspiration, the subject is asked to take a deep inspiration. This records the **inspiratory reserve volume (IRV)**. Following a normal expiration, the subject is again asked to make a deep expiration. This records the **expiratory reserve volume (ERV)**. The lung volumes and capacities have been explained at the beginning of this chapter under the heading 'Ventilation'.

2 *Forced vital capacity.* The simplest and the easiest test of ventilatory functions is the **forced expiratory volume (FEV)**. The subject is asked to breathe out forcibly after a maximal inspiration and the volume expired is measured. The volume expired in the first 1 s of the expiration is designated FEV_1 and the total volume expired is the **forced vital capacity (FVC)**. It is called forced vital capacity because of the forced expiration.

The volume exhaled can be measured by recording the volume expired against time, using a bell-type spirometer. The record obtained is called a **spirogram** (Fig. 6.24).

In a normal subject the FEV_1 is about 4.2 litres and the FVC about 5.0 litres. This means that the FEV_1 is 84% of the FVC (Fig. 6.24A). In general, this ratio is always more than 80%. An FEV_1 less than 80% of the FVC is abnormal (Fig. 6.24B).

FEV_1, FVC and FEV_1% give very useful information for the assessment of **obstructive** and **restrictive** impairments, e.g. as are seen in patients suffering from *bronchial asthma*, *chronic bronchitis* and *emphysema* (obstructive lung diseases) and from *fibrotic conditions* of lungs, including pneumoconiosis (restrictive lung diseases).

Another important piece of information can be obtained from this spirogram. The time taken for the expiration of the FVC is not 2 s (Fig. 6.24B) but 4 s. This is due to the increased resistance offered by the bronchi to the flow of air, because of their narrowing, which is the primary pathology in obstructive lung diseases. The measurement of time for a particle of gas to flow out of the lungs is called transit time. The *mean transit time* (MTT) in normal persons is always less than 3 s. Measurement of MTT is suggested by some to be a sensitive indicator of airways disease.

Figure 6.24C shows the spirogram of another patient. The FEV_1 in this patient is 2.7 litres, the FVC is 3.0 litres and the FEV_1% is 90%. This is typical of restrictive lung disease. In this patient the FVC is comparatively less. Although the FEV_1 is less than the normal, the FEV_1% of the FVC is normal.

FEV_1 and FVC measurements are repeated in patients suspected of obstructive lung disease after giving the patient a bronchodilator (salbutamol 1% for 3 min through a nebulizer). Improvements in both FEV_1 and FVC indicate reversibility and confirm the occurrence of bronchospasm in these patients.

3 *Peak expiratory flow rate (PEFR).* Another important forced expiratory manoeuvre, which is rapid and can be performed at the bedside, is the measurement of the **PEFR**. The subject, after making a full inspiration, exhales forcibly through a flowmeter (e.g. Wright flowmeter, Fig. 6.25). In normal persons with a maximum effort, the PEFR goes up to 8–12 litres/s. In athletes and trained young men, it can go as high as 20 litres/s. PEFR is decreased in patients suffering from bronchial obstruction. If airway obstruction is suspected, reversibility is tested by repeating the test after giving a bronchodilator. If reversibility is positive, airway spasm is confirmed. A PEFR record of the patient gives useful information on the progress or deterioration of the patient's condition.

4 *Forced expiratory flow 25–75 (FEF25–75).* This pulmonary function index is calculated from the spirogram obtained by using the bell-type spirometer. The patient, after full inspiration, forcibly exhales. The volume exhaled

Fig. 6.25 Wright peak flowmeter.

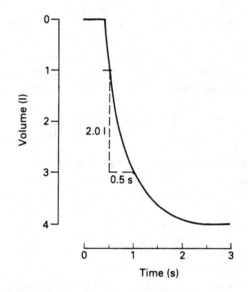

Fig. 6.26 Peak expiratory flow 25–75 recorded by a bell-type spirometer. FEF25–75 in this case = 4 litres/s.

is recorded against time on a moving drum, in the same way as is done to record the FEV. The middle half of the total spirogram (25–75%) is marked out and the time taken for this volume to be exhaled is measured (Fig. 6.26). The **FEF25–75** is the volume divided by time in seconds. Normally FEF25–75 is 3–5 litres/s.

There is generally good correlation between FEV_1 and FEF25–75 in patients suffering from obstructive lung

Fig. 6.27 Flow–volume loop in a normal subject. FVC, forced vital capacity; PIFR, peak inspiratory flow rate; PEFR, peak expiratory flow rate; MEF50, maximum expiratory flow at 50% of FVC—normal = 4–6 litres/s; MEF25, maximum expiratory flow at 25% of FVC—normal = 2–4 litres/s; RV, residual volume.

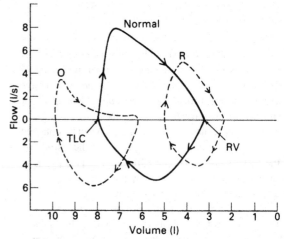

Fig. 6.28 Flow–volume loops in restrictive lung disease (R) and obstructive lung disease (O), compared with a normal subject. TLC, total lung capacity; RV, residual volume.

diseases. FEF25–75 has the advantage of avoiding measurements during the effort-dependent first quarter of FVC. Like other spirometric indices, FEF25–75 is modified by age, sex and body size.

5 *Flow–volume loops.* Special electronic equipment is required to record the flow–volume loops. The subject performs the same forced expiratory manoeuvre after full inspiration as for the FEV. Instead of using the bell-type spirometer, the flow and volume are simultaneously recorded on the x–y recorder. Usually flow is recorded along the y axis and volume along the x axis (Fig. 6.27). An important feature of the flow–volume loop is that it is impossible to get outside the loop, no matter how much or how long the expiratory effort. It also shows the inspiratory loop, which is not shown in spirograms.

Recording of flow–volume loops is one of the ventilatory function tests, which is routinely used in most pulmonary investigation hospital laboratories. This technique measures all of the ventilatory parameters described above. In particular, it measures the following:

1 Forced vital capacity expiration (FVC).
2 Forced vital capacity inspiration (FCI).
3 Peak expiratory flow rate (PEFR).
4 Maximum expiratory flow at 50% of FVC (MEF50). Normal value: 4–6 litres/s.
5 Maximum expiratory flow at 25% of FVC (MEF25). Normal value: 2–4 litres/s.
6 Peak inspiratory flow rate (PIFR).

7 Maximum inspiratory flow rate at 50% of vital capacity.
8 Maximum inspiratory flow rate at 25% of vital capacity.

MEF50 and MEF25 are effort-independent flow rates. In obstructive airway diseases, these parameters are significantly decreased (Fig. 6.28). In restrictive lung diseases, the loop becomes elliptical. The FVC and FEV_1 are decreased. All the flow parameters are decreased but their ratio to the FVC does not change.

Inspiratory flow loops are useful in upper airways obstruction, such as tracheal obstruction, laryngeal obstruction due to inflammation or neoplasm or obstruction of the larynx by inflammation of the epiglottis. In all these conditions the inspiratory loops are flattened.

In upper airways obstruction the expiratory loops are also flattened. This reduces the utility of the inspiratory loops in diagnosis as compared with the expiratory loops.

Patients who record obstructive types of flow–volume loops are given bronchodilators (salbutamol 1% for 3 min) and repeat the test to see reversibility.

MEF50 and MEF25 reduction in the presence of normal FVC and FEV_1 also indicates small or peripheral airways obstructive disease.

6 *Test of uneven ventilation and closing volume.* Uneven ventilation is best tested by the **radioactive xenon** technique. This test requires a gamma camera and radioactive xenon; it is used for research and a very few selected patients. The routine test is the **single-breath nitrogen test**. The advantage of this test is that, besides measuring the uneven ventilation, the closing volume can also be measured simultaneously. To perform this test, pure

Fig. 6.29 Single-breath N_2 method. CV, closing volume; RV, residual volume.

oxygen, a rapid nitrogen analyser and a recorder are used; the latter records nitrogen concentration against lung volume. The subject takes a full inspiration of pure oxygen, followed by slow expiration (the flow should not be more than 0.5 litre/s). The rapid nitrogen analyser analyses the concentration of nitrogen near the mouth. Four phases are recorded (Fig. 6.29). Phase 1 is expired from the anatomical dead space, so it contains pure O_2. It is every small. Phase 2 is also short. In this phase nitrogen concentration rises rapidly as the dead space and alveolar gases are expired. Phase 3 is a plateau of N_2 concentration because it is the alveolar gas. Phase 4 shows a rapid rise in N_2 concentration. This signals the onset of closure of airways.

Phase 3 in normal subjects is almost flat. In patients with uneven ventilation, this phase rises steadily and the slope is the measure of inequality of ventilation. It is expressed as the percentage increase in nitrogen per litre of expired volume (0.70% increase per litre).

In patients with weak airways due to destruction of lung parenchyma, as in *emphysema* and *obstructive airway disease*, the closing of the airways takes place early and the closing volume, which is the volume of phase 4, is increased.

7 *Helium dilution technique (closed circuit method)* (Fig. 6.30). This method is used for measurement of **total lung capacity** (TLC) and residual volume. Helium is poorly diffusible through the alveolar capillary membrane. The subject rebreathes into a spirometer containing a known volume of a known concentration of helium in oxygen for a few minutes. The final concentration of helium in the spirometer is measured by a helium analyser.

Example:

If the initial volume of the helium–oxygen mixture =

Fig. 6.30 Helium dilution technique using the closed-circuit method.

Fig. 6.31 Sequence of events in body plethysmography (body box). (a) Before the mouthpiece shutter is closed. (b) Inspiration with the mouthpiece shutter closed.

2 litres, the initial concentration of helium = 8%, the final concentration of helium = 4% and the TLC to be measured = x litres:

$$2 \times \frac{8}{100} = (x + 2) \times \frac{4}{100}$$
$$16 = 4x + 8$$
$$4x = 8$$
$$x = 2 \text{ litres}$$

The residual volume (RV) can be obtained by subtraction (TLC – FEV = RV).

In obstructive lung disease the TLC and RV are normal or higher than normal, but in restrictive disease TLC is decreased. In emphysema the RV is much higher than normal.

8 *Body plethysmography (body box)* (Fig. 6.31). The tech-

niques for measurement of **residual volume** and **functional residual capacity** assume free communication of all parts of the lung with the atmospheric air for efficient and complete dilution and washout of either helium or nitrogen. If there is obstruction to any part of the lung, these techniques will give low values. To obtain true values of all the air in the lungs, whether or not they are in free communication with the atmosphere, the body plethysmograph is used. The principle used is based on **Boyle's law** for gases, which relates gas pressure to gas volume:

$$P^1 V^1 = PV$$

The subject sits within the box and the door is tightly closed. The subject breathes air around him/her through a mouthpiece mounted with a shutter that is electrically controlled. At the end of normal expiration (when measuring the functional residual capacity), the shutter is closed and the subject inspires against this obstruction. Figure 6.31 demonstrates the events before and after closing the mouthpiece shutter; at the end of expiration the intra-alveolar pressure (P) is atmospheric as there is no gas flow. The thoracic gas volume (V) at the end of expiration, or functional residual capacity, is unknown. The mouthpiece shutter is then closed and the subject inspires against the obstruction. The new thoracic volume will then become $\Delta V + V = V^1$. The pressure of the new gas volume, V^1, recorded in the mouthpiece at the end of the inspiration, will drop to P^1.

The increase in thoracic volume ΔV is determined by the rise in the plethysmographic pressure, which is calibrated with volume change.

Since P, P^1 and ΔV are known, V (the functional residual capacity) can be worked out from Boyle's law:

$$PV = P^1(\Delta V + V)$$

The total lung capacity is measured, using the helium dilution technique, and is usually measured simultaneously with the single-breath method used for calculation of the diffusion capacity of the lung for CO (see below).

Gas diffusion

Diffusion capacity of the lung is defined as the total volume of a gas that diffuses through the lung alveolar–capillary membrane per unit time per unit partial pressure difference of the gas. It is recorded in ml/min/mmHg partial pressure (see Table 6.3).

The rate of transfer of gas across the pulmonary membrane depends upon the surface area of the pulmonary membrane, the partial pressure difference across the pulmonary membrane, the pulmonary membrane thickness, the molecular weight and the solubility coefficient of the gas. Other factors which offer serious limitations to the study of oxygen (O_2) diffusion across the pulmonary membrane are the pulmonary blood flow and the haemoglobin concentration in the blood. In order to minimize the effects of these latter factors, O_2 is not used for the study of diffusion; instead, carbon monoxide (CO) is used, because CO transfer is only *diffusion-dependent* and is not affected by perfusion. The diffusion capacity for O_2 is calculated from a measurement of the diffusion of CO. In essence the method depends on the patient breathing a small amount of CO and the partial pressure of the gas is measured in a sample of alveolar air.

Two techniques are used:

1 *Single-breath technique.* The subject takes a full inspiration of gas mixture (10% helium, 0.3% CO in air) and holds his breath for 10 s and then exhales. The first 1 litre or so is discarded (dead-space volume) and, out of the remaining, 1 litre is collected (alveolar air) and analysed for CO and He concentrations. From the difference of helium concentration in the inspired and expired air and from the volume of air inspired, the total lung capacity (TLC) is calculated:

$$C_1 \times V_1 = C_2 \times (V_1 + V_2)$$

where C_1 and V_1 are concentration of He and volume of inspired air, C_2 is the concentration of He in expired air, and V_2 is the total lung capacity. The diffusion capacity for CO (DL_{co}) is calculated by dividing the volume of CO taken up in the lungs per minute (V_{CO}) by the partial pressure of alveolar CO (PA_{co}) as follows:

$$DL_{co} = \frac{V_{CO}}{PA_{co}}$$

The alveolar partial pressure of CO is taken as the driving force because the alveolar capillary blood CO concentration (in non-smokers) is negligible. In young men at rest, the DL_{co} is about 17 ml (min) mmHg. This value is multiplied by a factor of 1.23 to obtain the O_2 diffusion capacity.

Breath-holding may be difficult for some patients. In such cases, the steady-state technique is used.

2 *Steady-state technique.* The principle of the technique is the same as for the single breath. In this technique the subject breathes 0.25% CO and 6% He in air steadily until the rate of CO uptake becomes constant. When this steady state is reached, the alveolar air is collected and analysed and calculated as for the single-breath method.

Arterial blood gases. Full investigations of a patient with pulmonary disease are never satisfactory without the determination of the arterial blood gases. Arterial blood is taken by arterial puncture, e.g. the radial, brachial or femoral artery, with a syringe in which the dead space is filled with heparin. The blood obtained is immediately analysed in an arterial blood gas analyser. If the blood cannot be analysed promptly after collection, it must be kept in ice-water at 4°C for not more than half an hour. In no case should it be kept for more than an hour before analysis.

The most serious outcome of pulmonary diseases is hypoxia. One of the important causes of hypoxia is hypoventilation, which is well illustrated by the CO_2 gas equation:

$$Pco_2 = \frac{\dot{V}CO_2}{VA} k$$

where $\dot{V}CO_2$ is CO_2 output, VA is alveolar ventilation and k is a constant. This relationship shows that, if alveolar ventilation is halved, Pco_2 is doubled. Similarly, the relationship of pH to Pco_2 can determine the degree of hypoventilation. A crude but reliable relationship has been observed. For every 10 mmHg rise in Pco_2, the pH drops by roughly 0.1. Thus, from looking at pH only, one can guess the degree of hypoventilation when the drop in pH is entirely due to hypoventilation.

Determination of arterial blood gases before and after exercise or after treatment with 100% O_2 can give a fairly good idea about other causes of hypoxia. If, after moderate physical exercise, hypoxia is increased, it indicates either a diffusion defect or ventilation/perfusion imbalance or both. Hypoxia due to diffusion defects and hypoventilation are easily corrected by 100% O_2 therapy. If Po_2, after therapy, fails to rise to normal levels, hypoxia is most probably due to a shunt.

Test for elastic properties of the lungs
Compliance is the change in volume of the lung per unit change in pressure. In order to measure compliance, one has to know the intrapleural pressure. Direct measurement of the intrapleural pressure is difficult. Instead, intraoesophageal pressure (which is not identical to the intrapleural pressure but reflects intrapleural pressure changes fairly well) is measured.

The subject swallows a small balloon at the end of a rubber tube which is placed halfway between the pharynx and the stomach. The balloon is filled with a few millilitres of air. The rubber tube is connected to a pressure-measuring device. The subject inspires air from a spirometer to total lung capacity and expires in steps of 500 ml through a valve connected with an automatic shutter. After each step the lungs are relaxed with the glottis open and the oesophageal

pressure is measured. The pressure measured is plotted against the volume to get the pressure–volume curve. The slope of the curve represents the compliance (see Fig. 6.7).

One of the factors which affect the compliance of the lungs is the lung size. Compliance is directly related to the size of the lungs. For this reason the compliance per unit volume of lung, which is known as the *specific compliance*, is calculated. Large lungs show large compliance; if the elastic properties of the lungs are affected, the specific compliance of the same large lung is decreased.

Sometimes compliance is measured during inspiration and expiration by measuring the oesophageal pressure at the end of inspiration and expiration. This measurement, which is known as dynamic compliance, is sensitive and decreases significantly in patients with increased airway resistance.

Test of airway resistance
Airway resistance is measured by finding the pressure difference between the mouth and the alveoli and the rate of air flow, using the pressure, resistance and flow relationship expressed by Ohm's law:

$$\frac{\text{Airway}}{\text{resistance}} = \frac{\text{Mouth pressure} - \text{alveolar pressure}}{\text{Flow of air}}$$

Flow of air and mouth pressure are easy to measure, but the measurement of alveolar pressure requires the use of the body plethysmograph. The subject sits in the body box connected to the pneumotachograph head, which measures the air flow. A side tube from the mouthpiece is connected to a transducer, which measures instantaneous mouth pressure. Before inspiration the pressure in the box is atmospheric. When the subject inspires, the alveolar pressure falls as the gas expands due to change in volume of the chest. This increases the pressure in the box, from which the change in the volume of the lungs can be determined. The change in the volume of the lungs due to inspiration can be converted to alveolar pressure change, using Boyle's law, if the initial lung volume is known.

Test of ventilation/perfusion relation
Unequal ventilation can be tested by the nitrogen washout test described earlier. The distribution of blood in the lungs is tested by injecting albumin labelled with radioactive iodine or technetium. The radioactivity of the lung is measured by a gamma camera. The photograph of radioactivity shows directly the distribution of blood in the lungs. Instead of radioactive albumin, radioactive xenon dissolved in saline can also be used. From the numerical

data of radioactivity, the results can be expressed as blood flow per unit volume of the lungs.

The ventilation can be measured by using radioactive xenon gas. The subject takes a single breath or series of breaths of radioactive xenon, after which the radioactivity is measured by a gamma camera, and the results are expressed as ventilation per unit lung volume.

Further reading

1 Guyton, A.C. & Hall, J.E. (1996) Respiration. In: *Textbook of Medical Physiology*, 9th edn, pp. 477–536. Saunders, Philadelphia.
2 Levitzky, M.G. (1990) *Pulmonary Physiology*. McGraw-Hill, New York.
3 West, J.B. (1995) *Respiratory Physiology—The Essentials*, 5th edn. Williams & Wilkins, Baltimore.

7 / Nutrition and Metabolism

Objectives

On completion of the study of this section, the student should be able to:

1 Understand the functions of essential nutrients required for maintenance of health and identify their sources.

2 Become familiar with major diseases caused by nutritional deficiencies so as to further his/her knowledge and skills in their diagnosis and management during his/her clinical studies.

3 Understand the concept of the metabolic rate so as to explain variations of energy expenditure and to describe the energy requirements of individual patients.

4 Comprehend the basic metabolic concepts which underlie different physiological states so as to predict nutritional needs.

5 Develop a comprehensive understanding of the integration of metabolic processes so as to relate metabolism to the state of nutrition.

Introduction

Maintaining the human body in a constant state of health requires a continuous supply of nutrients. Some of these nutrients are consumable, i.e. they are used up. Examples of these are **fats** and **carbohydrates**, which are mainly catabolized to provide *energy*, normally in the form of adenosine triphosphate (ATP), for work as well as for vital life processes at the cellular level (e.g. ion transport, maintenance of cell membrane potentials and chemical synthesis). Fats (triacylglycerols) and carbohydrates (glycogens) are also forms of energy storage in the body, which are mobilized when required. Other nutrients, such as **proteins,** are essential components of the structure of living cells. Many important enzymes and hormones are made up of protein or polypeptide molecules.

To a certain extent, the sources of energy are interchangeable, but excess quantities of fat cannot be oxidized without the provision of minimal amounts of carbohydrate or protein.

In adults and in children, cells are continuously renewed and in this process some protein losses are incurred. On the other hand, growing children and pregnant mothers are forming new cells for new tissues and growth of organs.

Following injury or disease, cells which have been damaged will have to be replaced. Proteins are made of **amino acids**; however, some amino acids cannot be synthesized in the human body (i.e. **essential amino acids**). It is clear, therefore, that a continuous supply of dietary protein is important in order to supply the essential amino acids. It is also pertinent to note that some specialized carbohydrates and lipid molecules are components of cell membranes and some hormones and enzymes.

In addition to the above, the body requires a supply of **minerals** and **trace elements**, which take part in the structure of specialized molecules in the human body. We also need a continuous supply of a group of substances known as **vitamins**. These substances, more often than not, cannot by synthesized in the human body and must be present in the diet. They play numerous biochemical roles and their deficiency earn cause serious disease conditions (such as corneal opacity or xerophthalmia, rickets, beriberi and scurvy), characterized by tissue damage, failure of growth and impairment of specific metabolic processes.

A proportion of any meal can be described as inert, having no nutritive value. This is because it is not absorbed. Many plant polysaccharides, such as cellulose, fall into this category, now collectively known as **nonstarch** polysaccharides (NSP) fall into this category. They are not attacked by the host's digestive enzymes, or preferably NSP which also includes a group of nondigestible food components such as pectins, β-glucans and gums (e.g. gum arabic and guar gum), although some digestion by bacterial enzymes occurs. However, evidence suggests that **dietary fibre** (e.g. cellulose) is of considerable value in the diet. How and why does fibre in the diet exert its beneficial effects? This is not entirely clear, but it is established that molecules of NSP are strong adsorbing agents. They adsorb large quantities of water and also possibly toxic molecules which may be produced by the flora of the digestive tract. The adsorption of large amounts of water is also very important, and this leads to a much larger *faecal mass* and therefore easier transit through the intestines and easier expulsion. NSP are also found to decrease plasma low density lipoprotein cholesterol due to decreased absorption of bile acids. This leads to synthesis of new bile acids from cholesterol.

Nearly all food contains small quantities of toxic substances. They can be added during processing, for example, to preserve the food, or gain entry to the food incidentally, for example, during crop spraying or treatment with fertilizers.

Water is not strictly a nutrient but it is required as a solvent for body fluid components. Water constitutes over 60% of body weight; and therefore water intake is vital for replacement of losses through the skin and urinary system. Water is also a by-product of metabolism. A balance between water intake and water loss is essential for maintenance of the constancy of the internal environment. The delicate balance is of particular importance in hot environments, where evaporative water losses in sweating are an essential mechanism for heat dissipation.

This chapter deals with the nutrients and their sources, physiological roles and requirements. The main focus is to correlate the physiological state with variations in requirements and adjustments in underlying metabolism, so as to understand the changes which occur under physiological conditions, stress and relevant clinical situations.

Physiology of feeding

Food intake is regulated over long periods of time with such precision that a person can maintain his/her body-weight for 20 years or more within a few kilograms. The precision of this regulation becomes clear if it is realized that during the same period the individual would have consumed at least 4 tons of the essential nutrients, not considering the water intake. If his/her variation of body-weight was within 4 kg, then the precision of the control system is 10^{-3}. These calculations are based on a diet giving about

10 MJ/day (2400 kcal) and consisting of about 400 g carbohydrate, 60 g fat and 80 g protein.

Appetite and hunger

Appetite can be defined as the desire to eat. It may be influenced by the taste and smell of food and may be greater for some food items than others. There is reason to believe that appetite is increased for substances deficient in the body at any one time. An example of this is salt appetite under conditions of excessive sweat losses of NaCl. There is evidence in animals and in humans that appetite for foods already eaten during a meal is less than that for new food items. Preference for new items is probably a biological mechanism to ensure that a variety of foods is consumed. In prosperous societies, however, it can lead to overeating due to the availability of a large variety of food items.

The feeling of hunger is one of the important physiological stimuli for the appetite. The feeling of satiety is experienced after feeding. There are neurons in the hypothalamus which have been designated as the **feeding centre** in the lateral hypothalamus and as the **satiety centre** in the ventromedial nucleus. In hungry animals these neurons are stimulated by the sight and smell of food and they also display specific responses to different food items. Stimulation of the feeding centre neurons results in promotion of eating behaviour, while injury or damage results in severe loss of appetite (**anorexia**). On the other hand, stimulation of the satiety centre results in loss of appetite and its destruction causes overeating (**hyperphagia**). The latter is the underlying pathology in what is known as **hypothalamic obesity**. There is evidence that the hyperphagia of hypothalamic obesity is partly explained by hypersecretion of insulin, due to stimulation of the vagi during the cephalic phase of gastrointestinal stimulation.

Hypoglycaemia is usually associated with hunger and hyperglycaemia with satiety. However, hunger can occur with hyperglycaemia, as in diabetes mellitus. A theory which has been advanced for the regulation of feeding is known as the *glucostatic hypothesis*. The cells in the satiety centre have a high rate of glucose utilization and, unlike other parts of the nervous system, their glucose uptake can be influenced by insulin. When their glucose utilization is high, satiety is experienced, but, when utilization falls, hunger is felt. Thus, a high arteriovenous concentration difference of glucose (high utilization) is associated with satiety, while a low concentration difference is associated with hunger. This hypothesis explains the presence of hunger with hyperglycaemia in diabetes. In this case, there is decreased utilization of glucose by the neurons in the satiety centre. However, the precise mechanism for

Table 7.1 Carbohydrate contents of cereals and cereal foods.

	Percentage by weight
Wheat	69
Sorghum (durra)	74
Rice	87
Millet (*Pennisetum* species)	75
Maize	64
Barley	69
Cassavas	35
Potatoes	18
Sweet potatoes	28
Yams	27
Bread	45–60
Porridge (sorghum species)	17
'Kisra' (sorghum species)	42

Table 7.2 Carbohydrate contents of some pulses and seeds.

	Percentage by weight
Beans	54
Lentils	57
Peas	50
Soya beans	24
Groundnuts	19

Table 7.3 Fructose and sucrose contents various fruits.

	Percentage by weight
Apples	15
Apricots	6
Bananas	16
Dates, fresh	38
Dates, dried	63
Grapes	15
Guavas	16
Mangoes	16
Oranges	12
Pears	27

the maintenance of body-weight is not fully understood. There seems to be a relationship between a set point for body-weight and feeding behaviour in the normal control mechanism.

The nutrients

Sources and physiological roles
The main nutrient sources of energy are carbohydrates and fats. Although proteins can also be used to supply energy, it is good dietary planning to avoid this. Proteins are more expensive than carbohydrates. It is important to ensure that children receive adequate energy in order to spare dietary protein for growth. Excess energy intake is the main cause of overweight and all the attendant diseases associated with it, such as diabetes mellitus, hypertension and coronary heart disease.

Carbohydrates
The body tissues require a constant daily supply of carbohydrates, in the form of glucose, in all metabolic reactions. Comparatively little is stored. Approximately 100 g of glycogen is stored in the liver and about 225 g in the muscles, and there is about 10 g of glucose in the blood. For most individuals, the supply available from storage depots would be insufficient for 1 day's need. The principal function of dietary carbohydrate is to serve as a major source of energy for the body. When metabolized, carbohydrates yield 4 kcal or 17 kJ/g.

Carbohydrates are available in the form of starches and sugars. Starch is contained in cereals, roots and stems (Table 7.1). Pulses and seeds also have appreciable amounts of carbohydrate (Table 7.2). Sugar is found in sugar cane and sugar beet. Sugar cane contains 10% sugar (sucrose), while sugar beet contains 6% sugar (sucrose and fructose). Refined sugar intake is blamed for the causation of overweight, dental caries, hyperlipidaemia and atherosclerosis. However, the evidence for the latter is inconclusive. Fruits contain various amounts of sugar. Fructose and sucrose are contained in many fruits (Table 7.3). Although NSP are not digested they are subjected to bacterial fermentation in the large intestine and some may be absorbed in the form of short chain fatty acids with the production of gas.

Fats
Butter, animal fat and vegetable oils are almost pure fat; they provide the highest amount of energy per gram (9 kcal = 38 kJ), which is more than twice the amount of energy supplied by each gram of carbohydrate. Because of the high energy content and low solubility of fats, they are used as a storage form of energy. Not only ingested fat but carbohydrate and amino acids not immediately used by the tissues are converted to fat and stored in the adipose tissue. Fat sources provide 5–20% of the energy content of diets in the poorer parts of Africa, Asia and Latin America. They may provide up to 80% of the energy intake in more affluent societies. This is simply explained by the fact that fats and oils are expensive and their intake tends to be

Table 7.4 Examples of plant food with high fat content.

	Percentage by weight
Groundnuts	44
Sesame	51
Soya beans	24

Table 7.5 Essential and non-essential amino acids.

Essential amino acids	Non-essential amino acids
Valine	Glycine
Lysine	Alanine
Threonine	Serine
Leucine	Cystine
Isoleucine	Tyrosine
Tryptophan	Proline
Phenylalanine	Hydroxyproline
Methionine	Citrulline
Histidine	Arginine
	Glutamine
	Aspartate
	Glutamate

Table 7.6 Protein contents of some animal and plant foods.

	Percentage by weight
Animal foods	
Beef	18–32
Veal	21
Lamb	18–29
Pork	13–33
Poultry	17–30
Fish	17–19
Egg	13
Milk (cow)	3.5
Plant foods	
Beans (various types)	24
Peas	22
Soya beans	37
Chick-peas	19
Groundnuts	26
Sesame	20
Cereals	7–16

influenced by the income in various communities. Excessive fat consumption, especially of the saturated types, results in hyperlipidaemia and the risks of atherosclerosis, coronary heart disease and hypertension. Some plant foods with a high fat content are shown in Table 7.4.

Energy can also be obtained from ingested alcohol (7 kcal = 30 kJ/g).

Protein

The primary structure of proteins is the number, type and order of amino acids. Proteins vary in size from relatively small polypeptides to very complex molecules with several hundred thousand amino acid units. There are nine amino acids that are classified as essential, since they must be supplied in the food. Body synthesis of these amino acids is lacking or so limited as to be insufficient to meet metabolic needs (Table 7.5). Histidine was first found to be required by infants; however, recent work in humans suggests that it may also be essential for adults. Without an adequate supply of the **essential amino acids**, protein cannot be synthesized or body tissue maintained.

The other amino acids, which can be synthesized by the body in adequate amounts for normal function, are termed non-essential (see Table 7.5). This is not to suggest that these amino acids are not essential constituents of the proteins, but rather that it is not essential to include them in the diet since the tissues can synthesize their own supply from carbohydrate, far and other amino acids.

The main sources of animal protein are meats (mainly muscle). The protein contents of some animal foods are shown in Table 7.6. All meats have large amounts of water, from 60 to 75% of their weight. Dried meat and dried fish have very little water and therefore their protein content is very high, up to 70%. The protein contents of some commonly used pulses and legumes are shown in Table 7.6.

Although the protein content of cereals is low compared with other seeds, it is important to note that large amounts of cereals are usually consumed for their carbohydrate content. Therefore, the amount of protein consumed in cereal foods constitutes a significant amount of the total daily protein intake. This is of particular importance in poorer parts of the world, where 80–90% of the energy comes from cereal foods. It has been estimated that in some developing countries 90% of the protein intake comes from staple cereal foods.

Proteins of plant origin, however, are deficient in one or more of the essential amino acids. They are therefore of lower quality than animal proteins. *Amino acid* (or *chemical*) *scores* can be calculated for the most deficient (or most **limiting**) amino acid to describe the quality of any protein source. The amino acid score is calculated as follows:

$$\text{Amino acid score} = \frac{\text{mg of amino acid in 1 g of test protein} \times 100}{\text{mg of amino acid in 1 g of reference protein}}$$

Table 7.7 Water-soluble and fat-soluble vitamins required in the human diet and their sources.

	Sources
Water-soluble vitamins	
Vitamin B₁ (thiamine)	Thiamine is mainly found in the germ of cereals and seeds. Yeast, liver and meats are rich sources
Vitamin B₂ (riboflavine)	Milk, organ meats, eggs, cereals
Vitamin B₆ (pyridoxine)	Cereals, liver, yeast
Nicotinamide (or niacin)	Meats, liver, pulses
Pantothenic acid	Liver, kidney, egg yolk, milk
Biotin	Egg yolk, liver, kidney, meat
Vitamin B₁₂ (cobalamin)	Liver, meat
Folic acid (folacin)	Green leafy vegetables, meat, liver
Vitamin C (ascorbic acid)	Green peppers, chili (fresh), guavas, citrus fruits and parsley
Fat-soluble vitamins	
Vitamin A (retinol)	Milk and butter are good sources; also liver, kidney, egg yolk
Carotene (vitamin A precursor)	A yellow pigment found in vegetables and fruits. It can be converted in the body to retinol. One microgram of retinol equals 6 µg of carotene
Vitamin D (calciferol)	A rich source is fish-liver oil. Diet is not an important source of vitamin D. Most of it is synthesized in the skin from 7-dehydrocholesterol (provitamin D₃) by the effect of ultraviolet light. The liver hydroxylates the vitamin to 25-hydroxycholecalciferol and the kidney makes the active form 1,25-dihydroxycholecalciferol under the effect of parathyroid hormone. For this reason, vitamin D₃ is now viewed as a prohormone
Vitamin E (α-tocopherols)	Vegetable oils, meats, eggs, leafy vegetables
Vitamin K (several naphthoquinones)	Fresh leafy vegetables, liver, fish-liver oil

This score is a crude way to evaluate the percentage of adequacy of the protein because it does not take into account the digestibility of the protein, the availability of the amino acids, the utilization of those amino acids by the human body or the ability of that protein to support cellular synthesis. However, it can be used to calculate dietary protein requirements of a mixture of proteins compared with a reference protein; for example, if egg or milk protein requirement is 30 g/day and the amino acid score of the dietary proteins available is 60%, then the required amount of this mixture would be [(30 × 100)/60] = 50 g/day. As will appear later in this chapter, other factors also influence the requirements of dietary protein.

Vitamins

In addition to adequate energy and protein intake, there are certain substances which are required in minute amounts to achieve normal growth of the young and to maintain health in adults. These substances, which are known as vitamins, mainly act as coenzymes or a prosthetic group of enzymes responsible for promoting essential chemical reactions in tissue metabolism. They are often called accessory food factors in view of the fact that they do not supply calories or contribute appreciably to body mass. The exact mode of action of some vitamins is not yet clear but clinical conditions due to deficiency are well known. Vitamins regulate metabolism, help convert fat and carbohydrate into energy and assist in the formation and maintenance of bones and tissues. As these substances cannot be synthesized in the body, a constant supply of dietary vitamins is essential. Table 7.7 gives a list of the main vitamins required in human diets and their sources.

Vitamins are complex chemical substances with known chemical structure and most of them have been synthesized. Specific biochemical roles have been described for most vitamins. For specific biochemical actions, a textbook of biochemistry should be consulted. The following is a brief description of their roles in metabolism and associated deficiencies.

Water-soluble vitamins

Vitamin B₁. The active form, thiamine pyrophosphate, is an important coenzyme in mammalian tissues and required in the oxidative decarboxylation of pyruvate, oxoglutarate and 2-oxo acids derived from methionine, threonine, leucine, isoleucine and valine. In addition, it acts as a coenzyme for the transketolase reaction in the pentose phosphate pathway. Thiamine is needed for the metabolism of carbohydrates, fats and proteins. However, all the evidence from the effects of thiamine deficiency link it with disturbance of carbohydrate metabolism, especially in the brain. Thiamine requirement is linked to carbohydrate intake. Its deficiency causes dry or wet *beriberi* and gastrointestinal disturbances.

Vitamin B₂. This vitamin maintains the health of mucous membranes. It is required for the synthesis of two coenzymes: flavin mononucleotide (FMN) and flavin adenine dinucleotide (FAD). These, in turn, form the prosthetic groups of several different enzyme systems (the flavoproteins), which catalyse oxidation–reduction reactions in the cells and function as hydrogen carriers in the mitochondrial electron transport system. They are also coenzymes of several dehydrogenases and enzymes of oxidative deamination of amino acids. Vitamin B_2 deficiency leads to inflammation of the tongue (*glossitis*) and ulcerations at the angle of the mouth (*angular stomatitis*).

Vitamin B₆. This is rapidly converted in the body into the coenzymes pyridoxal-5′-phosphate and pyridoxamine phosphate. They form the prosthetic groups of enzyme–coenzyme systems in the pathways of energy production and amino acid and fat metabolism. In addition, vitamin B_6 catalyses the synthesis of *tryptophan* and its conversion into nicotinamide. It is also concerned with the synthesis of haemoglobin. It is therefore important for growth. Deficiency causes *anaemia*, irritability and convulsions. Deficiency in some patients can be associated with oral contraceptives and some drugs.

Nicotinamide. This is necessary for formation of nicotinamide adenine dinucleotide (NAD) and nicotinamide adenine dinucleotide phosphate (NADP) (oxidative coenzymes). Deficiency causes *pellagra*, with skin, neurological and gastrointestinal manifestations. Its role in the prevention of pellagra is not fully understood.

Pantothenic acid. This is incorporated in coenzyme A (CoA) and is thus essential in the intermediary metabolism of carbohydrate, fat and protein. No deficiency has been described in humans. It is widespread in foods and is synthesized by intestinal bacteria. There is no known deficiency disease.

Biotin. This forms part of several carboxylase enzymes. Absorption is inhibited by raw egg white (avidin). It is synthesized by intestinal bacteria and daily requirements are minute. It is an essential coenzyme for fatty acid synthesis

and oxidation. Its deficiency results in lethargy, loss of appetite, nausea, dermatitis and muscle pain.

Vitamin B₁₂. This vitamin is essential for normal function in the metabolism of all cells, especially for those of the gastrointestinal tract, bone marrow and nervous tissue, and for growth. It is involved in protein, fat and carbohydrate metabolism. It is necessary for the maturation of red blood cells and maintains the myelination in the nervous system. It is the only vitamin not yet synthesized. Failure to absorb vitamin B_{12} because of the absence of the **intrinsic factor** in the gastric secretion (e.g. due to surgical resection of the intrinsic factor-secreting portions of the stomach or the absorbing surfaces of the ileum) results in a deficiency state. The latter produces a **megaloblastic** maturation of the red cells in the marrow, with a resulting macrocytic anaemia and a leucopenia with hypersegmented polymorphonuclear leucocytes.

Folic acid (pteroylglutamic acid). This is important in the synthesis of deoxyribonucleic acid (DNA), purines, haem and some amino acids; hence it has an important role in the growth and maturation of red and white blood cells. Deficiency causes poor growth, *megaloblastic anaemia* and *sprue*.

Vitamin C. This vitamin functions as a cofactor or a coenzyme and is required for a number of hydroxylation and oxidative reactions. It is required for the production and maintenance of collagen, a protein substance found in all fibrous tissues (connective tissue, cartilage, bone matrix, tooth dentin, skin and tendon). The integrity of cellular structure depends on it. It maintains the health of capillaries via the synthesis of collagen; the latter promotes healing of wounds, fractures and bleeding gums and decreases liability to infection. Vitamin C also facilitates removal of iron from ferritin. Its deficiency causes *scurvy*.

Fat-soluble vitamins

Vitamin A. Retinol is required for the formation of the pigment rhodopsin (visual purple), which is needed for vision in dim light. The vitamin is also required for normal growth and for maintenance of healthy epithelial tissue. In addition, vitamin A (retinol) also appears to play a role in fertility and various metabolic pathways (e.g. cholesterol synthesis, mucopolysaccharide synthesis). Deficiency causes *night-blindness* and *xerophthalmia*, which may progress to corneal opacity and blindness.

Vitamin D. The active form of vitamin D_3 (1,25-dihydroxycholecalciferol) is essential for normal growth and development and is important for the formation of normal bones and teeth. Along with parathyroid hormone and calcitonin, vitamin D has an important role in the maintenance of appropriate serum levels of calcium and phosphorus to support normal mineralization of bone. The active form of vitamin D_3 acts on the gut to promote absorption of calcium and phosphate and on bone to increase calcium and phosphate mobilization. Its deficiency causes *rickets* and *osteomalacia*.

Vitamin E. This vitamin acts on the germinal epithelium, and deficiency causes infertility, red-cell fragility and muscular dystrophy in animals. It protects cell membrane lipids from oxidation, thus maintaining low cellular peroxide levels. In humans, deficiency can develop in association with defective lipid absorption or transport. Selenium also acts as an antioxidant and therefore decreases vitamin E requirements. Deficiency takes months to develop because vitamin E stores are high.

Vitamin K. Normal fat absorption is necessary for vitamin K absorption. Adequate intake is required for synthesis of *prothrombin* and other coagulation factors (VII, IX and X) in the liver. Deficiency is characterized by tendency to bleed. Patients with biliary obstruction, which leads to failure of fat absorption, may develop vitamin K deficiency and therefore tend to bleed. Such patients require vitamin K injections before surgery. A water-soluble analogue (K_3) is available for clinical use. Vitamin K also plays a significant role in calcification.

Minerals

Calcium and iron have well-known roles in human and animal nutrition. Other minerals are needed in varying amounts. Those required in minute quantities (less than 100 mg/day) are referred to as trace elements. Some trace elements have attracted attention and acquired significance in human nutrition. The following account describes the main sources and physiological roles of minerals and trace elements.

Calcium

Calcium is the most abundant mineral in the human body and is required throughout life, but especially during periods of growth, pregnancy and lactation. The main source of calcium in the human diet is milk (160 mg/100 g) and cheese (400–1200 mg/100 g). Smaller amounts of calcium are also found in cereals and seeds. Sesame is a rich source, containing about 1200 mg/100 g. High phytic acid, oxalic acid and fibre content in the diet interferes with absorption. Calcium is absorbed mainly in the duodenum and jejunum, because of the lower pH of intestinal contents. Vitamin D is essential for its absorption, which is also enhanced by dietary protein and the presence of lactose.

Calcium is required for mineralization of bone. It is also an important constituent of body fluids, where it mediates several physiological functions in the extracellular fluid as well as intracellularly. These functions are discussed in relation to the physiology of the different organs. The calcium turnover is shown in Fig. 7.1. The regulation of the plasma calcium level will be discussed with parathyroid function (Chapter 9).

Fig. 7.1 An overview of calcium turnover and exchange in the body.

Fig. 7.2 An overview of iron turnover and exchange in the body.

Phosphorus

Milk and its products are the main source of phosphorus in the human diet. Cow's milk has a higher phosphorus concentration than human milk. When diluted, cow's milk has a lower calcium/phosphorus ratio than human milk. This can lead to lower calcium absorption in infants fed on diluted cow's milk. Phosphorus absorption is in the jejunum and is affected by the same factors as calcium.

Phosphorus is needed in the formation of bone. Its reabsorption in the kidney is reciprocally related to that of calcium. A constant Ca : P ratio in tissue fluids is maintained by parathyroid hormone acting on bone and kidney. Hyperphosphataemia lowers the Ca : P ratio and can lead to tetany. Failure to reabsorb phosphorus in the renal tubules leads to hypophosphataemia, which can cause osteomalacia and rickets. Phosphorus and calcium contribute to the regulation of the conversion of vitamin D into its active form *calcitriol* (see Chapter 9). Phosphorus plays important roles in energy metabolism (ATP), in phosphate buffers and in phospholipids.

Iron

The adult male and non-menstruating female loses approximately 1.0 mg/day of iron. Of this amount, 50–60% is lost from the gastrointestinal tract and excreted in the bile or lost by shedding of mucosal cells. The remaining 40–50% is lost from the skin and the hair and in the urine. Iron is obtained from meat, cereals, pulses and vegetables. Red meats contain 2–3 mg/100 g in the form of haem. White meats contain 0.5–1 mg/100 g and liver has 7–10 mg/100 g. 'Hilba' (fenugreek seed) has a very high content—22 mg/100 g of dry seeds—and pulses have 2–9 mg/100 g. Iron is absorbed mainly in the duodenum and upper jejunum in the ferric state. The oxidation of ferrous to ferric iron is accomplished by means of vitamin C, HCl and an NADH-dependent flavoprotein. Absorption depends on a protein receptor, apoferritin, found in the intestinal mucosa. The rate of absorption seems to be controlled by the amount of iron accepted by the intestinal mucosa in response to the body's requirement. The latter is reflected by the amount of available iron in the blood. There is no specific mechanism for adjusting the rate of excretion of iron; therefore, the iron content of the body is regulated by the rate of absorption. Normally only about 10% of dietary iron is absorbed. The absorption of iron may be interfered with in the presence of phytic acid and oxalate, which are usually found in whole-cereal flour and other plant foods. That is why iron from plant sources (non-haem iron) is poorly absorbed.

Iron is required for synthesis of haemoglobin, myoglobin and the cytochrome oxidase enzymes. Haemoglobin contains about 67% of body iron, and about 30% is found in the storage forms of ferritin and haemosiderin. Figure 7.2 gives an overview of iron turnover.

Table 7.8 Recommended daily allowances (RDA).

	Body-weight (kg)	Energy (kcal)	Energy (MJ)	Protein (g)	Vit. A (retinol) (µg)	Vit. D (µg)	Thiamine (mg)	Riboflavine (riboflavin) (mg)	Niacin (mg)	Folic acid (µg)	Vit. B$_{12}$ (µg)	Ascorbic acid (mg)	Calcium (g)	Iron (mg)
Children														
1	7.3	820	3.4	14	300	10.0	0.3	0.5	5.4	60	0.3	20	0.5–0.6	5–10
1–3	13.4	1360	5.7	16	250	10.0	0.5	0.8	9.0	100	0.9	20	0.4–0.5	5–10
4–6	20.2	1830	7.6	20	300	10.0	0.7	1.1	12.1	100	1.5	20	0.4–0.5	5–10
7–9	28.1	2190	9.2	25	400	2.5	0.9	1.3	14.5	100	1.5	20	0.4–0.5	5–10
Male adolescents														
10–12	36.9	2600	10.9	30	575	2.5	1.0	1.6	17.2	100	2.0	20	0.6–0.7	5–10
13–15	51.3	2900	12.1	37	725	2.5	1.2	1.7	19.1	200	2.0	30	0.6–0.7	9–18
16–19	62.9	3070	12.8	38	750	2.5	1.2	1.8	20.3	200	2.0	30	0.5–0.6	5–9
Female adolescents														
10–12	38.0	2350	9.8	29	575	2.5	0.9	1.4	15.5	100	2.0	20	0.6–0.7	5–10
13–15	49.9	2490	10.4	31	725	2.5	0.9	1.4	16.4	200	2.0	30	0.6–0.7	12–24
16–19	54.4	2310	9.7	30	750	2.5	0.9	1.4	15.2	200	2.0	30	0.5–0.6	14–28
Adult man (moderately active)														
	65.0	3000	12.6	37	750	2.5	1.2	1.8	19.8	200	2.0	30	0.4–0.5	5–9
Adult woman (moderately active)														
	55.0	2200	9.2	29	750	2.5	0.9	1.3	14.5	200	2.0	30	0.4–0.5	14–28
Pregnancy (latter half)														
		+350	+1.5	38	750	10.0	+0.1	+0.2	+2.3	400	3.0	50	1.0–1.2	
Lactation (first 6 months)														
		+550	+2.3	46	1200	10.0	+0.2	+0.4	+3.7	300	2.5	50	1.0–1.2	

Based on *Human Nutritional Requirements* (1974) WHO Monograph Series No. 61, Geneva.

Nutritional requirements

In the previous pages, we described the nutrients, their roles and their sources. The requirements of the human body for each of the nutrients vary with many factors. Body size is the main determinant of energy and protein requirements. However, other factors, such as age, sex and physiological state (such as periods of rapid growth, pregnancy, lactation and old age), all have an influence of nutritional requirements.

The term minimum nutritional requirement refers to the physiological amount of a nutrient used daily by the body to maintain health, growth and a general state of well-being compatible with work and leisure. Over short periods of time this can come from body stores and should therefore be replaced from the diet. If the diet does not supply these minimum requirements, the stores become depleted and nutritional deficiency diseases appear. However, recommended nutritional allowances are estimates based on food intake surveys and experimental studies. There are wide variations between individuals and populations. Therefore, an average estimate is given for a large group (e.g. children in the age-group 1–3 years, male adolescents 13–15 years,

etc.). These allowances are recommended by governments and international organizations and are usually 20% above the average for any group, allowing for a safety margin in nutritional advice and planning.

Recommendations in the USA and Europe greatly exceed surveyed nutrient intakes in developing countries. This brings up the concept of adaptation to the levels of nutrient intake available in any given community. In some societies children and adults do not attain their maximum growth potential (height and weight). They therefore adapt to the lower intake by decreasing the attained weight and height but manage to maintain health compatible with work and reproduction. Therefore, physiological nutritional requirements are not always possible to attain in developing countries. Increasing the energy intake in such communities has been found to increase productivity. Whether the recommended allowances are true requirements is difficult to say. These estimates can be considered as guidelines for nutritional planning and decision-making by the physician. They give a good margin of safety. The needs of an individual may depart significantly from the recommended average for his weight, age and sex. Table 7.8 gives the

Table 7.9 Energy cost of physical activity.

Classification of workloads	kJ	kcal	W
Very light	< 10	< 2.5	< 170
Light	10–20	2.5–4.9	170–350
Moderate	21–30	5.0–7.4	350–500
Heavy	31–40	7.5–9.9	500–650
Very heavy	41–50	10–12.5	650–800
Exceedingly heavy	> 50	> 12.5	> 800

Very light work	*Light work*	*Moderate work*
Most office jobs	Driving	Digging
Sitting, writing or reading	Electrical work	Shovelling
Needlework	House cleaning	Mechanical repairs
Cooking	Operating machines	Walking
Playing a musical instrument	Carpentry	Cycling up to 16 kph
		Tennis

Heavy work	*Very heavy work*	*Exceedingly heavy work*
Carrying loads	Fast swimming	Felling trees
Swimming	Sprinting	High performers in competitive athletics, e.g.
Cycling at > 16 kph	Cross-country running	long-distance running
Walking uphill	Hill climbing	
Jogging		
Football		

Definitions
Kilocalorie (kcal) = amount of heat energy required to raise the temperature of 1 kg water by 1°C
　　　　1 kcal = 4.184 kJ
　　Kilojoule (kJ) = amount of energy required to move 1 kg mass 1 m by a force of 1 newton (N)
　　Watt (W) = the power resulting from the exertion of 1 kJ energy for 1 s
　　　　1 W = 0.06 kJ/min
　　　　　　= 0.0144 kcal/min

recommended allowances as given by the United Nations Food and Agriculture Organization (FAO) and the World Health Organization (WHO).

Energy requirements

The requirements of an individual depend on five variables: body-weight, physical activity, body composition, age and climate.

1 *Body-weight.* A large person needs more energy to move about, to climb stairs, etc. Energy expenditure experiments show that the energy required for a given task varies directly with body-weight. Furthermore, the energy needed for maintenance of body functions at resting or basal conditions varies directly with body-weight, which is representative of active cell mass.

2 *Physical activity.* Occupational and recreational work are more variable than other daily activities. A person working as a manual labourer needs more energy than an office clerk. A person who swims or plays football in his/her leisure time spends more energy than one whose hobby is reading or music. Table 7.9 gives the energy cost of various occupational and leisure activities.

3 *Body composition.* Lean body tissues have a higher metabolic rate than fat. Therefore, the higher the fat content, the lower the energy requirement. This factor is responsible for the sex difference in basal metabolic rate (BMR) often described in textbooks.

4 *Age.* Two factors are responsible for the effect of age: physical activity and the basal metabolic rate, both of which decrease with age. Children are very active, while elderly people tend to decrease their physical activity and eventually retire. The basal metabolic rate is high in children and decreases with age. It depends on many factors, such as body composition and active cell mass.

5 *Climate.* Extremes of climatic conditions tend to restrict physical activity (behavioural adaptation). The BMR is also found to vary with climate. It is lower in people living in hot environments. This means that at rest they produce less heat. We therefore consider this as a physiological adaptation.

Protein requirements

The economy of protein metabolism is such that daily protein turnover is about seven times the amount of amino acids required per day. This emphasizes that proteins are constantly broken down and the amino acids are reutilized. The reutilization is incomplete and this is why dietary amino acids are required. There is an obligatory loss of amino acid nitrogen, which has to be replaced to maintain nitrogen balance. The obligatory (or endogenous) nitrogen loss in a 65 kg man is 3.5 g/day, which is equivalent to 22 g of protein. This can be taken as the minimum protein requirement. Estimates of protein requirements are largely based on nitrogen balance studies. Additional amounts of protein are required for normal growth in infants, children and adolescents and during pregnancy and lactation. During the first 3 months of life, an infant needs 2.4 g/kg body-weight. Between the ages of 3 and 12 months, it falls to between 1.85 and 1.44 g/kg. Adequate energy is required for protein utilization in growth. In adolescents, increasing the energy intake was found to decrease oxidation of amino acids and enhance protein synthesis.

Infants and children

Infancy is defined as the 1st year of life. During this period, the infant doubles its weight at best and at 1 year his/her weight may be three times the birth weight. This rapid growth rate requires relatively high nutritional requirements. Energy needs are determined by his or her basal metabolism, rate of growth, body size, age and activity. Enough calories must be provided to ensure growth and to spare protein from being used as energy. The best way to determine the adequacy of infants' energy intakes is to carefully monitor their gain in height and weight. Energy needs are supplied by carbohydrate and fat in milk during the first 6 months. Thereafter, energy also comes from supplementary feeding in the form of cereals and other strained and cooked foods, including meat, vegetables and fruits, which also supply additional protein, minerals and vitamins.

There is a relative decrease in the energy requirements with age. Obviously, the quantities recommended increase with age because of the increase in body-weight. Protein requirements during infancy, when there is rapid growth, are higher on a per kilogram basis than those of the adult or older child. Nitrogen from protein must be provided for the

Table 7.10 The relationship between infant's age, energy requirements and protein requirements.

Age (months)	Energy requirements		Protein requirements	
	(kJ/kg)	(kcal/kg)	(g/kg)	(g/day)
0–3	485	116	2.20	11
3–6	415	99	1.85	13
6–9	400	95	1.65	14
9–12	420	101	1.50	14

formation of new tissues, the maturation of tissue and the maintenance of tissues. Recommended protein requirements show a similar pattern to energy (Table 7.10).

These protein requirements are based on high-quality protein, e.g. egg white. If poorly digestible or lower-quality protein is used, then corrections will have to be made. It is essential to supply adequate energy intake for protein utilization.

Minerals are essential for new tissues, in particular calcium and iron. Milk provides the required calcium. After the 6th month, supplementary iron is necessary. It should be remembered that cow's or goat's milk has a high phosphorus content compared with human milk; this may lead to hypocalcaemia. To treat this, the Ca : P ratio in the feeds should be raised to 4 : 1. Hypocalcaemia is also associated with Mg deficiency and may give rise to tetany. Low serum Mg is also encountered in protein–energy malnutrition (PEM). Copper deficiency may be due to prolonged parenteral treatment, chronic diarrhoea and other diseases. It causes anaemia, loss of appetite and retardation of growth. Zinc deficiency has been reported in association with protein depletion. The daily requirement for infants is 3–5 mg.

Sodium and potassium are found in milk and other infant foods. These can easily be lost in diarrhoea and vomiting. Gastroenteritis (inflammation of the gastrointestinal tract) is a common condition in out-patients and paediatric wards. Therefore, dehydration is a common occurrence. In addition to the fluid loss, there is also loss of electrolytes and shifts of fluid between the intracellular and extracellular compartments. To prevent the occurrence of hypertonic dehydration or hypokalaemia, attention should be given to replacement fluid therapy, either oral or intravenous. Giving normal infant foods may be dangerous, as this can increase the tonicity of extracellular fluid, which may lead to convulsions and loss of consciousness.

Vitamin requirements during infancy are met by milk and supplementary feeding; therefore, vitamin deficiencies

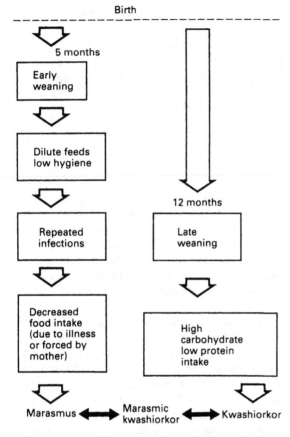

Fig. 7.3 Diagrammatic scheme of the causation of protein–calorie malnutrition. (Based on Maclaren, D.A. (1966) A fresh look at protein–calorie malnutrition. *Lancet* **ii**, 485–8.)

are uncommon. However, some infants who are breast-fed may develop vitamin K deficiency in the first few days after birth, giving rise to haemorrhagic disease of the newborn. Vitamin D is needed for calcium metabolism and skeletal growth in children. Since this nutrient is also synthesized in the skin, the amount required from dietary sources is dependent on factors such as geographical location and time spent out of doors. Children living in tropical areas may need no dietary vitamin D. In temperate zones, however, some dietary source is needed. Other fat-soluble vitamin deficiencies are seen with children who have malabsorption of fat, e.g. steatorrhoea. Recommended daily intakes are given in Table 7.8. Of particular importance is vitamin C. Milk is a poor source of this vitamin. Therefore, a mixed diet should aim at providing it for infants and children.

Protein–energy malnutrition (PEM) (Fig. 7.3) occurs in developing countries due to food shortages, poor nutritional

education, recurrent infection or a combination of these factors. Typically it affects children under 5 years old.

Marasmus is the name given to protein and energy deficiency. This is seen in infants and children when there is a general shortage of food. It can be seen in adults also in famine situations. Poverty and poor housing conditions, as in slums and unauthorized settlements around big cities, predispose to PEM. Repeated infections, especially of the respiratory system and the gastrointestinal tract, early weaning and enforced dietary restrictions during such illnesses are among the common causes of this disorder. Misinformed mothers may stop breast-feeding too early if a second pregnancy occurs.

The victims of this disease are emaciated, i.e. they lose subcutaneous fat and suffer severe muscle-wasting. They have a typical skin-and-bone appearance. Infants exhibit an anxious facial expression. These children get diarrhoea and gastroenteritis, leading to severe dehydration. The abdomen is often distended with gas. The child is usually severely underweight. Height is less affected (Fig. 7.4a).

Kwashiorkor is the name given to PEM when the disease is due to protein deficiency associated with adequate energy intake. It affects children of 2–4 years old when the food supplements contain energy-rich but low protein contents. The typical example of kwashiorkor is the sugar baby of Jamaica. An abundance of sugar combined with poor protein foods leads to the development of a typical kwashiorkor picture (Fig. 7.4b).

The child usually has oedema, enlargement of the liver and muscle-wasting but abundant subcutaneous fat. Although growth is retarded, weight is less severely affected because of the oedema. The child is apathetic and does not cry often, unlike the anxious marasmic child. In kwashiorkor there are skin lesions and the hair is thin, depigmented and easy to pluck. There is anaemia. Impaired intestinal absorption may lead to vitamin and mineral deficiencies.

The term marasmic kwashiorkor is given to a mixture of the above two extremes of PEM when various degrees of protein and energy deficiencies occur. A PEM marasmic child fed on sweetened drinks develops kwashiorkor signs, while a protein-deficient child who is too weak or apathetic to take adequate amounts of food develops marasmic signs. In clinical practice, then, these children are simply diagnosed as PEM.

Nutrition in physiological stress

There are times when the physiological nutritional requirements are increased; therefore, dietary deficiencies are more likely to occur. Three such states will be presented:

(a)

(b)

Fig. 7.4 (a) A child with marasmus. (b) A child with kwashiorkor. (Reproduced with permission from R.G. Whitehead, Director, Dunn Nutrition Centre, Cambridge, UK.)

adolescence, pregnancy and lactation. Average recommended allowances for these states will be found in Table 7.8. It should be noted, however, that individual requirements may be significantly different, depending on the nutritional status of the subject before the physiological demand has increased.

Adolescence

The adolescent period is associated with rapid physical growth (growth spurt), sexual maturation and psychological stresses. There is an increase in energy requirements due to the rapid physical growth and increased physical activity, particularly in adolescent boys. Adolescent girls tend to store fat, which is considered as a secondary sexual characteristic of the female body. Protein requirements increase and should supply 12–15% of the total energy. Carbohydrates should supply about 50% and fat about 30–45% of the daily energy intake.

Calcium requirements increase dramatically by about 400 mg/day, due to rapid skeletal growth in boys and girls. Iron intake should be particularly monitored, as anaemia can easily occur due to the rapid increase in muscle mass and blood volume. Females are more likely to become

deficient due to menstrual losses (15–30 mg/period) and the possibility of pregnancy, especially in societies where early marriage is common. An additional 10–15 mg/day of iron is recommended for females and 5–10 mg/day for males. These represent about 80% more for boys and 120% more for girls.

As to the need for vitamins in adolescence, high amounts of thiamine, riboflavine (riboflavin) and niacin are recommended because of the high energy requirements. In most cases, because of increased energy intake, the intake of B vitamins will also increase.

Pregnancy

The fetus, placenta and maternal response to pregnancy constitute the three factors which determine the nutritional needs. If pregnancy occurs before the age of 17 years, the additional demands of adolescence may compromise the growth of both mother and fetus. The nutritional status and therefore the nutrient reserves of the mother before gestation are an important determinant of her nutritional requirements.

The daily energy requirements of pregnancy increase by about 1.5 MJ on average per day—about 10–15%

Table 7.11 Nutritional allowances of the pregnant mother compared with non-pregnant requirements.

	Non-pregnant	Pregnant
Energy (MJ)	9.2	10.7
Protein (g)	29	35
Calcium (mg)	200	400
Iron (mg)	14–28	14–28
Vitamin A (retinol) (µg)	750	750
Vitamin D (µg)	2.5	10
Vitamin B_1 (mg)	0.9	1.0
Vitamin B_2 (mg)	1.3	1.5
Niacin (mg)	14.5	16.8
Vitamin C (mg)	30	50
Vitamin B_{12} (µg)	2.0	3.0
Folic acid (µg)	200	400

more than the previous requirement. This is due to a general increase in the basal metabolism, energy storage and energy expenditure. As anticipated from the physiological changes of body composition, most of the energy intake goes into the fat stores during the second trimester. This period is usually associated with a good appetite and rapid weight gain. During the third trimester more energy expenditure is associated with the mother's movement, due to the increased body-weight. At this stage, energy is needed to spare protein for fetal growth. However, the total energy requirements may not increase very much because at this stage most mothers tend to keep their physical activities to a minimum.

Additional protein is obviously needed during pregnancy to support the synthesis of maternal and fetal tissues, and needs increase as pregnancy proceeds. The recommended daily intake of protein during pregnancy increases by 6 g/day. Table 7.11 gives the nutritional requirements during the latter half of pregnancy as recommended by the WHO. Other authorities recommend 20 g/day. During the first trimester little extra protein is required. Protein is required mainly for the growth of the uterus and the fetus, both of which are greatest during the third trimester. Protein is also required for growth of the breasts and the increased blood volume. Adverse results of protein deficiency during pregnancy are difficult to separate from the effects of energy deficiency in clinical situations. Almost all cases of limited protein intake are accompanied by limitation in availability of energy; under such conditions, decreased birth weight and greater incidence of pre-eclampsia have been reported.

The mother's diet should supply adequate iron throughout pregnancy. During the first trimester a normal diet will give the required iron supply. A marginally adequate diet,

however, will not be satisfactory during the second and third trimesters. It is therefore advised that iron therapy (30–60 mg/day) should be given to mothers in developing countries throughout pregnancy to build up maternal stores and to prevent iron-deficiency anaemia. This is essential for the extra maternal haemoglobin, fetal blood and liver stores and maternal stores of iron to meet delivery losses and to prepare for lactation. An anaemic woman is clearly less able to tolerate haemorrhage with delivery and she is more prone to develop puerperal infection.

The mother needs calcium, mainly for the growth and calcification of fetal bones. This is most active during the third trimester. During early pregnancy, most of the extra calcium requirements can be provided from the mother's bones. Milk is a good source of both calcium and protein. All mothers should be advised to take 0.5 litres of milk per day, especially during the second and third trimesters. This amount provides an extra 17 g of protein and 600 mg of calcium. The recommended daily allowance is 1000–1200 mg. As only about 30% of the dietary calcium is absorbed, this intake should provide an adequate margin of safety.

The vitamin requirements of pregnant women are only moderately increased. Therefore, a normal balanced diet is usually adequate. However, in developing countries vitamin supplements are usually given as part of antenatal care when the economic status of the family is poor. Table 7.11 indicates the marked increase in vitamin D requirements during pregnancy to increase the absorption and use of calcium and phosphorus. This supply can normally be synthesized in the body if adequate exposure of the skin to sunlight is ensured. This is important to facilitate the absorption of calcium and for active calcification in the fetal skeleton. Interest in vitamin K in pregnancy largely centres on haemorrhagic disease of the newborn due to vitamin K deficiency. Parenteral vitamin K is often administered to parturient women since the newborn has a sterile gut and bacterial synthesis of vitamin K is thus an unreliable source in the neonatal period. Ascorbic acid deficiency has not been shown to affect the course or outcome of pregnancy in humans. However, because low plasma levels of ascorbic acid have been reported to be associated with premature rupture of the membranes, as well as pre-eclampsia, questions have arisen about its possible association with these conditions. Folic acid demands increase by 100%, mainly for maternal haemopoiesis and fetoplacental growth. Folate deficiency will lead to megaloblastic anaemia, which frequently occurs in pregnancy.

Intrauterine nutrition is an important prerequisite for fetal development and attaining a good weight at birth. It should be emphasized that fetal stores of minerals and

Table 7.12 The relationship between milk production and age of lactating baby.

Age of baby (months)	Milk production (ml)
1	500
2	800
3	900
4–6	900–1000
7–9	1000–1200
10–12	1300–1500

vitamins are used during the early postnatal period. In particular, good iron stores are necessary for the prevention of anaemia during infancy. For the first 6 months, the baby depends on these stores because milk is a poor source of iron. More information on the fetoplacental unit will be found in Chapter 15.

An important aspect of fetal growth during the last trimester is the rapid growth of the fetal brain. It has a maximum growth rate about the 34th week of pregnancy. Therefore, adequate nutrition at this critical stage is of vital importance for intrauterine brain development.

Lactation
The nutritional requirements of lactating mothers are similar to those during pregnancy. Milk production is the main concern. Table 7.12 shows that the quantity of milk produced increases as the baby grows.

One litre of milk has about 2.7 MJ (650 kcal) of energy. The metabolic energy cost of its production is estimated at about 1.6 MJ (400 kcal). However, the total recommended daily energy intake is 2.1 MJ (500 kcal). It is assumed that the extra energy will come from the body stores of fat deposited during pregnancy (about 4 kg). The daily energy intake of the mother will depend on the amount of milk she is producing and the state of her body stores.

The WHO recommends an additional protein intake of 17.5 g during the first 6 months and 13 g thereafter. Some other authorities recommend an additional 20 g daily. The amounts of calcium and iron required during lactation are the same as those required by the pregnant mother. Vitamin C should be increased to 50–60 mg/day. Vitamin A (retinol) recommended intake should be increased by 400 µg. The vitamin B group is also marginally increased above those required for pregnancy, except folic acid, which is about 300 µg/day compared with 200 µg in non-pregnant women and 400 µg during pregnancy.

Lactating mothers should take adequate amounts of fluid, especially in hot weather, to ensure adequate milk production. Breast-feeding mothers should be discouraged from dieting to control body-weight. They should also be advised that use of oral contraceptives may suppress lactation, especially in the first 6–10 weeks after giving birth.

Energy metabolism

The term metabolism means 'change'. It is used to describe enzyme-catalysed chemical reactions in which large molecules are broken into smaller ones (catabolism) and others in which smaller molecules are used for the synthesis of larger and more complex ones (anabolism).

In general, *catabolic* or degradative processes produce energy, whereas *anabolic* or synthetic processes consume energy but result in storage or growth. The body requires energy for the generation of heat, for exercise and locomotion, for the synthesis of new tissues and for various cellular activities, such as maintenance of ionic gradients, processes of secretion and detoxification. To provide these energy needs, various tissues oxidize glucose (from carbohydrate), free fatty acids (FFAs) and ketone bodies (from fat) and amino acids (from proteins). These energy-containing substrates or metabolic fuels are provided as a mixture to tissues in the bloodstream and their oxidation is linked to the generation of a limited number of high-energy compounds, of which ATP is the most important. It is extremely important to appreciate that ATP does not function as a simple store of chemical energy in the cell. In combination with adenosine diphosphate (ADP), ATP functions as an energy transfer system in the cell; the generation of ATP from ADP during the oxidation of fuels (e.g. glucose) conserves chemical energy, which is utilized in a number of processes (Fig. 7.5).

Since the human digestive system does not provide a continuous supply of nutrients at a rate suitable for requirements, the ability to survive depends on systems for storage of metabolic fuels when they are in excess and their release as required. The metabolic fuels, such as glucose, FFAs and amino acids, cannot be stored as such to any great extent, due to osmotic problems. Instead, they are stored in the form of macromolecules in *adipose tissue* (as triacylglycerol), in *liver* and *skeletal muscle* (as glycogen) and in skeletal muscle (as proteins); however, the available metabolic fuels are related to body composition (Fig. 7.6). In addition, metabolic fuels are found in the circulation as their constituents: carbohydrate, mainly as glucose but also (as in exercise) lactate and pyruvate; fats as FFAs and glycerol; and protein as amino acids (mainly alanine and glutamine) (see Fig. 7.6).

The biochemical pathways for the transformation of energy are outside the scope of this book. However, the following section will deal with the rate of liberation of energy in the whole body and its regulation.

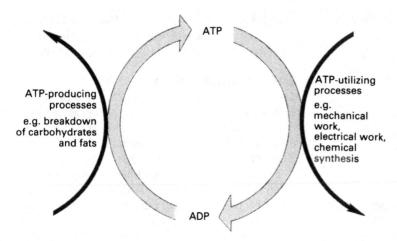

Fig. 7.5 The ATP–ADP cycle. (Redrawn from Weatherall, D.J., Ledingham, J.G.G. & Warrell, D.A. (eds) (1987) *Oxford Textbook of Medicine*, 2nd edn. With permission from Oxford University Press, Oxford.)

Fig. 7.6 Diagrammatic presentation of the available metabolic fuels in the normal adult. (Redrawn from Weatherall, D.J., Ledingham, J.G.G. & Warrell, D.A. (eds) (1987) *Oxford Textbook of Medicine*, 2nd edn. With permission from the Oxford University Press, Oxford.)

The metabolic rate

The amount of energy released in the body varies with the amount of work performed and the amount of heat produced. Any excess energy intake will go into the body stores, i.e. there is no significant excretion of energy-containing compounds under physiological conditions. However, the utilization of energy as external work is not so efficient (see Chapter 13). It has been found that the rate of energy

metabolism is directly related to *oxygen consumption*. The uptake of oxygen by the subject is used in measuring the *metabolic rate*, as will be described later in this section.

The production of CO_2 varies with the fuel being utilized. Thus, when glucose is the only source of energy being used at a certain time, the ratio of CO_2 produced to O_2 consumed during a given interval of time is equal to 1 (i.e. $(CO_2/O_2) = 1$). This ratio is known as the **respiratory quotient (RQ)**. In the case of glucose oxidation, it can be appreciated from the chemical reaction:

$$C_6H_{12}O_6 + 6\,O_2 \rightarrow 6\,CO_2 + 6\,H_2O + energy$$

$$RQ\ (ratio) = \frac{6}{6} = 1.00$$

When fatty acids are used for energy production, the RQ is found to be 0.70. The RQ also goes under another name, the *respiratory exchange ratio (R)*. The RQ for protein is 0.82. It appears from this description that the mixture of fuels (*the metabolic mixture*) being used at a given time will determine the RQ. We also know that the energy released by carbohydrates, fats and proteins is different. In the human body, 1 g of carbohydrate or protein yields 17 kJ (4 kcal) and 1 g of fat yields 39 kJ (9 kcal). The relevance of the RQ to energy metabolism is that it can be used to arrive at an energy equivalent for the O_2 utilized. Figure 7.7 gives the energy equivalent of 1 litre of O_2 utilized at different respiratory quotients, i.e. with different metabolic mixtures. In this case, the non-protein RQ is used, which means that the energy due to protein is deducted by calculation of the amount of protein used, as indicated by urinary nitrogen.

The basal metabolic rate (BMR)

The rate of energy release at basal conditions is known as the **BMR**. A person is described to be in a basal state when

RQ   kJ

Energy equivalent for one litre of oxygen

Fig. 7.7 Nomogram for determination of the energy equivalent of O_2 at different RQs.

he/she is fully rested, at least 12 hours after the last meal. Measurement of the BMR gives the minimum energy expenditure of the individual and allows comparisons to be made with normal values.

Basal metabolism represents the energy used for the vital physiological processes of the body, such as the work of the heart, respiration, brain and all the continuing cellular activities, such as synthesis of protein and the all-important active transport of ions and compounds across cell membranes.

The conditions for measuring the BMR are:
1 A good night's sleep, i.e. physical rest.
2 Last meal 12 hours before measurement.
3 The patient should be in a comfortable room temperature (no sweating or shivering or extra cardiovascular work).
4 The patient should be mentally relaxed.
A good night's sleep ensures physical and mental rest. Explaining the procedure to the patient is important so as not to cause anxiety before and during measurement. A comfortable room temperature will avoid activation of mechanisms associated with temperature regulation.

The reason for having the last meal 12 hours before-hand is that food intake is associated with stimulation of secretion, gut movement and absorption processes, all of which increase energy release. Even more important is the metabolic energy release in the liver stimulated by

Fig. 7.8 Nomogram for determination of body surface area. A line joining the height and weight values of the subject crosses the middle scale and the value of body surface area is read in m^2.

incoming food substances. The increase in energy production after food intake is known as the **specific dynamic action (SDA)**. It is specific because each food substrate has a specific effect, e.g. protein increases the BMR by 30% of its energy content; carbohydrates and fats have an SDA of 6 and 4%, respectively.

Factors affecting the BMR. The BMR is usually expressed as kcal/m^2/hour. The unit of surface area of the body (m^2) provide a means of allowing comparisons to be made between individuals of different size. The surface area can be obtained from a nomogram (Fig. 7.8) based on height and weight. Using this unified expression, it has been found that animals of different size have closely similar BMRs.

Pulley

Bell cylinder

O₂

Valve

Water seal

CO₂ absorber

Mouth piece

Valve

Rotating drum

Kymograph

Fig. 7.9 The Benedict–Roth spirometer used for measuring O_2 consumption by the closed-circuit method.

This makes physiological sense because the area of the skin is closely related to the amount of heat loss. Using this expression, it was found that **age** and **sex** were factors which affect the BMR. Small infants have a higher BMR than children and adults. The BMR also falls in old age.

Females have lower BMRs than males. However, the sex difference disappears if the BMR is expressed in terms of kcal/kg lean body mass/hour. The *lean body mass* is used instead of surface area. Women have more fat than men and, as fat has a lower metabolic rate than lean tissues, their BMR appears lower when this is not taken into account. Therefore, there is no real sex difference but a difference due to **body composition**.

Other factors include the **emotional state** (level of catecholamines), **climate**, state of the **menstrual cycle**, **pregnancy**, **lactation**, **body temperature** and level of **thyroid hormones** (see Chapter 9).

Measurement of the metabolic rate

Direct calorimetry. This method directly measures the heat produced by the body during a given period of time. The subject sits inside a specially designed heat-insulated chamber (**body calorimeter**). The heat gained by the chamber is measured. This method is difficult and was used in the early days of research on energy metabolism.

Indirect calorimetry. Indirect methods use the measurement of O_2 consumption for calculation of energy expenditure. A closed-circuit method employs a floating cylinder filled with oxygen at atmospheric pressure, from which the subject breathes. Expired air, which contains both O_2 and CO_2, is returned to the cylinder through appropriate valves (Fig. 7.9). The passage of expired air goes through a small cylinder of *soda lime*, which absorbs the CO_2. Thus, when the subject continues to breathe in and out of this system, the amount of oxygen decreases gradually with each breath. This decrease is recorded graphically on a moving *kymograph*. Thus, a record of O_2 consumption per unit time is obtained. You may have the opportunity of seeing this simple method in your practical physiology course.

An open-circuit method is also used. The subject in this case breathes in *atmospheric air* and breathes out into a special large bag, in which all the expired air is collected over 5–10 min. The volume of expired air is then measured by a gas flowmeter. This is the **Douglas bag** method. A sample of the expired air is then collected from a side tube and analysed. O_2 consumption and CO_2 production can be calculated by comparison with the atmospheric air which was inspired. Other open circuits are now available which make it possible for a working man/woman to carry a small instrument into which he/she breathes out his/her expired air. The instrument measures the volume of expired air and the O_2 utilization directly. This has made it much easier to measure the metabolic rate under ambulatory and field conditions.

Metabolic homoeostasis: an integrated approach

The human body, like all biological systems, requires a regular intake of nutrients, which come from plant and animal origins. Feeding is regulated by the need for exogenous energy and other nutrient sources. The intake of food takes place at mealtimes over short periods of time. Between meals, the body cells rely on endogenous stores of nutrients, which are mobilized and used according to the *state of metabolism* at any particular time.

Short-term changes in the metabolic state of an individual are brought about by three main variables: (i) food intake or its absence; (ii) the level of metabolic activities; and (iii) physical muscular activity. Quantitative and qualitative changes in metabolism take place rapidly with the **intake of food, fasting, starvation** and **muscular exercise**. Physiological states during **periods of growth, pregnancy** and **lactation** have a long-term influence on the state of nutrition and metabolism.

Under pathological conditions, certain changes also occur in the metabolic state of the individual, e.g. *liver disease, specific nutritional deficiencies, surgery* and *endocrine disorders*. Some diseases exert greater demand on one or more of the nutrients and thus lead to nutritional or metabolic abnormalities, e.g. loss of glucose in diabetes and albumin in renal diseases. Drug or hormone therapy, on the other hand, may also influence the state of metabolism of the patient so as to require nutritional and metabolic adjustments.

This section deals with the dynamic changes and physiological mechanisms which regulate the responses of the body to food intake and deprivation. It also addresses the needs of the body under steady physiological states and ageing.

Metabolic responses to feeding

The metabolic changes related to feeding may precede the entry of food into the mouth. The awareness of a coming meal and the sense of food in the mouth induce changes, such as delivery of saliva and gastric juice and secretion of gastrointestinal hormones. During feeding there is a large *positive fuel surplus* absorbed from the gastrointestinal tract. Immediately following a meal, absorption of various nutrients results in elevated blood levels of glucose, blood lipids and amino acids. The high circulating levels of glucose stimulate insulin secretion and decrease that of glucagon. The latter is particularly evident after a carbohydrate-rich meal. Absorbed carbohydrate, mainly in the form of glucose, passes first to the liver via the portal system. The liver removes about 60–80% of carbohydrate and stores some as glycogen (via enhanced hepatic **glycogenesis**) for later use, and converts the rest to fatty acids and triacylglycerols. The latter two are then secreted as very-low-density lipoproteins (VLDL), whose fatty acids are subsequently stored in adipose tissue. The rest of the glucose (20–40%) enters the peripheral tissues, where it is stored as glycogen or oxidized to provide chemical energy in the form of ATP.

Meanwhile, the *fat component* of the meal is absorbed and then released, mainly as *chylomicrons*, which reach the systemic circulation via the thoracic duct to be stored in adipose tissue. In adipose tissue, triacylglycerol uptake from chylomicrons and from VLDL is stimulated by the activation of lipoprotein lipase. At the same time, the high insulin and glucose levels inhibit triacylglycerol breakdown by the hormone-sensitive lipase and enhance esterification of fatty acids. This leads to a marked decrease in the release of FFAs and consequently decreased circulating levels of FFAs.

Amino acids are not stored as such but are utilized in protein synthesis, which is increased due to the inhibition of hepatic *gluconeogenesis* following a meal. This effect is related to the high plasma insulin/glucagon concentration ratio. The increase in insulin concentration antagonizes the action of glucagon on the liver so that gluconeogenesis is decreased. At the same time, excess amino acids are oxidized in the liver, with the exception of branched-chain amino acids (leucine, isoleucine and valine), which tend to be broken down in extrahepatic tissues, mainly skeletal muscle.

The overall effect of the meal is therefore to promote *storage* of carbohydrate as glycogen in liver and muscle, storage of triacylglycerols in liver and particularly in adipose tissue, and incorporation of amino acids

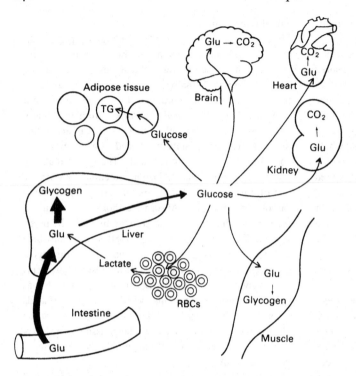

Fig. 7.10 Glucose utilization by various tissues after absorption from the small intestine. The thickness of lines indicates the flux through that route. TG, triacylglycerols; RBCs, red blood cells.

as protein, probably in all tissues. The metabolic changes in response to feeding are summarized in Fig. 7.10.

After a carbohydrate-rich meal, the RQ will rise and approach unity, reflecting suppression of fatty acid oxidation and increased use of glucose. If the meal is rich in fat, the rate of digestion, absorption and processing of lipids to produce chylomicrons is considerably slower than the digestion of carbohydrate and absorption of glucose. A problem may arise after a meal that contains much protein and little carbohydrate, due to the fact that insulin secretion under these conditions could result in *hypoglycaemia*. The decreased blood glucose is due to the inhibition of glucose production and facilitation of glucose utilization. This is normally prevented by the additional secretion of *glucagon* in response to a high-protein meal. The **absorptive phase** during and after a meal proceeds smoothly into the **post-absorptive phase**.

Metabolic responses to fasting and starvation

For simplification, the metabolic responses to starvation can be divided, into three phases: **postabsorptive phase**, **short-term starvation** and **long-term starvation**. These periods are characterized by specific metabolic changes but the transition from one to another is gradual. In practice the effects of starvation are rarely as simple as described below, since flood deprivation usually occurs against a background of injury or infection, or as part of protein–energy malnutrition or famine.

Postabsorptive phase

The postabsorptive phase starts 2–3 hours after oral glucose intake. However, a mixed meal containing protein, fibre and fat delays gastric emptying and takes longer to digest and absorb from the intestine. The postabsorptive phase in this case starts 4–6 hours after the meal.

During this phase nutrients come from the body stores, i.e. the liver and adipose tissue. This process of mobilization is triggered by the falling blood glucose. Insulin secretion is decreased and glucagon is increased. This pattern of hormone secretion leads to increased **glycogenolysis** and decreased glycogen synthesis (Fig. 7.11). **Gluconeogenesis** increases, drawing upon alanine as a main source of glucose synthesis in the liver. Tissues which depend almost entirely on glucose as a source of energy continue to use blood glucose, irrespective of the metabolic changes that take place during absorption or in the postabsorptive phase. It is pertinent to note that the liver is responsible for almost all of the glucose output in the postabsorptive state, most of which comes from *gluconeogenesis* (about 75%) and the rest from *glycogenolysis*.

In adipose tissue, the falling insulin and glucose concentrations decrease triacylglycerol synthesis and increase

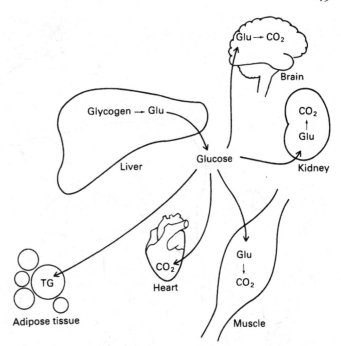

Fig. 7.11 Glucose utilization during the postabsorptive phase.

lipolysis, resulting in the enhanced release of FFAs. These are used to provide the energy needs of most tissues, such as skeletal muscle and the heart, thus sparing more glucose for other tissues. By the end of an overnight fast, the body will be oxidizing mainly fat, as indicated by an RQ value in the range of 0.7–0.8, although the brain will still be using glucose almost exclusively. However, the rate of lipolysis and the decrease of insulin secretion in the postabsorptive phase is not sufficient to stimulate hepatic conversion of free fatty acids to ketone bodies.

Release of amino acids will start to occur, mainly related to a marked decrease in the synthesis of muscle proteins under the influence of low insulin levels. In skeletal muscle, amino acids will begin to provide a source of energy (although not a major one), and alanine, together with glutamine, will predominate. These amino acids are taken up in the splanchnic circulation, where they contribute to hepatic *gluconeogenesis*, supplementing glucose production by glycogen breakdown.

The postabsorptive phase normally extends for 6–8 hours and ends when another meal is taken, or it may extend for 16–40 hours, as during fasting. The *Ramadan* fast lasts about 15 hours in the tropics. Therefore, it can be considered as a postabsorptive state with little or no effects attributable to starvation. As a matter of fact, the Ramadan fast enables endocrine and metabolic mechanisms,

stimulated during the postabsorptive state, to function to a fuller extent, unhampered by the introduction of meals at short intervals.

Short-term starvation

The metabolic changes that occur during periods of short-term starvation (2–7 days) are a continuation and acceleration of the processes that started during the postabsorptive period. The metabolic changes occurring in short-term starvation are summarized in Fig. 7.12.

During this period, the progressive decline in blood glucose and insulin concentrations, accompanied by elevated glucagon secretion, leads to increasing *release of amino acids* (mainly as glutamine and alanine) from muscle and increasing *lipolysis* in adipose tissue. Alanine, removed by the liver, lactate, produced by erythrocytes and other tissues, and glycerol, released by *lipolysis*, all contribute to an increasing rate of hepatic *gluconeogenesis*. During this period, gluconeogenesis is two to three times greater than during the postabsorptive period and is responsible for virtually all of the glucose released by the liver. Estimation of glucose production from various gluconeogenic precursors during this period of starvation is presented in Table 7.13.

The increase in gluconeogenesis during short-term starvation is associated with an increase in protein degradation and thus a substantial *negative nitrogen balance*

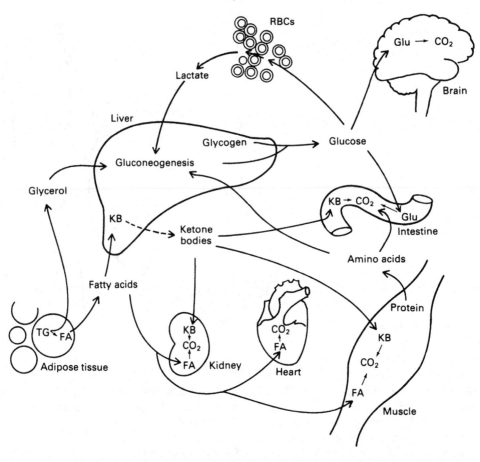

Fig. 7.12 Pattern of fuel utilization during short-term starvation. FA, fatty acids; KB, ketone bodies; RBCs, red blood cells; TG, triacylglycerols.

Table 7.13 Approximate estimates of gluconeogenic precursors during starvation in humans.

| | Glucose produced each day (g) | | |
| | Duration of starvation | | |
Gluconeogenic precursors	1 day	2–4 days	Several weeks
Lactate	40	40	40
Glycerol	20	20	20
Amino acids	60	50	15
Total glucose produced from above precursors	120	110	75
Glucose available for brain (from gluconeogenic precursors)	80	65	35
Brain energy needs (glucose equivalents)	100	100	100

Data taken from Cahill *et al.* (1966) *J. Clin. Invest.* **45**, 1751–69; Owen *et al.* (1969) *J. Clin. Invest.* **48**, 574–83; Owen *et al.* (1979) *Adv. Exp. Med. Biol.* **111**, 119–88.

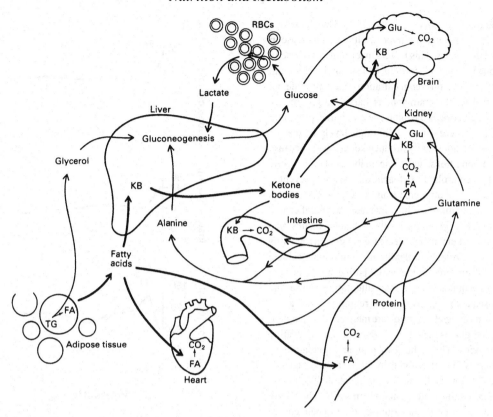

Fig. 7.13 Pattern of fuel utilization during prolonged starvation. The thickness of lines is approximately proportional to the flux through the route. FA, fatty acids; KB, ketone bodies; RBCs, red blood cells; TG, triacylglycerols.

exists, with most of the nitrogen being excreted as urinary urea. The liver at this stage takes up increasing quantities of FFAs released from adipose tissue. An increasing proportion of FFAs, under the influence of the low insulin/glucagon concentration ratio, will be channelled into oxidation, leading to increased *ketogenesis*. As a result, plasma levels of *ketone bodies* are increased. At this stage, ketone bodies will begin to provide a significant contribution to energy needs of various tissues, including muscle and brain. In fact, oxidation of ketone bodies may provide as much as 10–20% of the energy requirement of the brain.

Thus, the overall metabolism during short-term starvation is characterized by high rates of protein catabolism, gluconeogenesis and ketogenesis to meet the body's energy needs.

Long-term starvation

The metabolic changes that occur during long-term starvation (2–6 weeks) account for the ability of the body to survive prolonged periods without any caloric intake. These changes include decreased rate of protein breakdown and nitrogen excretion and increased dependence on triacylglycerol from adipose tissue for energy (Fig. 7.13).

In prolonged starvation, *hepatic glucose production* decreases from about 200 g/day during the postabsorptive period to about 50 g/day during prolonged starvation, with about 75% of hepatic glucose being derived from non-amino acid sources (i.e. lactate, pyruvate and glycerol). At the same time, *renal gluconeogenesis* becomes an important source of carbohydrate, contributing about 40 g/day (derived from amino acids), with excess nitrogen being secreted as ammonia rather than urea. Consequently, nitrogen loss progressively decreases during prolonged starvation. Moreover, since the demand for glucose is decreased during this period, the rate of *release of amino acids* from muscle is also decreased, eventually to about one-third of that in the postabsorptive state.

The increased rate of *lipolysis* of adipose tissue triacylglycerol appears to be brought about mainly by the very low insulin concentration in prolonged starvation, since sympathoadrenal activity is decreased. The increased delivery of fatty acids to the liver results in an increase in the rate of *ketogenesis*. This results in a progressive rise in blood ketone body concentrations to a steady level around 8–9 mmol/litre. At this concentration, they provide an important fuel for the brain and, as starvation progresses, they displace glucose as the main energy source, providing 60–80% of its energy needs. The high levels of plasma *ketone bodies* do not usually produce ketoacidosis because under these conditions, unlike in diabetes, ketone body production is controlled. Ketoacidosis is also prevented by the production of ammonia from renal gluconeogenesis (mainly from glutamine), which increases the renal capacity to excrete H⁺. The high levels of ketone bodies also appear to contribute to the decrease in gluconeogenesis associated with prolonged starvation, by inhibiting muscle proteolysis. Therefore, ketone bodies both decrease hepatic glucose production and serve as an alternative fuel for the brain. Consequently, the two major requirements for survival during prolonged starvation are met, namely, maintenance of blood glucose levels (Fig. 7.14) and conservation of body proteins. This control of protein degradation by fat oxidation is also illustrated in the terminal stages of starvation. As mobilizable fat supplies eventually run out, a *preterminal* rise in protein catabolism starts. The ability to withstand prolonged starvation is thus dependent on the initial amount of adipose tissue.

Among other hormones, beside insulin and glucagon, that are important in the adaptation to starvation are *thyroid hormones*, *growth hormone* and *cortisol*. Starvation causes a dramatic decrease in plasma levels of free tri-iodothyronine (fT_3) and a corresponding increase in reverse tri-iodothyronine (rT_3) concentrations. The decrease in thyroid hormones is probably responsible for the decrease in the *basal metabolic rate* that usually occurs with prolonged starvation. In addition, both growth hormone and cortisol appear to contribute to the maintenance of blood glucose and FFA mobilization.

Manifestations of starvation observed in famine victims include loss of subcutaneous fat, severe muscle-wasting and loss of elasticity of the skin. The skin becomes a dull colour and may show areas of pigmentation. The immune response is diminished and *white-cell production* is decreased. The decreased body defences make starvation

Fig. 7.14 Changes of the concentrations of: (a) plasma glucose; (b) insulin; and (c) glucagon during a period of prolonged fasting. (Based on Marliss *et al.* (1970) *J. Clin. Invest.* **49**, 2256.)

patients more exposed to infection, e.g. diarrhoeal diseases, amoebiasis, tuberculosis and pneumonia. The body defences are also decreased due to impairment of the *immune response* and decreased numbers of white blood cells. Another cause of death is shock from decreased blood volume. This may be related to *hypoalbuminaemia* due to diminished albumin production, which lowers the plasma colloid osmotic pressure, causing fluid to move from the blood to the interstitial space (famine oedema).

Further reading

1 Garrow, J.S. & James, W.P.T. (Eds) (1993) *Davidson and Passmore's Human Nutrition and Dietetics*, Part 1: *Physiology*, 9th edn, pp. 12–263. Churchill Livingstone, Edinburgh.

8 / Gastrointestinal Physiology

Objectives

On completion of the study of this section, the student should:

1 Become familiar with significant structural features of the gastrointestinal tract so as to relate structure to function.

2 Differentiate between the various types of intestinal movements so as to comprehend their role in digestion and to interpret symptoms and signs related to gut motility.

3 Understand the neurological and hormonal mechanisms which control the digestive functions, in particular:

  (a) Control of salivary secretions.

  (b) Control of gastric secretions.

  (c) Control of secretions of pancreatic juice.

  (d) Control of formation and release of bile.

  (e) Control of secretion of intestinal juice.

4 Apply the above knowledge in selecting methods for assessment of the functions of the stomach, pancreas, liver and gall-bladder.

5 Understand the processes of digestion and absorption of various food substances so as to give appropriate dietary advice to patients.

6 Understand the functions of the colon in order to explain clinical problems such as diarrhoea and constipation.

Introduction

Food consists mostly of complex substances such as carbohydrates, lipids, proteins, vitamins and minerals. Before they can be absorbed into the body, carbohydrates, fats and proteins have to be broken down or modified to simpler forms. It is the function of the gastrointestinal tract to *secrete enzymes* which break down the complex food materials into simple forms, a process referred to as *digestion*, and then to convey the end-products to the bloodstream, the process being referred to as *absorption*. While the food is being processed, it needs to be mixed and propelled along the tract, and this is achieved by various types of coordinated movement (*motility*). The functions of motility, secretion, digestion and absorption of food are integrated at each level of the gastrointestinal tract. To understand these functions, the reader will follow the path of food from the mouth to the anus, rather than deal with each of the major functions separately, i.e. motility, secretion and absorption throughout the tract.

Anatomical considerations

The gastrointestinal tract is simply a tube with muscle walls throughout its length; it is lined by an epithelium which is adapted for the function of the various parts of the tract. The salivary glands, the liver and the pancreas pour their secretions into the gut lumen. Basically, the tube is composed of four layers (Fig. 8.1), which are, from within outwards:

1 The mucosa, consisting of the lining epithelium, interepithelial connective tissue or lamina propria and a layer of longitudinal smooth muscle, the muscularis mucosae.

2 The submucosa, containing, in addition to connective tissue, the blood-vessels and lymphatics and a network of neurons and nerve fibres referred to as the **submucous** or **Meissner's plexus**.

3 The intestinal muscle layers consist generally of inner circular and outer longitudinal layers. This basic arrangement may be modified, e.g. the longitudinal layer is modified into the taeniae coli in the large intestine. The circular layer is modified in certain places to form sphincters. Except for the muscle in the upper third of the oesophagus

and in the external anal sphincter, which is striated, the muscle in the rest of the alimentary tract is smooth. Between the two external muscle layers lies the **myenteric (Auerbach's) plexus**, containing a network of neurons and fibres.

4 The serosa provides an outer fibrous coat and continues on to the mesentery and the peritoneal lining of the abdominal cavity.

Blood supply

The gut is well supplied with blood. Blood from the stomach, most of the intestine, the pancreas and the spleen drains via the portal vein into the liver, and the combined vascular bed of these organs comprises the splanchnic circulation. The splanchnic vascular bed receives about 25–30% of the cardiac output.

Control of gastrointestinal functions

Generally, secretion and motility in the gastrointestinal tract are controlled by nervous and hormonal mechanisms, which are closely integrated so that control may better be described as neurohormonal.

The enteric nervous system (ENS)

Mechanical and chemical changes in the gut are conveyed to the central nervous system via *visceral afferent* fibres travelling in the vagi and spinal nerves, while *efferent* fibres reach the gut in sympathetic and parasympathetic nerves.

   Sympathetic fibres pass in the splanchnic nerves, which synapse in the ganglia in front of the aorta, and postganglionic fibres reach the gut. Most of the **parasympathetic**

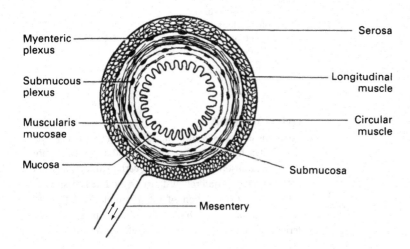

Fig. 8.1 Diagram of a transverse section through the gut to show the layers in the gut wall.

outflow to the gut is in the vagi, which provide fibres to the gut from the oesophagus down to the middle of the transverse colon. The remaining part of the colon, rectum and anal canal receive parasympathetic fibres in the pelvic splanchnic nerves. All the parasympathetic fibres are preganglionic; they synapse with postganglionic neurons in the submucous and myenteric plexuses, and short postganglionic fibres reach glands and smooth-muscle cells of the gastrointestinal tract. Some of the postganglionic sympathetic fibres end on intestinal smooth-muscle cells but many fibres end on cholinergic neurons of the intrinsic nerve plexuses. They release noradrenaline, which inhibits the release of acetylcholine from the intrinsic neurons.

Thus, according to the classical concept of the autonomic nervous system, the neurons and nerve fibres in the wall of the gut (*intrinsic neurons*) are merely parts of the system consisting of sympathetic (noradrenergic) fibres and parasympathetic (cholinergic) neurons. In addition to these, the intrinsic nerve supply, consisting of the **submucous** and **myenteric plexuses**, contains many other types of neurons, some of which release serotonin (5-hydroxytryptamine (5-HT)) as transmitter (serotoninergic) and some release peptides (peptidergic), which include vasoactive intestinal peptide (VIP), substance P and gastrin-releasing peptide (GRP). Other neurons release nitric oxide (NO), which is formed from L-arginine by the enzyme nitric oxide synthase. The two plexuses are interconnected with many interneurons so that the total number of neurons in the gut is about 100 million, i.e. about the same number of neurons as in the spinal cord. These neurons have a high degree of functional independence from the central nervous system. When all the extrinsic nerves of the gut are cut, gut neurons are able to maintain the complex functions of secretion and motility on their own. The view now is that the neurons and fibres in the wall of the gut, collectively referred to as the ENS, are more than a station in the autonomic nervous system; they constitute a gut **'mini-brain'** that communicates with the central nervous sysem through the extrinsic autonomic nerves.

In general, stimulation of the extrinsic *parasympathetic* nerves to the gut results in increased motility, relaxation of sphincters, stimulation of secretion and vasodilatation. Stimulation of the *sympathetic* nerves inhibits motility, contracts sphincters and causes vasoconstriction; secretion is not necessarily inhibited, however, and on some occasions may be modestly stimulated.

On the other hand, the intrinsic nerves have important functions. **Meissner's plexus** subserves sensory functions, including responses to stretch and chemical composition of gut contents in contact with the epithelium. Stimulation of this submucous plexus leads to increased blood flow and increased exocrine and endocrine secretions. **Auerbach's plexus** (myenteric plexus) is mainly concerned with regulation of gut motility, e.g. peristalsis.

The gut as an endocrine organ

The gut occupies a unique position in endocrinology. In 1902, Bayliss and Starling discovered and isolated for the first time a substance from the upper intestine which stimulated exocrine secretion of the pancreas. They called this substance **secretin**. They introduced the word 'hormone' (Greek for 'I arouse to activity'), which was later used to describe secretions of endocrine glands.

Endocrine cells are found scattered in the wall of the gut from the stomach to the colon in order to cater for the changing needs of secretion and motility; if collected together, their mass would be greater than any of the familiar endocrine glands. All the known gastrointestinal hormones are **peptides**. Many of the endocrine peptide-containing cells also contain an amine, such as serotonin, dopamine or histamine. When an amine is absent, the enzyme that forms it (amino acid decarboxylase) may be present; the cell takes up the amino acid and decarboxylates it to form the amine. This has led to the hypothesis that all gut endocrine cells possess the APUD property (amine precursor uptake and decarboxylation). Many peptides and amines found in the gut endocrine cells are also present in neurons in the gut and the brain.

The gut produces numerous peptides, only four of which have established status as gastrointestinal hormones. These are: secretin, gastrin, cholecystokinin-pancreozymin (CCK-PZ or CCK) and glucose-dependent insulinotropic peptide (GIP). The remaining peptides have various pharmacological effects still under investigation. Since their physiological role is not yet fully understood, they may be referred to as 'candidate' hormones.

There are three ways in which a gastrointestinal peptide may act:

1 *Endocrine*: the peptide is released into the blood, through which it reaches its target organ or cell to act (e.g. gastrin, secretin).

2 *Paracrine*: the peptide is released into the interstitial fluid and diffuses along it to act on a neighbouring target cell (e.g. somatostatin).

3 *Neurocrine*: the peptide acts as a neurotransmitter in this case, i.e. it is released from a nerve ending into a junctional cleft to act on a target cell (e.g. vasoactive intestinal peptide (VIP), gastrin-releasing peptide (GRP)).

In all cases, the target cells possess receptors which are specific for the peptide.

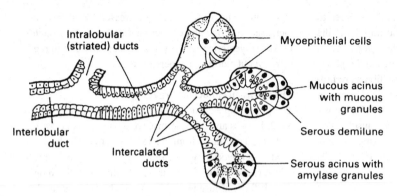

Fig. 8.2 Diagram of the acini and ducts of the submandibular salivary gland and the types of lining cells.

Mastication, saliva and deglutition

Mastication

Solid food is broken down by the process of mastication (chewing). Mastication also stimulates the secretion of saliva and helps to mix it with the food particles to produce a bolus which can then be swallowed. Mastication is started voluntarily but continues as an involuntary reflex. The contact of the food particles with the teeth and gums induces reflex opening of the jaws followed by closure; this produces rhythmic closure and opening at about one cycle per second. Considerable force can be applied to crush solid pieces of food; the molars can exert a force of more than 100 kg. When the bolus is of suitable consistency and size, it will be swallowed.

Salivary glands

Anatomical considerations

Most of the saliva in the mouth comes from three major pairs of glands, the **parotid, submandibular** and **sublingual** glands, which discharge their secretions into the mouth through ducts.

A small amount of saliva comes from small salivary glands scattered in the mucosa of the mouth and pharynx.

Salivary glands are typical exocrine glands. The basic secretory units are the acini, which are drained by intercalated ducts. These join to form intralobular or striated ducts, which lead to the interlobular ducts, which drain into the main duct opening into the mouth (Fig. 8.2).

There are two types of cells in the acini: *serous cells*, which contain granules and secrete electrolytes, water and the enzyme ptyalin (salivary amylase), and larger *mucous cells*, which secrete mucus. An acinus may be purely serous or purely mucous or may be mixed. In humans, the parotid

gland is purely serous, while the submandibular and sublingual glands are mixed.

The cells lining the intralobular ducts deserve a special mention; their basal membrane is extensively folded and they contain a lot of mitochondria, features which give the basal part of these cells a striated appearance and account for the name of **striated ducts**. As evidenced by the high content of mitochondria, these cells are metabolically very active; they are, in fact, mainly responsible for active transport of electrolytes which modify the composition of the primary acinar secretion. Myoepithelial cells are found between the basement membrane and the cells lining the lumen of acini and intralobular ducts. When stimulated, these cells contract and increase salivary flow.

Nerve supply

Salivary glands receive sympathetic and parasympathetic nerves. The sympathetic nerves originate in the upper four thoracic segments of the spinal cord, synapse in the superior cervical ganglion and reach the three pairs of salivary glands in company with the arteries. The parasympathetic supply originates in two salivary nuclei in the brainstem: the superior and inferior salivary nuclei. From the inferior salivary nucleus, fibres leave the medulla in the glossopharyngeal nerve (IX) and synapse in the otic ganglion, and postganglionic fibres reach the parotid glands. Fibres from the superior salivary nucleus leave in the facial nerve (VII), enter the chorda tympani branch and synapse in the submandibular ganglion, and postganglionic fibres supply both the submandibular and the sublingual glands.

Effects of nerve stimulation. Stimulation of the **parasympathetic** (cholinergic) nerves leads to a lot of watery secretion and marked vasodilatation. If atropine is given first, the secretion is blocked but the vasodilatation is largely unaffected. This atropine-resistant vasodilatation

is partly cholinergic and partly non-cholinergic. Although the cholinergic component is unusual in not being blocked by atropine, it can be blocked by botulinum toxin. The non-cholinergic mechanism may be mediated by vasoactive intestinal peptide (VIP). Furthermore, activation of parasympathetic nerves leads to release of the enzyme kallikrein from active gland tissue. Kallikrein acts on α_2-globulin in the interstitial fluid surrounding the gland cells to produce a vasodilator peptide called bradykinin. An injection of atropine is usually given preoperatively in order to inhibit salivary secretion while the patient is under general anaesthesia. A side-effect of atropine-like drugs or anticholinergic drugs is suppression of salivary secretion, leading to a dry mouth.

Stimulation of the **sympathetic** nerve supply will cause vasoconstriction and usually a small amount of viscous secretion. While there is general agreement that parasympathetic pathways operate during natural stimulation of salivary secretion, there is doubt whether the sympathetic nerves contribute under normal circumstances. It seems reasonable to assume that parasympathetic nerves stimulate the serous cells to produce a watery secretion and the sympathetic nerves act on the mucous cells to secrete saliva of high mucus content.

Composition and functions of saliva

About 1 litre of saliva is produced per day. It is hypotonic, with a specific gravity of about 1.003 (range 1.002–1.010) and pH that ranges from 6.2 to 7.4, increasing with the rate of secretion. Mixed saliva contains about 0.5% of solids, which are inorganic and organic in nature. The inorganic constituents include Na^+, Cl^- and HCO_3^-, the concentration of each being dependent on the rate of flow of saliva (Fig. 8.3). Potassium is found at a fairly constant concentration of 20 mmol/litre, making saliva one of the extracellular fluids with an unusually high potassium content. The concentration of calcium is 1.5 mmol/litre and phosphorus 5.5 mmol/litre. The organic constituents include mucin, the enzymes amylase, lingual lipase, kallikrein, lysozyme and carbonic anhydrase, and glycoproteins, mostly with the same specificity as the ABO blood group antigens found in red cells. About 80% of people have these antigens in their saliva and are described as secretors. Saliva also contains some disintegrating cells, from lining mucosa and glands, and microorganisms.

The secretion of electrolytes and water in saliva occurs in two stages. There is first a primary secretion in the acini, which is secondarily modified at the level of the striated ducts. The primary acinar secretion is approximately isotonic and has an electrolyte composition similar to

Fig. 8.3 Relationship of electrolyte concentrations to the rate of flow of saliva from the human parotid gland after parasympathetic stimulation. (After Thysen, J.H. (1954) *American Journal of Physiology* **178**, 155–9.)

that of plasma. It has recently been shown that a chloride pump exists in the basolateral membrane of acinar cells, which actively transports Cl^- from the blood into the acinar lumen, to be followed by Na^+, K^+ and water. HCO_3^- is actively secreted by both the acinar and the striated duct cells. At the striated duct, Na^+ is reabsorbed, unaccompanied by water, and K^+ is secreted; this process is influenced by aldosterone. While a relatively constant amount of K^+ is secreted, irrespective of the rate of flow, less and less Na^+ is reabsorbed as the rate of flow of saliva increases. This pattern of electrolyte exchange, unaccompanied by water movement at the level of the striated ducts, results in the production of a hypotonic saliva and explains the changes in electrolyte concentrations in relation to the rate of secretion of saliva (Fig. 8.3).

The functions of saliva

1 Saliva moistens and lubricates food and thus facilitates swallowing.

2 Saliva has a digestive function. Ptyalin is an amylase with optimum pH of 6.8. It breaks down starch to dextrins, maltotriose and maltose. **Ptyalin** is considered of minor physiological importance, as the food stays in the mouth for a short time. However, the action of ptyalin continues in the stomach for about half an hour and is arrested only when gastric acid penetrates the food mass. Salivary amylase may also be important for digesting away some of the food debris between the teeth. The serous salivary glands on the tongue secrete a **lipase** that breaks down triglycerides into monoglycerides and fatty acids. The action of lingual lipase may also continue in the stomach after food is swallowed.

3 Saliva keeps the oral mucosa constantly moist and in this way also helps the movements of the tongue and lips in speech.

4 Saliva is important for protection of the oral mucosa; its cleansing and washing effects are reinforced by the presence of the enzyme lysozyme, which is bactericidal. Saliva also contains immunoglobulin A (IgA) and lactoferrin, which deprives bacteria of iron.

5 By acting as a solvent, saliva is important for the sense of taste. Any substance must first dissolve in saliva before it can be sensed by the taste buds.

6 Buffering action of saliva: saliva neutralizes any acids that may result from bacterial action, and swallowed saliva may help to neutralize gastric HCl in the empty stomach. The buffers in saliva include bicarbonate, phosphate and mucin. The concentration of bicarbonate is increased as the rate of salivary flow rises in response to eating.

7 Saliva serves as a vehicle of excretion for substances like lead, mercury, fluorides and iodides. In parts of the world where the fluoride content of the soil and drinking-water is high, fluoride may be deposited on the teeth.

If the salivary glands are congenitally absent or destroyed by disease or irradiation, xerostomia (dry mouth) results. In this condition, swallowing and speech are difficult and the patient has to take frequent sips of water. Loss of the cleansing and protective functions of saliva also leads to degeneration of the oral epithelium.

Control of salivary secretion

While other secretions in the gut are controlled by nervous and hormonal mechanisms, salivary secretion is controlled exclusively by nervous mechanisms. Secretion of saliva is essentially mediated by nervous reflexes.

The presence of food in the mouth stimulates general receptors and, especially, taste receptors. Sour-tasting substances, such as lemon, are particularly effective stimulants of salivary secretion. Impulses travel along afferent nerves to the **salivary nuclei** in the brainstem and possibly to sympathetic centres. Efferent impulses travel along autonomic nerves to the salivary glands. This reflex is innate and is not acquired by learning (non-conditioned).

Secretion of saliva may also occur by **conditioned reflexes**, resulting from seeing, smelling, hearing or even thinking about appetizing food. In this case, initial impulses arise in the parts of the brain concerned with these special sensations and stimulate the salivary centres. Pavlov, at the end of the nineteenth century, demonstrated the conditioned reflexes in dogs with salivary fistulae. The secretion of saliva in response to bell-ringing without presentation of food demonstrated the conditioned reflex.

In humans, mouth-watering on seeing or thinking of food provides evidence of this psychic reflex.

Occasionally, secretion of saliva may continue even after food has been swallowed. This occurs when the food contains irritant substances or when there is nausea. The receptors for this reflex are in the stomach and upper intestine. Secretion of saliva is reduced during sleep, dehydration or severe mental stress.

Deglutition (swallowing)

The oesophagus

The oesophagus is a tube that connects the pharynx to the cardiac part of the stomach. It is 25–35 cm long, traversing the thorax except for the lowest 2–3 cm, which are in the abdomen. The oesophagus is lined with stratified squamous epithelium.

In humans, the muscle in its wall is striated in the upper third, smooth in the lower third and mixed in the middle. Both the upper and lower ends are guarded by sphincters. There is a definite anatomical band about 3 cm long at the upper end, forming the *cricopharyngeal sphincter*. At rest, the upper sphincter is closed at a pressure of 40–100 mmHg.

At the lowest 3 cm resides the *lower oesophageal sphincter* (LOS). There is no definite thickened band at the lower end but the presence of the LOS can be demonstrated physiologically. If a perfused thin polythene tube connected to a manometer is gradually withdrawn from the stomach through the oesophagus, a band of pressure of about 15–35 mmHg will be recorded as the tip of the catheter traverses the region of LOS. Both sphincters are normally closed. They open only to allow a bolus to pass through.

The swallowing centre

A collection of neurons in the floor of the fourth ventricle in the medulla controls and coordinates the process of deglutition. Afferent impulses from the pharynx and oesophagus travel to the swallowing centre in the V, IX and X cranial nerves and efferent impulses pass down the V, IX, X and XII cranial nerves to the muscles in the tongue, pharynx, larynx and oesophagus. The vagal nuclei are particularly important as they supply the striated muscle of the pharynx and upper oesophagus as well as the smooth muscle in the oesophagus.

Swallowing

The swallowing process is considered in three stages: buccal, pharyngeal and oesophageal. The buccal stage is

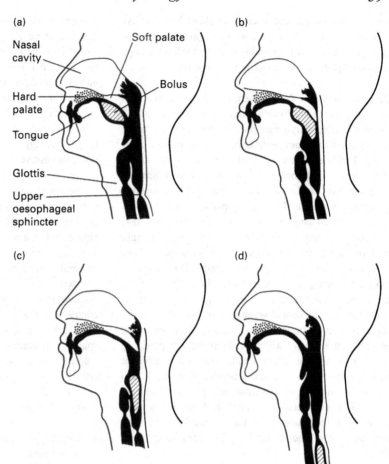

(a)

Nasal cavity

Soft palate

Hard palate

Bolus

Tongue

Glottis

Upper oesophageal sphincter

(b)

(c)

(d)

Fig. 8.4 Events during the stages of swallowing. (a) The bolus is propelled into the pharynx by the tongue after its tip is placed on the hard palate. (b) Contractions of the distal part of the tongue propel the bolus further into the oropharynx, which is now separated from the nasopharynx. (c) The bolus is entering the oesophagus through the relaxed upper oesophageal sphincter with the glottis closed and the epiglottis bending over it. (d) The bolus is now in the oesophagus and is propelled along by peristaltic contractions.

voluntary but both the pharyngeal and oesophageal stages are reflex. (See Fig. 8.4.)

Buccal stage. Pieces of food are collected by the tongue into a bolus (Fig. 8.4). The tip of the tongue is pressed against the hard palate, thus creating a chamber between the tongue and the palate. Contraction of the mylohyoid and styloglossus muscles causes the tongue to move upward and backward. It propels the bolus towards the pharynx. The soft palate rises and the posterior pharyngeal wall moves forward as a result of the contraction of the superior constrictor muscle of the pharynx. They meet and close off the nasopharynx.

Respiration is inhibited during swallowing. The larynx starts to rise, signalling the end of the buccal stage. From this moment onwards, the process of swallowing becomes involuntary. The rise of the larynx helps to push it off the path of the bolus. During the buccal stage, the lips and jaws are closed. It is very difficult to swallow when the jaws are

apart. During dental operations saliva cannot be swallowed and it collects in the mouth, from which it has to be removed by suction.

Pharyngeal stage. This requires highly coordinated muscle contractions to propel the bolus to the upper end of the oesophagus while avoiding the entrance to the air passages at the larynx. The movements are coordinated by the swallowing centre in the medulla. The tongue moves further backward and pushes the bolus against the epiglottis, which bends over the larynx and divides the bolus into two parts. The epiglottis is not essential for swallowing and can be removed without a significant effect on the process. The opening of the larynx is closed by contraction of the muscles surrounding its girdle, and the vocal folds are approximated.

The bolus is propelled downwards by the contraction of the middle and inferior constrictors of the pharynx and reaches the upper end of the oesophagus. The *cricopharyngeal* sphincter relaxes for about 1 second. As soon as the bolus enters the oesophagus, the cricopharyngeal sphincter closes, the vocal folds open, the larynx drops and the epiglottis returns to its previous position.

Oesophageal stage. With efferent impulses descending in the vagi from the swallowing centre, the contraction which closes the cricopharyngeal sphincter proceeds down the oesophagus as **primary peristalsis**, which propels the bolus along. Peristalsis consists of enlargement of the lumen at the level of the bolus and ahead of it, accompanied by contraction above the bolus, which is thus propelled down the oesophagus. This primary peristaltic wave travels down the oesophagus at about 4 cm/s for solid food. It is coordinated locally by the myenteric plexus. In the upright position liquids fall by gravity to the lower part of the oesophagus ahead of the peristaltic wave. If the bolus is too big or sticky, or if there is material regurgitated from the stomach, its progression down the oesophagus is helped by development of **secondary peristalsis**. Secondary peristalsis is initiated by localized distension of an oesophageal segment, which sends afferent impulses in the vagi to the medullary swallowing centre. Efferent vagal impulses cause secondary peristalsis, which is also locally coordinated by the myenteric plexus. Thus, the main difference between primary and secondary peristalsis is in their mode of initiation: the first follows a normal swallow, the second from localized oesophageal distension.

Vagal impulses relax the LOS ahead of the peristaltic wave. The bolus enters the stomach and the sphincter then closes rather slowly, taking 7–10 s.

Difficulty in swallowing is termed **dysphagia**. Swallowing may be investigated radiologically by a barium swallow. It may also be studied by oesophageal manometry, which records pressure changes in the oesophagus during swallowing.

Competence of the gastro-oesophageal junction. Except for the short abdominal segment, pressure in the oesophagus is the same as intrathoracic pressure, i.e. mostly negative, so that pressure in the stomach is always higher than in the oesophagus. It is therefore necessary to have a barrier at the gastro-oesophageal junction; otherwise, gastric contents will be regurgitated or refluxed (pushed back) into the oesophagus. As the lining mucosa of the oesophagus is not adapted to dealing with corrosive gastric hydrochloric acid and pepsin, reflux will cause inflammation (reflux oesophagitis); the patient experiences a painful burning sensation in the chest (heartburn).

Competence of the gastro-oesophageal junction is now believed to be almost entirely due to the physiological sphincter at the lower end of the oesophagus. Mechanical factors, such as the acute angle of entry of the oesophagus into the stomach and the valve-like action of mucosal folds at the cardio-oesophageal junction, seem to be unimportant. The antireflux function of the lower oesophageal sphincter has been shown to be due to its *resting pressure* (15–35 mmHg), its *intra-abdominal length*, which is exposed to positive intra-abdominal pressure, and its *overall length*.

The lower oesophageal sphincter is under neural and hormonal control. Between swallows, tonic vagal cholinergic impulses maintain contraction to keep the sphincter closed; but, during swallowing, efferent impulses in the vagus are inhibitory, i.e. cause the sphincter to relax, the transmitter probably being nitric oxide (NO), although vasoactive intestinal peptide (VIP) may also be involved. The hormone gastrin, released from the stomach by food, contracts the LOS. Secretin and CCK, released from the upper intestine, oppose the action of gastrin and relax the sphincter. Secondary oesophageal peristalsis may be considered as a second line of defence since it helps to clear refluxed material back into the stomach.

In the disease **achalasia**, the resting pressure of the lower oesophageal sphincter is high and it fails to relax on swallowing, thus resulting in functional obstruction. In addition, oesophageal peristalisis is weak or absent, the oesophagus dilates and food accumulates in it. The patient complains of dysphagia and aspiration of retained oesophageal contents may occur. The condition is due to loss of inhibitory myenteric neurons containing VIP and nitric oxide, especially in the lower part of the oesophagus.

The stomach

Anatomical considerations

The stomach is a fibromuscular bag situated between the oesophagus and the small intestine. It is approximately J-shaped with anterior and posterior surfaces and rather sharp sides, known as the greater and lesser curvatures. The area of the gastro-oesophageal junction is also known as the cardia. The fundus is the dome-shaped part of the stomach above an imaginary horizontal line from the cardia to the greater curvature, and it usually contains swallowed air (Fig. 8.5). The stomach wall has three layers of muscle: an outer longitudinal, a middle circular, which thickens to form the pyloric sphincter, and an inner oblique, extending from the cardia to the greater curvature.

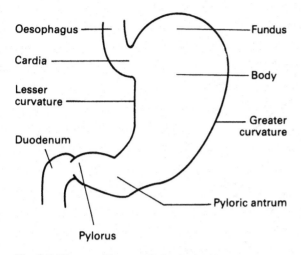

Fig. 8.5 Diagram of the stomach showing its parts.

Fig. 8.6 Diagram of a main gastric gland showing the various types of cells.

The innervation of the stomach consists of its autonomic nerve supply as well as the intrinsic nerve plexuses. Postganglionic sympathetic fibres reach the stomach from the coeliac plexus. Preganglionic parasympathetic fibres are supplied by the right and left vagi. They synapse with the neurons in the submucous and myenteric plexuses, and short postganglionic fibres reach the gastric glands and smooth muscle. There are also reflex arcs entirely within the wall of the stomach.

Histologically, the gastric mucosa may be divided into three major areas:

1 *The cardiac area* accounts for about 10% of the lining mucosa. Most of the cells in the cardiac glands secrete mucus.

2 *The main gastric area* includes the mucosa of both the fundus and the body and accounts for 70–80% of the gastric mucosa. The pits are short and the gastric glands are long and tubular, consisting of isthmus, neck and body or base (Fig. 8.6). Usually four gastric glands open into a single pit. These glands secrete all the constituents of gastric juice. The parietal (or oxyntic) cells are most numerous in the isthmus and neck regions but are also seen in the body of the gland. Parietal cells secrete hydrochloric acid. They also secrete the intrinsic factor.

Chief or peptic cells are serous cells found in the body. They contain zymogen granules, which are the source of the gastric pepsinogens. There are also endocrine cells, which may secrete peptides or amines, such as histamine. Mucous neck cells are found in the neck and isthmus regions; they secrete mucus and pepsinogen.

The gastric epithelium has great powers of repair. Every minute it replaces about half a million cells lost from the surface. The surface epithelial cells have a lifespan of a few days, while the parietal, chief and endocrine cells live for a few months.

3 *The pyloric area* constitutes about 15% of the gastric mucosa. Most of the cells in the gastric glands are mucous cells. The endocrine cells or G cells, which secrete gastrin, are found in the pyloric glands.

Functions of the stomach

1 The stomach stores food and regulates its passage to the small intestine. It enables the body to take large amounts of food at mealtimes. In its absence, food has to be taken more frequently.

2 The stomach secretes gastric juice, which liquefies and partly digests food to produce semifluid chyme, which is suitable for further intestinal digestion and absorption.

3 It has a protective function. Hydrochloric acid kills ingested bacteria and thus limits their entry to the small intestine. Vomiting is a protective mechanism whereby harmful ingested material is thrown out.

Parietal cell

Fig. 8.7 Schematic representation of the process of production of hydrochloric acid by the parietal cell. CA, carbonic anhydrase; CM, carrier mechanism; ✶, active transport.

4 The stomach produces the intrinsic factor, a mucoprotein necessary for the absorption of vitamin B_{12}.

5 Gastric hydrochloric acid is necessary for the absorption of iron in the upper intestine.

6 The stomach has been found to have an endocrine function. It produces a number of peptides, including gastrin, glucagon, somatostatin, substance P, VIP and GRP.

Gastric juice

Humans secrete 2–3 litres of gastric juice per day. The main components of gastric juice are hydrochloric acid, digestive enzymes, mucus and the intrinsic factor.

Hydrochloric acid

Gastric acid is secreted by the parietal cells. These are pyramidal in shape, with the apical membrane invaginated to form an intracellular canalicular system (Fig. 8.7). Mitochondria account for about 40% of the cytoplasm, which also contains flavoproteins, cytochrome oxidase and carbonic anhydrase. When the cell is inactive, there are numerous tubulovesicles in the cytoplasm. When it is actively secreting, these vesicles seem to merge with the canaliculi, which become extensive and display microvilli.

At maximum rates of secretion, gastric juice has a pH

of 0.9 and the following electrolyte composition: $H^+ = 140$ mmol/litre; $K^+ = 15$ mmol/litre; $Na^+ = 10$ mmol/litre; and $Cl^- = 165$ mmol/litre, balancing the three cations. As the pH of the plasma is 7.4, it is obvious that the parietal cell has to concentrate H^+ more than 10^6 times in order to secrete it into gastric juice. The numerous mitochondria and enzymes of the parietal cell provide it with the means to perform this task. H^+ and Cl^- ions are transported across the canicular membrane into the canaliculi and hence the lumen of the gastric gland.

As shown in Fig. 8.7, a likely source of H^+ in the parietal cell is from the dissociation of intracellular water into H^+ and OH^-. Another source may be H^+ resulting from oxidation of substrates like glucose. As the mucosal side is always electronegative in relation to the serosal side, H^+ is not transported across the canalicular membrane against an electrical gradient, but it is transported against a huge concentration gradient.

H^+ is transported across the canalicular membrane by an adenosine triphosphate (ATP)-driven pump, which exchanges H^+ with K^+. This pump has been called H^+, K^+ adenosine triphosphatase (ATPase). It can be inhibited by a drug called omeprazole, which is consequently a very strong inhibitor of gastric acid secretion. OH^- will tend to accumulate in the cytoplasm, but it is neutralized by combination with carbonic acid (H_2CO_3) to give H_2O and HCO_3^-. H_2CO_3 can be readily formed from CO_2 and H_2O under the influence of carbonic anhydrase, which is abundant in the parietal cell. HCO_3^- diffuses from the cell to the plasma and Cl^- enters via a carrier mechanism that facilitates the exchange between the two ions. Cl^- can also enter the cell in company with Na^+, which is then pumped out by Na^+, K^+ ATPase. Cl^- is transported across the canalicular membrane into the lumen, while K^+ is returned to the inside by H^+, K^+ ATPase.

It has recently been shown that the tubulovesicles in the cytoplasm in the unstimulated or resting parietal cell contain H^+, K^+ ATPase. Under stimulation by neural or hormonal mechanisms, the tubulovesicles fuse with the apical membrane, thus placing H^+, K^+ ATPase in parallel with K^+ and Cl^- channels and leading to HCl secretion, with K^+ being recycled back to the cytoplasm.

The maximum amount of HCl that can be secreted in response to a stimulus such as pentagastrin or histamine—the maximum acid output (MAO)—is directly proportional to the number of parietal cells or parietal cell mass (PCM). The normal stomach has about 10^9 parietal cells, which have the capacity to secrete up to about 20 mmol H^+ per hour.

During the height of gastric acid secretion, the blood leaving the stomach has more HCO_3^- and less Cl^-, and its pH shifts slightly to the alkaline side. The excess HCO_3^- is finally excreted in urine. This may follow the ingestion of a meal, and has been described as the postprandial alkaline tide. In persistent vomiting, this situation is perpetuated, leading to *metabolic alkalosis*. In addition, there are dehydration and loss of Na^+ and K^+ ions.

Normally, gastric hydrochloric acid activates pepsinogen to pepsin and provides the suitable acidic medium for the action of pepsin. HCl also plays an important role in stimulating the secretion of pepsinogen. Its protective role in killing ingested bacteria has already been referred to. Its presence is also important for the absorption of non-haem iron in the duodenum: HCl dissolves iron, enabling it to form soluble complexes with ascorbic acid and protein–SH groups, which reduce ferric iron (Fe^{3+}) to the better-absorbed ferrous iron (Fe^{2+}).

Enzymes

Rennin, which clots milk, has been found in the calf stomach. It is absent from the stomach of the human infant and adult. The fundic mucosa of the human stomach secretes a **lipase** that hydrolyses triglycerides to monoglycerides and fatty acids. Its activity is equivalent to about one-fifth of that of pancreatic lipase. However, the main enzyme secreted into gastric juice is **pepsin**. The gastric glands secrete seven types of **pepsinogens**, which have been divided into two groups, I and II, subsequently renamed A and C, respectively. Group A pepsinogens consist of five components and are secreted by the chief cells and mucous neck cells. Group C comprises the two remaining components, which arise from these cells and other cells in the cardiac, antral and Brunner's glands.

The inactive pepsinogens are activated in the lumen by hydrochloric acid to pepsin and, once activated, they can activate more pepsinogen, i.e. *autocatalysis*. The pH optima of the pepsins are 1.5 to 3.5. Pepsins clot milk and break down proteins into peptones and polypeptides. They are particularly important for the breakdown of collagen and therefore the breakdown of connective tissue in meat. The digestion of protein by pepsin is not essential. If the stomach is removed, protein digestion can be initiated and maintained by pancreatic proteolytic enzymes.

Mucus

Mucus is an important constituent of gastric juice. It is present as a gel on the surface of the mucosa and protects the lining of the stomach against mechanical and chemical injury. By lubricating and facilitating the mixing of chyme, it protects the lining of the stomach against mechanical injury. It protects the mucosa against chemical injury by acting as a physical barrier to HCl and pepsin; it also neutralizes the acid and thus arrests the action of pepsin as well. The surface epithelial cells secrete HCO_3^-, which contributes to the protective role of mucus.

Gastric mucus is a glycoprotein with a large carbohydrate component. In about 75% of people, described as secretors, the carbohydrate part has the same antigenic specificity as the ABO antigens. It is noteworthy that people with group O are more susceptible to duodenal ulceration than other groups. The secretion of mucus is stimulated by mechanical and chemical irritation of the mucosa and is increased after either sympathetic or parasympathetic stimulation.

Intrinsic factor

Gastric parietal cells secrete a glycoprotein with a molecular weight of 45 000, which combines with ingested *cyanocobalamin* or vitamin B_{12} (the extrinsic factor) and the complex is absorbed in the terminal part of the ileum by receptor-mediated endocytosis. The intrinsic factor–cyanocobalamin complex binds to specific receptors on enterocytes in the ileum and cyanocobalamin traverses the cell to the blood. It seems that the role of the intrinsic factor is to stimulate endocytosis of cyanocobalamin. Neural or hormonal stimulation of gastric secretion will also increase the secretion of the intrinsic factor. The main defect in **pernicious anaemia** is atrophy of the gastric mucosa, including loss of parietal cells, leading to achlorhydria (absence of acid secretion) and deficiency of the intrinsic factor, which result in malabsorption of vitamin B_{12} and megaloblastic anaemia. Megaloblastic anaemia also results some years after total removal of the stomach. Secretion of the intrinsic factor is thus the only essential function of the stomach.

Control of gastric secretion

Gastric secretion is controlled by neural and hormonal mechanisms, which are so integrated and interrelated as to warrant the use of the term neurohormonal. The control mechanisms are excitatory, followed by inhibitory means to limit the secretion. Secretion is usually considered in three phases, which correspond to the site where the stimuli to secretion start. These phases partly overlap and are also integrated.

Cephalic phase

The cephalic phase can occur by conditioned and non-conditioned reflexes. In the **non-conditioned** reflex, presence of food in the mouth stimulates gustatory and other receptors and afferent impulses travel to the vagal nucleus in the medulla; efferent impulses reach the stomach in the vagus nerves to cause secretion. The **conditioned reflex** follows psychic stimulation by seeing, smelling, hearing or thinking of appetizing food. Afferent impulses impinge on the vagal centre, which sends impulses to the gastric glands through the vagi (Fig. 8.8).

Vagal impulses descending to the stomach release acetylcholine, which directly stimulates gastric glands to secrete gastric juice. Vagal impulses also release the hormone **gastrin** from the pyloric antrum, through a non-cholinergic mechanism via release of **gastrin-releasing peptide (GRP)**. Thus, during the cephalic phase, the gastric glands are stimulated by the vagi both directly and indirectly through release of gastrin, which enters the blood to stimulate the glands.

The cephalic phase of gastric secretion is affected by emotional factors. Chronic stress stimulates and acute stress, such as a sudden fright, reduces gastric acid secretion. All of these effects reach the stomach through the vagi, and this provides the rationale for surgical vagotomy to reduce gastric acid secretion as a treatment for patients with peptic ulcer.

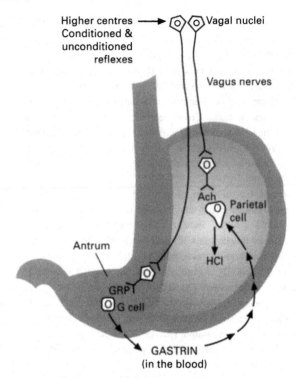

Fig. 8.8 Mechanisms mediating the cephalic phase of gastric acid secretion.

Gastric phase

The gastric phase is mediated by nervous and hormonal mechanisms.

Distension of the stomach stimulates gastric secretion via *long vagovagal reflexes* and also by *short intramural cholinergic reflexes*. In the long reflex, both the afferent and efferent components travel in the vagi. Efferent vagal impulses act on gastric glands through acetylcholine and also release gastrin. In the short reflex, receptors that respond to stretch discharge to neurons in the nerve plexuses of the gastric wall, and efferent fibres stimulate the gland cells by releasing acetylcholine. Gastrin may also be released by reflexes entirely within the wall of the stomach (Fig. 8.9).

Gastrin is secreted by flask-shaped G cells in the pyloric antrum and upper intestine. Gastrin is released by *distension* and by peptides and L-amino acids resulting from the digestion of proteins. Alcohol and caffeine may also release gastrin, but carbohydrates and fats are poor releasers. Vagal excitation releases gastrin, whatever the phase of gastric secretion. Gastrin is a peptide that exists in many forms and whose occurrence in tissues and the blood has been investigated by radioimmunoassay. The

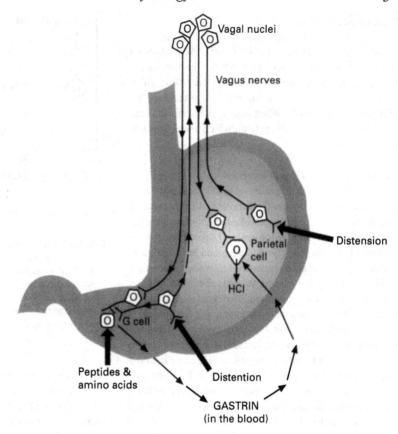

Fig. 8.9 Neural and hormonal mechanisms that stimulate acid secretion during the gastric phase.

physiological forms of gastrin have either 17, 34 or 14 amino acid residues, and each may occur in sulphated or non-sulphated types. The activity of gastrin resides in the four C-terminal amino acids (Trp–Met–Asp–Phe–NH$_2$). Pentagastrin, which is widely used in gastric function tests, is a synthetic peptide with β-alanine added at the N terminus.

Actions of gastrin. When given in pharmacological doses, gastrin has a wide variety of multiple effects. Gastrin is a strong stimulus of gastric acid secretion but it also stimulates the secretion of pepsin and the intrinsic factor. Gastrin also stimulates intestinal secretion, pancreatic secretion of enzymes and bicarbonate and biliary secretion of bicarbonate and water. It contracts the LOS, stimulates gastric motility (but slows gastric emptying), stimulates intestinal motility and relaxes the ileocaecal sphincter. Gastrin has a trophic effect on the mucosa of the stomach, small intestine and colon. Of all these effects, the physiological ones are: stimulation of gastric acid secretion and pancreatic enzyme secretion and the trophic effect.

Gastrin is degraded and excreted by the kidneys. It is also catabolized by the small intestine and gastric fundus.

Rarely, a pancreatic islet cell grows into a tumour that secretes gastrin, called a **gastrinoma**. The gastrinoma results in a syndrome of hypergastrinaemia, excessive basal and stimulated gastric acid hypersecretion, peptic ulceration and diarrhoea (*Zollinger–Ellison syndrome*). The tumour may more rarely occur in the stomach or duodenum.

Intestinal phase

Distension and the presence of protein digestion products in the upper intestine result in gastric acid secretion from denervated gastric mucosa after a latent period of 1–3 hours. Since gastrin is found in the upper intestine, this phase may partly be mediated by direct release of **intestinal gastrin** by food. In addition, another peptide, named **entero-oxyntin**, may be released from the intestine by food and reaches the stomach through the blood to stimulate gastric acid secretion. Amino acids absorbed from the small intestine into the blood may also contribute to mediation of the intestinal phase.

Pepsinogen secretion

Pepsinogen secretion is strongly stimulated by vagal excitation and to a lesser extent by gastrin. Acid plays an
important role in pepsin secretion and its digestive action.
Acid in the lumen excites a local cholinergic reflex, which
stimulates pepsinogen secretion and also potentiates the
effects of other stimuli. When acid is delivered into the
upper intestine, it releases secretin, which also stimulates
pepsinogen secretion.

Histamine and gastric acid secretion

Histamine is a potent stimulant of gastric acid secretion.
This effect of histamine on the parietal cell is not blocked
by conventional antihistamines like mepyramine maleate,
i.e. the receptors involved are not H_1 receptors, which
mediate effects such as vasodilatation and bronchial constriction; they have been termed H_2 receptors. H_2 receptor
blockers have been developed; they include cimetidine and
ranitidine, both potent inhibitors of gastric acid secretion,
and both are being used for the treatment of peptic ulcers.

Even though the effect of histamine on gastric acid
secretion has been known since 1920, it is still not certain
how it works. **Enterochromaffin-like (ECL) cells** in the
lamina propria form and store histamine. It has been proposed that acetylcholine and gastrin release histamine from
these cells. The released histamine diffuses to the parietal
cell to act on the H_2 receptor to stimulate secretion of
hydrochloric acid. Work on the isolated parietal cells has
shown that the parietal cell has receptors for histamine, for
acetylcholine and for gastrin and that these receptors interact in various combinations to augment the actions of each
other. It may be that gastrin and acetylcholine both release
histamine from its cell and interact with it on the parietal
cell. The second messenger for the action of histamine
on the parietal cell is cyclic adenosine monophosphate
(cAMP). Gastrin and acetylcholine act through the release
of intracellular Ca^{2+}. The mutual potentiation between
these messengers explains the interactions among the three
secretagogues.

Role of inhibitory mechanisms in the control of gastric acid secretion

In addition to excitatory mechanisms, there are inhibitory
mechanisms, which limit gastric acid secretion:
1 Emotions, such as acute fear and the feeling of nausea,
reduce gastric acid secretion. These effects are probably
mediated by reduction in the normal **vagal tone** to the
stomach.
2 In the pyloric antrum, when the pH drops to 2.5 or less,
acid secretion is reduced. Acid in the antral lumen inhibits

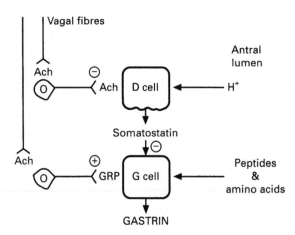

Fig. 8.10 Mechanisms that regulate release of gastrin from
G cells in the antrum.
Note: (i) H^+ in the antrum releasing somatostatin from D cells,
which inhibits release of gastrin, is the mechanism of the negative
feedback drop that restrains acid secretion; (ii) suppression of
somatostatin release by vagal excitation contributes to the
mechanism of vagal release of gastrin.

release of gastrin. This is the basis of a negative feedback
loop whereby excess acid leads to a reduction in the amount
of secreted acid. D cells in the stomach and the intestine
secrete **somatostatin**, a peptide originally isolated from the
hypothalamus. Somatostatin inhibits gastric acid secretion
both by directly inhibiting the parietal cell and by inhibiting
release of gastrin from G cells. It has been proposed that
acid releases somatostatin from antral D cells, which then
diffuses to nearby G cells to inhibit release of gastrin (Fig.
8.10). In hypo- or achlorhydria, the negative feedback loop
is interrupted; gastrin release continues unchecked, leading
to hypergastrinaemia. This occurs in pernicious anaemia
and may follow vagotomy. Whenever the antrum or part of
it is excluded from the path of acid chyme, as may happen
after a gastrojejunostomy, hypergastrinaemia also results,
which can lead to gastric acid hypersecretion and peptic
ulceration.
3 The presence of acid, fat and hypertonic solutions in the
upper intestine inhibits gastric acid secretion. These effects
are mediated mainly by hormonal mechanisms.
(a) It has been postulated that a hormone, called **bulbogastrone** is released from the duodenal bulb to inhibit
gastric acid secretion. Another hormone, called **enterogastrone**, has been postulated to inhibit both gastric acid
secretion and motility when released from the upper
intestine. Neither bulbogastrone nor enterogastrone has
yet been obtained in pure form and the term 'entero-

gestrone' is now applied to any agent from the small intestine which inhibits gastric acid secretion. A peptide with 43 amino acid residues can be released from the small intestine by glucose and fats. One of its early discovered effects was inhibition of gastric acid secretion and it was thus called **gastric inhibitory peptide (GIP)**. However, later work has shown GIP to be a potent releaser of insulin from the β cells of pancreatic islets, and it is now believed that GIP is the physiological insulin releaser of the small intestine and its name has been changed to glucose-dependent insulinotropic peptide, with the same acronym of GIP.

(b) Acid and digestive products of proteins and fats release the hormones **secretin** and **cholecystokinin (CCK)** from the mucosa of the upper intestine into the blood, from where they stimulate pancreatic secretion. Both hormones can also act on the stomach. Secretin is a potent inhibitor of gastric acid secretion and it inhibits release of gastrin from the antrum. In small doses, CCK stimulates gastric acid secretion but in higher doses it inhibits stimulation of gastric acid secretion by gastrin. It has recently been shown that the inhibitory effects of secretin and CCK are mediated through release of somatostatin from D cells, which diffuses to inhibit the parietal cells as well as the release of gastrin from G cells. Thus, secretin and CCK normally released from the intestine may contribute to intestinally initiated mechanisms that limit gastric acid secretion.

(c) **Pancreatic glucagon** is also secreted by A cells in the stomach and duodenum, and a substance that cross-reacts with some of the antiglucagon antibodies has been found in the rest of the small intestine and is called glucagon-like immunoreactive factor (GLI) or **glicentin**. In addition to its effects on carbohydrate metabolism, glucagon is a good inhibitor of gastric acid secretion in humans.

(d) Other peptides inhibitory to gastric acid secretion include **neurotensin, vasoactive intestinal peptide (VIP)** and **somatostatin**.

(e) Certain types of **prostaglandins** inhibit gastric acid secretion in humans.

Tests of gastric secretory function

After an overnight fast, basal acid secretion is collected for 1 hour. It amounts to 1–4 mmol H^+ per hour, but it is very variable between individuals and even in the same individual at different times. Gastric acid secretion is maximally stimulated by an injection of pentagastrin (6 μg/kg) or histamine (0.04 mg/kg, accompanied by an H_1 receptor blocker), and the **maximum acid output** (MAO) is then

determined. MAO is higher in men than in women and it tends to decline after the age of 50. It also correlates with parameters of body build, such as body-weight, lean body mass and height. The MAO is directly proportional to the parietal cell mass.

Acid secretion is usually absent (achlorhydria) in **pernicious anaemia** and may be reduced (hypochlorhydria) in gastric carcinoma. One-third of patients with **gastric ulcer** have reduced acid secretion and the rest secrete within the normal range. About one-sixth to one-third of the patients with **duodenal ulcer** are acid hypersecretors while the rest secrete within the normal range. Basal acid secretion in the **Zollinger–Ellison syndrome** (gastrinoma) is so high that it amounts to over half of the maximally stimulated output, which is also greatly increased.

After an operation of vagotomy for treatment of peptic ulcer, it is desirable to know whether the vagotomy has been complete. This is assessed by the *insulin hypoglycaemia test*. Insulin at 0.2 U/kg is injected intravenously to reduce glucose to about 2.78 mmol/litre (50 mg/100 ml). The hypoglycaemia stimulates the vagal centre and, if the vagi are intact, gastric acid secretion is stimulated after a latent period of about 40 minutes. Lack of an acid response indicates that the vagotomy is complete.

Absorption in the stomach

A small amount of water is absorbed in the stomach. Alcohol is also partly absorbed in the stomach. Undissociated organic acids, such as acetyl salicylic acid or aspirin, may be absorbed, and generally lipid-soluble substances or drugs can be absorbed in the stomach.

Gastric motility

When the electrical activity of the smooth muscle in the wall of the stomach is explored by microelectrodes, it is found that the fundus is electrically silent but that two types of potentials may be recorded from the rest of the stomach: slow spontaneous waves of depolarization followed by repolarization, occurring at the rate of three per minute and referred to as slow waves or **basal electric rhythm (BER)**, and **action potential spikes**, superimposed on the slow waves and occurring in association with contractions. BER is responsible for coordination of contractions and determines their frequency. It originates in a group of smooth-muscle cells, located high on the greater curvature and considered as the pacemaker, and sweeps along the stomach to the pylorus.

During the *interdigestive period* bursts of depolarizations, accompanied by peristaltic contractions, pass along the stomach. Such activity occurring in the empty stomach is referred to as the **migrating motor complex** (MMC). The MMC moves on along the whole length of the small intestine to reach the ileocaecal valve after 1.5–2 hours. When the cycle reaches the ileocaecal junction, a new wave of MMC starts in the stomach. As soon as food is ingested, the activity of the MMC is terminated. The function of the MMC is to sweep remnants in the stomach and small intestine into the colon. It is evident that periods of fasting are associated with such waves.

The motility function of the stomach after food is taken is best appreciated by recognizing two distinct motor regions: the proximal and the distal stomach.

The proximal stomach

As food enters the stomach, the proximal region (fundus and upper third of body) relaxes in order to accommodate the incoming food (**receptive relaxation**). This is mediated through a vagovagal reflex, the efferent arm of which is inhibitory to the musculature of the upper stomach and non-cholinergic. Recent evidence has indicated that the transmitter may be **nitric oxide**. Thus, the first function of the proximal stomach is receiving and storing ingested food.

In addition, there are slow sustained tonic contractions in the proximal stomach that slowly push contents towards the distal region and duodenum. These contractions actually provide the pressure gradient for the emptying of liquids and liquefied chyme from the stomach into the duodenum, which is the second major function of the proximal region.

The distal stomach

The main activity in the distal stomach (lower two-thirds, of the body, antrum and pylorus) is **peristalsis**, whereby grinding of solids and liquefaction of chyme occur and chyme is propelled to the duodenum. Peristaltic contractions are initiated by distension and mediated by a cholinergic vagovagal reflex.

The pylorus is an atypical sphincter in that it is open for the greater part of the time and closes only when a peristaltic contraction passes over it. When this happens, the stomach is closed off from the duodenum, retropulsion of antral contents occurs and time is afforded for grinding of the solids in chyme to reduce their size to particles that are small enough to pass through the lumen of the pylorus when it relaxes (< 0.25 mm in diameter).

Gastric emptying occurs through coordination of the contractions of the antrum, pylorus and duodenal bulb, these being referred to as the *gastroduodenal pump*. As gastric contents are propelled into the distal stomach, the

Fig. 8.11 An illustration showing that liquids are emptied at a faster rate than solids, which require more time to be broken down into small particles (based on Camilleri, M. *et al.* (1985) *Am. J. Physiol.* **249**, G580–G585).

antrum, pylorus and proximal duodenum are relaxed. Chyme which has been liquefied or is already in liquid form passes readily into the duodenum, being pushed along by the tonic contraction of the proximal stomach. The terminal antrum then contracts, further aiding the propulsion of liquid chyme. This is followed by contraction of the pylorus, which closes off the stomach and arrests emptying to allow grinding of solids in chyme. The proximal duodenum next contracts, moving contents just emptied further into the distal duodenum and jejunum. The antrum, pylorus and duodenal bulb then relax and the sequence is repeated.

Control of gastric emptying

The rate of gastric emptying depends mainly on the activity of the gastroduodenal pump and to a lesser extent on duodenal resistance to oncoming chyme.

Liquids are emptied rapidly from the stomach and, irrespective of their starting volume, are all emptied at the same rate. Digestible solids are emptied more slowly and indigestible solids, such as plant fibres, are emptied at very slow rates (Fig. 8.11).

When chyme arrives in the duodenum, its chemical characteristics affect various duodenal receptors and the effect is then conveyed to the stomach to inhibit its motility and the activity of the gastroduodenal pump, i.e. *negative feedback control*.

Hypertonic chyme slows down the rate of gastric emptying. This is mediated by **osmoreceptors** in the duodenum and jejunum.

The arrival of *acid chyme* in the duodenum (pH less than 6) inhibits gastric motility and increases duodenal motility, leading to increased duodenal resistance. The result is marked inhibition of gastric emptying. Excess acid in the duodenum acts on **receptors** which are sensitive to changes in pH.

The presence of emulsified fat and, to a lesser extent, peptides and amino acids in the duodenum slows the rate of gastric emptying.

There are duodenal receptors which respond to *distension*. Duodenal distension inhibits contractions of the pyloric antrum and slows gastric emptying.

All of these feedback mechanisms are conveyed from the upper intestine to the stomach by **neural** and **hormonal** means.

The nervous pathways may be via a long vagovagal reflex whereby the efferent vagal impulses are inhibitory to gastric motility. In addition, these effects may be mediated by an inhibitory enterogastric reflex, whose centre is probably in the coeliac ganglion.

Since these effects still occur after denervation of the stomach and upper intestine, hormonal mechanisms must contribute. It has been postulated that a hormone, called **enterogastrone**, is released from the upper intestine by acid, fat and hypertonic solutions. It inhibits gastric motility (and acid secretion) and thus slows gastric emptying.

The intestinal hormone **secretin** inhibits gastric motility, while **CCK** stimulates it, but both contract the pylorus, thereby increasing its resistance, and thus slow gastric emptying. Although **gastrin** stimulates gastric motility, it also stimulates intestinal motility and thus increases duodenal resistance, and, when the gastrin-stimulated acid reaches the duodenum, it releases secretin and CCK. Therefore, the net effect of gastrin is slowing of gastric emptying (Fig. 8.12).

Emotions also affect the rate of gastric emptying. Fear prolongs while excitement speeds up gastric emptying.

After truncal vagotomy, the activity of the gastroduodenal pump is reduced, leading to slowing of gastric emptying and dilatation of the stomach. This is usually avoided by performing a pyloroplasty (enlargement of the pyloric canal) or joining the stomach directly to the jejunum (gastrojejunostomy) at the same time.

Vomiting

Vomiting is mainly a protective mechanism by which the stomach removes from the digestive tract harmful or potentially harmful materials. *Irritation* or *overdistension*

Fig. 8.12 Control of gastric motility and gastric emptying. The figure illustrates the neural mechanisms mediating receptive relaxation of the proximal stomach and peristalsis in the distal stomach. It also illustrates the neural and hormonal mechanisms that mediate upper intestinal inhibitory effects on gastric emptying. Solid lines indicate stimulatory effects, while interrupted lines indicate inhibitory effects on motility. NO, nitric oxide; ACh, acetylcholine; NA, noradrenaline (norepinephrine).

of the stomach or duodenum is normally the strongest stimulus for vomiting to occur. Substances that induce vomitting are called **emetics**. Vomiting may also accompany movement, and some people seem to be especially prone to *motion sickness*. Vomiting may occasionally follow disgusting or shocking sights or smells.

A collection of neurons present bilaterally in the medulla oblongata is referred to as the **vomiting centre**. It controls and integrates the process of vomiting. The centre receives afferent impulses from the stomach and duodenum in both the vagi and the sympathetic nerves. There are also afferents from the pharynx; the receptors concerned are very potent. Mechanical stimulation of the pharynx easily induces vomiting, and this may be useful in emergency situations when a poisonous substance has accidentally been ingested. Efferent impulses travel from the vomiting centre in the V, VII, IX, X and XII cranial nerves plus the spinal nerves to the diaphragm and abdominal muscles.

Vomiting is usually preceded by **nausea** and retching. A deep breath is taken, the glottis is closed and the soft palate rises to close off the nasopharynx; the cricopharyngeal sphincter then opens. This is immediately followed by violent contractions of the *diaphragm* and *abdominal muscles*. In the meantime, the fundus and body of the stomach are *relaxed*. Reverse peristalsis, usually starting at the angular notch, directs chyme towards the cardia. Sometimes antiperistalsis may even start in the lower intestine. The most important factor for expelling chyme from the stomach, however, is the squeezing of the stomach between the diaphragm and the abdominal muscles. Intragastric pressure rises sharply and propels chyme towards the cardia. The *lower oesophageal sphincter relaxes* and gastric contents are expelled through the oesophagus to the outside. Vomiting is normally accompanied by salivation and slowing of the heart. Skin vasoconstriction and sweating may occur.

Emetics, such as warm salt and water or mustard and water or *copper* and *zinc sulphates*, when taken by mouth, induce vomiting. They act on receptors in the stomach and duodenum which discharge to the vomiting centre. Other emetics, such as *morphine, apomorphine, digitalis* derivatives and *tartar emetic*, act centrally on an area in the floor of the fourth ventricle called the **chemoreceptor trigger zone**. This zone discharges to the vomiting centre. In *motion sickness*, initial impulses arise in the labyrinth and reach the chemoreceptor trigger zone through the cerebellum. Psychic stimuli arise in the frontal cortex of the brain and impulses pass directly to the vomiting centre.

The exocrine pancreas

The main source of digestive enzymes in the body is the exocrine pancreas.

Anatomical considerations

The greater mass of the pancreas is composed of acinar gland tissues, which produce pancreatic juice. Dispersed among the acini are the endocrine islets of Langerhans, which secrete insulin, glucagon and somatostatin.

The cells lining the acini are **serous cells** containing zymogen granules, which are the precursors of the enzymes of pancreatic juice. The endoplasmic reticulum is extensive and contains numerous ribosomes, which form the enzyme proteins.

The duct system of the pancreas is the same as in salivary glands. Cells of intercalated ducts often extend into the central part of the acinus and are referred to in this position as **centroacinar** cells. In over 70% of people, the main pancreatic duct joins with the bile-duct at the **ampulla of Vater** (Fig. 8.13), the opening of which, into the duodenum, is surrounded by the **sphincter of Oddi** (the choledochoduodenal sphincter).

Preganglionic parasympathetic fibres arrive in the vagus to synapse with ganglion cells around the larger ducts; postganglionic fibres supply the acini. The sympathetic fibres accompany the blood-vessels and visceral afferent fibres run with sympathetic nerves.

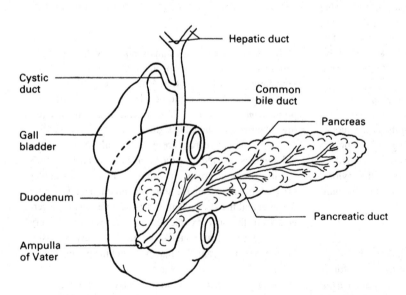

Fig. 8.13 Anatomical relationships of the pancreas, liver, gall-bladder and associated ducts with the duodenum.

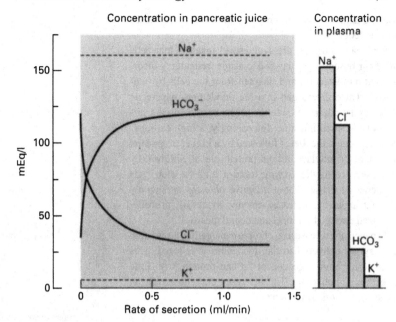

Fig. 8.14 Concentrations of the major ions in pancreatic juice as its secretory rate is increased. Note the reciprocal relationship between Cl⁻ and HCO₃⁻.

Composition and functions of pancreatic juice

The volume of pancreatic juice secreted per day is about 1.2–1.5 litres. Pancreatic juice is isotonic, with a specific gravity of 1.008–1.030; it has an alkaline pH of about 8. It has 1% inorganic materials (electrolytes) and 1–2% organic materials, mostly enzymes.

Electrolytes

The electrolytes are produced by **centroacinar** and **duct cells**. They include the cations Na^+, K^+ and Ca^{2+} and the anions HCO_3^- and Cl^-. The greater bulk of the electrolytes is in the form of $NaHCO_3$. When pancreatic secretion is stimulated, the concentrations of Na^+ and K^+ are near to their level in the blood and remain fairly constant, but HCO_3^- and Cl^- vary with the rate of flow of secretion. HCO_3^- concentration rises and that of Cl^- drops as the rate of flow increases, such that their sum remains constant (see Fig. 8.14). Apparently, the primary secretion of centroacinar cells consists of $NaHCO_3$; the duct cells reabsorb HCO_3^- in exchange for Cl^-. At very low rates of flow, a large amount of HCO_3^- is reabsorbed in exchange for Cl^-, making their concentration near to those in the blood. When the rate of pancreatic secretion is high, there is less time for this exchange, so that the concentration of HCO_3^- increases at the expense of Cl^- (Fig. 8.14).

$NaHCO_3$ in pancreatic juice makes a major contribution to the neutralization of acid chyme, along with bile and duodenal secretion, in order to create a suitable medium for the action of pancreatic enzymes.

Enzymes

The pancreas secretes enzymes that act on all the major types of foodstuffs. The protein-splitting enzymes include **trypsin, chymotrypsin, elastase** and **carboxypeptidase**. They are all secreted in an inactive precursor zymogen form, which is converted to the active enzyme in the intestinal lumen. All pancreatic enzymes are proteins. Trypsinogen is activated into trypsin by the enzyme **enteropeptidase** (enterokinase), secreted by duodenal mucosal cells. Once trypsin is produced, it acts similarly to activate chymotrypsinogen to chymotrypsin, proelastase to elastase and procarboxypeptidase to carboxypeptidase. Thus, the activation of trypsinogen by enteropeptidase is the key to activation of the pancreatic proteases, and enteropeptidase is considered the most important enzyme in intestinal juice.

Trypsin, chymotrypsin and elastase are *endopeptidases*, splitting proteins into shorter peptide chains. Carboxypeptidase is an *exopeptidase*, which splits off amino acids at the C terminus of the peptides.

Starch is split by **pancreatic amylase** at 1,4-glucosidic bonds to maltose, maltotriose and α-dextrins. **Pancreatic lipase** is the most important fat-splitting enzyme. In the presence of bile salts and colipase, which is also secreted by the pancreas, it breaks down triglycerides into fatty acids and monoglycerides. Other lipolytic enzymes are **cholesterol esterase**, which liberates cholesterol and **phospholipase A₂**, which is responsible for breaking down phospholipids into lysophospholipids and fatty acids.

Nucleic acids are broken down by **pancreatic nucleases** into nucleotides.

Pancreatic enzymes are synthesized inside acinar cells by the ribosomes of the endoplasmic reticulum, incorporated into vacuoles and secreted from the cells by exocytosis. Once discharged into the duodenum, pancreatic enzymes are adsorbed on to the **glycocalyx** lining the surface of the small intestine. Interestingly, a high carbohydrate content in the diet is followed by a higher proportion of pancreatic amylase, a high-protein diet is followed by increased proteolytic enzymes and a high-fat diet leads to increased lipase. These *adaptive changes* are mainly brought about by increased enzyme synthesis, probably mediated through hormonal and neural means.

In pancreatic disease, e.g. chronic pancreatitis, the amount of enzymes delivered to the duodenum is reduced. This leads to impaired digestion of fat and protein, with little effect on carbohydrate. The increased excretion of fat in the stools is termed **steatorrhoea**.

Control of pancreatic secretion

Like gastric secretion, pancreatic secretion is regulated by neurohormonal mechanisms and may be considered to occur in three phases: cephalic, gastric and intestinal.

Cephalic phase

The cephalic phase is mediated by the vagus nerve. In animals direct stimulation of the vagus leads to pancreatic secretion which is viscous and *rich in enzymes*. In humans, the sight or smell of appetizing food, as well as its presence in the mouth, is followed by secretion of pancreatic juice containing both enzymes and electrolytes, with the enzymes forming the greater portion. Vagal excitation during the cephalic phase releases, first, acetylcholine, which directly acts on pancreatic acinar and duct cells, and, secondly, **gastrin** from the antrum of the stomach, which also stimulates pancreatic secretion (Fig. 8.15).

Gastric phase

When food reaches the stomach, it activates both neural and hormonal mechanisms. Gastric distension stimulates the pancreas through *long vagovagal reflexes* and also via local *gastropancreatic reflexes*. Gastrin is released from the antrum by distension acting through vagovagal and intramural reflexes and by peptides and amino acids bathing the antral lumen.

Intestinal phase

The intestinal phase is the main phase of pancreatic secretion. Gastric acid, amino acids or fatty acids, on reaching

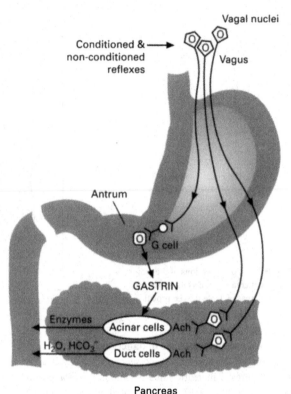

Fig. 8.15 Mechanisms that mediate the cephalic phase of pancreatic juice secretion.

the upper intestine, stimulate secretion from the pancreas. This effect is mediated mainly hormonally. It is now established that the intestinal phase of pancreatic secretion is mainly mediated by two hormones released from the upper intestine: **secretin** and **cholecystokinin**-pancreozymin (CCK) (Fig. 8.16).

Release and effects of secretin

Secretin is released into the blood from S cells in the upper intestinal mucosa, mainly by acid (pH 4 or less) and to a lesser extent by amino acids and fatty acids. Secretin is a peptide with 27 amino acid residues similar in sequence to pancreatic glucagon, GIP and VIP. Its effects are as follows:

1 Secretin acts on centroacinar and duct cells in the pancreas to stimulate secretion of *bicarbonate and water*.

2 It similarly acts on biliary duct cells to stimulate hepatic bile flow and bicarbonate secretion. The stimulation of fluid and electrolyte secretion by secretin in both the pancreas and the biliary system is mediated by cyclic adenosine monophosphate (cAMP).

Fig. 8.16 Release and actions of secretin and CCK during the intestinal phase of pancreatic juice secretion. LAA, L-amino acids; FA, fatty acids.

3 Secretin also augments the action of CCK in stimulating pancreatic enzyme secretion.
4 In the stomach, secretin inhibits gastric acid secretion and the release of gastrin, but it stimulates pepsin secretion.
5 It inhibits gastric motility, contracts the pylorus and thus slows gastric emptying.
6 Secretin relaxes the LOS.
7 Secretin inhibits intestinal motility and contracts the ileocaecal sphincter.

Vasoactive intestinal peptide (VIP)
VIP is found in certain neurones and endocrine cells throughout the intestine; it also stimulates secretion of water and bicarbonate from the pancreas, but it is a weaker stimulus than secretin. VIP has 28 amino acid residues similar in sequence to glucagon and secretin.

Release and effects of CCK-PZ
Pancreatic enzyme secretion is stimulated by an upper intestinal hormone, which was originally called pancreozymin. Later work showed that the activity of pancreozymin and that of another hormone that was shown to contract the gall-bladder and which was called cholecystokinin (CCK) were found in one and the same intestinal

peptide, now referred to as cholecystokinin-pancreozymin (CCK-PZ) or simply CCK. CCK is released from I cells in the upper intestine, mainly by L-amino acids and fatty acids and to a lesser extent by HCl. Release of CCK, however, is suppressed by bile acids. Since CCK stimulates release of bile acids into the duodenum, this strongly suggests that bile acids exert negative feedback control on CCK release.

CCK is a peptide existing in many forms—with 8, 12, 33, 39 or 58 amino acid residues. The last five amino acids at the C terminus are the same as in gastrin and the physiological activity resides in the last eight C-terminal amino acids. All forms of CCK are sulphated. Its effects are as follows:
1 CCK acts on pancreatic acinar cells to stimulate *secretion of enzymes*, but it also augments the stimulation of water and bicarbonate secretion by secretin.
2 CCK has a trophic effect on the pancreas.
3 It contracts the gall-bladder, relaxes the choledocho-duodenal sphincter and causes discharge of bile into the intestine.
4 In small doses CCK stimulates gastric acid secretion but in higher doses it inhibits gastrin-stimulated secretion.
5 Although CCK stimulates gastric motility, it contracts the pylorus, thereby slowing gastric emptying.

6 It antagonizes the action of gastrin at the LOS and thus relaxes it.

7 CCK stimulates intestinal motility.

8 CCK has been found in enteric neurons and the brain, especially the cerebral cortex, and evidence has been presented that it may be concerned with the mechanism of satiety.

Although CCK may act through cAMP, its second messenger in stimulating enzyme secretion from acinar cells seems to be mainly Ca^{2+}. Another potent enzyme stimulant is acetylcholine, which also acts through Ca^{2+}.

A peptide isolated from the intestine specifically stimulates secretion of chymotrypsinogen from the pancreas; it has been called **chymodenin**. Its presence raises the possibility of the presence of more enzyme-specific hormones.

During all phases of pancreatic secretion, there is close integration between neural and hormonal stimuli. Vagal stimulation potentiates the responses of the pancreas to secretin and CCK. The mutual potentiation between secretin and CCK is considered an important factor in the physiological response to food.

Tests of pancreatic function

Recently, direct cannulation of the pancreatic duct through a duodenoscope has been achieved and pure pancreatic juice collected. The parameters determined are usually the volume of secretion and bicarbonate and amylase or trypsin outputs. The capacity of the pancreas to secrete can be assessed after an injection of secretin, followed 30 minutes later by an injection of CCK. The pancreas may also be challenged indirectly by introducing food, acid or amino acid solutions into the upper intestine. If the response is reduced, it may indicate either pancreatic disease or abnormal intestinal mucosa, as in **coeliac disease**, resulting in reduced hormone release.

Pancreatic function can also be assessed by determining faecal fat excretion over a 24-hour period. Normally, about 5 g of fat are excreted per day. In severe pancreatic juice deficiency, up to 50 g of fat may be excreted per day (steatorrhoea).

The liver

Anatomical considerations

The liver weighs about 1.5 kg in the adult. Its basic architectural unit is the lobule (Fig. 8.17), composed of many cellular plates radiating between the central vein and the portal tracts. The hepatic plates are two cells thick. Between the cells there are bile canaliculi, which drain into biliary ducts, and between the plates are found the blood sinusoids. The hepatic sinusolids are lined by endothelial cells and macrophage cells called Kupffer cells. The sinusoids receive blood from branches of the portal vein and branches of the hepatic artery. There is a very narrow space between the endothelial lining of the sinusoids and the hepatic cells, called the space of Disse. This space connects directly with a terminal lymphatic, which drains into a lymphatic vessel in the portal tract. There are large pores in the endothelial lining of the sinusoids, about 1 µm in diameter. These pores are large enough to allow protein molecules to pass through with lymph. Lymph leaving the liver has a protein concentration almost as high as that of the plasma.

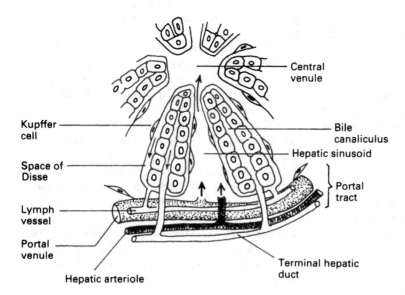

Fig. 8.17 Microscopic structure of hepatic lobule. For details, see text.

Hepatic circulation

For more details on the hepatic circulation, see Chapter 5.

The liver has a dual blood supply, from the portal vein and the hepatic artery. The portal vein is formed by the confluence of the superior mesenteric and splenic veins. It therefore drains the stomach, the small intestine, part of the colon, the pancreas and the spleen. The branches of the portal vein drain into the sinusoids. The hepatic artery arises from the coeliac axis. It supplies the bile-ducts and other structures in the portal tracts and also gives branches that open into the sinusoids. The central veins drain the lobules and collect to form the hepatic vein, which leaves the liver to join the inferior vena cava.

Blood flow through the portal vein is about 1 litre per minute and about 500 ml per minute flows through the hepatic artery. Total hepatic blood flow is thus about 1.5 litres/min. This is approximately 30% of the blood volume and explains why the liver is one of the important blood reservoirs in the body.

Constriction or obliteration of the hepatic vascular channels may follow fibrosis of the liver parenchyma, occurring in liver cirrhosis or hepatic schistosomiasis, raising portal pressure to 20 or 30 mmHg (portal hypertension). In portal hypertension collateral channels to the systemic circulation enlarge and the vessels become tortuous (varices).

The liver forms about 1 ml of lymph per minute, containing about 6 g of protein/100 ml. This is equivalent to between a third and one-half of lymph formed in the whole of the body at rest.

Accumulation of fluid in the peritoneal cavity is called **ascites**. It occurs readily when hepatic venous pressure rises to partially obstruct drainage of blood from the liver. Transudation of fluid into lymph takes place and this leaks through the liver surface into the abnormal cavity. This fluid is almost pure plasma, containing protein with a concentration of 80–90% of that in plasma. The high protein content also creates an osmotic gradient, which attracts more water. In portal hypertension, back pressure on gut capillaries causes oedema of the wall of the gut and fluid exudation into the peritoneal cavity. Since the liver forms the plasma proteins, disease or partial destruction of the hepatocytes leads to hypoproteinaemia, which also contributes to ascites formation.

Functions of the liver

The functions of the liver are so numerous that it is convenient to group them under three subheadings: vascular, secretory and metabolic functions:

1 *Vascular functions*:

  (a) *Storage*. Since the liver blood flow is 30% of blood volume, it is one of the important reservoirs of blood in the body. In the case of strenuous exercise or haemorrhage, part of the hepatic blood is diverted towards the exercising muscles or the vital organs, respectively.

  (b) *Antigen clearance*. The liver filters blood coming from the gut. Kupffer cells in the liver sinusoids belong to the macrophage or reticuloendothelial system. They remove bacteria, debris, particulate matter or any other antigens contained in the blood arriving from the gut.

2 *Secretory functions*. The liver continuously secretes bile, which, after storage and concentration in the gall-bladder, is discharged into the duodenum.

3 *Synthesis function*. The liver synthesizes many useful substances such as albumin and the coagulation factors. Hepatic failure therefore results in hypoalbuminaemia and bleeding disorders.

4 *Metabolic functions*. The liver has a central role in the metabolism of the major types of foodstuffs as well as substances of endogenous or exogenous origin. Details about these metabolic processes may be obtained by reference to specialized texts.

The most serious complication of **hepatic failure** is hepatic encephalopathy. This is probably due to accumulation of substances toxic to the brain, such as *ammonia*, mercaptans, phenols and amines derived from bacteria in the gut. Ammonia is mostly produced by intestinal bacteria and the ability of hepatocytes to detoxicate it to urea is greatly impaired. Other toxins are also derived from gut bacteria. Ammonia combines with *glutamate* in the brain where it gives rise to glutamine and leads to glutamate depletion. Since the latter is the main excitatory transmitter in the brain, its depletion could account for the neuroinhibition of hepatic encephalopathy.

Tests of liver function

Liver function tests are mainly based on assessment of the synthetic, secretory or excretory functions of the liver.

The synthetic functions are assessed by determination of the concentration of the plasma proteins and prothrombin time.

The secretory function may be assessed by determination of bile acids in serum. The role of the liver in bilirubin metabolism may be assessed by estimation of serum bilirubin and other related tests, such as determination of urinary excretion of conjugated bilirubin and urobilinogen.

The excretory function can be assessed after administration of the dye bromsulphthalein (BSP). BSP is conjugated with glutathione in the hepatocytes and excreted in bile. BSP is administered intravenously and its plasma level is determined 45 minutes later. Normally, not more than 5%

Table 8.1 Composition of human bile (mmol/litre).

	Hepatic bile	Gall-bladder bile
Water	98.0%	89.0%
Total solids	2–4%	11.0%
Bile salts	26	145
Bilirubin	0.7	5.0
Cholesterol	2.6	16
Phospholipids (lecithin)	0.5	4.0
Na^+	145	130
K^+	5	12
Ca^{2+}	5	23
Cl^-	100	25
HCO_3^-	28	10
pH	8.3 ± 0.3	7.3 ± 0.3

of BSP should be retained. Alkaline phosphatase, is normally excreted in bile. In biliary obstruction its plasma level rises. For more details of liver function tests, a specialized textbook should be consulted.

The biliary system

Bile is secreted continuously by the hepatocytes. As bile is needed in the intestine only when food is ingested, it needs to be stored between meals. The gall-bladder has a capacity of 30–50 ml. It *stores* and *concentrates* bile and *regulates* its *discharge* into the duodenum. The cystic duct leading from the gall-bladder joins the common hepatic duct to form the common bile-duct, which opens into the duodenum in company with the pancreatic duct at the **ampulla of Vater** (see Fig. 8.13). The opening into the duodenum is guarded by the **choledochoduodenal sphincter**.

Composition and functions of bile

Bile is a viscous golden-yellow or greenish fluid with a bitter taste. It is iso-osmotic with plasma and slightly alkaline. The liver produces about 5 litres of bile per day but only 500–600 ml are poured into the duodenum daily. The composition of the human bile from the liver and in the gall-bladder is given in Table 8.1. It is clear from this table that the gall-bladder not only stores bile but also concentrates it. Concentration is achieved through active absorption of Na^+, Cl^- and HCO_3^- by the lining epithelium, with associated passive water movement out of the lumen. The drop of pH of gall-bladder bile is due to the reduction of the concentration of $NaHCO_3$. The gall-bladder epithelium also secretes mucus, which increases the viscosity of bile.

Neutralization of acid chyme

$NaHCO_3$ in bile is responsible for its alkaline reaction and participates with pancreatic and duodenal secretions in the neutralization of acid chyme delivered from the stomach.

Fat digestion and absorption

The bile salts are essential for the *emulsification* and *absorption* of fats. Since absorption of the fat-soluble vitamins is closely related to the absorption of fats in general, bile salts are also important for the absorption of vitamins A, D, E and K.

The bile salts are the sodium and potassium salts of the bile acids. These are steroid acids, synthesized in the liver from cholesterol by the enzyme cholesterol 7α-hydroxylase. The principal primary bile acids are **cholic acid** and **chenodeoxycholic acid**. They are conjugated in the hepatocytes with glycine and taurine, to give **glycocholic** and **taurocholic acids** respectively.

Enterohepatic circulation of bile acids.
About 20–30 g of bile acids are poured into the duodenum per day. Some of the bile acids are deconjugated and dehydroxylated in the 7α position by the intestinal bacteria. Dehydroxylation results in the production of the **secondary bile acids**, i.e. deoxycholic and lithocholic acids. The intestine thus contains both conjugated and unconjugated primary and secondary bile acids. On reaching the terminal ileum, 90% of the bile acids are absorbed by secondary active transport, i.e. cotransported with Na^+, which is pumped out by Na^+, K^+ ATPase in the basolateral border of the enterocyte, and reach the liver through the portal vein. In the liver cells, the bile acids are reconjugated and resecreted in bile.

In the small intestine cholic acid is absorbed faster than chenodeoxycholic acid, and conjugated bile acids are absorbed better than unconjugated bile acids. Some unconjugated bile acids are absorbed passively in the colon and also reach the liver through the portal vein. About 0.6 g of unconjugated dehydroxylated bile acids are lost in the faeces daily. These are replaced by new synthesis from cholesterol in the liver, so that the total bile acid pool is maintained constant at 2–4 g. Since the amount of bile acids poured into the duodenum each day is 20–30 g, the daily turnover of the total bile acid pool through the enterohepatic circulation must be 6–10 times.

The presence of bile acids in portal blood as a result of the enterohepatic circulation is essential for stimulating and maintaining the secretion of bile by the hepatocytes. If the enterohepatic circulation is interrupted (e.g. due to obstruction by disease or surgical removal of the terminal ileum), bile flow is markedly decreased. Synthesis of bile acids in the hepatocytes and of cholesterol in the liver and intestinal mucosa is increased. Despite this, however, the output of bile acids into the duodenum is reduced. Deficiency of bile acids leads mainly to defective fat digestion and absorption and **steatorrhoea** (excessive fat in the stool). Absorption of fat-soluble vitamins is also reduced. Excess amounts of bile acids entering the colon may result in diarrhoea (see below).

Functions of the bile acids

1 In the intestinal lumen the bile acids are essential for **emulsification** of fats. They enter into the formation of **mixed micelles**, needed for absorption of lipids and fat-soluble vitamins.

2 Bile acids have a negative feedback effect on the release of CCK from its cells in the upper intestine and thus contribute to the regulation of pancreatic secretion and the discharge of bile into the intestine.

3 They have a negative feedback effect on the synthesis of cholesterol by the intestinal mucosal cells.

4 In the liver, bile acids are important for stimulating bile secretion and flow (choleresis), but they have a negative feedback effect on the synthesis of bile acids from cholesterol and also on hepatic synthesis of cholesterol. Bile acids in the liver also take part in the formation of *micelles*, which render cholesterol soluble in bile.

5 In the colon, bile acids inhibit reabsorption of water and electrolytes, stimulate motility and may cause diarrhoea.

Excretory function of bile

Bile is a medium for excretion of bile pigments, cholesterol and many drugs, e.g. penicillin, toxins, various inorganic substances, such as copper and zinc, and dyes, such as bromsulphthalein.

The principal bile pigment, **bilirubin**, is conjugated with glucuronic acid in hepatocytes to form bilirubin diglucuronide, thereby rendering it water-soluble. The conjugated bilirubin is actively secreted by the liver cells into the bile canaliculi independent of the secretion of bile acids. The colour of bile is due to bilirubin.

About 1–2 g of **cholesterol** appears in bile per day. Cholesterol is water-insoluble; it is solubilized by incorporation in micelles, along with the bile acids and **phospholipid**. The micelles remain stable so long as the concentrations of bile acids, phospholipids and cholesterol remain within certain limits. If the relative concentration of any of the constituents alters, cholesterol may be precipitated out of solution. In people who produce bile with a high concentration of cholesterol, **cholesterol gallstones** may form in the gall-bladder.

Fig. 8.18 The relationship between bile flow and bile acid secretion in humans. The dotted line is extrapolated to give the bile acid-independent secretion. (From data by Sherstan, T., Nilsson, C.S., Cahlin, E., Filipson, M. & Brodin-Persson, G. (1971) *European J. Clin. Invest.*, **1**, 242–7.)

Control of the biliary system

There are two aspects of control of the biliary system to consider:

1 Secretion of bile by the liver cells (**choleresis**).

2 Contraction of the gall-bladder with relaxation of the choledochoduodenal sphincter to pour bile into the duodenum (**cholecystokinesis**).

The human liver secretes bile at a pressure of about 25 cm H_2O. Between meals, the choledochoduodenal sphincter is normally closed, offering a resistance of about 30 cm H_2O. Bile secreted by the liver is thus diverted to the gall-bladder during the interdigestive periods. Pressure in the lumen of the gall-bladder varies between 0 and 16 cm H_2O.

Control of choleresis

In the **hepatocytes**, the main driving force for bile secretion is the active transport of organic anions, especially *bile acids*, into the canaliculi, with water flowing passively along the osmotic gradient created. In the **biliary ducts**, *bicarbonate* is secreted independently of bile acid secretion and is followed passively by water. Total bile flow is thus due to two components: bile acid-dependent and bile acid-independent components.

Bile acid-dependent component. There is a direct linear relationship between the rate of bile flow and bile acid secretion (Fig. 8.18). After cannulation of the bile-duct during a surgical operation on a man, bile acids were introduced into the duodenum through a tube. Bile was collected from the cannula and its flow rate and bile acid output were determined. The exogenous bile acids were incorporated into the **enterohepatic circulation** and produced the increase in bile secretion. This *bile acid-dependent component* depends mainly on the integrity of the enterohepatic circulation. At least 90% of the rate of secretion of bile acids is determined by the rate of clearance of reabsorbed bile acids from the portal vein. The remaining 10% is due to synthesis of new bile acids by hepatocytes. As mentioned previously, interruption of the enterohepatic circulation results in markedly reduced choleresis.

Bile acid-independent component. With reference to Fig. 8.18, the regression line does not pass through the origin. When extrapolated, it intercepts the *y* axis at about 0.2 ml/min. This means that, when the rate of bile acid secretion is zero, there would still be some bile flow, i.e. the *bile acid-independent component*. This fraction of bile secretion is due to secretion of HCO_3^-, followed by water, by the biliary duct cells. It depends on active sodium transport, since it is blocked by inhibition of Na^+, K^+ ATPase. Pure stimulation of this component may actually lead to reduction in the concentration of bile acids in bile.

The bile acid-independent fraction of bile secretion is stimulated by the hormones **secretin glucagon**, **CCK** and **gastrin**. They all stimulate the secretion of HCO_3^- and passive H_2O transfer by the biliary duct cells. Vagal stimulation also stimulates bile flow. The effect is mediated mainly indirectly, through stimulation of gastric acid secretion, which leads to release of secretin and CCK. All substances that stimulate hepatic secretion of bile or choleresis are termed **choleretics**.

Control of the discharge of bile into the intestine
Contraction of the gall-bladder is followed almost immediately by relaxation of the choledochoduodenal sphincter. The sphincter is kept closed by cholinergic mechanisms (which can be blocked by atropine) and relaxed by the hormone CCK. The passage of a peristaltic wave down the duodenum also causes opening of the sphincter of Oddi, which allows bile in the bile-duct to enter in spurts during periods of duodenal relaxation, stopping during contraction. This mechanism may be of value after cholecystectomy.

Discharge of bile into the duodenum is regulated by nervous and hormonal mechanisms. The nervous component is mediated by the **vagus nerve** and follows psychic influences and food ingestion. During this cephalic phase, bile is discharged for only a brief period into the duodenum.

The main pouring of bile occurs when chyme reaches the upper intestine and the mechanism is mainly hormonal, being mediated by **CCK**. The presence of digestive products of fats and proteins, i.e. fatty acids and L-amino acids, releases CCK from the upper intestine into the blood. CCK contracts the gall-bladder and relaxes the choledochoduodenal sphincter, thereby discharging bile into the duodenum. Both vagal excitation and secretin augment the action of CCK on the gall-bladder. $MgSO_4$ contracts the gall-bladder and discharges bile into the intestine because it releases CCK. Generally, substances that lead to the pouring of bile into the intestine by contracting the gall-bladder and relaxing the sphincter are called **cholagogues**.

Radiological test of biliary function
The function of the gall-bladder and biliary ducts may be assessed radiologically (cholecystography) after oral or intravenous administration of a radio-opaque substance which is excreted by the liver into the bile, e.g. tetra-iodophenolphthalein or iopanoic acid. A non-functioning gall-bladder fails to show the opaque material in its cavity. Gallstones show as filling defects. The function of the gall-bladder may be evaluated further by giving a cholagogue and assessing its contraction. The cholagogues used include ingestion of a fatty meal or administration of $MgSO_4$, **CCK** or **caerulein**. Caerulein is a peptide with 10 amino acids. It has all the properties of gastrin and CCK and is used in cholecystography to contract the gall-bladder. Ultrasonography may also be used to detect gallstones and measure the contractility of the gall-bladder.

Jaundice
An increase of the bile pigment bilirubin in plasma (normal 0.5 mg/dl) to about 2.5 mg/dl or more results in yellow pigmentation of the skin, sclera and mucous membranes. If this is due to obstruction of the bile-duct, it is known as **obstructive jaundice**. Excessive haemolysis of red blood cells (RBCs) can also lead to jaundice, even with normal liver and biliary function. This type is known as **haemolytic jaundice**. It is due to formation of bilirubin in excess of the liver capacity to excrete it. In obstructive jaundice the bilirubin is conjugated and therefore gives a direct reaction with the van den Bergh test. In haemolytic jaundice most of the bilirubin is non-conjugated and bound to plasma protein. Therefore, the protein needs to be precipitated by ethanol before the van den Bergh test is applied. The test is said to be indirect. This is one way to differentiate between the two types of jaundice. A third type is **hepatic jaundice**. In this case there is severe damage to the liver cells, caused by disease, and any of the

Fig. 8.19 Diagram of longitudinal section of two villi to show the histological organization of the mucosa of the small intestine (*right*) and the blood supply (*left*).

following processes may be reduced: uptake, conjugation or active secretion of bilirubin into the bile canniculus. Normal amounts of bilirubin fail to be excreted and therefore accumulate and give rise to jaundice.

The small intestine

In the small intestine the digestion of food materials is completed and the products of digestion are absorbed. The small intestine is, in fact, the main site of absorption of nutrients in the body.

The small intestine extends from the pylorus to the caecum. It is arbitrarily divided into the duodenum, jejunum and ileum. The jejunum is taken as the upper two-fifths of the intestine below the duodenum. The ileum is the remaining three-fifths. The most prominent histological feature in the intestinal mucosa is the presence of the **villi**, small finger-like projections about 1 mm in height. In humans and some animals, there are **mucosal folds** up to 1 cm in height and about 5 cm in length. In addition, the epithelial cells lining the villi have numerous **microvilli**. The mucosal folds, villi and microvilli enormously increase the intestinal surface available for absorption. The total surface area has been estimated to be about 300 square metres.

Between the bases of the villi are found the intestinal glands (**crypts of Lieberkühn**), which secrete intestinal juice (succus entericus). **Brunner's glands** are found in the submucosa of the duodenum. Their secretion reaches the lumen through ducts that penetrate the mucosa to open at the base of the crypts. Lymphoid tissue is found throughout the small intestine, but in the ileum it is aggregated into prominent nodules called **Peyer's patches**.

The lamina propria constitutes the connective-tissue core of the villus. It contains a central arteriole that breaks up into looping capillaries that connect to venules, a single lymph vessel (lacteal), nerve fibres, smooth-muscle cells that extend along the villus and many mononuclear cells, including lymphocytes, plasma cells and macrophages (Fig. 8.19). In the crypts, the lining epithelial cells include the following types: (i) undifferentiated, actively dividing cells, frequently seen in mitosis; (ii) mucus-secreting **goblet cells**; (iii) various epithelial endocrine cells; and (iv) **Paneth cells** containing large eosinophilic granules. Although Paneth cells have been shown to contain lysozyme and immunoglobulins, their precise function still remains uncertain. The epithelial cells lining the villi include: (i) the digestive absorptive columnar cells, with microvillous brush border, called enterocytes; (ii) mucus-secreting goblet cells; and (iii) a few endocrine epithelial cells.

It has been shown that the actively proliferating cells in the crypts migrate on to the villus, taking 2–5 days. In the process these cells become differentiated into the enterocytes, and digestive enzymes appear in their brush border. The microvilli of the enterocytes are covered by a layer of **glycocalyx**, which is a complex of polysaccharide and protein. Glycocalyx mainly adsorbs pancreatic enzymes and seems to place the final products of digestion in a strategically advantageous position for absorption.

Cells are constantly shed from the tips of the villi and are replaced by upward-migrating, actively proliferating cells of the crypts. The intestinal epithelium is thus one of the most actively proliferating tissues in the body. In humans 50–200 g of gastrointestinal mucosa are renewed daily. Agents that inhibit mitosis, such as ionizing radiation and cytotoxic drugs, lead to flattening of the mucosa as cells extruded from the tip are unreplaced.

Intestinal secretion

Brunner's glands in the duodenum secrete an alkaline fluid that contains mucus but no enzymes.

The intestinal crypts secrete about 1 litre per day of intestinal juice or **succus entericus**. This has a pH of 6.5–7.6 and 1.6% of solids, 0.6% organic and 1% inorganic. Intestinal juice is a turbid fluid with a fishy odour. Most of the enzymes are found either in the brush border or in the cytoplasm of the enterocyte and are thus present in only trace amounts as a result of disintegration of desquamated mucosal epithelial cells in the lumen. The enzymes that are actually secreted into the lumen are **enteropeptidase** (enterokinase) and **amylase**.

As mentioned earlier, enteropeptide activates trypsinogen to trypsin and thereby holds the key to activation of all the pancreatic proteolytic enzymes. Enteropeptidase is, in fact, the most important enzyme secreted in intestinal juice. When it is congenitally deficient, protein digestion is severely impaired.

Succus entericus participates in the neutralization of acid chyme delivered from the stomach. Its enzymes complete the digestion of food materials.

Digestion in the small intestine

The polypeptides resulting from the action of the pancreatic *endopeptidases* (trypsin, chymotrypsin and elastase) are further attacked by the *exopeptidases*. These are the carboxypeptidases of pancreatic juice, which split off the terminal amino acids with the free carboxyl group, and the aminopeptidases of the succus entericus, which split off the terminal amino acids with the free amino group. The result is a mixture of **amino acids** and **oligopeptides**, i.e. tetra-, tri- and dipeptides. The short peptides are taken up by the brush border of the enterocyte, where they are broken down by **oligopeptidases**. Some of the di- and tripeptides are, however, absorbed intact into the cytoplasm of the enterocyte, where they are hydrolysed by **intracellular di- and tripeptidases** to their constituent amino acids.

The nucleotides resulting from the action of the **nucleases** are hydrolysed further by the **nucleotidases** and **nucleosidases** of intestinal juice to a mixture of purine and pyrimidine bases, phosphoric acid and pentose sugars.

Lipase of succus entericus acts like pancreatic lipase to split triglycerides into fatty acids and monoglycerides, but is considered of less importance than pancreatic lipase.

Maltose, resulting from the action of salivary, pancreatic and intestinal amylase on starch, is broken down by **maltase** in the brush border of the enterocyte to two molecules of glucose. The disaccharides sucrose and lactose (milk sugar) taken with the food are hydrolysed, respectively, by **sucrase** and **lactase** in the brush border of the enterocyte. Sucrose is broken down to glucose and fructose, and lactose to glucose and galactose. All the disaccharidases are developed at the time of birth but a decrease in the activity of lactase occurs after weaning in most species. In humans, regression of lactase activity occurs, but there are ethnic differences in the extent of the decline. In northern European populations, for instance, the decline is quite slow. Deficiency of a disaccharidase may be inherited or may be secondary to small-bowel disease. It leads to malabsorption of the corresponding sugar. The unabsorbed disaccharide is broken down by intestinal bacteria to lactic and other acids and this results in distension, flatulence and osmotic diarrhoea. Milk or *lactose intolerance* is found in a high proportion of the population in Africa and Asia and may constitute a problem in nutrition.

Deficiency of a specific disaccharidase may be investigated by giving a test dose of the disaccharide, followed by monitoring of blood glucose level. Failure of the blood glucose level to rise is indicative of the disaccharidase deficiency. Clinically, disaccharidase deficiency is indicated by the occurrence of diarrhoea. Disaccharidase enzymes may also be estimated directly on samples of intestinal mucosa obtained by peroral biopsy.

A summary of digestive enzymes and their actions is given in Table 8.2.

Dietary fibre

Fibres of plant origin are mostly carbohydrates. They are not hydrolysed by pancreatic or intestinal enzymes in humans. They include cellulose, hemicellulose, lignin and various gums and pectic substances. They pass unchanged

Table 8.2 Summary of digestive enzymes.

Source	Enzyme*	Substrate	Catalytic products
Salivary glands	Ptyalin (amylase)	Starch	Dextrins, maltotriose and maltose
	Lingual lipase	Triglycerides	Monoglycerides and fatty acids
Stomach	Pepsins	Proteins	Peptones and polypeptides
	Gastric lipase	Triglycerides	Monoglycerides and fatty acids
Pancreas	Trypsin	Proteins and polypeptides	Peptides
	Chymotrypsin	Proteins and polypeptides	Peptides
	Elastase	Elastin and other proteins	Peptides
	Carboxypeptidase A	Polypeptides	Carboxy-terminal amino acids with aromatic or aliphatic side-chains
	Carboxypeptidase B	Polypeptides	Carboxy-terminal amino acids with basic side-chains
	Colipase	Fat droplets	Facilitates exposure of active site of pancreatic lipase
	Pancreatic lipase	Triglycerides	Monoglycerides and fatty acids
	Cholesterol esterase	Cholesterol esters	Cholesterol
	Phospholipase A_2	Phospholipids	Fatty acids, lysophospholipids
	Pancreatic amylase	Starch	Dextrins, maltotriose and maltose
	Ribonuclease	RNA	Nucleotides
	Deoxyribonuclease	DNA	Nucleotides
Small intestine	Enteropeptidase	Trypsinogen	Trypsin
	Aminopeptidases	Polypeptides	N-terminal amino acids
	Oligopeptidases	Di-, tri- and tetrapeptides	Amino acids
	Maltase	Maltose	Glucose
	Lactase	Lactose	Glucose and galactose
	Sucrase	Sucrose	Glucose and fructose
	Nucleotidases and nucleosidases	Nucleotides and nucleosides	Pentoses, purine and pyrimidine bases and phosphate

* All the proteolytic enzymes are secreted in inactive zymogen form. The pepsinogens are activated to pepsins by HCl. Trypsinogen is activated to trypsin by enteropeptidase; trypsin activates the zymogen forms of the rest of the proteolytic enzymes, as well as procolipase to colipase and prophospholipase A_2 to phospholipase A_2. RNA, ribonucleic acid; DNA, deoxyribonucleic acid.

to the lower small intestine and colon, where they are metabolized by bacteria to short-chain fatty acids and the gases carbon dioxide, hydrogen, hydrogen sulphide and methane, leading to an increase in osmolality and greater bulk of colonic contents. This stimulates motility, leading to reduced transit time and greater amounts of stools. Natural food, which is nearer to the diets of rural populations, has a high fibre content. In contrast, the refined food of the industrialized or urban societies is low in fibre. Epidemiological evidence has been presented to suggest that consumption of low-fibre diets is associated with constipation, diverticulosis, colonic cancer, irritable bowel syndrome, haemorrhoids, appendicitis, gallstones, hypertension, coronary heart disease and diabetes mellitus, all of which have a high prevalence in Europe and North America. A shift to more natural, moderately high-fibre diets is now advocated. As more and more people urbanize

in the developing countries, they would do well to avoid repeating the experience of the developed countries.

Control of intestinal secretion

Brunner's glands in the duodenum are stimulated mainly by hormones. **Secretin** can cause secretion but a hormone which specifically stimulates Brunner's gland has been postulated; it is called **duocrinin** and is still known only in crude extract form. **Vagal stimulation** can cause secretion but the role of the vagus is probably minor since denervation of a duodenal segment has very little effect on its response to food.

Secretion of intestinal juice is very low in the interdigestive period. The most important stimulus is the presence of food in the lumen of the intestine. Distension, as well as tactile and irritating stimuli, evoke considerable secretion from intestinal glands through local neural reflexes.

Secretion of electrolytes and water in the intestinal lumen is mainly due to active secretion of Cl⁻ through a specific channel activated by cAMP. Cl⁻ is followed by passive diffusion of Na⁺ and water. Activation of the Cl⁻ channel by cAMP occurs under physiological conditions after a meal, through the action of a gastrointestinal peptide, e.g. VIP, or neurotransmitters. The toxin of the cholera vibrio produces profuse secretion through activation of adenylate cyclase and increasing the concentration of cAMP. Indeed, death in cholera is due almost entirely to the dehydration and shock due to severe diarrhoea. If the water and electrolyte losses are promptly replaced, the patient can be saved.

Vagal stimulation is an unreliable stimulus of intestinal secretion, but parasympathomimetic drugs stimulate secretion. Sympathetic stimulation exerts an inhibitory influence on intestinal secretion. Section of the splanchnic nerves is followed by secretion, called *paralytic secretion*. This may also be contributed to by vasodilatation consequent on loss of sympathetic vasoconstrictor tone.

The hormones **gastrin**, **CCK**, **secretin** and **glucagon** stimulate intestinal secretion. It has been postulated that a hormone, called **enterocrinin**, is released from the intestinal mucosa into the blood by chyme to stimulate secretion of succus entericus; it is still known only in crude extract form. **Vasoactive intestinal peptide (VIP)** stimulates intestinal secretion. A tumour that produces VIP may rarely arise from a cell in the pancreatic islets; it has been called a *vipoma*. It causes a syndrome of severe watery diarrhoea, hypokalaemia and achlorhydria (WDHA syndrome or *pancreatic cholera*).

Intestinal absorption

Although a small amount of water is absorbed in the stomach and substantial amounts of sodium and water are absorbed in the colon along with folic acid, some amino acids and short-chain fatty acids, the main site of absorption of nutrients is the small intestine. To be absorbed, a substance traverses an unstirred water layer (UWL), a glycocalyx layer and the brush border, cytoplasm and basolateral borders of the enterocyte. After passing through the basement membrane, it enters either a capillary, subsequently passing into the portal circulation, or the lacteals into lymph to eventually reach the systemic circulation through the thoracic duct. The mechanism of transport may be **passive diffusion** along an electrochemical gradient, or may be **carrier-mediated**. When carrier-mediated transport is along an electrical or chemical gradient, it is called **facilitated diffusion**; no direct energy input is required. When a carrier transports a substance against an electrical or chemical gradient, energy input is required and the process is called **active transport**. Active transport is fastest, followed in descending order by facilitated diffusion and passive diffusion. Some large substances may be absorbed by **endocytosis**.

Absorption of carbohyrates

Digestion of starch and disaccharides ends in the hexose monosaccharides glucose, galactose and fructose. Complete digestion of nucleic acids produces pentose sugars. Glucose and galactose are actively transported and fructose is transported by facilitated diffusion, while the pentoses are passively absorbed.

There is experimental evidence that shows a direct link between the absorption of glucose and that of sodium. The presence of sodium in the gut lumen increases the rate of glucose absorption. Inhibition of the sodium pump, e.g. by **ouabain**, reduces the rate of glucose absorption. Administration of substances that block the release of metabolic energy, such as **dinitrophenol**, as well as that of the glycoside **phloridzin**, inhibits the rate of glucose

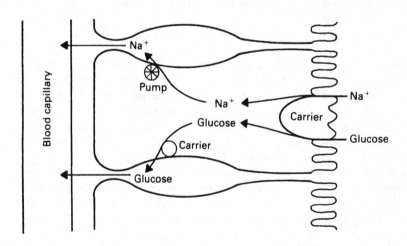

Fig. 8.20 Diagram showing the cotransport of sodium and glucose by the absorptive cells of the small intestine. Details are in the text.

absorption. These findings lend support to the model shown in Fig. 8.20. There is a membrane carrier protein in the brush border for **cotransport** of glucose and Na^+ to the inside of the cell (sodium–glucose cotransporter, SGLT 1), where they are released. Glucose is further transported by **facilitated diffusion** across the basolateral membrane by another carrier (glucose transporter 2 (GLUT2)). The sodium is actively extruded across the basolateral membrane out to the *intercellular space* by the sodium pump, i.e. Na^+, K^+ ATPase. This creates a gradient for the entry of Na^+ across the luminal membrane and is the step that requires direct input of energy. Dinitrophenol and ouabain inhibit the transport of sodium to the outside of the enterocyte and consequently the absorption of glucose as well. Indeed, intestinal absorption of glucose is one of the best examples of **secondary active transport**, i.e. secondary to the action of Na^+, K^+ ATPase. Phloridzin acts by competing with glucose for the carrier at the brush border. Since the carrier has more affinity for glucose than for galactose, the latter is transported more slowly.

Fructose is partly converted to glucose and lactate within the enterocyte, creating a steep inward concentration gradient. In addition, there is a specific membrane carrier for fructose so that it is transported by **facilitated diffusion**. The *pentoses*, being transported by **passive diffusion** have the slowest rate of absorption, followed in ascending order by fructose, galactose and glucose. All of these monosaccharides enter portal blood to reach the liver for further metabolic processing.

In a mixed meal, usually all the digestible carbohydrates are absorbed. The bulk of carbohydrate absorption occurs in the upper intestine.

Absorption of proteins

Digestion of proteins results in the liberation of amino acids and short peptides. *Di- and tripeptides* are, in fact, absorbed faster than their constituent amino acids. As explained previously, they are hydrolysed by brush-border and cytoplasmic oligopeptidases. Amino acids are absorbed according to their optical isomerism: D-amino acids are transported by passive diffusion but the naturally occurring L-amino acids are transported by several *active transport* mechanisms. The active absorption of L-amino acids, like that of glucose, is sodium-dependent; the presence of sodium accelerates the rate of amino acid transport. There seem to be separate mechanisms for the transport of basic, acidic and neutral amino acids. A fourth mechanism transports imino acids, such as proline, hydroxyproline and glycine. Small peptides have separate carriers, which may provide additional mechanisms in case the amino acid transport systems are saturated under physiological condi-

tions. As the amino acids accumulate within the enterocyte, they passively diffuse into the blood to enter the portal circulation.

Even whole proteins and polypeptides may be absorbed. In infants, protein antibodies from maternal colostrum enter the enterocyte probably by pinocytosis and exit by exocytosis into the blood. In this way *passive immunity* is conferred on the infant. The ability of the enterocyte to absorb whole proteins declines with age but small amounts may be absorbed in adulthood, thus providing the basis for the occurrence of food allergies. The intestine is one of the entry sites for protein antigens.

About 85–90% of ingested protein is usually absorbed and most of the absorption of protein materials occurs in the upper intestine. It is noteworthy that most of the protein in stools comes not from the diet but from cellular debris and intestinal bacteria.

The purine and pyrimidine bases resulting from the digestion of nucleic acids are absorbed by active transport.

Absorption of fats

Triacylglycerols, along with some monoglycerides and fatty acids, resulting from the action of lingual and gastric lipases, are delivered in crude emulsion form into the duodenum. In the upper intestine, bile salts and lecithin emulsify the fat mixture further and pancreatic lipase attacks the fat globules at their interface with water in the presence of colipase and bile salts. Colipase is secreted by the pancreas; it binds to the surface of fat droplets, displacing the emulsifying agents and allowing lipase to anchor to the droplet. The triglycerides are consequently hydrolysed to fatty acids and monoglycerides.

With the presence of bile salts and monoglycerides, **mixed micelles** are produced. These are stable water-soluble structures 3–10 nm in diameter that can incorporate other lipid components within them. Essentially, molecules are aggregated in a micelle in such a way that water-soluble hydrophilic polar groups, i.e. hydroxyl and carboxyl groups, are facing the outer side of the micelle while fat-soluble hydrophobic hydrocarbon chains are facing the interior of the micelle. In addition to the basic building-blocks of the micelle, i.e. the bile salts and monoglycerides, long-chain fatty acids, cholesterol and fat-soluble vitamins are incorporated into the interior of the micelle. In this way, these hydrophobic compounds are made water-soluble. The mixed micelles enter the **unstirred water layer** (UWL) immediately adjacent to the intestinal epithelium and make contact with the brush border of the enterocyte.

The **monoglycerides, long-chain fatty acids** and **cholesterol**, being lipid-soluble, enter the enterocyte by passive diffusion, although recent evidence has indicated use of carrier-mediated transport. The bile-salt micelles diffuse back into the chyme to pick up more monoglycerides, fatty acids and cholesterol and bring them into contact with the enterocyte. Thus, the bile salts seem to perform a transfer function through the UWL that helps the absorption of monoglycerides, long-chain fatty acids, cholesterol and probably also **fat-soluble vitamins**. The **bile salts** are absorbed actively in the terminal ileum to enter the portal circulation and reach the liver, from which they are resecreted into bile in the upper intestine (*entero-hepatic circulation*).

The **monoglycerides, long-chain fatty acids** and **cholesterol** that enter the enterocyte are re-esterified to triglycerides and cholesterol esters. They are then surrounded by a layer of lipoprotein, cholesterol and phospholipid to form **chylomicrons**. These enter the lacteals and leave the intestine in lymph to reach the systemic circulation through the thoracic duct.

The fatty acids with more than 10–12 carbon atoms are considered long-chain and are incorporated into the chylomicrons, as just explained. **Short-chain fatty acids** with less than 10–12 carbon atoms are directly absorbed into the enterocyte by secondary *active sodium-dependent transport* mechanism; they pass directly to the liver in portal blood.

Most absorption of fat occurs in the upper intestine, although substantial absorption takes place in the ileum. In a mixed meal about 95% of the fat is absorbed. The stools contain about 5 g of fat per day, which is equivalent to about 5% of the stool bulk, but most of this fat is derived from cellular debris and remnants of intestinal bacteria rather than from the diet. Defective assimilation of fats leads to increased excretion of fat in the stools, well in excess of 5 g/day. The stools are also pale, greasy and bulky with an offensive smell. This condition is called **steatorrhoea**. Steatorrhoea may result either from maldigestion (e.g. deficiency of pancreatic lipase or bile salts) or malabsorption due to diseased intestinal mucosa, e.g. in the **coeliac syndrome**.

Absorption of vitamins

Absorption of the fat-soluble vitamins A (retinol), D, E and K is tied to that of fat. If fat absorption is deficient, absorption of the fat-soluble vitamins will also be defective. Conditions which lead to steatorrhoea may be accompanied by symptoms of fat-soluble vitamin deficiencies.

Absorption of vitamin B_{12} (cyanocobalamin) requires the presence of a glycoprotein secreted by the parietal cells of the gastric mucosa; it has been called the intrinsic factor. It combines with vitamin B_{12} derived from food (the extrinsic factor) and the complex is absorbed in the terminal ileum. Probably the intrinsic factor stimulates endocytosis of cyanocobalamin after the complex is bound to specific receptors on the enterocyte.

It is now realized that the intestinal absorption of the water-soluble vitamins, a diverse group of chemical substances, does not mainly occur by passive diffusion. Except for pyridoxine and *p*-aminobenzoic acid, both of which are absorbed by passive diffusion, the rest are absorbed by carrier-mediated transport. Although there are minor species differences, ascorbic acid, biotin, inositol, nicotinic acid and thiamine are absorbed by active transport, while choline, folic acid and riboflavine are absorbed by facilitated diffusion.

Absorption of water and electrolytes

Secretions from salivary glands, stomach, bile, pancreas and intestine add up to a total of 7 litres/day. Ingested water is about 2 litres/day (may be much more in hot climates). Out of this daily input of 9 litres of water, a negligible amount is absorbed in the stomach. Net daily absorption in the small intestine is about 7.5–8 litres and in the colon about 1 litre. The remainder is excreted in the stools, 150–200 ml/day. Thus, about 98% of the water entering the lumen of the alimentary tract each day is reabsorbed. This huge internal turnover of water amounts to about 20% of the total amount of water in the human body. Also it should be remembered that water moves freely in and out of the lumen of the small intestine depending on the osmotic pressure of its contents. It is thus easy to understand that persistent vomiting or diarrhoea can readily result in dehydration and this is especially true in infants and young children.

Part of the **sodium** in the lumen of the small intestine can move passively in either direction across intestinal epithelium, following water movement, depending upon the osmotic gradient. The other part moves across the luminal border of the small intestine and colon along a concentration gradient created by **Na^+, K^+ ATPase**, which is located at the *basolateral membrane* of the epithelial cells. Such actively absorbed sodium in the small intestine facilitates the absorption of glucose, amino acids and short-chain fatty acids. In turn, the presence of glucose facilitates the absorption of sodium. This is the basis of the proved benefit of oral administration of both NaCl and glucose in diarrhoeal diseases, e.g. cholera. In the colon, active absorption of sodium is followed by passive water absorption.

For the most part, **potassium** moves across intestinal epithelium by diffusion. Since the gut lumen is electronegative in relation to the blood, net movement of potassium occurs into the lumen. A small component of potassium is actively secreted into the lumen as part of mucus. The net loss of potassium to the lumen of the small and large intestines explains why *hypokalaemia* readily develops in diarrhoea.

In the ileum and colon, **chloride** is actively reabsorbed in exchange for bicarbonate, which tends to make the lower intestinal contents more alkaline.

Malabsorption syndromes

There are a variety of conditions which lead to defects of digestion and absorption. Some common examples are as follows:

1 Failure of absorption of fats, carbohydrates and proteins leads to loss of weight and *malnutrition*.

2 Malabsorption of carbohydrates usually leads to diarrhoea of the osmotic type. The action of colonic bacteria on the unabsorbed carbohydrate results in gas formation, *flatulence* and abdominal distension.

3 Malabsorption of bile acids and fatty acids leads to diarrhoea with frequent loose motions.

4 Impaired fat digestion leads to a high fat content of the stool, which becomes bulky, foul-smelling and frothy (*steatorrhoea*).

5 Vitamins and minerals may fail to be absorbed in a variety of conditions, leading to specific deficiencies, e.g. *tetany* and *osteoporosis* in the case of Ca^{2+}, Mg^{2+} and P malabsorption; *anaemia* in the case of iron, folate or B_{12} malabsorption; and a *tendency to bleed* or to bruise easily when there is failure to absorb vitamin K, as in obstructive jaundice.

Movements of the small intestine

The functions of movements of the small intestine are the *mixing* and churning of chyme to aid digestion and absorption and the *propulsion* of chyme along to the colon.

Study of the electrical activity of the smooth muscle in the small intestine indicates that in the duodenum, just above the opening of the bile and pancreatic ducts, there is a **'pacemaker'** region from which small-bowel slow waves, also called basal electric rhythm (BER), start and move caudally. These are spontaneous cyclic waves of smooth-muscle depolarization and repolarization, which are responsible for the coordination of intestinal movements. Their frequency gradually declines as they move caudally; they are about 12/min in the duodenum and 8/min in the ileum. Spikes of action potentials associated with contractions are superimposed on the depolarization phase of the slow waves.

During the *interdigestive* period, the migrating motor complex (MMC), originating in the stomach, travels along the small intestine down to the ileocaecal junction. As previously explained, the MMC consists of bursts of depolarization accompanied by peristaltic contractions. The cycle of MMC may be considered as consisting of three phases: phase I is characterized by absence of contractions, phase II by irregular contractions and phase III by a burst of regular, large-amplitude contractions. The function of the MMC is to propel any remnants in the stomach and small intestine into the colon during the interdigestive period.

Two other types of movement will be described below: a mixing movement (**segmentation**) and a propulsion movement (**peristalsis**).

Segmentation contractions (Fig. 8.21a)

Segmentation contractions are ring-like contractions of the circular muscle layer appearing at regular intervals along a

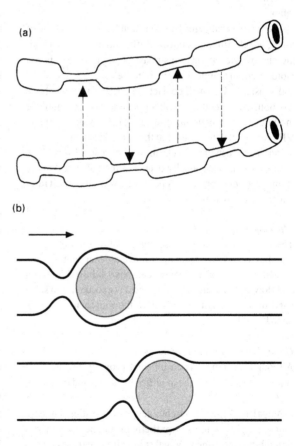

Fig. 8.21 (a) Diagram showing segmentation contractions of the small intestine. Relaxed segments between the dotted lines have become contracted and vice versa. (b) Diagram showing a bolus distending a segment of intestine, causing a peristaltic wave of contraction.

length of the small intestine. Soon they disappear and are replaced by another set of ring contractions, arranged such that the parts that were contracted become relaxed and those that were relaxed become contracted. Although segmentation contractions are primarily mixing movements; they may also have a propulsive effect on contents. Segmentation contractions persist after extrinsic denervation, but disappear after destroying the *intrinsic nerve plexus* in the small intestine.

Peristalsis

Peristaltic waves also occur in the oesophagus, stomach, colon and ureters. Peristalsis consists of a travelling wave of contraction above the bolus preceded by relaxation at the bolus site and below it (Fig. 8.21b). It persists after *extrinsic denervation* and is abolished after destruction of *intrinsic nerves*. It is controlled by an intramural myenteric reflex.

The reflex is triggered by distension leading to release of 5-HT, which stimulates intrinsic afferent neurons. Ascending cholinergic interneurons relay the signal to excitatory motor neurons, inducing them to release acetylcholine and substance P, which contact the circular muscle above the bolus. Descending cholinergic interneurons activate inhibitory motor neurons to release nitric oxide (NO) and VIP, which relax the muscle at the bolus site and below it.

Peristalsis usually travels in an oral–caudal direction. Antiperistalsis occasionally occurs in the colon and in the stomach during vomiting. A peristaltic wave travels at rates which vary between 2 and 25 cm/s.

Movements of the villi

The villi move during digestion. They do not move together, each villus seeming to move independently of the others. The villus movement consists of fast shortening and slow lengthening. The movement is executed by a short band of muscle that extends from the muscularis mucosa on to the villus.

Control of intestinal movements

Although movement is an inherent property of intestinal smooth muscle, it may be modified by neural and hormonal factors.

Vagal excitation and cholinergic stimulation increase motor activity, while **sympathetic** or adrenergic stimulation inhibits movement. Vagal stimulation increases movement of the villi, while sympathetic stimulation makes them pale and motionless. In addition to acetylcholine and noradrenaline (norepinephrine), other effects on intestinal smooth muscle may be mediated by **serotonin** (5-HT) or

substance P, which cause contraction, and by **VIP** or **nitric oxide**, which produce relaxation.

In humans, sympathectomy does not affect intestinal movements. Vagotomy is followed by *transient hypomotility*; normal motility is restored after a mean time of 10 hours. Inhibition of intestinal peristalsis, largely mediated through a nervous reflex, is termed **paralytic** or **adynamic ileus**. The inhibition may be initiated by excessive irritation of the intestine during abdominal operations, by intestinal overdistension, by peritonitis or even by renal, vesical or skin irritation. The efferent arm of the inhibitory reflex is in the sympathetic nerves to the intestine.

The hormone **gastrin** stimulates intestinal motility and relaxes the ileocaecal sphincter. **CCK** also stimulates intestinal movements. Conversely, **secretin** inhibits intestinal motility and contracts the ileocaecal sphincter. **Motiline** is a peptide containing 22 amino acids secreted by cells in the duodenum. It stimulates intestinal motility and seems to regulate interdigestive MMC activity.

There is experimental evidence indicating that chyme releases a hormone from the upper intestine that specifically stimulates movements of the villi; it has been called **villikinin**. The chemical nature of villikinin awaits final clarification.

The colon

The large intestine has a wider diameter than that of the small intestine. It starts with the **caecum** and continues as the ascending, transverse and descending colon. The **sigmoid colon** leads to the **rectum** and **anal canal** in the pelvis. One prominent morphological feature of the colon (Fig. 8.22) is that the outer longitudinal layer is modified to form three longitudinal bands, called **teniae coli**, visible on the outer surface. Since the muscle bands are shorter than the length of the colon, the colonic wall is sacculated and forms **haustra**. The mucous membrane of the colon lacks villi and consists of simple short glands lined mostly by mucus-secreting goblet cells. There are scattered *lymphoid nodules*, especially prominent in the caecum and appendix. In humans, the colon has a length of about 150 cm and a capacity of between 0.9 and 1.8 litres.

Secretion

Secretion in the colon is mainly **mucus**; no digestive enzymes are secreted by the colon. The mucus helps to lubricate faeces and neutralize any acids present; colonic contents have a pH of about 8. It also protects against irritants and provides a binding medium for faecal matter. The main stimulus to mucus secretion is the contact of the glands with colonic contents. In addition to direct

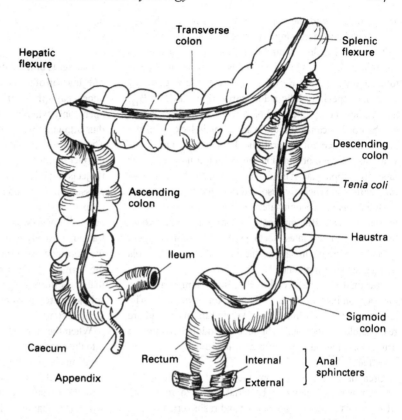

Fig. 8.22 The human colon.

stimulation of the gland cells, further secretion may occur via a reflex pathway involving the **parasympathetic** pelvic splanchnic nerves. Parasympathomimetic drugs, e.g. pilocarpine, stimulate colonic secretion and this stimulation can be blocked by atropine.

Absorption in the colon

From 0.5 to 1.5 litres of water is absorbed from the chyme delivered to the colon each day. The intestinal chyme is thus transformed into *semisolid faeces* with a net loss of water from the gut of 150–200 ml/day. Thus, the principal substance absorbed in the colon is water. **Na$^+$, K$^+$ ATPase** at the *basolateral membrane* of colonic epithelial cells pumps Na$^+$ to the intercellular spaces and the blood. This creates a concentration gradient for Na$^+$ to enter the cells. About 60 mmol of sodium is actively absorbed daily and water follows along the osmotic gradient created. **Potassium** is secreted into the lumen of the colon, while **chloride** is reabsorbed in exchange for **bicarbonate**, which is secreted into the lumen. Persistent diarrhoea therefore results in dehydration, hypokalaemia and metabolic acidosis due to loss of HCO$_3^-$ from the gut. Some absorption of nutrients does take place in the colon. Folic acid, some

amino acids and short-chain fatty acids resulting from the bacterial fermentation of carbohydrates are absorbed. In addition, certain drugs, e.g. steroids, aspirin, anaesthetics, sedatives and tranquillizers, may be absorbed by the colonic epithelium. However, carbohydrates, whole proteins and fats cannot be absorbed, so that it is not possible to maintain nutrition adequately by rectal instillation. The considerable absorptive capacity of the colon is nevertheless useful clinically, as it provides a convenient route of drug administration, i.e. by rectal enema, especially in children.

Intestinal bacteria

At birth, the intestine is sterile and the newborn baby passes a greenish, semifluid material called meconium. This is derived from amniotic fluid swallowed by the fetus while in the uterus. Meconium consists mainly of carbohydrate substances and the green colour is due to unreduced bile pigments. Bacteria are ingested and gain access to the intestine a few days after birth and thereafter stay throughout life. It is well recognized that the colon contains a **bacterial flora**, but recently it has been realized that the small intestine also contains bacteria. Apparently some bacteria escape destruction by gastric hydrochloric acid and gain access to the upper intestine, from which they spread caudally, increasing in numbers as they do so.

The intestinal flora should be viewed as living in symbiosis with the host. On the whole, its effects are beneficial to the body. Vitamin K and a number of the B group of vitamins, especially **folic acid, biotin, thiamine** and **B$_{12}$**, are synthesized by intestinal bacteria. Vitamin B$_{12}$ cannot be absorbed because the intrinsic factor is lacking in the colon. Evidence for absorption of vitamin K and other vitamins has been obtained in rats, which usually eat their faeces (coprophagia). It is now realized that in humans only **folic acid** is significantly absorbed from the colon.

Bile acids are deconjugated and dehydroxylated by intestinal bacteria. Bile pigments are similarly broken down by bacteria in the intestine to produce **stercobilinogen**, which is excreted in faeces, the brown colour of stools being due to this pigment.

Intestinal bacteria decarboxylate some amino acids to produce amines such as histamine and tyramine. The amines **skatole** and **indole** are excreted in faeces and are responsible for its smell. The level of indole excretion in urine is used as an index of bacterial activity in the small intestine.

Urea diffuses slowly from the blood into the colon, where it is broken down by bacterial urease to **ammonia**. Most of this ammonia is absorbed and reconverted to urea in the liver. The large intestine is a major source of ammonia in the body. Since accumulation of ammonia seems to be an important factor in causing hepatic encephalopathy, the management of hepatic failure includes administration of poorly absorbed antibiotics, e.g. neomycin, in order to sterilize the gut.

Bacterial fermentation of undigested carbohydrates, mostly in the form of dietary fibre, in the human colon may produce short-chain fatty acids and several gases: **carbon dioxide, hydrogen sulphide, hydrogen** and **methane**, which come out in flatus. It is important to remember, however, that normally about half of the quantity of flatus is nitrogen, mainly derived from swallowed air.

The presence of intestinal bacteria is important for the normal development of the gut and the *immune system*. This was shown by maintaining animals in germ-free environments. In germ-free animals, the immune system is hypoplastic. There are fewer lymphocytes and plasma cells and the concentration of immunoglobulins is greatly reduced. Furthermore, the gut in these animals becomes enlarged, with poor epithelium and villi.

A surgical blind loop may lead to stasis and overgrowth of bacteria within the loop. The bacteria deconjugate and dehydroxylate bile acids and bind vitamin B$_{12}$, lead-

ing to steatorrhoea and macrocytic anaemia (blind-loop syndrome).

Movements of the colon

The junction of the ileum with the caecum is guarded by the **ileocaecal sphincter**. The sphincter remains closed and opens only when an intestinal peristaltic wave reaches it, thus allowing ileal contents to pass briefly into the colon. The safety of the ileocaecal junction is further ensured by the fact that the end of the ileum containing the sphincter projects slightly into the caecum; in this way, when the pressure in the colon rises, it tends to squeeze the ileum to keep it shut, but, when ileal pressure increases, the ileal end will open. Muscle of the ileocaecal sphincter is contracted by **acetylcholine, α-adrenergic** stimulation and the hormone **secretin**. **Beta-adrenergic** stimulation and the hormone **gastrin** relax the sphincter. It is noteworthy that the effects of gastrin and secretin on the ileocaecal sphincter are opposite to their effects on the lower oesophageal sphincter.

When the stomach fills, and especially when it empties into the duodenum, a fast peristaltic wave is initiated in the small intestine passing along to the ileum; the ileocaecal sphincter relaxes briefly, allowing chyme to pass through into the caecum. This is termed the **gastroileal reflex**, which is probably mediated by the **vagus**.

Movements of the colon consist of *segmenting* contractions, which are non-propulsive, and *peristalsis*, which propels colonic contents towards the rectum. Occasionally *antiperistalsis* may be seen, starting at about the junction of the ascending and transverse colon and travelling towards the caecum. Antiperistalsis mixes contents and probably helps absorption of water.

Segmental contractions produce localized pressure waves and are probably partly responsible for haustral contractions. They serve to mix contents and aid absorption.

A special type of peristalsis occurs only in the colon; it is called **mass movement** or mass action contractions. These are powerful contractions advancing rapidly along the colon. They are preceded by sudden disappearance of haustral contractions, allowing rapid advance of colonic contents. Mass movements push faeces into the rectum, which is usually empty. The rectum is distended and the process of **defecation** may thereby be initiated. The contractions normally occur one to three times a day and are usually not felt by the subject.

Transit time through the intestine

If a barium meal is radiologically followed through the intestine, it will be seen to reach the caecum in about 4

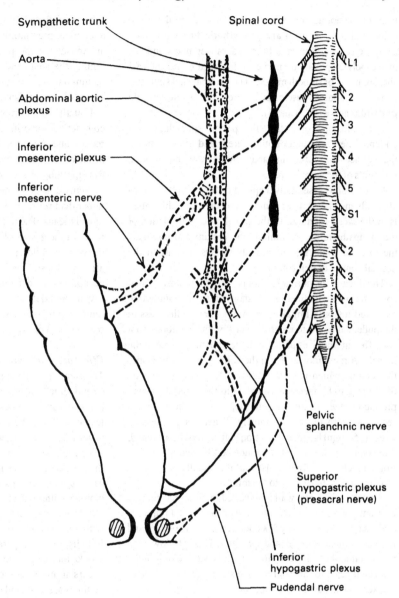

Sympathetic trunk

Spinal cord

Aorta

Abdominal aortic plexus

Inferior mesenteric plexus

Inferior mesenteric nerve

L1

2

3

4

5

S1

2

3

4

5

Pelvic splanchnic nerve

Superior hypogastric plexus (presacral nerve)

Inferior hypogastric plexus

Pudendal nerve

Fig. 8.23 The nerve supply of the distal colon and rectum in humans. (Redrawn from Garry, R.C. (1934) *Physiological Reviews*, **14**, 107. With permission from the American Physiological Society.)

hours, but it will be 8–9 hours before all the meal enters the colon. The front of the meal reaches the hepatic flexure in 6 hours, the splenic flexure in 9 hours and the pelvic colon in 12 hours. Transit is greatly slowed down between the pelvic colon and the anus. After 3 days, about three-quarters of the meal will have been expelled, with one-quarter still remaining in the rectum. These times may be longer for ordinary food. When small coloured beads or melon seeds are swallowed with a meal, about 70% of them are recovered from the stools in 72 hours, but complete recovery

of the seeds takes more than a week. Thus, remnants from a meal may still have to be excreted in the stools 1 week after its ingestion. There is great individual variation in transit time.

Defecation

The nerve supply of the distal colon and rectum is shown in Fig. 8.23. **Sympathetic** fibres originate in the lower thoracic and upper two lumbar segments of the spinal cord and traverse the sympathetic chain to form plexuses on the front of the aorta, from which fibres proceed to the distal colon and the rectum. **Parasympathetic** fibres originate from the second, third and fourth sacral segments and run in the pelvic splanchnic nerve to the rectum and internal anal sphincter of smooth muscle. The external anal sphincter consists of striated muscle and is innervated by the **somatic pudendal** nerve (S2, 3 and 4).

It should be noted that the pelvic splanchnic and pudendal nerves contain both efferent and afferent fibres that connect the rectum and anal sphincters with the sacral segments of the spinal cord.

Defecation is essentially a **spinal reflex**, which is normally influenced by higher centres. The centre of this reflex is in the sacral segments of the spinal cord. Stimulation of the sympathetic nerves inhibits the rectum and contracts the internal sphincter but probably plays no part in the normal control of defecation.

The rectum is normally empty and the external anal sphincter is maintained in a state of tonic contraction mediated reflexly. Impulses from muscle spindles pass in the pudendal nerve to enter the cord by the S2 dorsal root and efferent impulses pass out in the pudendal nerve to the muscle. A mass movement in the colon pushes faeces into the rectum, which is thus distended. Normally distension of the rectum by faeces is signalled to the cerebral cortex, producing the desire to defecate, which occurs when rectal pressure reaches 18 mmHg. When rectal pressure rises to 55 mmHg, the defecation reflex may be initiated. However, the spinal reflex cannot be allowed to operate immediately; the subject must wait for socially convenient circumstances, like going to the toilet.

Stretch of the rectal wall is signalled to the spinal cord by afferent fibres in the *pelvic splanchnic nerve*, and impulses in the same nerve cause reflex contraction of the rectum and relaxation of the internal anal sphincter. This is followed by reduction in the number of tonic impulses travelling in the pudendal nerve to the external anal sphincter; the sphincter relaxes and faeces leave the rectum.

When the situation is not convenient for defecation, the tonic contraction of the external anal sphincter is voluntarily maintained or even increased, which leads to accommodation of the rectum to distension and return of the tonic contraction of the internal anal sphincter. When proper circumstances are available, the tonic contraction of the external sphincter is lifted and the spinal reflex for evacuating the rectum operates unhindered. In infants the reflex proceeds unhindered (automatic) due to lack of cortical voluntary control.

Expulsion of faeces from the rectum is assisted by voluntary straining: a deep breath is taken and then expelled against a closed glottis. Straining greatly raises intra-abdominal pressure. In addition, contraction of the levator ani muscle in the pelvic floor helps to expel faeces by pulling the anal canal over the faecal mass. Not only the rectum but the large intestine up to the middle of the transverse colon may also be evacuated.

Usually ingestion of a meal is followed by a *mass action* contraction wave in the colon that pushes faeces into the rectum and produces the desire to defecate. This response of the colon, which may be initiated by gastric filling, gastric emptying, filling of the small intestine or even somatic movement, is better described as the **gastrocolic response** rather than reflex, as it is mediated by both neural and hormonal means. The hormone involved may be **gastrin**. As a result of the gastrocolic response, defecation after meals is the rule in children and some people habitually defecate after breakfast. However, in adults, cultural factors, habit, occupation and personal circumstances alter the gastrocolic rhythm and determine the time of defecation. It is well to remember that there is a wide range of normal bowel habit; once every 3 days as well as three times a day is normal.

Effect of spinal-cord lesions on defecation

Transection of the spinal cord is followed by a period of **spinal shock**, during which the rectum and sphincters are paralysed and patulous, leading to retention of faeces. If the lesion is above the sacral segments (upper motor-neuron lesion), tone returns and the spinal reflex of defecation starts to operate without interference from higher centres, after the period of spinal shock is over. The rectum is described as *automatic*. In this case, when it fills, it automatically empties without the patient being aware of the act.

Lesions that destroy the sacral cord or its connections with the rectum produce a lower motor-neuron lesion. Initially, there is paralysis similar to that during spinal shock, but, after some time, tone returns and evacuation occurs at intervals; the rectum is described as *autonomous* in this case (i.e. independent of central neural control). Apparently, evacuation is brought about by reflex arcs entirely confined to the wall of the rectum. Whenever a person loses control over the act of defecation, he/she is said to have *faecal incontinence*.

Congenital megacolon (Hirschsprung's disease)

Children affected by this disease have severe constipation and abdominal distension. The basic defect is congenital absence of ganglion cells in both the myenteric and submucous plexuses, especially those containing VIP and nitric oxide, commonly in the rectum and sigmoid colon. Loss of inhibitory tone in the aganglionic segment makes it narrow and devoid of propulsive activity; this leads to distension and dilatation of the colon proximal to the affected segment. The condition is treated by surgical removal of the aganglionic segment.

Faeces

The amount of stools passed in 24 hours varies from 80 to 200 g. The brown colour of stools is due to stercobilinogen, derived from bacterial degradation of bile pigments. The smell of faeces is due to the amines *skatole* and *indole* and to gases produced by carbohydrate fermentation, such as hydrogen sulphide. All are produced by the action of intestinal bacteria. The faecal reaction is slightly alkaline on the surface (pH 7–7.5).

About 75% of the stool is water; the rest consists of organic and inorganic solids. Organic material consists mainly of desquamated epithelial cells, bacteria, mucus and remnants of digestive enzymes. Most of the nitrogenous material, 1–2 g/day, is thus derived from non-dietary sources. Fat in the stools is also mostly non-dietary, amounting to about 5 g/day. In steatorrhoea up to 50 g may be lost per day. Inorganic material in faeces consists mainly of calcium and phosphates. Undigested plant fibres, such as fruit seeds and skin, may be seen in stools.

It is important to realize that more than half the stool is actually derived from the remnants of intestinal epithelium, digestive enzymes and intestinal bacteria and their products. The stools are thus not simply the unabsorbed food remnant. The most convincing proof of this fact is that during starvation faeces, although small in amount, are still passed.

Further reading

1 Ganong, W.F. (1999) Section V. Gastrointestinal function. In: *Review of Medical Physiology*, 19th edn, pp. 447–491. Appleton & Lange, Stamford, Connecticut.

2 Johnson, L.R. (1997) *Gastrointestinal Physiology*, 5th edn. Mosby-Year Book, St Louis, Baltimore, Boston.

3 Chang, E.G., Sitrin, M.D. & Black, D.D. (1996) *Gastrointestinal, Hepatobiliary and Nutritional Physiology*. Lippincott-Raven, Philadelphia, New York.

9 / The Endocrine System

Objectives

On completion of the study of this chapter, the student should be able to:

1 Describe the neural and hormonal control of the pituitary gland by the hypothalamus and other parts of the nervous system so as to investigate patients with endocrine disorders.

2 Describe the chemical nature and metabolism of the hormones secreted by the endocrine glands in order to use appropriate methods of investigation and therapy.

3 Explain the control and actions of hormones secreted by the major endocrine organs in the human body so as to interpret the manifestations of endocrine disorders.

4 Describe and start to recognize the manifestations of clinical endocrine disorders so as to reach an early diagnosis.

5 Explain the basis of commonly used tests of endocrine functions.

The endocrine glands

Together with the nervous system, the endocrine glands constitute the control systems in the body. They provide the necessary communication for distant control of body functions and homoeostatic regulatory mechanisms. The nerves conduct impulses to distant organs and therefore provide a fast means of communication. The endocrine glands secrete **hormones** directly into the bloodstream. These hormones are special chemical substances which act on specific receptors in distant organs or tissues.

Neuroendocrine relationships

The endocrine glands can be considered as a system which functions in close harmony with the nervous system. This is because the pituitary gland is closely connected with the **hypothalamus** at the base of the brain. The hypothalamus, in turn, receives information from almost all other parts of the brain directly or indirectly. (Figure 9.1 gives a diagrammatic representation of the connections of the hypothalamus.) It is therefore in a position to be influenced by incoming information, whether somatic, visceral, psychic or emotional.

The hypothalamus influences the pituitary gland through two distinct mechanisms:

Fig. 9.1 Diagram of the hypothalamus and the pituitary gland showing major tracts and the nuclei closely related to the pituitary glands.

1 Direct **neural tracts** from the hypothalamic nuclei to the posterior pituitary (neurohypophysis).

2 Secretion of **releasing hormones** (RH) or **inhibitory hormones** (IH), which are carried to the anterior pituitary (adenohypophysis) by means of the **hypothalamohypophyseal portal vessels** (Fig. 9.2). The RH and IH are specific for the individual hormones of the anterior pituitary gland.

The anterior pituitary gland is closely controlled by the *releasing* or *inhibitory hormones* of the hypothalamus. Most other endocrine glands function under the control of the anterior pituitary hormones. The thyroid gland is controlled by the **thyroid-stimulating hormone** (TSH), the adrenal cortex by the **adrenocorticotrophic hormone** (ACTH) and the gonads (ovaries and testes) by the **follicle-stimulating hormone** (FSH) and **luteinizing hormone** (LH). **Growth hormone** (GH) and **prolactin** (PRL) act on tissues rather than on specific endocrine glands.

The only two major endocrine glands not under the control of the trophic hormones of the anterior pituitary are the **parathyroid glands** and the **islets of Langerhans** of the pancreas. These are directly controlled by the chemical substrates they regulate, i.e. blood calcium and blood glucose, respectively.

The control of the neurohypophysis and the adrenal medulla deserves a special place in this description of neuro-endocrine interrelations. The neurohypophysis acts as a storage organ for the granules of hormones secreted in the hypothalamic nuclei. Release of these hormones requires stimuli, which act via the hypothalamohypophyseal tracts. The adrenal medulla, on the other hand, receives its nerve supply from the sympathetic neurons in the spinal cord (preganglionic fibres). These neurons have connections with the hypothalamus. Therefore, whenever there is massive sympathetic activity, e.g. 'fight or flight', the adrenal medulla is also stimulated.

The anterior pituitary gland

The anterior lobe of the pituitary gland (adenohypophysis) is the larger of the two glands. Its embryological origin is from the roof of the primitive mouth (Rathke's pouch). It consists of cells which take acid stain (40%) or basic stain (10%) or do not take any (50%). Hence the names **acidophil**, **basophil** and **chromophobe** cells, respectively. More recently, the cells have been classified on the basis of the hormones they secrete. Table 9.1 gives the hormones secreted by each of the cell types.

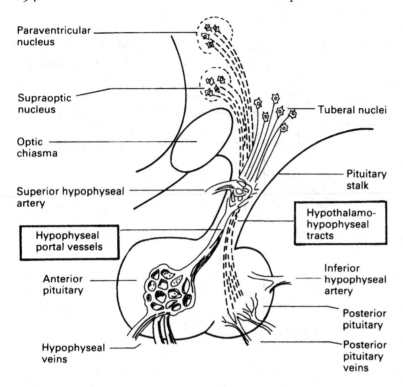

Fig. 9.2 The pituitary gland and its connections with the hypothalamus. Note the hypothalamohypophyseal portal vessels to the anterior pituitary and the hypothalamohypophyseal tracts to the posterior pituitary.

Table 9.1 Cell types of the anterior pituitary and the hormones they produce.

Cell type	Stain	Hormone	Molecule	Mol.wt/daltons
Somatotropes	Acidophilic	Growth hormone (GH)	Protein	22 000
Mammotropes	Acidophilic	Prolactin (PRL)	Protein	23 000
Corticotropes	Basophilic or chromophobe	ACTH	Polypeptide	4 500
Thyrotropes	Basophilic	TSH	Glycoprotein	28 000
Gonadotropes	Basophilic	LH	Glycoprotein	28 000
		FSH	Glycoprotein	35 000

The blood supply of the anterior pituitary comes from the superior hypophyseal arteries, which are branches of the internal carotid arteries. These hypophyseal arteries supply the primary capillary plexuses of the hypothalamo-hypophyseal portal vessels, which travel down the pituitary stalk (see Fig. 9.2). The portal vessels therefore constitute the main blood supply of the anterior pituitary. They transport the releasing hormones to the adenohypophysis. The capillaries in the anterior pituitary form sinusoids similar to those seen in the liver, thus providing close contact between the blood and the glandular cells. The hormones of the anterior pituitary are carried via the hypophyseal veins. The blood supply of the posterior pituitary gland comes from the superior and inferior hypophyseal arteries.

Hormones of the anterior pituitary

The four trophic hormones come from *basophil cells* and they control three endocrine organs: the thyroid, the adrenal cortex and the gonads. The following description of the individual hormones will be given under the following subheadings: chemistry and degradation, control of secretion, actions of the hormone and abnormalities.

Thyroid-stimulating hormone (thyrotrophin) (TSH)

Chemistry and degradation

TSH is a glycoprotein of molecular weight 28 000 daltons and comprises two subunits, one (α) that is common to LH, FSH and human placental lactogen (HPL) and one (β) that

Table 9.2 Hormones of the hypothalamus.

Hypothalamic hormones	Molecule	Nuclei
Thyrotrophin-releasing hormone (TRH)	Tripeptide	Paraventricular and dorsomedial
Corticotrophin-releasing hormone (CRH)	Polypeptide (41)	Paraventricular
Gonadotrophin-releasing hormone (GnRH)	Decapeptide	Preoptic area and arcuate
Growth hormone-releasing hormone (GHRH)	Polypeptide (40, 44)	Arcuate
Growth hormone inhibitory hormone (somatostatin)	Peptide (14)	Ventral
Prolactin inhibitory hormone (PIH)	Dopamine	Arcuate
Prolactin-releasing hormone (PRH)	Polypeptide	Ventral

The figures in brackets indicate the number of amino acids in polypeptide hormones.

expresses TSH hormone bioactivity. It has no species specificity, so that TSH extracted from ox or pig is found to be active in humans. Its half-life is about 60 min. The kidney has been found to be more able to break it down than the liver.

Control of secretion

TSH is controlled by the anterior part of the median eminence of the hypothalamus, which releases **thyrotrophin-releasing hormone** (TRH) (Table 9.2):

1 TRH is controlled by **negative feedback** according to the level of the hormones of the thyroid gland, i.e. thyroxine and tri-iodothyronine (T_4, T_3).

2 The effect of TRH on the pituitary can be blocked by T_4 and T_3 by decreasing TRH-binding sites on anterior pituitary cells. This may be the main site of the negative feedback mechanism (Fig. 9.3).

3 There seems to be a **circadian rhythm** (diurnal rhythm), with maximum secretion before or at midnight and minimum values at about 11 a.m. This is probably mediated by a similar TRH rhythm.

4 The effect of environmental temperature on TSH secretion has been shown in animals and in infants but there seems to be little effect in adults. However, there is a long-term effect of heat and cold on thyroid function. Thus, acclimatization to heat (when living in a hot climate) leads to slightly lower thyroid function and acclimatization to cold is associated with thyroid activity in the upper levels of normal.

5 There is evidence that TSH release can be blocked by stress, somatostatin, dopamine and glucocortoids.

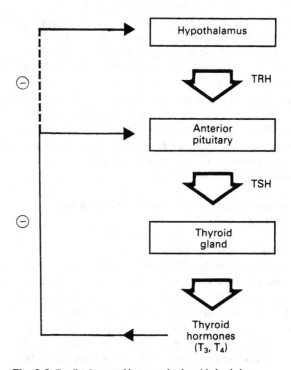

Fig. 9.3 Feedback control between the thyroid gland, the anterior pituitary and the hypothalamus. The solid arrow indicates that the main feedback is exerted on the pituitary, with a minor control mechanism on the hypothalamus indicated by the broken arrow.

Actions of TSH

Thyrotrophic hormone, as the name implies, is important for the growth and development of the thyroid gland.

The actions of TSH are mediated by cyclic adenosine monophosphate (AMP) via receptor sites on thyroid cells. TSH accelerates the process of iodine trapping and therefore its concentration by the thyroid gland. It is also concerned with the synthesis of the thyroid hormones and their release. Thus, TSH specifically accelerates oxidative coupling of thyroid hormone precursors. It also activates the proteolytic enzymes, which release the thyroid hormones from their storage form in the thyroglobulin molecules. (For more detail see the section on thyroid hormone synthesis and release, pp. 206–210.)

Abnormalities of TSH

Primary pituitary deficiency or excess of TSH is rare. Thyroid disease, however, is common and this is usually due to diseases of the thyroid gland itself. Therefore, high or low TSH is usually secondary to thyroid disease. In hyperthyroidism and thyrotoxicosis the TSH levels are found to be low due to the negative feedback effect of the excess T_3 and T_4. In hypothyroidism the levels of TSH are high due to diminished thyroid hormone levels and therefore absence of the negative feedback.

However, in the case of endemic goitre (due to iodine deficiency), the blood levels of TSH are found to be elevated, which explains the enlargement of the thyroid gland. The function of the thyroid gland in endemic goitre is usually within the normal range.

Adrenocorticotrophic hormone (corticotrophin) (ACTH)

Chemistry and degradation

ACTH is a polypeptide of a relatively small molecular weight, 4500 daltons, consisting of a single chain of 39 amino acids. ACTH is one of a family of related peptides that are derived from a larger precursor glycoprotein, of molecular weight 31 000 daltons, called **pro-opiomelanocortin** (POMC), which is a megamolecule the products of which also include α-melanocyte-stimulating hormone (**α-MSH**) and **endorphin**. The half-life of ACTH is short and estimated to vary between 5 and 15 minutes. The degradation of ACTH takes place in the blood. Little is known of the sites of ACTH breakdown.

Control of ACTH

1 The secretion of ACTH, like TSH, is under the control

Fig. 9.4 Feedback control of ACTH. The main feedback is shown to be on the hypothalamus, with a minor control mechanism on the anterior pituitary.

of a releasing hormone from the hypothalamus. **Corticotrophin-releasing hormone** (CRH) is under the control of circulating adrenal glucocorticoid hormones by means of a negative feedback mechanism. As shown in Fig. 9.4, the negative feedback works mainly on the hypothalamus but it can also work directly on the anterior pituitary.

2 ACTH is rapidly released in response to physical or emotional stress and hypoglycaemia. This response to stress is part of the general preparation to counteract injury, infections and various other stressful conditions.

3 It is also known that there is a **circadian rhythm** of ACTH secretion, which results in high levels of ACTH, and therefore cortical steroids, in the morning and low levels in the evening and during the night. This rhythm is related to the pattern of sleep and is reversed in workers who are on night duty.

4 Stimulation of arterial baroreceptors inhibits CRH release. This effect is mediated through the nucleus of the tractus solitarius in the medulla. Table 9.3 gives a summary of the control of ACTH secretion.

Table 9.3 Control of adrenocorticotrophic hormone (ACTH).

Stimulus	Effect
1 Stress Physical, surgery, trauma Pyrogens Emotional strain Cytokines Hypoglycaemia	Release of neurotransmitters and peptidides in the hypothalamus to release CRH*
2 Diurnal rhythm	Effect via hypothalamic neurons to release CRH
3 Cortisol	Negative feedback on hypothalamic CRH and decreasing its effect on anterior pituitary cells. Inhibition of synthesis of POMC

* Vasopressin (antidiuretic hormone [ADH]) enhances the effect of corticotrophin-releasing hormone (CRH). POMC, pro-opiomelanocortin.

Actions of ACTH

ACTH is necessary for the healthy growth and repair of the adrenal cortex and for maintaining healthy vascularity of the gland. In cases of ACTH deficiency, the adrenal cortex atrophies and its blood-vessels disappear. Conversely, ACTH excess causes hypertrophy.

ACTH influences the adrenal cortex to stimulate the synthesis and release of cortisol and the other glucocorticoids. It increases the number of mitochondria in the adrenal cortical cells. It acts on adenylate cyclase and a protein kinase to increase the lipid content of the adrenal cortex. Free cholesterol is also increased. ACTH decreases the ascorbic acid content of the adrenal cortex; this effect was once used as a method for biological assay of the hormone.

ACTH has a melanocyte-stimulating action which is believed to cause pigmentation of the skin in conditions where high ACTH levels are found, e.g. destruction of the adrenal cortex (Addison's disease). Its absence, on the other hand, as in panhypopituitarism, is associated with pallor of the skin.

Several other effects of ACTH have been described, e.g. stimulation of insulin secretion and mobilization of free fatty acids (FFAs) from adipose tissue. The physiological significance of these actions remains to be explained.

Abnormalities

High ACTH is found in Addison's disease due to the absence of the negative feedback from the glucocorticoids

of the adrenal cortex. High levels are also found in basophil adenomas of the anterior pituitary. This is associated with hypersecretion of glucocorticoids, leading to what is known as *secondary Cushing's disease*.

However, in *primary Cushing's disease*, when an adrenal adenoma is responsible for high levels of glucocorticoids, ACTH secretion is inhibited by negative feedback. Measurement of plasma ACTH is therefore required to differentiate between primary and secondary Cushing's disease.

Gonadotrophic hormones

The gonadotrophic hormones are follicle-stimulating hormone (FSH) and luteinizing hormone (LH), which control both male and female gonadal functions.

Chemistry and degradation of FSH

Human FSH is a double-chain glycoprotein of molecular weight 35 000 daltons. It is species-specific and therefore only human FSH can be used for the treatment of patients. The half-life of human FSH is about 3 hours. It is probably broken down in the liver. FSH appears in the urine in appreciable amounts. Urinary excretion reflects the blood levels and production by the anterior pituitary. It is secreted in large amounts during the menopause and therefore menopausal women's urine contains high concentrations.

Control of FSH

Only small amounts of FSH can be detected during childhood. At puberty, the secretion of gonadotrophins is stimulated by specific gonadotrophin-releasing hormones (GnRH) under the influence of the nervous system, i.e. the stimulus is neural in origin and its initiation depends on the development of the nervous system and its maturation during adolescence.

After the establishment of puberty, the regulation of FSH depends upon the following:

1 The level of ovarian oestrogens has a negative feedback effect on pituitary FSH-releasing hormone (Fig. 9.5). The sharp fall of oestrogens in the middle of the cycle triggers a small but significant mid-cycle peak of FSH (Fig. 9.6).

2 In the male there is a negative feedback control with testicular testosterone from the Leydig cells.

3 Inhibin is a polypeptide, secreted by the seminiferous tubules and the Sertoli cells, which inhibits FSH secretion. It is also secreted by the granulosa cells in females.

4 FSH itself has an inhibitory effect on the hypothalamic RH, i.e. there is a short-loop feedback mechanism between the pituitary and the hypothalamus (see Fig. 9.5).

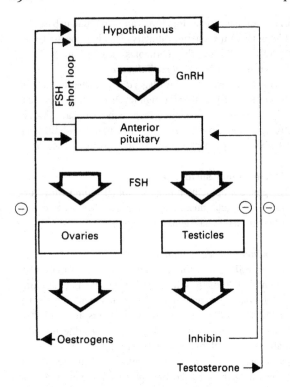

Fig. 9.5 Diagrammatic representation of the negative feedback between ovarian and testicular hormones and FSH.

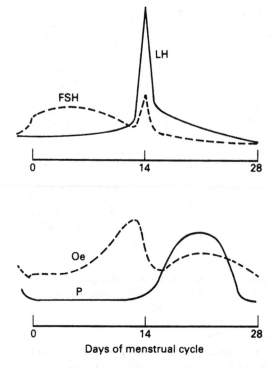

Fig. 9.6 The diagram shows the cyclic nature of secretion of the pituitary gonadotrophins and the ovarian sex hormones. FSH, follicle-stimulating hormone; LH, luteinizing hormone; Oe, oestrogens; P, progestogens.

Actions of FSH

1 FSH is responsible for the growth and maturation of a crop of primordial follicles in the ovaries up to their maturation towards the middle of the menstrual cycle. The Graafian follicles produce oestrogens, which are responsible for proliferation of the endometrium during the first half of the cycle. Oestrogens are also responsible for the development of the female genital tract and secondary sex characteristics in adolescent females.

2 Together with LH, FSH stimulates ovulation. This occurs at the time of the mid-cycle peaks of the gonadotrophic hormones.

3 In males, FSH is responsible for the growth and development of the seminiferous tubules and it stimulates spermatogenesis. This effect requires LH for full development and function. For more detail see Chapter 14.

Chemistry and degradation of LH

LH is a double-chain glycoprotein of low molecular weight, about 28 000 daltons, with a half-life of about 1 hour. It is filtered by renal glomeruli and appreciable amounts appear in the urine during the 3–4 days at mid-

cycle. During the menopause, large amounts of LH can be recovered from the urine.

Control of LH secretion

Small amounts of LH are found in childhood. Like FSH, it increases at the onset of puberty, presumably triggered by a hypothalamic clock, and is secreted in a pulsatile manner (2–3 h) under the influence of GnRH.

LH secretion during the menstrual cycle is regulated as follows:

1 There is a large mid-cycle peak of secretion, which seems to be stimulated by a *positive feedback* mechanism associated with the high level of preovulation oestrogens (see Fig. 9.6).

2 LH is inhibited by *negative feedback* associated with progesterone levels (Fig. 9.7).

3 LH secretion can act on the hypothalamus to inhibit further GnRH secretion by a *short-loop negative feedback* (Fig. 9.7).

4 17-Beta-oestradiol decreases the level of LH secretion but, if it is administered during the follicular phase, it increases the responsiveness of the pituitary to GnRH.

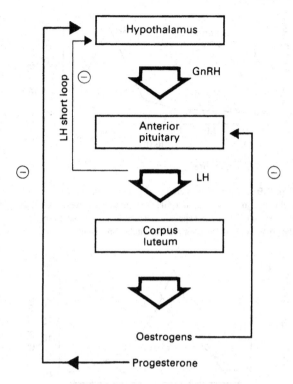

Fig. 9.7 Feedback between the ovarian hormone progesterone and hypothalamic control of LH secretion. A short-loop feedback is also shown to exist between the pituitary and the hypothalamus.

Actions of LH

LH acts synergistically with FSH in the promotion of the growth and maturation of the ovarian follicles. During the middle of the cycle a sharp increase in LH release (about 20-fold) is responsible for ovulation.

LH also maintains the corpus luteum during the secretion phase of the menstrual cycle. Towards the end of the cycle luteolysis occurs and results in a drop in the levels of both oestrogens and progesterone, which come from the corpus luteum. This marks the end of the menstrual cycle (see Fig. 9.6). For more detail see Chapter 14.

Abnormalities of the gonadotrophic hormones

FSH and LH are affected by emotional and psychological factors. Disturbances of fertility and the menstrual cycle have been reported at times of war and stress. In some women, emotional stress may result in amenorrhoea (absence of cyclic bleeding).

In the absence of the mid-cycle peak of LH and FSH, there is the usual menstruation but there is no ovulation (anovular cycle). This is a known cause of infertility. Some drugs are now known to stimulate LH secretion,

e.g. clomiphene (clomifene), which can be used in some cases of infertility.

Failure of secretion results in delayed puberty or hypogonadism. Precocious (premature) puberty, on the other hand, can occur as a result of premature release of gonadotrophins, associated with disorders involving the posterior hypothalamus or due to tumours of the pineal body (gland). Damage to the hypothalamus can also lead to cessation of gonadotrophic hormone secretion and consequently gonadal atrophy.

Growth hormone (GH)

Growth hormone, or somatotrophin, is secreted throughout life. The name growth hormone is misleading, as it implies its secretion during the growth periods. During childhood and adolescence, it is concerned with the regulation of metabolism and attainment of the growth potential of the child. In adult life, however, it works in concert with other hormones in the short-term day-to-day regulation of energy metabolism. GH stimulates the mobilization of fat and inhibits glucose utilization. Therefore, it shifts energy metabolism towards the use of FFAs rather than glucose. It also has an anabolic effect on protein utilization in the repair process of tissues.

Chemistry and degradation of GH

GH is a peptide hormone consisting of 191 amino acids in a single chain, with two intramolecular disulphide bridges. Two forms have been described in plasma. Its molecular weight in humans is 20 000 or 22 000 dalton. It is species-specific and therefore only human or synthetic GH can be used in the treatment of cases of its deficiency. Its half-life is short (20–30 min), which necessitates half-hourly serial sampling in its investigation.

Control of GH secretion

Like most of the peptide hormones, GH is stored in vesicles and secreted by the process of exocytosis in response to appropriate stimuli. The hypothalamic control is achieved by means of GH-releasing hormone (GHRH) (or **somatocrinin**) and GH inhibitory hormone (GHIH) (or **somatostatin**). The latter has also been identified in the D cells of the islets of Langerhans, where its physiological significance is associated with insulin and glucagon regulation. The overall regulation of GH secretion is summarized in Fig. 9.8. GHRH and GHIH are involved in the control of GH secretion by the anterior pituitary. Both peptides interact with membrane receptors on the somatrophic cells of the anterior pituitary gland to effect the changes in GH release. GHRH effects are calcium-dependent and may

Fig. 9.9 The pattern of secretion of growth hormone during and following glucose absorption. GH (solid line) is suppressed during the absorptive phase and appears as a distinct peak burst during the postabsorptive phase of glucose intake (broken line).

Fig. 9.10 The secretion of growth hormone after protein intake. PAN, plasma amino nitrogen, indicating the absorption of amino acids. Note the secretion of GH during the absorptive phase of protein intake.

Fig. 9.8 Regulation of growth hormone by the anterior pituitary gland. Negative and positive feedback mechanisms are indicated, bearing in mind that GH has a pulsatile release pattern of short durations. GHIH, growth hormone inhibitory hormone; GHRH, growth hormone-releasing hormone.

involve adenylate cyclase. GHIH effects require changes in calcium and cyclic AMP concentration to inhibit the release of GH. In addition to the hypothalamic input to the somatotropes, feedback effects of GH and of somatomedins participate in the regulation of GH secretion.

The secretion of growth hormone takes place in discrete pulses, so that basal levels are usually very low. The pattern of its secretion is found to occur as follows:

1 GH is released under conditions of lack of glucose. Hypoglycaemia (e.g. after insulin therapy) is a strong stimulus, which acts by stimulating GHRH secretion. On the other hand, glucose intake and hyperglycaemia inhibit GH secretion.

2 GH appears in the postabsorptive phase following glucose intake (Fig. 9.9). During starvation or continued fasting, GH is secreted periodically every 2–3 hours. The nature of the triggering mechanism for these peaks is not clear.

3 Muscular exercise in the postabsorptive state results in GH secretion. This effect is found to be abolished if glucose is taken at the same time.

4 Intake of protein or amino acids results in the secretion of GH. This response is also inhibited by concomitant glucose intake (Fig. 9.10).

5 During sleep GH is found to be released several times. The levels of these peaks are higher and occur with greater frequency in children than in adults.

6 Stress conditions, e.g. due to trauma or emotion, are found to stimulate GH secretion.

7 Glucagon, lysine-vasopressin and L-dopa have also been found to stimulate the release of GH. The physiological significance of these responses is not fully understood.

8 On the other hand, cortisol, FFAs, GH and, of course, glucose are found to inhibit its secretion. Prolonged corticosteroid administration in children leads to stunted growth.

Actions of GH

In addition to the promotion of growth, GH has several short-term effects on the utilization of amino acids, glucose and FFAs. Its long-term effect on somatic growth depends on **somatomedin C**, which is secreted by the liver in response to GH. Somatomedin C is also known as **insulin-like growth factor I** (IGF-I). IGF-I is responsible for the effect of GH on bone growth. However, a direct effect of GH on bone cartilage makes epiphyseal stem cells responsive to IGF-I. Somatomedins have been described to inhibit secretion of GH by stimulating GHIH release. They may also act directly to inhibit the effect of GHRH on the pituitary. Growth stops once the epiphyses of the long bones close. The growth-promoting action of GH also requires normal thyroid function and insulin. The sex hormones are also necessary for growth during adolescence.

Its short-term metabolic effects are as follows:

Protein metabolism. GH stimulates the transport of amino acids into the cells. Their incorporation during protein synthesis is also stimulated. Generally, GH causes a positive nitrogen balance and net protein anabolism, which is known as the protein-sparing action of GH.

Carbohydrate metabolism. GH inhibits peripheral utilization of glucose by muscle and adipose tissues. This is opposite to the action of insulin (insulin antagonism) and increases hepatic glucose output (diabetogenic effect). Abnormal GH secretion or prolonged administration therefore causes a type of diabetes mellitus.

Fat metabolism. GH mobilizes FFAs from adipose tissue stores. This action depends on a hormone-sensitive tissue lipase. This results in an increase in FFA levels during fasting, during muscular exercise and in the postabsorptive phase of glucose intake. GH also increases the oxidation of FFAs in muscle. Table 9.4 gives a summary of the effect of GH.

In conclusion, it is clear that the effects of GH lead to a net anabolic effect on protein metabolism, shifting of energy metabolism towards the utilization of FFAs and sparing of glucose. Therefore, in adults this hormone is concerned with the short-term regulation of metabolism, while during childhood and adolescence the same metabolic effects take place, in addition to skeletal growth.

Abnormalities of GH secretion
Deficiency of GH in childhood results in retardation of somatic growth but it has no effect on mental development. The child becomes a dwarf, with height much below that expected for its age (Fig. 9.11). In some cases of **dwarfism**, there is normal GH secretion but a deficiency of somatomedins. In a rare type of dwarfism (**Laron dwarf**), there is a lack of GH receptors.

Table 9.4 Effects of growth hormone.

On metabolism
Protein
Positive nitrogen balance (anabolic)
Decreased protein catabolism
Decreased plasma amino acids
Decreased blood urea
Increased plasma phosphate
Increased excretion of 4-hydroxyproline during growth
Increased transport of amino acids into cells
Increased protein synthesis through increased transcription of DNA to RNA and increased translation of RNA
Net protein anabolic effects lead to growth in children and replacement of tissue wear and tear and adults
Fat
Increased FFA mobilization (catabolic)
Increased FFA utilization; shift of energy metabolism to fat
Carbohydrate
Decreased sensitivity to insulin, conservation of glucose
Decreased utilization of glucose, hyperglycaemia leading to stimulation of insulin secretion, excess GH, diabetogenic effect
On growth
Increase in size and length of bones before closure of epiphyses
Growth of all organs and tissues
Stimulation of formation of growth factors in liver and other tissues
Somatomedin C (IGF-I) secretion by liver essential for bone growth
Growth factors promote protein synthesis

DNA, deoxyribonucleic acid; GH, growth hormone; RNA, ribonucleic acid.

Deficiency in adult life is not fully understood. There is reason to believe that some cases of obesity may be associated with decreased GH secretion. Growth hormone deficiency in adults is one of the earliest manifestations of hypothalamic disease.

Excess of GH before or during adolescence results in an abnormal stimulation of skeletal growth and a pituitary giant (**gigantism**). During adult life, after skeletal maturation, the effect of hypertension results in acromegaly. This condition is characterized by enlargement of certain bones, such as the jawbone, the frontal bone and the bones of the hands and feet. The skin of the face is thickened and the tongue is enlarged. Some internal organs, such as the liver and spleen, are also enlarged.

Fig. 9.11 The girl on the left has isolated GH deficiency. The age difference with her sister is 18 months. (Reproduced with permission from Edwards, C.R.W. & McNicol, G.P. (eds) (1986) *Integrated Clinical Science*, p. 31. William Heinemann Medical Books, London.)

GH is found to be secreted continuously (i.e. it loses its periodic pattern of release) and fails to be suppressed by glucose intake. This continuous secretion eventually results in diabetes mellitus, which is resistant to insulin therapy.

Prolactin (PRL)

Chemistry

Prolactin (PRL) (or mammotrophin), also known as lactogenic hormone, is chemically similar to GH. Human PRL is a single-chain polypeptide with a molecular weight of about 22 500 daltons. Its half-life is 15 min, it is secreted in a pulsatile manner, and blood levels are higher at night and during sleep.

Control

1 PRL seems to be continuously inhibited by a hypothalamic inhibitory hormone (PIH). It is therefore stimulated by abolishing the release of PIH in the hypothalamus. PRL is at its highest at term. Immediately following labour, the hormone drops rapidly to a basal level during the first few days.

2 There are discrete bursts of release, giving rise to high plasma concentrations every time there is stimulation of the nipples during suckling. Therefore, a PRL-releasing hormone (PRH) has also been postulated to explain this phenomenon (see Table 9.2). When the mother stops breast-feeding, the PRL level gradually decreases and eventually stops.

3 Other stimuli, such as muscular exercise, sleep and stress (physical or emotional), seem to work through the hypothalamus.

4 Hypothalamic TRH stimulates PRL secretion as well as the secretion of TSH.

5 PRL has a short-loop negative feedback inhibitory effect on the hypothalamus to stop its own release.

L-Dopa inhibits PRL secretion. There is evidence that **dopamine**, which is found in the hypothalamus, is PIH. Chlorpromazine, which blocks dopamine, is found to stimulate PRL release. Bromocriptine inhibits PRL release by stimulation of dopamine receptors.

Actions of prolactin

PRL acts on the breast to produce milk. The continued secretion during pregnancy causes growth of the mammary gland tissue but does not stimulate the production of milk. This is because of the inhibitory effect of the large amounts of oestrogens and progesterone secreted by the placenta.

After delivery, PRL initiates and maintains milk production. A burst of secretion of PRL is produced during each suckling. This prepares the milk for the next feed.

PRL release during breast-feeding exerts an inhibitory effect on the ovaries and suppresses the menstrual cycle in about one-half of lactating mothers. It seems to decrease the sensitivity of the ovaries to gonadotrophins. Breast-feeding, which stimulates PRL release, can be regarded as a physiological mechanism leading to birth control and spacing of pregnancies.

It is believed that PRL also acts centrally, probably on certain areas of the limbic system, to produce the characteristic maternal and nursing behaviours in the mother.

Abnormalities of prolactin secretion

Hyperprolactinaemia is found in cases with acidophil or chromophobe adenoma of the pituitary gland. Prolactin-secreting adenoma is a common anterior pituitary tumour, which occurs more often in women than in men. It causes infertility in both. Hyperprolactinaemia is not always associated with **galactorrhoea** (abnormal production of milk). On the other hand, cases of galactorrhoea have been described without elevation of blood PRL levels.

Hypersecretion of PRL occurs as a result of hypothalamic pituitary disorders, including section of the pituitary stalk and therefore interference with the production or transport of PIH. Hypersecretion is associated with **secondary amenorrhoea** and infertility. Treatment with bromocriptine or other dopamine agonists is used in such cases.

Deficiency can occur as an isolated pituitary PRL deficiency or as part of **panhypopituitarism**.

Abnormalities of the anterior pituitary

Several clinical syndromes are known to be associated with disorders of the pituitary or the hypothalamus. The predominant clinical features depend upon the position of the lesion and the hormone or group of hormones which are affected most.

Hypopituitarism

Hypopituitarism is usually due to destruction of the anterior pituitary by disease, radiation or total removal by surgery. The gonadotrophins are usually affected first. Evidence of TSH and ACTH involvement appears later. In children the predominant feature is failure to grow.

Sheehan's syndrome (Simmond's disease) is hypopituitarism due to destruction of the adenohypophysis in women, following severe post-partum haemorrhage. Loss of pubic and axillary hair is noted, together with lack of lactation. There is generalized weakness (asthenia) and loss of vigour, with hypothyroidism developing later. The menstrual cycle stops. The severity of this condition depends on the extent of pituitary destruction.

Hypothalamic hypopituitarism results from lesions in the hypothalamus and failure to produce the hypothalamic releasing or inhibitory hormones. This is secondary hypopituitarism, which will respond to administration of releasing hormones, such as TRH or gonadotropin releasing hormone (GnRH).

Hypopituitarism in children leads to stunted growth (**dwarfism**). However, there are different types of dwarfs. Isolated GH deficiency will lead to dwarfism and will respond to human GH therapy (see Fig. 9.11). Some dwarfs, however, secrete GH but seem to have a faulty response. IGF-I is responsible for the growth-promoting effect on cartilage and bone. One type of dwarfism seems to have a deficiency of IGF-I production. A hypothalamic defect which results in failure of secretion of GnRH results in **hypogonadism** associated with obesity. This is known as **adiposogenital syndrome** or **Fröhlich syndrome**.

Panhypopituitarism is a term given to a generalized hypofunction of the pituitary. In this condition, most, if not all, of the pituitary hormones are involved. Therefore, the clinical manifestations will include adrenal and thyroid deficiencies, as well as dwarfism and hypogonadism.

Pituitary tumours

An adenoma of the pituitary is a benign tumour, which may be minute in size but, nevertheless, gives rise to overproduction of a particular hormone. Adenomata have been described as arising from acidophil, basophil and chromophobe cells. Therefore, the clinical manifestations of the tumours will depend on the hormone or hormones involved. Thus, acromegaly, hyperprolactinaemia and Cushing's syndrome can be produced. The tumour may also enlarge and press on neighbouring structures, such as the *optic chiasma*. This leads to bilateral temporal hemianopia and progressive blindness. This is particularly common with chromophobe adenoma.

The pineal body

The pineal body has been found to secrete certain transmitters which influence hypothalamic and therefore pituitary functions. **Melatonin**, a derivative of serotonin, is released by the pineal body. This hormone suppresses the release of GnRH and causes inhibition of secretion of gonadotrophins. In young animals, this leads to failure of sexual maturation. Melatonin is rapidly removed from the blood and metabolized in the liver.

On the other hand, the pineal body receives neural messages from parts of the central nervous system, particularly the hypothalamus. Sympathetic nerves to β-adrenergic receptors on pineal cells activate cyclic AMP and melatonin synthesis and secretion.

Sympathetic supply to the pineal gland responds to diurnal light and dark variation. There is marked secretion during the evening and night, which returns to a low basal secretion by day. The night secretion of melatonin is higher in children. It is twice the level in adolescence and more than 10 times that in adults. This steady decrease in melatonin secretion with age is difficult to explain and its functional significance in the regulation of human reproduction remains to be explained.

The posterior pituitary gland

The posterior pituitary (neurohypophysis) develops from the neural tube of the embryo, i.e. it has the same embryogenic origin as the nervous system—hence the name neurohypophysis. It has direct nerve tract connections with the hypothalamus, mainly with the supraoptic nucleus and the paraventricular nuclei.

It is responsible for the storage of hormones synthesized in **magnocellular neurons** in the hypothalamus. **Antidiuretic hormone** (ADH), also known as **arginine vasopressin**, is mainly produced in the **supraoptic nucleus** of the hypothalamus. The hormone **oxytocin** is mainly produced in the **paraventricular nuclei**. These hormones (in a larger polypeptide precursor) travel down the nerve fibres (axoplasmic flow) and remain as storage granules in the nerve endings within the neurohypophysis until they are released by specific stimuli.

Antidiuretic hormone (ADH)

The name vasopressin has also been given to ADH because of the powerful vasoconstrictor effect of the hormone.

Chemistry and degradation

ADH (vasopressin) consists of a chain of nine amino acids (nanopeptide). Synthetic vasopressin is now available. There are slight species-specific differences in molecular structure. The half-life of the hormone is about 5 minutes. It is degraded mainly in the liver and the kidneys.

Control of ADH release

The release of ADH, stored in the nerve endings in the posterior pituitary, is stimulated by nerve impulses, originating in the hypothalamus, which travel down the same neurons and release the hormone. The hormone is released into the blood by exocytosis of the secretory granules. The main physiological stimuli known to result in its secretion are as follows:

1 *An increase in the osmotic pressure of the extracellular fluid (ECF)*. This occurs in states of dehydration, due either to excessive water loss or to water deprivation. High osmotic pressure stimulates **osmoreceptors** in the anterior hypothalamus. These receptors are located near the supraoptic nucleus and the impulses generated in them stimulate the release of ADH. A very small change in the ECF osmotic pressure—1%—is detected by the osmoreceptors and results in regulation of ADH (Fig. 9.12). If it is noted that the osmotic pressure of ECF is only 290 mosmol/litre, then it is realized that this is a very sensitive mechanism. The hypothalamic centres are also

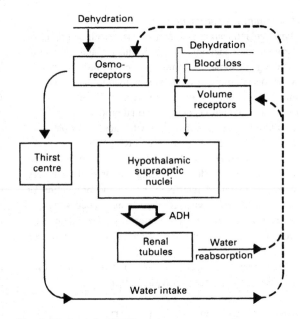

Fig. 9.12 Control of ADH by volume receptors and osmoreceptors. Dehydration is seen to work through both mechanisms.

responsible for initiating the sensation of thirst. This sensation, however, requires a bigger rise in the osmotic pressure.

2 *A fall in blood volume*. This occurs in conditions leading to dehydration or after blood loss. Haemorrhage initially causes a fall in the blood pressure in the venous system. If the cardiac output is decreased, arterial blood-pressure will also fall. It is believed that there are **volume receptors** situated in the low-pressure system of the great veins and the right atrium. One of the earliest responses to haemorrhage is ADH release. Afferent impulses travel through the vagus nerve and are relayed in the vagal nuclei to the hypothalamus. The response to volume receptor stimulation is more powerful than that due to osmoreceptors, i.e. hypovolaemia will stimulate ADH secretion even if the ECF is hypotonic. Both mechanisms tend to release ADH, which, in turn, causes the kidney tubules to reabsorb water. The volume of urine is consequently greatly decreased and water is retained in the body so as to correct the volume and osmolality of the extracellular fluid.

3 *Arterial blood pressure*. In response to hypotension **arterial baroreceptors** decrease their output to the vasomotor centre. Hypotension after haemorrhage is the most potent stimulus to vasopressin release. High plasma levels of the hormone are reached, which cause vasoconstriction as well as conservation of water.

4 *Age*. With advancing years the secretion of vasopressin increases in response to plasma osmotic pressure. On the other hand, the renal response to the antidiuretic effect is decreased. These changes render elderly subjects more likely to develop water retention and hyponatraemia.

5 *Other stimuli*. ADH is released by stimuli like pain, emotional stress and physical trauma. Drugs such as morphine, barbiturates and nicotine also stimulate the release of ADH. Its secretion is inhibited by alcohol—hence the diuretic and dehydrating effect of alcohol consumption.

The ADH response is an important mechanism in the concentration of urine in humans and other mammals living in hot, arid environments. It is noticeable that the kidney produces a small volume of concentrated urine in the hot summer months when compared with the winter. It is important to remember this fact when dealing with patients with renal disease. A high concentration of urine leads to deposition of solids and crystallization of certain salts, such as oxalates, in the urinary tract and may lead to infection.

Actions of ADH

ADH increases the water permeability of the collecting ducts of the kidney. This effect is mediated by V_2 **receptors** which increase intracellular cyclic AMP. Cyclic AMP activates a protein kinase that phosphorylates certain membrane proteins; this results in an increase in the permeability of the luminal membrane to water by insertion of water channels in the luminal membrane. These are protein molecules (**aquaporins**), which become inserted by exocytosis from the cytoplasm to increase the permeability of the luminal membrane to water. Since the interstitial fluid in the renal medulla is *hypertonic*, water quickly passes out of the tubules and is reabsorbed into the blood. The urine becomes more concentrated and smaller in volume.

ADH also increases the permeability of the collecting ducts to urea. This also helps the reabsorption of water.

The hormone decreases the blood flow in the renal medulla. This helps to maintain the hyperosmolality of the peritubular fluid.

In doses bigger than those normally released by the posterior pituitary, ADH causes generalized vasoconstriction and a rise in arterial blood pressure. This vasoconstrictor effect is mediated by V_1 **receptors**, which apparently increase intracellular calcium ions. Acute blood loss results in vasopressin release and elevation of blood pressure. ADH, however, is of doubtful significance in the short-term regulation of normal arterial blood pressure. The well-known cardiovascular reflexes are more important in this respect.

Abnormalities

1 Lack of ADH results in the production of large volumes of dilute urine, which leads to thirst and excessive drinking (polydipsia). This condition is known as **diabetes insipidus**. It is usually due to a lesion in the hypothalamus. Removal of the posterior pituitary or pituitary stalk section usually produces a transient type of the disease.

2 ADH secretion increases after **surgical operations**, leading to abnormal water retention and therefore lowering of sodium concentration in the ECF (hyponatraemia). This is due to dilution of the ECF rather than a sodium deficit.

3 In **congestive heart failure** there seems to be an abnormal release of ADH, in spite of the increased blood pressure central venous pressure. The volume receptor mechanism fails to suppress ADH secretion. Another explanation of water retention due to ADH is the increased half-life of the hormone in congestive heart failure. This is probably due to diminished degradation of the hormone by the liver and the kidneys.

Oxytocin

Chemistry and degradation

Oxytocin is also a nanopeptide hormone. Synthetic oxytocin is available for therapeutic use. Its half-life is 1–4 minutes and it is mainly degraded by the liver and kidneys. There are synthetic analogues used in clinical practice. It causes ejection of milk from the lactating breasts and contractions of the uterus during labour. Its chemical structure is similar to that of ADH. It is produced mainly in the paraventricular nuclei of the hypothalamus but it has been demonstrated in other parts of the central nervous system, where its function is believed to be as one of the neuropeptide transmitters.

Control of oxytocin release

1 Oxytocin is released by stimulation of the nipples of the lactating mother. Its main action in this case is to eject milk and therefore facilitate breast-feeding. Milk ejection is a **neurohumoral reflex**. The afferent part of the reflex is the somatic pathway for touch sensation and the efferent part is via the hormone oxytocin. Oxytocin release may take place without stimulation of the nipples, e.g. in response to visual or auditory stimuli from the baby.

2 Distension of the uterus and stretching of the cervix stimulates oxytocin release. During childbirth this hormone facilitates contraction of the uterine muscles, which leads to the gradual expulsion of the fetal head through the birth canal (see Chapter 15).

3 During coitus, stimulation of the vagina and the genital organs may bring about oxytocin release. In the female sexual orgasm, oxytocin is released and, if there is lactation, milk may be ejected. There are also repeated contractions of the uterus and the fallopian tubes, which may help the sperm to travel up the female genital tract.

4 Psychological and emotional factors, such as fear, may inhibit the release of oxytocin. Anxiety, pain and sympathoadrenal stimulation release oxytocin and alcohol inhibits its secretion.

Those stimuli that release oxytocin seem to work at the level of the hypothalamic nuclei. Impulses from the paraventricular nuclei travel in the hypothalamohypophyseal tracts to release the stored hormone from the nerve endings in the neurohypophysis directly into the bloodstream.

Actions of oxytocin

Two main physiological actions are known:

1 *Ejection of milk.* This is brought about by contraction of the **myoepithelial cells** of the ducts of the mammary gland. The hormone does not stimulate milk production; it only helps the ejection of the milk during suckling.

2 *Contraction of the uterus.* This is an important action during labour. The pregnant uterus becomes more sensitive to the action of oxytocin towards the end of pregnancy. It has been found that oestrogens make the uterine muscles more sensitive to oxytocin, while progesterone decreases this sensitivity. At term, there is a rapid fall in the mother's serum progesterone level and therefore increased uterine sensitivity to oxytocin. (For more detail see Chapter 15.)

Abnormalities

There is no known clinical condition related to an abnormality of oxytocin secretion. Synthetic preparations of oxytocin are widely used in obstetrics to *induce labour* and to promote uterine contraction during childbirth. This shortens the duration of labour and helps prevent maternal and fetal distress.

The thyroid gland

Anatomical considerations

The thyroid is the largest single endocrine gland. It weighs 20–25 g but it varies with age, sex and physiological condition, such as pregnancy and lactation.

The thyroid gland is the only endocrine gland that does not store its hormone within the cell but in follicular cavities surrounded by the cells.

The main histological feature is the thyroid follicle, which is a spherical structure formed of a single layer of

Fig. 9.13 Diagram showing: (a) the normal microstructure of the thyroid follicles; (b) smaller follicles lined with columnar epithelium in hyperthyroidism; and (c) the flattened epithelium with wide follicles full of stored colloid in hypothyroidism.

epithelial cells, which surround a cavity filled with a colloid material. The type of epithelial cells forming the follicles varies according to the activity of the gland (Fig. 9.13). With normal activity the cells are cubical. With increased activity they become tall and columnar and microvilli can be seen projecting into the colloid. With deceased activity they become flat cells. The quantity of colloid material in the cavity of the follicle also varies with the activity of the gland. A few **clear cells** or C cells may be seen in the walls of the follicles but they have no contact with the cavity of the follicle. They are therefore also referred to as the parafollicular cells. They produce the hypocalcaemic hormone, **calcitonin**.

Hormones of the thyroid

The gland produces **thyroxine** (levothyroxine) (T_4), **tri-**

Fig. 9.14 Diagram of thyroid gland cell showing the steps of thyroid hormone synthesis: (1) iodine trapping, showing iodide pump (IP); (2) thyroglobulin synthesis; (3) oxidation of iodide to iodine; (4) iodination of tyrosine molecules within the thyroglobulin molecule to give monoiodotyrosine (MIT) and di-iodotyrosine (DIT) at the apical border of the cell; (5) coupling of MIT and DIT to give T_3 and T_4, still within the thyroglobulin molecule in the colloid; (6) pinocytosis of thyroglobulin; (7) proteolysis of thyroglobulin and release of T_3 and T_4.

iodothyronine (T_3) and **calcitonin**. Calcitonin is concerned with calcium metabolism and will be considered with the parathyroid hormone and the control of plasma calcium.

Iodine forms an integral part of the thyroxine and tri-iodothyronine molecules. Iodine is taken in food and in drinking-water. A minimum daily intake of about 100–150 μg (in the form of potassium or sodium iodide) is required for normal thyroid function. The iodide is easily absorbed in the intestine to circulate in plasma in a concentration of about 0.3 μg/100 ml; 30–50% of iodide circulating in blood is taken up by the thyroid, while the rest is lost in urine. The thyroid can therefore remove iodide from blood against a concentration gradient ranging from about 40 times in a normal gland to several hundred times in an overactive gland. This selective uptake of iodide by the thyroid gland, or iodide trapping, can be achieved only by active transport (iodide pump). Also, as the follicular cell has a resting membrane potential of –50 mV, the iodide pump has to work against electrical and concentration gradients. Various other tissues can also trap iodide, particularly the salivary and mammary glands, but the thyroid contains 90–95% of body iodide.

Stages of synthesis of thyroid hormones (Fig. 9.14)

Thyroglobulin synthesis
Thyroglobulin is a large protein synthesized by the endoplasmic reticulum of the thyroid cells and secreted into the colloid. Its molecular weight is 660 000 daltons. The importance of thyroglobulin lies in the fact that it has 140 molecules of the amino acid **tyrosine**, which is used for thyroid hormone synthesis. The synthesis of thyroid hormones takes place within the thyroglobulin molecules in the colloid.

Oxidation of iodide
The trapped iodide ions are oxidized into iodine in the thyroid cell by means of peroxidase enzyme. The oxidized form is capable of combining with tyrosine.

Iodination of tyrosine
The tyrosine molecules on the surface of thyroglobulin are iodinated to give **monoiodotyrosine** (MIT) and **di-iodotyrosine** (DIT). This iodination process is rapid and it occurs as soon as the thyroglobulin is synthesized and

during its passage through the cell membrane into the follicles of the thyroid.

Coupling of MIT and DIT

The next stage is condensation or the coupling reactions of iodotyrosines (MIT and DIT) to give iodothyronines. This is a slow process, which starts in a few minutes but continues for several days within the follicular colloid. When one MIT and one DIT molecule are coupled, **tri-iodothyronine** (T_3) is formed and, when two DIT molecules are coupled, **thyroxine** (levothyroxine) (**tetraiodothyronine, T_4**) is formed. The *coupling reactions* take place on the surface of the thyroglobulin molecule and, in the same way as MIT and DIT, both T_4 and T_3 are attached to the thyroglobulin molecule by peptide linkages.

The active thyroid hormones, T_3 and T_4, and their inactive precursors, MIT and DIT, are stored in the colloid of the thyroid follicles. They can only be released from the colloid by proteolysis of thyroglobulin.

Release of T_3 and T_4

In the thyroid cells, the next step results in the release of T_3 and T_4 from the thyroglobulin molecule. First, thyroglobulin is taken up by the cells by pinocytosis. There are proteases present in an inactive form, but, when activated, they break the peptide linkages between the thyroglobulin molecules and the iodinated compounds. MIT, DIT, T_4 and T_3 are set free. T_3 and T_4 leave the follicle by their concentration gradient to reach the rich capillary network around the follicles.

In the thyroid cell there is another enzyme, *deiodinase*, which only acts on iodinated tyrosines (MIT and DIT) after they are released from their attachment with the thyroglobulin molecule. Deiodinase has no effect on T_4 and T_3. The iodine released by deiodinase from MIT and DIT is reused for iodination of tyrosine and represents a significant source of iodine. Very minute amounts, if any, of MIT and DIT escape deiodination and appear in the circulation. Considerable loss of MIT and DIT in urine may occur if the enzyme deiodinase is congenitally deficient, which results in a type of goitre that occurs in siblings.

Figure 9.14 illustrates the various steps of thyroid hormone synthesis. Drugs such as perchlorate and thiocyanate interfere with iodide trapping. *Thiouracil* and related compounds inhibit iodination and coupling reactions and, as such, can be used to treat hyperthyroidism. Propylthiouracil also inhibits conversion of T_4 to T_3.

Transport and degradation of thyroid hormones

T_4 and T_3, once they reach the circulation, are transported

Table 9.5 The proportions of T_3 and T_4 bound to different plasma proteins.*

Binding protein	T_3 (% bound)	T_4 (% bound)
TBG	46	67
TBPA	Trace	20
Albumin	53	13

* Data from Ganong, W.F. (1999) *Review of Medical Physiology*, 19th edn. Appleton & Lange, Stamford, Connecticut.

in blood attached to plasma proteins, namely, **thyroxine-(levothyroxine)-binding globulin** (TBG), **thyroxine-(levothyroxine)-binding prealbumin** (TBPA), also known as **transthyretin**, and **thyroxine(levothyroxine)-binding albumin** (TBA). The proportions of the hormones passed to each of these proteins depend on their affinities for the hormone (Table 9.5). TBG has a high affinity for T_4 and therefore it binds more T_4 than T_3. Albumin has a higher concentration in plasma than TBG and therefore it has a high capacity to bind T_4 and T_3 but it has less affinity. The normal plasma levels are 60–160 nmol/litre for T_4 and 1.2–2.8 nmol/litre for T_3. The half-lives of T_4 and T_3 are about 9 and 1.5 days, respectively. Only minute amounts of the hormones are found free within plasma. The physiological actions of T_3 and T_4 and their negative feedback with TSH are due to the free fractions.

Most of T_4 is deiodinated in the liver, kidneys and other tissues to give active T_3 **(3,5,3-tri-iodothyronine)** and an inactive form known as **reverse T_3 (rT_3)** or 3,3,5-tri-iodothyronine. Further deiodination takes place, resulting in iodotyrosines (MIT and DIT). In the pituitary and brain, T_4 is deiodinated to T_3 intracellularly. The conversion of T_4 to T_3 is decreased by hypermetabolic states, such as fever, trauma, burns and malignancies. Starvation depresses T_3 formation but increases rT_3 levels, and overfeeding increases T_3 and decreases rT_3.

Control of thyroid function

The function of the thyroid gland is controlled by the hypothalamopituitary axis. The hypothalamus produces a **thyrotrophin-releasing hormone** (TRH), which reaches the adenohypophysis via the hypophyseal portal vessels. Under the influence of TRH, the adenohypophysis produces **thyroid-stimulating hormone (TSH)**, which controls the function of the thyroid gland. The thyroid hormones circulating in blood regulate the release of TSH by a negative feedback control (see Fig. 9.3 and the section on the control of secretion).

TSH influences thyroid function in different ways.

Table 9.6 Summary of the effects of thyroid hormones.

On metabolism
Increased basal metabolic rate
Increased O_2 consumption
Calorigenic effect
Increased Na^+, K^+ ATPase activity
Fat mobilization
Increased absorption of glucose in the small intestine
Increased formation of LDL receptors

Growth and development
Normal skeletal growth
Mental development

Central nervous system
Brain development
Potentiation of catecholamines, enhanced alertness
Decreased reflex time

Cardiovascular system
Increased contractility of cardiac muscle and increased
 heart rate
Potentiation of catecholamines through increased
 numbers and affinity of β-adrenergic receptors

On reproduction
Normal gonadal function
Milk production

On bone marrow
Normal erythropoesis

LDL, low density lipoprotein.

It increases the vascularity of the gland to facilitate more efficient removal of the hormones from the gland. TSH stimulates the steps involved in the synthesis and release of thyroid hormones, from the process of iodide trapping to the activation of proteases which liberate thyroid hormones from their attachment to the thyroglobulin molecule into the colloid.

Actions of thyroid hormones (Table 9.6)
Although the thyroid gland produces more T_4 than T_3, the latter hormone is more potent and acts much faster than the former. T_3 enters the cell more easily than T_4. The latter is also transformed to T_3 in the cytoplasm. T_3 binds avidly to receptors on the cell nucleus and promotes messenger ribonucleic acid (mRNA) and ribosomal RNA (rRNA) synthesis. The nuclear receptors for thyroid hormones are considered as **nuclear transcription factors**. One such receptor (TRβ2) is found in brain cells only. Other receptors are found in almost all other body tissues. The vari-

ety of receptors and therefore transcription of a variety of enzymes explains the wide range of effects of the thyroid hormones:

1 *Effects on general metabolism*. Thyroid hormones have a **calorigenic action**. They stimulate oxygen consumption and energy expenditure by all active tissues of the body, with some exceptions, such as the brain, pituitary and testes. Because the metabolic rate of the body is accelerated, heat production will increase. In hyperthyroidism, heat loss mechanisms are stimulated, i.e. sweating and vasodilatation of skin vessels.

2 *Effects on growth and development*. Thyroid hormones are important for normal growth and development. This is clearly seen in congenital deficiency of thyroid hormones, resulting in the **thyroid dwarf (the cretin)**. GH can exert its full effect on skeletal growth only in the presence of adequate thyroid hormones.

3 *Effects on the nervous system*. Thyroid hormones are essential for the normal development and function of the central nervous system. **Mental retardation** is an important feature of **cretinism**. There are defective synaptic development and myelination in the brain. If treatment of cretinism is not started early after birth, mental retardation will persist.

In hyperthyroidism, the activation of the central nervous system may be due to potentiation of the effects of catecholamines, which stimulate the reticular activating system.

Deficiency of thyroid hormones later in life (myxoedema) depresses mental functions. The patient becomes mentally slow and forgetful. Reflex activities are also slowed down. The relaxation phase of a stretch reflex becomes significantly prolonged. Prolongation of the ankle jerk relaxation phase is a useful clinical sign in hypothyroidism.

4 *Effects on metabolism*. Since thyroid hormones are essential for normal growth, in physiological quantities they stimulate protein synthesis, but, in large amounts, because of the accelerated metabolic rate, thyroid hormones indirectly cause protein breakdown to provide fuel for the increased energy expenditure. The patients go into negative nitrogen balance. Catabolism of muscle protein leads to *muscle-wasting* and removal of bone protein results in hypercalcaemia, hypercalciuria and osteoporosis.

In carbohydrate metabolism, thyroid hormones are *hyperglycaemic* (diabetogenic) hormones. They increase blood glucose in several ways. They promote glucose absorption in the intestine and stimulate glycogenolysis and gluconeogenesis. They also promote degradation of insulin and increase peripheral glucose utilization. The accelerated energy expenditure is partly explained by increased Na^+, K^+ adenosine triphosphatase (ATPase) activity and mitochondrial protein synthesis.

In lipid metabolism, thyroid hormones decrease serum cholesterol levels. This is due to increased formation of low-density lipoprotein (LDL) receptors. Thus, in hyperthyroidism the serum cholesterol level is low or normal, while in hypothyroidism it is usually high. They also mobilize FFAs from adipose tissue.

5 *Effect on vitamin requirements.* Thyroid hormones promote conversion of β-carotene to vitamin A. They also facilitate absorption of vitamin B_{12}. Because thyroid hormones accelerate energy metabolism, there is a greater body requirement for vitamins of the B group, especially thiamine in hyperthyroid states.

6 *Water and mineral metabolism.* Thyroid hormones have a diuretic effect. There is an increase in the glomerular filtration rate (GFR) and an increase in renal excretion of sodium and calcium. Because of their catabolic effect on protein, potassium, creatine and uric acid, excretion is also increased.

7 *Effects on the cardiovascular system.* Thyroid hormones increase the chronotropic and inotropic effects of catecholamines on the heart. The number and affinity of β-adrenergic receptors are increased. Both the heart rate and the stroke volume are increased. As a result, cardiac output increases and systolic blood pressure rises. Vasodilatation is brought about by the stimulated heat-loss mechanism. This results in decreased peripheral resistance and the diastolic pressure tends to drop. Consequently, high pulse pressure is usually recorded and a collapsing pulse is detected. A high sleeping pulse is a clinical sign of hyperthyroidism, while low electrocardiogram (ECG) voltage is seen in hypothyroidism. The effects on the heart can be decreased by β-adrenergic blockers, e.g. propranolol.

8 *Effect on the alimentary tract.* Thyroid hormones increase the motility of the gastrointestinal tract and improve the appetite. Patients with hyperthyroidism have very good appetites and complain of *diarrhoea*, while those with hypothyroidism have poor appetites and are usually constipated.

9 *Effects on muscles.* Excessive production of thyroid hormones causes considerable muscle weakness (**thyrotoxic myopathy**) due to several reasons:

(a) Protein catabolism and muscle-wasting are important features of hyperthyroidism. There is also evidence that some changes take place in muscle myosin and ATPase activity and that there are decreased levels of muscle adenosine triphosphate (ATP).

(b) The water and electrolyte disturbance caused by abnormally high levels of thyroid hormones contributes to muscle weakness.

(c) Thyroid hormones increase the excitability of nervous tissue. Among the effects of this are the fine tremor and spontaneous twitches seen in hyperthyroidism. This continuous activity in the muscles ultimately leads to depletion of energy stores, fatigue and muscle weakness.

10 *Effect on gonads.* Thyroid hormones are essential for the normal development and function of the gonads. For instance, menstrual disturbances are seen in both hypo- and hyperthyroidism.

11 *Effect on mammary glands.* Thyroid hormones are important for maintenance of milk production, a fact sometimes made use of to increase milk production in dairy farming.

12 *Effects on bone marrow.* Thyroid hormones are important for bone marrow metabolism and for normal erythropoiesis. Hypothyroidism is characterized by anaemia due to depressed bone marrow activity, which can only be corrected by administration of thyroid hormones.

The actions of thyroid hormones can be well illustrated by considering the symptoms and signs of hypo- and hyperthyroidism.

Abnormalities of thyroid function

All thyroid disturbances are more common in females than in males.

Goitre

Goitre refers to any enlargement of the thyroid gland, with or without disturbance of function. There are many causes of goitre:

1 *Physiological goitre.* This is a diffuse moderate enlargement due to increased demand for thyroid hormones, as in puberty, pregnancy, lactation and chronic exposure to cold.

2 *Iodine deficiency.* Dietary iodine deficiency over a long period of time gives rise to **simple goitre**. This usually occurs in populations living in highlands far from the sea, where rainfall washes away the iodine content of the soil. Water and vegetables grown in these areas will be deficient in iodide. The condition is endemic; therefore, it is also referred to as '**endemic goitre**'. Several members of the family are usually affected. The size of the gland can be extremely large (Fig. 9.15), but there is no disturbance of function. The condition is a public health problem, which can be prevented by addition of iodide to table salt or cooking oil. Treatment of endemic goitre is surgical removal for cosmetic reasons and to avoid pressure on underlying structures, e.g. the trachea.

3 *Hereditary defect in thyroid hormone synthesis.* This may be due to hereditary deficiency of any of the enzymes concerned with thyroid hormone synthesis. Deficiency of these enzymes may lead to iodide trapping defect, iodine

Fig. 9.15 Patients with simple goitre in western Sudan. (Reproduced with permission from Bell, G.H., Emslie-Smith, D. & Paterson, C.R. (eds) (1980) *BDS Textbook of Physiology*, 10th edn. Churchill Livingstone, Edinburgh.)

organification defect, iodotyrosine coupling defect or deiodination defect. Consequently, low circulating thyroid hormone levels lead to increased production of TSH, which causes hypertrophy and hyperplasia of the gland. Since the condition is congenital, the child is a cretin with a goitre (a **goitrous cretin**). The condition is more common when the mother has endemic goitre.

4 *Excessive intake of goitrogens*, e.g. cabbage, turnip or drugs such as sulphonamides, thiocarbamides, perchlorate and thiocyanate, can suppress thyroid hormone synthesis and lead to goitre formation.

Hypothyroidism

Deficiency of thyroid hormone production may occur as a congenital abnormality due to congenital absence of the thyroid or congenital deficiency of any of the enzymes concerned with hormone synthesis (goitrous cretin). Hypothyroidism can also occur at adolescence or later in life.

Cretinism. When the deficiency is congenital, it is referred to as **cretinism**. The affected child is a **cretin**. Characteristically, the child is a mentally retarded dwarf. The features of cretins are so characteristic that they cannot be mistaken. The face is usually wrinkled and dry, the lips are thick and the tongue is large and usually protruding out of the mouth. Because of the enlargement of abdominal viscera and weak abdominal muscles, the belly is protruding, usually with an umbilical hernia (pot-belly).

It is very important to diagnose the condition soon after birth and immediately start the treatment; otherwise the mental retardation becomes irreversible.

Myxoedema. When deficiency of thyroid hormones is not congenital, the condition is referred to as **myxoedema**. It commonly occurs after the age of 50 but, if it occurs early in life, at adolescence, it is known as *juvenile myxoedema*. Myxoedema may be primary, due to damage of the thyroid, most commonly by an *autoimmune process*, or it may be due to surgical removal or radiation. It may be secondary to hypopituitarism. Thyroid autoimmune disease is triggered by thyroid damage or inflammation, leading to the release of appreciable amounts of thyroglobulin into the circulation and evokes specific antibody formation. These antibodies will reach the thyroid and destroy thyroid tissue.

The patient with myxoedema is usually overweight, with dry, thick, wrinkled skin, an expressionless face, thick lips and a large, thick tongue. The hair is dry, lustreless and easily lost from the scalp but, most characteristically, from the outer third of the eyebrows (Fig. 9.16).

Patients with myxoedema usually complain of intolerance to cold (due to their low metabolic rates). They are quite happy in a hot environment but feel cold in the slightest cool breeze. They are mentally depressed and forgetful; forgetting recent events or even the names of their close relatives. The appetite is poor and the patient is usually constipated. The pulse rate is slow (*bradycardia*) and there is low blood pressure. If the patient is still in the childbearing age, a common complaint is menstrual disturbances. The voice becomes hoarse and speech is slow and monotonous. Myxoedematous patients are usually weak and get tired very easily. They cannot cope with their normal household activities and spend most of their time in bed. Anaemia is a

Fig. 9.17 Photograph of a patient with hyperthyroidism. (Courtesy of Professor Khalil M. Salman, Dept. of Surgery, King Abdulaziz University Hospital, Jedda, Saudi Arabia.)

Fig. 9.16 Photograph of a patient with hypothyroidism. (Reproduced with permission from Emslie-Smith, D., Paterson, C.R., Scratchard, T. & Read, N.W. (eds) (1988) *BDS Textbook of Physiology*, 11th edn. Churchill Livingstone, Edinburgh.)

common finding in these patients. The duration of the ankle jerk is prolonged, particularly the relaxation phase of the reflex.

Hyperthyroidism (thyrotoxicosis)

Hyperthyroidism, which is characterized by high blood levels of thyroid hormones, can occur at an early age or it may occur later in life. The increased thyroid hormone secretion is due to abnormal **immunoglobulins** (IgG), known as **thyroid-stimulating immunoglobulins** (TSI). They seem to act by stimulating **TSH receptors** on the follicular cells. Due to the increased T_3 and T_4 output, TSH secretion is inhibited and its circulating level in thyrotoxicosis is usually low.

The patient usually complains of loss of weight, although she/he has a good appetite, and complains of weakness and tiredness after slight exertion. The patient is

nervous, anxious and easily excited and may often quarrel with family and children. There is a fine tremor, which can be seen in the outstretched hand.

The eyes may be protruding (**exophthalmos**) and the upper eyelids may be **retracted**, with the white sclera seen above the cornea, which gives the patient a startled look (Fig. 9.17). The exophthalmos is due to accumulation of mucopolysaccharides, fat and fluid behind the eyeball. The lid retraction is caused by increased tone in the levator muscle of the eyelid, due to potentiation of sympathetic activity by thyroid hormones. The syndrome of hyperthyroidism associated with exophthalmos and enlargement of the thyroid is known as **Graves' disease** or **exophthalmic goitre**.

Patients commonly complain of palpitations. The heart rate, the stroke volume and the cardiac output are all increased. The systolic blood pressure rises, while the diastolic blood pressure may fall due to vasodilatation. This may lead to *high cardiac output failure*. In some patients cardiac symptoms may be the only manifestation of thyroid disease. This should be remembered before they are referred to the cardiologist.

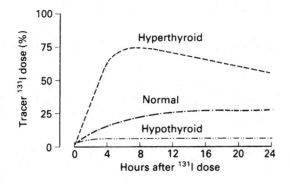

Fig. 9.18 Radioactive iodine uptake by the thyroid gland. The graph shows the percentage of the administered tracer dose taken up by the thyroid over a period of 24 hours in a normal person compared with hyper- and hypothyroidism.

Thyrotoxic patients usually have a wet, warm skin; the palms are wet and warm. In contrast, nervous sweating is associated with cold hands. Menstrual disturbances are frequent and diarrhoea is a common complaint.

Tests of thyroid function

A large variety of tests are used to assess thyroid function. Only some of these tests will be cited here:

1 Radioactive-iodine uptake (4- or 24-hour) and thyroid scanning are two tests that give a good indication of thyroid function and may assist in the diagnosis of the pathology of the condition. An oral dose of a radioactive isotope, such as ^{123}I or ^{131}I, is given and the uptake by the thyroid is measured. The uptake varies from one population to another, according to dietary iodine intake. High dietary iodine intake dilutes the test dose and may give misleadingly low radioactive iodine uptake values. The percentage of a dose of radioactive iodine is calculated and plotted against time. Figure 9.18 gives typical findings in cases of hyper- and hypothyroidism.

In thyroid scanning, after the administration of a dose of radioactive iodine, a graphic record of the density of isotope uptake (Fig. 9.19) is made by means of a scintiscanner. This test has the added value of detecting localized sites of activity (Fig. 9.20).

2 Estimation of serum T_3, T_4 and TSH: levels of total and free forms of T_3 and T_4, together with TSH, by radio-immunoassay or other methods in plasma, give a direct assessment of thyroid function. This is the test most used in clinical practice.

3 Measurement of protein-bound iodine (PBI) and of TBG is also used for assessment of thyroid function. The first is difficult and not specific and the second is influenced by a variety of drugs and physiological conditions.

The parathyroid glands and calcium homoeostasis

Extracellular Ca^{2+} is kept within a narrow range. The hormones concerned with its regulation are parathyroid hormone (PTH), *calcitonin* and *calcitriol*.

Anatomical considerations

The parathyroid glands are small, elongated nodules, usually four in number, embedded in the posterior surface of the lobes of the thyroid gland, one in relation to each pole. However, they may be less or more than four and may even be found in the mediastinum. They are 6 mm in length and weigh 20–50 mg. In contrast to their rich blood supply, the glands have a poor nerve supply, from branches of the superior and recurrent laryngeal nerves, which supply the blood-vessels.

In humans the parathyroid glands have two main types of cells. The **chief** (principal) cells form the major component of the cellular structure of the gland. They are small cells with poorly staining cytoplasm. They are the secretory cells of the gland. The less abundant cells are the oxyphil cells, which are seen only after puberty. The function of these cells has not yet been clarified.

Parathyroid hormone

Chemistry and degradation

PTH is a polypeptide with a molecular weight of 9500 daltons that is formed within the parathyroid cells as pre-pro-PTH (115 amino acids). Pre-pro-PTH is then converted to pro-PTH, from which PTH is formed (84 amino acids). In the circulation there is further cleavage, mainly in the liver, to form two fragments (C-terminal and N-terminal). Biological activity is associated with the N-terminal fragment. Degradation occurs mainly in the kidney. The C-terminal fragment has a longer plasma half-life (about 60 min) than the N-terminal fragment (about 5 min). Particularly high levels of PTH are found in patients with renal failure.

Control of secretion

1 The parathyroid glands are not under anterior pituitary control nor are they under nervous control. The main mechanism known to regulate PTH release is a negative feedback with plasma **ionized calcium** (Ca^{2+}). A decrease in plasma Ca^{2+} level stimulates the parathyroids to release PTH. Conversely, an increased plasma ionized calcium level decreases hormonal release.

2 Ionized magnesium has similar effects to Ca^{2+} but its physiological significance is unknown.

3 Stimulation of β-adrenergic receptors on parathyroid

(a)

(b)

Fig. 9.19 (a) Scintiscan of a normal thyroid gland using ^{99m}technetium pertechnetate (iodine analogue). It shows normal size and shape (butterfly appearance) of both lobes of the gland. The distribution of the tracer within the thyroid lobes is uniform and its concentration is within the normal limits. The time taken to obtain this image was 8 minutes. (b) Scintiscan of the thyroid gland in a patient showing symmetrical diffuse enlargement of both lobes of the gland. The distribution of the tracer is even and its concentration is increased. Note that the time required to obtain this image was only 1 minute. (Courtesy of Dr Tariq Al-Baghdadi, Nuclear Medicine, King Abdulaziz University Hospital, Jedda, Saudi Arabia.)

cells increases PTH secretion. This mechanism seems to modify the sensitivity of the gland to Ca^{2+}.

4 High levels of 1,25-dihydroxycholecalcifierol (calcitriol) inhibit PTH secretion. In this way it provides a negative feedback to the activation of vitamin D by the kidneys.

Under certain physiological conditions where there is an increased demand for calcium, such as pregnancy and lactation, the parathyroid glands hypertrophy and become more vascular and more active. Their hormone production consequently increases.

Actions of parathyroid hormone

PTH acts at different sites in the body to increase the level of plasma calcium:

1 In bone it promotes calcium reabsorption. This effect is achieved by activating **oesteoclasts**, by formation of new oesteoclasts and by retarding the conversion of oesteoclasts into oesteoblasts. As calcium is removed from bone, phosphate is removed too. The effects on bone are mediated by an increased production of cyclic AMP.

2 In the kidney its action is manifested in several ways:

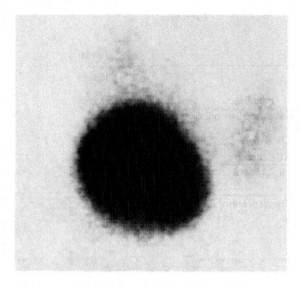

Fig. 9.20 Scintiscan of a toxic nodule of the thyroid gland. It shows an enlarged right lobe with a marked, localized, abnormally increased concentration of the tracer occupying its lower half. The upper part of the right lobe, as well as the normal-sized and shaped left lobe, are faintly visualized. The time required to obtain this image was only 1.5 minutes. (Courtesy of Dr Tariq Al-Baghdadi, Nuclear Medicine, King Abdulaziz University Hospital, Jeddah, Saudi Arabia.)

(a) It increases phosphate excretion by decreasing tubular reabsorption.

(b) It increases tubular reabsorption of calcium.

(c) It converts 25-hydroxycholecalciferol into active 1,25-dihydroxycholecalciferol (the active form of vitamin D_3) or **calcitriol**. Together with PTH it facilitates mobilization of calcium from bone and promotes intestinal calcium absorption. Calcitriol also facilitates active transport of Ca^{2+} from the osteoblasts to the extracellular fluid. Table 9.7 gives a summary of the regulation of calcitriol $(1,25\text{-}(OH)_2D_3)$.

Calcitonin

Calcitonin is the second hormone concerned with calcium homoeostasis. It is produced by **C cells** of the thyroid gland. It has the opposite effects to those of parathyroid hormone. Human calcitonin is a polypeptide consisting of 32 amino acids with a molecular weight of 3500 daltons.

The control of calcitonin secretion is stimulated by hypercalcaemia. It is released when there is a high Ca^{2+} level in the extracellular fluid, e.g. after a meal. Its secretion, in this case, is also stimulated by the gastrointestinal hormones **gastrin**, **cholecystokin** (CCK) and glucagon.

Table 9.7 Regulation of calcitriol $(1,25\text{-}(OH)_2D_3)$.

Increased by	Decreased by
Formation of calcitriol is catalysed by kidney enzyme 1α-hydroxylase, which is increased by: PTH low PO_4^{3-} Prolactin Calcitonin	High calcium through inhibition of PTH release Above also results in formation of inactive metabolite of calcitriol $(24,25(OH)_2D_3)$ Low PO_4^{3-} inhibits 1α-hydroxylase activity Acidosis Hyperthyroidism

Thus, it provides a second hormone for the regulation of the serum calcium level. However, this feedback mechanism is much faster than that of PTH and therefore it provides a short-term regulatory mechanism, e.g. preventing postprandial hypercalcaemia. It must be noted, however, that in the long term it is PTH which is more important in the regulation of serum calcium.

The actions of calcitonin produce a rapid decrease in serum Ca^{2+} concentration through the following mechanisms:

1 It suppresses osteoclastic activity in bone, leading to a decrease in calcium mobilization. This effect is more marked in children, because they have a greater osteoclastic activity due to rapid bone remodelling. In adults this is a weak effect, because the amount of calcium mobilized by oesteoclasts is much smaller. However, during pregnancy and lactation calcitonin may have a protective effect against excessive bone demineralization.

2 It increases the activity of oesteoblasts. This leads to increased mineralization of bone at the expense of extracellular fluid calcium concentrations.

3 In the long term, it decreases the number of oesteoclasts formed in the bone. The number of oesteoblasts is also decreased. Thus, its long-term effect is neutralized.

4 It has an inhibitory effect on the transport of calcium from the intracellular fluid to the extracellular fluid.

Regulation of plasma calcium level

The total body calcium in an adult man amounts to about 1200 g (30 000 mmol); 99% of it is found in bone while only 1% is found in soft tissues and body fluids. The skeleton is therefore an important store of calcium to be drawn from when the plasma calcium level tends to fall. In fact, there is continuous exchange of calcium between bone and blood. The exchangeable calcium pool in bone amounts

Source   Processing   Excretion

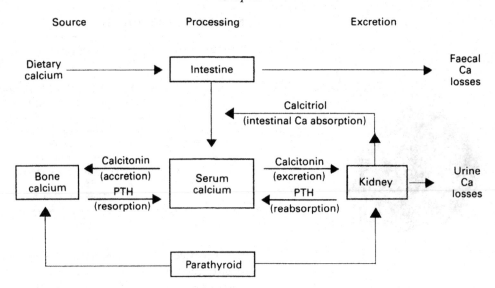

Fig. 9.21 Regulation of serum calcium level. Note that the main sites of regulation are: intestinal absorption, bone resorption and deposition and renal tubular reabsorption.

to about 4000 mg (100 mmol). The plasma calcium level ranges between 9 and 10.5 mg/dl (2.1 and 2.6 mmol/litre). About 50% is found in un-ionized complexes, mainly bound to plasma albumin. The rest is found in ionized form (1.00–1.3 mmol/litre). This range is kept reasonably constant by a delicate regulatory mechanism, which involves PTH, calcitonin, vitamin D and calcitriol.

The total body calcium is maintained within the normal limits by a balance of calcium intake and excretion (Fig. 9.21).

Absorption of calcium in the gastrointestinal tract is facilitated by **calcitriol**, formed in the kidney under the effect of PTH. However, absorption may be impaired by phytates, fats and oxalates, which form insoluble, poorly absorbed compounds of calcium. Gastrectomy renders the intestinal contents alkaline. Since calcium is more soluble in an acid medium, its absorption from the intestine will be impaired by gastrectomy.

In the kidney PTH stimulates tubular reabsorption of calcium. Only 150 mg of calcium is excreted in the urine per day.

The Ca^{2+} levels in the serum range between 1.0 and 1.3 mmol. The level remains reasonably constant. About 500 mg of calcium is mobilized and the same amount is deposited in bone every day. It appears from the above that calcium is added or taken from the plasma pool in such a way as to maintain a constant level (internal balance). Dietary intake, on the other hand, balances the calcium losses in faeces and urine (external balance).

Disturbance of parathyroid function

Hyperparathyroidism

Excessive production of PTH due to an active tumour or hyperplasia of the parathyroids leads to a series of disturbances in various organs and tissues:

1 Mobilization of calcium from bone leads to osteoporosis; the bones become weak and may fracture following minor trauma (pathological fractures). With excessive removal of calcium, the bones become fibrous, with formation of *bone cysts*, a rare condition called **osteitis fibrosa**. PTH stimulates the production of osteoclasts, which aggregate to form bony swellings (*osteoclastomas*).

2 In the kidneys, a raised plasma calcium level increases the filtered load of calcium and the tubular maximum is exceeded. The excess calcium is excreted in the urine, together with increased excretion of phosphate. The osmolar concentration of fluid in kidney tubules rises, leading to osmotic diuresis (polyuria.) Deposition of calcium phosphate crystals in the kidney ultimately leads to renal stone formation. The stones, which are characteristically calcium phosphate, are multiple and bilateral and tend to recur when removed. Kidney damage and renal failure are the final stages of the untreated condition.

3 Occasionally the presence of a high plasma calcium level may lead to abnormal calcification in soft tissues, such as muscles, cartilage, joint capsules and tendons.

4 Persistent hypercalcaemia leads to tiredness and mental confusion and which may result in coma and death.

5 High PTH is found in **renal failure** and in **rickets** (**secondary hyperparathyroidism**). This is due to long-standing low Ca^{2+} levels. There is hypertrophy of the parathyroid glands and lack of formation of calcitriol.

Diagnosis. Hyperparathyroidism may be suspected from the clinical picture. The diagnosis is confirmed if there are persistent high plasma calcium levels, especially if precautions are taken when blood samples are obtained from the patient. The main precaution is to take blood without using a tourniquet. It has been shown that using a tourniquet will raise the calcium level in the sample due to stasis of blood. The syringe and container used must be calcium-free. The diagnosis can be confirmed by the steroid suppression test. Giving hydrocortisone in daily doses of 40 mg for 8–10 days will suppress the plasma calcium level elevated by other conditions but not in hyperparathyroidism.

The development of radioimmunoassays for measuring PTH in plasma has made it possible for the direct diagnosis of dysfunction of parathyroid glands.

Hypoparathyroidism
Hypoparathyroidism is usually secondary to surgical removal or damage of the glands. It may also be due to an autoimmune process. The clinical picture is a result of a persistently low plasma calcium level. The presentation is that of latent or overt tetany.

Latent tetany is characterized by hypersensitivity (low threshold) of nerves and muscles, which can be demonstrated by two signs:
1 *Chvostek's sign.* Tapping the facial nerve at its emergence from the anterior border of the parotid gland in front of the ear causes contraction of the facial muscles.
2 *Trousseau's sign.* Carpal spasm can be demonstrated by arresting blood flow to the forearm by blowing a sphygmomanometer cuff above the systolic pressure and maintaining it for a few minutes. Characteristically, there will be flexion at the wrist, thumb and metacarpophalangeal joints with extension at the interphalangeal joints.

Pseudohypoparthyroidism is a congenital disease due to an abnormal reduction in PTH receptors with a normal secretion of PTH.

Tetany (latent or overt) may also result from lowering of plasma Ca^{2+} due to *alkalemia*, e.g. following hyperventilation or excessive vomiting. Hypocalcaemia can also be caused by a vitamin D deficiency in children or adults or in renal failure, due to a deficient production of calcitriol and the consequent poor intestinal absorption of calcium.

Long-standing hypocalcaemia may lead to overt tetany with spasm in the hands and feet (**carpopedal spasm**), spontaneous laryngeal spasms (laryngismus stridulus), convulsions and epileptic fits. Muscle cramps and muscle weakness are quite common. The patient may also present with **cataracts**, sometimes associated with mental retardation.

The endocrine pancreas
Diabetes mellitus is by far the most common endocrine and metabolic disorder encountered in medical practice. Insulin, the main hormone of the pancreas, is widely used in the treatment of diabetic patients.

The endocrine part of the pancreas consists of the **islets of Langerhans**. These are clusters of cells scattered between the acini of the exocrine pancreas. The islets are about 150 μm in diameter. They are richly supplied with blood-vessels. The cells of the islets consist of four main types: A cells (which constitute 20% of the islets' cells), B cells (about 75%) and D cells (3–5%). F cells (< 2%) constitute the remainder.

The A cells secrete the hormone **glucagon**. The B cells secrete **insulin**. The D cells secrete **somatostatin**. F cells release a hormone known as **pancreatic polypeptide** (PP), with, as yet, uncertain physiology.

Insulin
Insulin is the main hormone concerned with regulation of carbohydrate metabolism. In particular, insulin controls the level of blood glucose, glucose storage and utilization.

Chemistry and degradation of insulin
Insulin is a polypeptide consisting of 51 amino acids. Human insulin has a molecular weight of about 5800 daltons. The amino acid sequence has been worked out for human, bovine and porcine insulin. There are minor structural differences between species but their biological activity is similar. Human insulin is now prepared by biotechnology, which has decreased the use of animal insulins and therefore the formation of insulin antibodies.

The molecules of insulin consist of two chains: an **A chain**, consisting of 21 amino acids, and a **B chain**, consisting of 30 amino acids. The two chains are connected by two disulphide bridges. In the storage form, the molecule of **proinsulin** consists of a single chain (Fig. 9.22). The **C chain**, or **connecting peptide** (**C peptide**), consists of 31 amino acids. The C chain is removed before insulin is secreted by the B cells. The C peptide has no known function, but its blood levels indicate insulin secretion, because it is formed in equimolar quantities to insulin.

The half-life of insulin is about 5 minutes. It is carried into the pancreatic vein and goes through the portal vein to the liver before it reaches the systemic circulation. About

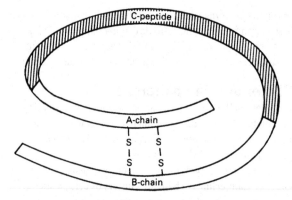

Fig. 9.22 The proinsulin molecule showing the insulin A and B chains connected by disulphide bridges. The C chain (connecting peptide) is shown as the shaded part of the proinsulin molecule. On cleavage of the C chain, equimolar quantities of insulin and C peptide are released from the B cells.

Fig. 9.23 Graph showing the normal pattern of insulin secretion stimulated by oral glucose intake.

half of it gets bound to liver cells. The insulin molecule then enters the cells by pinocytosis and is broken down by a proteolytic enzyme, which is also taken into the cell through the cell membrane. Almost all tissues bind and metabolize insulin. The kidneys also degrade significant amounts of insulin.

Regulation of insulin secretion

Insulin is found in plasma at a basal level (after an overnight fast) of about 5–10 μU/ml. Overweight and obese patients have higher-than-normal fasting levels. Its rate of secretion is markedly increased immediately after food intake.

1 The main stimulant to its secretion is *glucose*. Insulin secretion follows very closely the changes in the blood glucose level (Fig. 9.23). Entry of glucose into the B cells

does not depend on insulin. Unlike other cells in the body, B cells have glucose transporters in the cell membrane which do not require insulin for activation. It seems that glucose should be used by the B cells in order to stimulate insulin secretion. 2-Deoxyglucose (an unmetabolizable isomer of glucose) inhibits insulin secretion. There is an increase in intracellular Ca^{2+}, which is responsible for releasing insulin.

2 *Amino acids* in the diet are also a potent stimulus to insulin secretion. Both carbohydrate intake and protein intake stimulate the release of insulin. Together they have a synergistic action, which produces a marked increase in the amount secreted as a result of either alone.

3 The role of the autonomic nerve supply: there is evidence that stimulation of the right vagus nerve increases insulin secretion. This effect is blocked by atropine. Sympathetic stimulation, however, inhibits the release of insulin by means of an α-receptor mechanism.

4 The hormones of the gastrointestinal tract have been found to stimulate the secretion of insulin. Glucagon, gastrin, secretin and, in particular, glucose-dependent insulinotropic peptide (fomerly known as gastric inhibitory peptide) (GIP) all cause insulin release. GIP may be the main physiological gastrointestinal hormone responsible for insulin regulation after meals. It stimulates insulin secretion in very small amounts, similar to those normally found after a meal. These hormones potentiate the effect of glucose. Therefore, glucose taken by mouth results in far more insulin secretion than glucose given intravenously, although, in the latter instance, higher levels of blood glucose are attained.

5 The hormone **somatostatin**, secreted by D cells, inhibits the secretion of insulin. The physiological role of somatostatin, however, is not yet fully understood.

6 Insulin secretion is stimulated by a high level of *keto acids*, such as acetoacetic acid. This response helps to counteract further production of keto acids.

7 Many drugs have effects on insulin secretion. Sulphonylureas (e.g. **tolbutamide**) stimulate insulin secretion. Newer additions, such as **glibizide** and **gliburide**, stimulate insulin secretion and promote its action at the cellular level. These drugs have proved useful in treating patients who have some pancreatic insulin-secreting capacity left. Biguanides (e.g. **phenformin**) act by increasing glucose catabolism and decreasing its absorption in the intestine, but they have a tendency to produce lactic acidosis, which is an undesirable side-effect. Thiazide diuretics, however, inhibit insulin secretion. Diazoxide (once used for treatment of hypertension) is a potent inhibitor of insulin secretion.

Table 9.8 Summary of the effects of insulin.

On carbohydrate metabolism
Increases glucose entry in adipose tissue and muscle cells
Increases glycogen synthesis
Decreases gluconeogenesis
Decreases glucagon output from liver due to above two effects

On fat metabolism
Increases fatty acid, glycerol phosphate and triglyceride synthesis and therefore lipid deposition in adipose tissue cells and fat synthesis in liver
Inhibition of fat mobilization by inhibition of hormone-sensitive lipase
Activation of lipoprotein lipase
Decreased ketogenesis in liver

On protein metabolism
Increased amino acid uptake by cells
Increased protein synthesis
Decrease of glucogenic amino acid release from hepatocytes
Positive nitrogen balance through promotion of growth and decreased protein catabolism

On electrolytes
Uptake of K^+ into muscle and adipose tissue through an increase in Na^+, K^+ ATPase activity

The actions of insulin

The actions of insulin can be conveniently discussed in relation to glucose, amino acid and fat metabolism and in relation to electrolyte regulation. Specific insulin receptors have been demonstrated in many tissues, particularly in muscle, adipose tissue and liver. The binding of insulin to receptors on the cell membrane is a prerequisite for its intracellular actions.

Insulin receptors are genetically determined by a specific gene on chromosome 19. The intracellular sequence of events after the binding of insulin with the membrane receptor can be found in specialized texts. The receptor numbers and their affinity seem to be regulated. They increase in numbers in response to starvation and they decrease in obesity and in acromegaly. The affinity of insulin receptors increases in adrenocortical insufficiency and when insulin levels are low. On the other hand, affinity of receptors decreases when exposed to high glucocorticoid levels.

Table 9.8 gives a summary of the effects of insulin.

Actions on glucose metabolism. The strong hypoglycaemic action of insulin is the predominant effect, which results soon after the administration of the hormone. This hypoglycaemia is produced in several ways:

1 Insulin facilitates glucose uptake by many tissues. This is achieved by increasing the number of membrane **glucose transporters** (GLUT), which are membrane proteins the molecular structure of which is now known. One of these transporters ($GLUT_4$) is found intracellularly and becomes exteriorized on the cell membrane on exposure to insulin. The glucose transporters work through **facilitated diffusion**. Glucose transport into skeletal muscle and adipose tissue cells depends upon insulin. Some tissues do not need insulin for glucose entry into their cells, e.g. the liver, brain, kidneys, red blood cells and intestinal mucosa.

2 Insulin increases glycogen synthesis in the liver and in skeletal muscle.

3 Insulin decreases the glucose output from the liver by decreasing gluconeogenesis and by increasing glycogen synthesis.

4 Insulin increases the rate of utilization of glucose by skeletal muscle and by adipose tissues.

Actions on protein metabolism. Insulin is an anabolic hormone as far as protein is concerned. The following is a summary of its main actions:

1 It increases the uptake of amino acids by cells. In the liver and skeletal muscles, transport of amino acids into cells is greatly enhanced.

2 The hormone increases the rate of protein synthesis, especially in the liver and skeletal muscle. There is an increase in ribonucleic acid (RNA) formation and ribosomal protein synthesis by means of mRNA translation.

3 Protein catabolism is decreased. This leads to a positive nitrogen balance and decreased release of gluconeogenic amino acids.

Actions on fat metabolism. Insulin promotes storage of fat and decreases its utilization by the following actions:

1 It increases synthesis of FFAs in adipose tissue cells.

2 It increases the synthesis of glycerol phosphate.

3 It promotes the formation and deposition of triacylglycerols.

4 Insulin inhibits FFA mobilization from adipose tissue and therefore lowers the levels of circulating FFAs. Hormone-sensitive lipases are inhibited.

5 Ketone body formation (ketogenesis) in the liver is decreased and the uptake of ketone bodies by skeletal muscle is increased.

6 Insulin activates an enzyme (lipoprotein lipase) found on the surface of the endothelium of capillaries. It catalyses the catabolism of triacyclglycerol into FFA and glycerol.

Actions on electrolytes. Insulin increases the active transport of sodium and potassium across the cell membrane and there is an increase in the resting membrane potential. In the treatment of diabetic acidosis, insulin causes a net shift of K^+ from the extracellular to the intracellular fluid compartment. This may lead to the development of hypokalaemia, with its attendant serious complications.

On the other hand, K^+ depletion has been found to diminish insulin secretion, e.g. the thiazide diuretics may cause K^+ depletion and consequently decrease the secretion of insulin.

Abnormalities of insulin secretion

Diabetes mellitus is a syndrome due to an absolute or a relative deficiency of insulin secretion. **Type I**, or juvenile, diabetes mellitus mainly affects children and adolescents and is due to absolute or severe shortage of insulin. This makes it necessary for the patient to depend on insulin therapy—hence the name **insulin-dependent diabetes mellitus (IDDM)**. *Type II*, or maturity onset, diabetes mellitus, however, is usually of a less severe nature. The patient may require insulin or may not need it if the pancreas can be stimulated by oral hypoglycaemic agents—hence the name **non-insulin-dependent diabetes mellitus (NIDDM)**. Some patients may only require to adjust their diets so that the remaining insulin output is sufficient. The pathophysiology of NIDDM is heterogeneous. It is mainly due to decreased or delayed insulin secretion but the main defect is *insulin resistance*. In mild NIDDM the fault is a decreased number of insulin receptors; in others there is an abnormality in the receptors themselves or in the intracellular events following receptor stimulation. **Post-receptor insulin resistance** is believed to be the main defect in severe NIDDM. The disease may also be *secondary* to other endocrine disorders, such as excess GH, glucocorticoid and somatostatin secretions, which also cause different forms of insulin resistance.

The diabetic child fails to grow well. This is due to lack of the anabolic action of insulin which helps GH to achieve full utilization of the protein and energy intake. Insulin lack results in more catabolism of amino acids and decreased protein synthesis.

Diabetics suffer from persistent high levels of blood glucose (hyperglycaemia) even during the postabsorptive and fasting state. This is mainly due to increased basal and postprandial *hepatic glucose production*, associated with a deficient insulin response and decreased peripheral glucose utilization. Hyperglycaemia causes several complications. Glucose appears in the urine (**glucosuria**) when the blood glucose rises above the renal threshold and exceeds the transport maximum for its reabsorption. The excretion of

Fig. 9.24 Abnormalities of carbohydrate and fat metabolism in diabetes mellitus. The double-line arrows indicate increased formation of intermediates or end-products. The crossed arrows indicate impaired metabolic pathways.

glucose in the urine leads to osmotic diuresis, i.e. the glucose by its osmotic activity prevents reabsorption of water from the renal tubules. Thus, a large volume of urine is passed. The diuresis, or polyuria, leads to dehydration and thirst. The diabetic patient, therefore, needs to drink frequently. It is rather distressing to wake up several times at night to pass urine and to drink. This osmotic diuresis also leads to loss of electrolytes in the urine.

The metabolic abnormalities of diabetes mellitus are the result of the inability to utilize glucose. The fuel for energy alternatively comes from fat and protein. Fat mobilization results in loss of weight. The increased catabolism of FFAs leads to ketone body formation, **ketoacidosis**, due to accumulation of acetyl coenzyme A (acetyl-CoA) (Fig. 9.24). In some NIDDM patients the anticatabolic effects of insulin are still sufficient to prevent ketoacidosis, but its anabolic effects fail. The result is excessive hyperglycaemia and **hyperosmotic coma**.

The breakdown of protein corrects energy deficits due to loss of glucose in the urine. More amino acids are used to make glucose in the liver or catabolized to CO_2 and H_2O. Insulin insufficiency also results in decreased protein synthesis. The result of these abnormalities is muscle-wasting and further weight loss.

Insulin deficiency also leads to an increase in plasma lipoproteins. This causes **hyperlipidaemia** and consequently high cholesterol levels in the blood. The high cholesterol is associated with the development of atherosclerosis in diabetic patients.

Table 9.9 Metabolic abnormalities in diabetes mellitus due to insulin deficiency.

On carbohydrate metabolism
Decreased entry of glucose
Increased liver glucose output through gluconeogenesis
Decreased glycogen synthesis

On fat metabolism
Increased lipolysis
Increased formation of keto acids
Decreased synthesis of fatty acids
Decreased deposition of fat
Hyperlipidaemia due to decreased activity of lipoprotein
 lipase

On protein metabolism
Increased protein catabolism
Decreased entry of amino acids into cells
Decreased protein synthesis
Increased utilization of amino acids in hepatic
 gluconeogenesis. This may also be due to glucagon

On water and electrolytes
Osmotic diuresis
Dehydration due to polyurea
Na^+ and K^+ loss

Table 9.10 Some common long-term effects of diabetes mellitus.

Vascular pathologies	*Eye changes*
Atherosclerosis	Diabetic retinopathy
Ischaemic heart disease	Cataract
Cerebral stroke	
Ischaemia and gangrene of	*Nervous system*
the foot	Peripheral neuropathies
Microangiopathies	Autonomic insufficiency,
	diarrhoea
Diabetic nephropathy	
Glomerular damage	*Infections*
Renal failure	Skin infections
	Pulmonary tuberculosis
	Urinary tract infections

Electrolyte disturbances also occur in diabetic patients. Intracellular acidosis causes K^+ to leak into the extracellular fluid and become lost in the urine. On administration of insulin, K^+ enters the cells. **Hypokalaemia** occurs due to the presence of K^+ depletion. This is a serious effect of insulin administration in the management of diabetic acidosis, which may result in cardiac failure. Therefore, careful administration of K^+ has to be considered in cases of severe acidosis, as hyperkalaemia can be equally fatal.

Table 9.9 gives a summary of the effects of insulin deficiency.

Complications of diabetes mellitus. Long-standing diabetes mellitus inevitably leads to the development of vascular, renal and other pathologies. Table 9.10 gives a list of commonly encountered pathological changes and complications.

Glucagon
Glucagon is secreted by the A cells of the islets of Langerhans. In general, it exerts opposite effects to those of insulin. It plays important roles in the control of blood glucose and the regulation of fat and protein metabolism.

Chemistry and degradation of glucagon
Glucagon is a single-chain polypeptide hormone consisting of 29 amino acids. Its molecular weight is about 3500 daltons. In contrast to other peptide hormones, very few species differences are seen in the structure of glucagon. Glucagon-like substances have been identified in the mucosa of the gut. Its half-life in plasma is 3–6 minutes. Appreciable amounts of the glucagon secreted by the pancreas are taken up by the liver. The portal vein usually contains concentrations about twice the glucagon concentration in the peripheral circulation. The kidney also removes and degrades glucagon. It has been observed that the serum glucagon level is increased in patients with renal disease.

Control of secretion
1 Glucagon is mainly regulated by the blood glucose level. *Hypoglycaemia* results in glucagon secretion and hyperglycaemia inhibits its release.
2 Ingestion of protein or *amino acids* stimulates secretion of glucagon, which, in turn, promotes hepatic gluconeogenesis. Oral protein intake is a more potent stimulus, probably because of a stimulating action of the gastrointestinal hormones, such as **CCK** and **gastrin**. It is noteworthy that protein intake also stimulates insulin release; therefore, glucagon release will help prevent hypoglycaemia after a protein meal.
3 The hormone **somatostatin**, which is secreted by the D cells of the pancreatic islets, inhibits glucagon secretion as well as insulin. **Insulin** and **secretin** also inhibit glucagon secretion.
4 Sympathetic nerves cause release of glucagon. This is a β-receptor response. Its secretion is inhibited by an α-receptor mechanism but, during stress, the β receptors pre-

Table 9.11 Sites of action and effects of glucagon.

Site	Effect
Liver	Increased glycogenolysis
	Increased gluconeogenesis
	Increased lipolysis
	Increased ketogenesis
Adipose tissue	Increased lipolysis
Heart	Increased force of contraction
	Increased cardiac output
Pancreatic B cells	Increased insulin secretion

dominate. Vagal stimulation decreases glucagon secretion. It is possible that this vagal effect is activated by hypoglycaemia. Thus, hypoglycaemia not only stimulates the A cells directly but also works via the hypothalamus and relays to give vagal and sympathetic stimulation, both of which increase the release of glucagon.

5 Muscular exercise, pain, trauma, infection and other forms of physical stress increase glucagon secretion.

Actions of glucagon

The main action of glucagon is in the regulation of blood glucose. It safeguards against hypoglycaemia, while insulin prevents hyperglycaemia; however, glucagon has several other important actions:

1 It increases the blood glucose level by stimulating **glycogenolysis** (breakdown of glycogen) in the liver, but not in muscle. Therefore, its hyperglycaemic action depends on the presence of normal glycogen stores in the liver. Glucagon stimulates adenylate cyclase in liver cells, leading to activation of glycogen phosphorylase, which increases glycogen breakdown.

2 Protein breakdown in muscle is increased and protein synthesis in the liver is decreased. Glucagon increases gluconeogenesis by the conversion of some amino acids, lactate or pyruvate into glucose. It has a calorigenic action, which is probably due to deamination of amino acids.

3 Glucagon stimulates fat mobilization, acting via cyclic AMP. It therefore increases the level of FFAs in the blood and enhances keto acid formation. It also decreases triacylglycerol release from the liver and suppresses triacylglycerol synthesis in the liver.

Table 9.11 gives a summary of the sites of action and effects of glucagon. The mechanism of action of glucagon at the cellular level is summarized in Fig. 9.25.

Abnormalities of glucagon secretion

There is evidence that glucagon may play an important role in the pathogenesis of diabetes mellitus in some patients with this disease. It has been found that diabetic patients have higher than normal levels of glucagon in spite of the hyperglycaemia. This situation seems to be similar to that due to GH secretion in acromegaly; in both cases hyperglycaemia fails to suppress the release of the hormone.

Somatostatin

Somatostatin is a cyclic peptide, consisting of 14 amino acids with a molecular weight of 1640 daltons. It is produced by the D cells of the islets of Langerhans and intestinal mucosa. It is also produced in the hypothalamus,

Fig. 9.25 The mechanism of glucagon action on a target cell. AC, adenylate cyclase; cAMP, cyclic AMP; C, catalytic; Enzyme-P, phosphorylated enzyme; G, glucagon; I, inactive component; R, receptor.

where it is identified as the inhibitory hormone of pituitary growth hormone. It has also been found in other parts of the central nervous system as a neuropeptide which modifies the effect of neurotransmitters.

The control of somatostatin secretion is linked to food intake. Glucose, fat and protein all seem to increase its release. This effect is probably related to a β-adrenergic receptor mechanism. On the other hand, FFA and α-receptor stimulation inhibit its secretion. Like other peptide hormones, somatostatin appears to exert its effects through the adenylate cyclase system. However, evidence indicates that somatostatin effects on calcium permeability in target cells may be important in its mechanism of action.

Its physiological role in the inhibition of GH release is established. It also inhibits both insulin and glucagon secretion, but the physiological significance of this effect is not yet clear. However, there is evidence to indicate that somatostatin may be involved in the pathophysiology of diabetes mellitus and obesity.

Somatostatin is secreted by gastrointestinal mucosa, where it has been shown to decrease HCl secretion by inhibiting gastrin release. It also inhibits the secretion of other gut hormones, such as vasoactive intestinal peptide (VIP) and GIP.

The overall effects of somatostatin on gastrointestinal function are to decrease nutrient absorption as well as to inhibit digestion of nutrients. Motility of the stomach and small intestine is inhibited by somatostatin, and splanchnic blood flow is decreased.

Abnormalities

Tumours which secrete somatostatin give rise to hyperglycaemia and other features of diabetes mellitus. This condition is also associated with stagnation of bile and gallstone formation due to decreased gall-bladder contraction. Gastric motility and emptying are also decreased. These effects are due to inhibition of CCK release.

The adrenal gland

The adrenal gland is composed of two distinct glands, cortex and medulla, which in lower animals are anatomically separate. In spite of their close association in mammals, they are still totally different in development, structure and function.

Development

The adrenal cortex, which forms the outer part of the adrenal gland, develops from coelomic epithelium, while the medulla, which forms the central part of the gland, is of ectodermal origin, derived from the neural crest. The adrenal medulla, on the other hand, can be considered as a modified sympathetic ganglion, which receives preganglionic sympathetic fibres.

The adrenal cortex

Structure

The adrenal cortex is composed of large cells rich in cholesterol. The cells are arranged in three distinct layers (Fig. 9.26). The superficial layer lying immediately under the capsule is a thin layer of cells arranged in irregular groups and is referred to as the **zona glomerulosa**. It secretes the mineralocorticoids. The middle layer, **zona fasciculata**, which forms the bulk of the gland, is formed of long radial columns of cells. The inner layer lying next to the medulla, **zona reticularis**, is formed of a reticulum of branching and interconnected columns of cells. The two inner zones secrete the glucocorticoids and the adrenal androgens. The zona glomerulosa is responsible for regeneration of the adrenal cortical cells.

The blood supply of the adrenal cortex deserves special attention. It receives three arteries, which enter its capsule and form two plexuses within it. One plexus is subcapsular and the other is deeply situated in the zona reticularis. The latter plexus gives rise to venules, which penetrate into the adrenal medulla and drain into the medullary sinusoids. Thus, adrenal blood rich in glucocorticoids reaches the medulla and induces the synthesis of **phenylethanolamine-*N*-methyl transferase**, the enzyme required for adrenaline synthesis. However, the adrenal medulla also receives a direct blood supply from branches of suprarenal arteries, which pass through the cortex without giving branches.

Hormones of the adrenal cortex

The adrenal cortex is essential to life. Destruction of the glands is fatal unless replacement therapy is given. The adrenal cortex secretes steroid hormones, while, the medulla produces catecholamines. The cortex produces three main groups of steroid hormones, categorized according to their actions. The **glucocorticoids**, mainly **cortisol**, are concerned with regulation of metabolism. The **mineralocorticoids**, mainly **aldosterone**, are concerned with electrolyte regulation. The sex hormones are mainly **androgens**. Progesterone is found in the adrenal cortex as an intermediate product of the synthesis of glucocorticoids and mineralocorticoids.

Chemistry and metabolism of corticosteroids

Adrenal cortical hormones and gonadal sex hormones are

Adrenal
arteriole

Capsular arteriole   Medullary arteriole

Capsule

Zona
glomerulosa

Cortical
capillaries

Zona
fasciculata   } Cortex

Zona
reticularis

Medulla

Chromaffin
cells

Medullary vein (central vein)

Fig. 9.26 Cell layers of the adrenal cortex. (Reproduced from Borysenko, M. & Beringer, T. (1989) *Functional Histology*, 3rd edn. With permission from Little Brown & Co., Boston.)

synthesized from either acetate or cholesterol and proceed via various enzymatic steps (Fig. 9.27). The precise order in which these enzymatic actions take place is not known for certain. The molecular structure of the hormones is characterized by the **cyclopentanoperhydrophenanthrene** nucleus. C_{21} and C_{19} steroids contain 21 and 19 carbon atoms in their molecules, respectively, The gluco- and mineralocorticoids are C_{21} steroids. Androgens, such as **dehydroepiandrosterone** (DHEA), are C_{19} steroids. Figure 9.27 shows the pathways and enzymes for synthesis of the corticosteroids.

Cortisol in plasma is 90% bound to **transcortin**, an α-globulin, also known as **corticosteroid-binding globulin** (CBG). This binding makes the half-life of cortisol rather long (about 90 min) and little cortisol appears in the urine. Small amounts (6%) are loosely bound to *albumin* and the remaining 4%, which is metabolically active, circulates in the free form.

Cortisol is catabolized mainly in the liver by reduction and conjugation with glucuronic acid. It is also converted to cortisone, which has strong glucocorticoid activity but is physiologically insignificant because it does not reach the circulation. It is rapidly conjugated in the liver. The soluble conjugated products of glucocorticoids go into the circulation and are excreted in the urine.

Aldosterone synthesis occurs in the zona glomerulosa of the adrenal cortex. Progesterone is hydroxylated at the C_{21} position to form 11-deoxycorticosterone (DO^{21}), which is then hydroxylated at C_{11} to produce corticosterone. The conversion of the C_{18} methyl group of corticosterone to an aldehyde group leads to the formation of aldosterone (see Fig. 9.27). Aldosterone circulates in plasma weakly bound to *albumin* and more tightly bound to *transcortin* and a specific binding protein, **aldosterone-binding globulin**. Its half-life is about 20 minutes. The principal site of catabolism is the liver, where over 90% of aldosterone is cleared from the blood during a single passage. Measurements of 'urinary aldosterone' usually refer to

Fig. 9.27 Hormone synthesis in the adrenal cortex. The zona glomerulosa cannot convert corticosterone to cortisol. 1–5 indicate the enzymes responsible for hormone synthesis: (1) 17α-hydroxylase (lacking in zona glomerulosa); (2) 3β-dehydrogenase; (3) 21β-hydroxylase; (4) 11β-hydroxylase; (5) corticosterone methyloxidase.

conjugated aldosterone rather than to aldosterone itself, which is excreted in small quantities.

DHEA and **androstenedione** (adrenal androgens) have a more complex metabolism. DHEA is converted to androstenedione in the circulation. Androstenedione is also a precursor of **testosterone and oestrogens**. In adolescent females DHEA is responsible for the growth spurt and the growth of pubic and axillary hair. It is also necessary for the maintenance of sex drive in women. In menopausal women, it is the main source of oestrogens. DHEA and DHEA-sulphate, secreted by the adrenal cortex, are conjugated in the liver and excreted in urine.

Control of cortisol secretion

Secretion of cortisol is controlled by the hypothalamus via *corticotrophin-releasing hormone* (CRH) and by the adenohypophysis through *adrenocorticotrophic hormone* (ACTH). A negative feedback mechanism between cortisol and ACTH operates via the hypothalamus (see Fig. 9.4). There is a distinct diurnal variation in the release of cortisol, being highest in the early hours of the morning and lowest late at night (Fig. 9.28). Characteristically, the diurnal variation disappears with disturbance of adrenal cortical function, especially with hyperactivity.

Fig. 9.28 Diurnal variation in plasma cortisol levels. It depends on rhythmic release of CRH and ACTH and gives an example of circadian rhythms. The diurnal rhythm is reversed in persons on long-term night-work. (Reproduced with permission from Emslie-Smith, D., Paterson, C.R., Scratcherd, T. & Read, N.W. (eds) (1988) *BDS Textbook of Physiology*, 11th edn. Churchill Livingstone, Edinburgh.)

ACTH and cortisol are released in response to injury, hypoglycaemia and other stressful stimuli (see Table 9.3).

Actions of cortisol

Like other steroid hormones, cortisol enters the cell and induces protein enzyme synthesis. The hormone binds first to a cytoplasmic receptor. The receptor-bound steroid enters the nucleus, where transcription of mRNAs is increased. This results in the synthesis of the specific enzymes responsible for the numerous actions of cortisol in various tissues, many of which are part of the response to stress.

1 Cortisol is a *hyperglycaemic* hormone. It stimulates *gluconeogenesis*, i.e. the formation of glucose from non-carbohydrate precursors. This may be a direct effect, but it is mainly due to facilitation of the effect of glucagon and catecholamines. This is known as the *permissive role* of glucocorticoids. More glucose is also released from the liver.

Cortisol opposes the peripheral effects of insulin. It is one of the hormones known as insulin antagonists. The brain and the heart are not affected by the anti-insulin effect and therefore make use of the increased glucose supply. Overproduction of cortisol (Cushing's disease) leads to hyperglycaemia. The continuous stimulation of insulin production may ultimately lead to exhaustion of the B cells of the islets of Langerhans and result in frank diabetes mellitus (adrenal diabetes).

2 *Protein catabolism*: the gluconeogenic action of cortisol promotes protein breakdown in muscle, skin, connective tissue and bones, especially in the vertebrae and ribs. Therefore excess cortisol leads to retardation of growth, muscle-wasting, thinning of the skin and subcutaneous tissues and loss of connective tissue, especially in bone.

Although cortisol has an overall protein catabolic action, in the liver it increases protein synthesis.

3 Fat metabolism: cortisol mobilizes FFAs from adipose tissue and increases ketone-body formation in the liver. Under normal conditions fat catabolism and ketone body formation are not apparent because of the increase in glucose and insulin levels. Excess of cortisol leads to abnormal fat redistribution. It causes mobilization of fat from certain parts and deposition in others. Fat is deposited mainly in the trunk (truncal distribution) and removed from the limbs.

4 Effects on blood-vessels and water metabolism: cortisol makes blood-vessels more sensitive to catecholamines; it potentiates the pressor effect of adrenaline and noradrenaline on blood-vessels. It may therefore increase the effective glomerular filtration pressure, glomerular filtration rate (GFR) and water excretion. Patients with adrenal insufficiency cannot excrete a water load rapidly. There is usually a high level of ADH in these patients and a low GFR, both of which contribute to the above defect.

Glucocorticoids also increase the entry of tissue fluid into the capillaries, thus increasing plasma volume. Together with their potentiation of catecholamines, this effect is an important part of the stress responses which stimulate ACTH release. Both effects help to return the blood pressure back to normal.

5 Cortisol has a mild mineralocorticoid action in physiological doses, but in large quantities, as in adrenocortical overactivity, this effect may be significantly high.

6 The central nervous system requires an optimum supply of cortisol for normal function. Both excess and deficiency of cortisol may result in abnormal brain function, as shown by electroencephalogram (EEG) changes. Many patients with excess cortisol production (**Cushing's syndrome**) present with psychiatric manifestations and are mistakenly admitted to psychiatric hospitals.

7 Cortisol is anti-inflammatory and antiallergic. It suppresses or decreases inflammatory reactions and combats allergic reactions by inhibition of histamine release. Both of these effects are not seen with physiological amounts of the hormone but can be effectively demonstrated with therapeutic doses.

In therapeutic doses it destroys fixed lymphoid tissues and decreases formation of antibodies. Thus, it suppresses the immune response: hence its use in organ transplantation to prevent graft rejection. The patient, however, becomes more susceptible to infection.

8 Cortisol stimulates erythropoiesis and increases neutrophil and platelet counts, while it decreases the lymphocyte, eosinophil and basophil counts.

Control of aldosterone secretion

Aldosterone is mainly regulated via the renin–angiotensin system (see Fig. 10.10). ACTH plays a minor role in its control. The following are the main factors which stimulate aldosterone release:

1 The **renin–angiotensin system**: renin is an *enzyme* released by the juxtaglomerular cells of the kidney glomeruli and regulates aldosterone secretion through the action of angiotensin II. It acts on a plasma α_2-globulin (**angiotensinogen**) to convert it to **angiotensin I**. *Converting enzymes*, mainly formed in the lungs, convert angiotensin I into **angiotensin II**. Angiotensin II plays a role in aldosterone synthesis (Fig. 9.27) and stimulates the zona glomerulosa of the adrenal cortex to release aldosterone. Several physiological mechanisms activate the renin–angiotensin system:

(a) **Sodium depletion**: low levels of sodium in the distal tubules result in stimulation of the juxtaglomerular apparatus to release renin.

(b) Low renal blood flow: **renal ischaemia** due to low blood pressure, as in hypovolaemia due to haemorrhage or dehydration, results in the release of renin. The juxtaglomerular cells, in this case, act as baroreceptors.

(c) There is an increase in renin and consequently aldosterone secretion in the upright position.

(d) In the recumbent position, e.g. patients in bed, there is a diurnal rhythm, with a high level in the early hours of the morning.

2 A small increase in **plasma K^+** (1 mmol/litre) exerts a direct stimulating effect on the adrenal cortex to release aldosterone, while depletion of body K^+ is associated with decreased secretion. This regulatory action by K^+ appears to occur at the zona glomerulosa cell and appears to act independently of the renin–angiotensin system. Hyperkalaemia acts on the glomerulosa cells by opening voltage gated Ca^{2+} channels.

3 Several stimuli, such as trauma, surgery and anxiety, release aldosterone and cortisol from the adrenal cortex. This effect is due to secretion of ACTH from the anterior pituitary. Haemorrhage and hypovolaemia, on the other hand, do not depend on ACTH in stimulating aldosterone secretion; they act through the renin–angiotensin mechanism.

Actions of aldosterone

The main action of aldosterone is to conserve sodium and therefore maintain blood volume. In its absence, sodium is rapidly lost from the body, leading to fatal sodium depletion within a few days. Na^+ is actively absorbed in the proximal tubules of the kidneys. This is largely independent of aldosterone. The adjustment of Na^+ reabsorption takes place in the distal tubules, where the effect of aldosterone is exerted.

The mechanism of action of aldosterone depends on the hormone entering the cell and attaching itself to a cytoplasmic receptor. The hormone–receptor complex migrates to the nucleus and synthesis of mRNA is stimulated. This leads to increased ribosomal protein synthesis. The way in which protein synthesis is related to Na^+ reabsorption is not fully understood. However, the action of aldosterone may be produced by one or more of the following mechanisms: (i) provision of energy for ATP synthesis; (ii) a direct increase of active transport of Na^+ (sodium pump); and (iii) an increase in the number of open Na^+ channels in the lumenal membrane of the distal tubular cells. The end result is net transport of Na^+ from the tubular lumen to the renal interstitial fluid and consequently to the blood. The protein synthesis explains the delay of about 10–30 min before an administered dose shows its effect.

Another, unexpected, mechanism serves the purpose of ensuring both a rapid and a specific response to aldosterone. In this, aldosterone acts on a memberance (not a cystosolic receptor which binds neither cortisol nor spinolactone (a drug which competes with aldosterone for binding to cytoplasmic receptors)). The binding of aldosterone to this receptor produces a rapid activation of a Na^+/H^+-exchanger channel.

Common abnormalities of adrenocortical function

Adrenocortical overactivity (Cushing's syndrome). Excessive adrenocortical hormone secretion in about 75% of cases results from abnormal ACTH production (*secondary Cushing's syndrome, bilateral adrenal hyperplasia*). Excess ACTH is either produced by an adenoma of the anterior pituitary or from an extrapituitary origin, such as bronchogenic carcinoma. About 25% of cases are due to a secreting tumour of the adrenal cortex (*primary Cushing's syndrome*). In this case the ACTH is low, due to negative feedback by cortisol.

Cortisol and androgens are the main hormones that are produced in excess. Aldosterone excess is less evident, as it is mildly influenced by ACTH. The clinical features of Cushing's syndrome are therefore the result of excess cortisol and excess androgen production. Figure 9.29 shows a typical patient with Cushing's syndrome, with central obesity, 'moon' face and thin extremities.

The excess glucocorticoid effects of cortisol result in the following:

1 Increased hepatic gluconeogenesis, leading to *hyperglycaemia*: this effect depends on whether or not adequate insulin is available. If there is adequate insulin, fat synthesis will increase, leading to obesity, which is a cardinal sign of Cushing's syndrome. If there is an inadequate supply of insulin, hyperglycaemia and the inhibitory effect of cortisol on peripheral glucose uptake will lead to glucosuria and ultimately to frank insulin-resistant diabetes mellitus (*adrenal diabetes*) with ketoacidosis.

2 The *obesity* of Cushing's syndrome has a characteristic distribution, which is truncal or centripetal. Fat is mainly deposited in the anterior abdominal wall, causing abdominal protrusion, in the supraclavicular region, giving the patient a hump (buffalo hump), and in the face, which becomes round (moon face). In contrast, the limbs are thin because of reduced fat content and muscle-wasting.

Fig. 9.29 A patient with Cushing's syndrome. (Reproduced with permission from Burke, C.W. (1987) Adrenocortical disease. In: Wetherall, D.J., Ledingham, J.G.G. & Warrell, D.A. (eds) *Oxford Textbook of Medicine*, 2nd edn. Oxford University Press, Oxford.)

3 Protein depletion, due to protein catabolism in the skin and connective tissue, leads to the following:

(a) The skin becomes thin and paper-like.

(b) *Purple striae* appear, mainly in the abdomen, buttocks, thighs and shoulders, due to stretching of the skin.

(c) The face, especially in fair-coloured patients, becomes red, as the capillaries start to show more clearly through the thin skin (*plethoric face*). Patients with Cushing's syndrome have a greater tendency to develop polycythaemia, which adds to the redness of the face.

(d) Because the skin is thin and capillaries are weak, the patients easily *bruise* with the slightest knock and may develop *petechial haemorrhages*.

4 Removal of protein from bone: excess cortisol leads to removal of protein matrix from bone (*osteoporosis*). It is more evident in vertebral bodies, which tend to collapse, giving rise to back pain and deformity (*kyphosis*). Osteoporosis is also quite common in ribs, which become weak and easily fractured, commonly following a spasm of coughing (*cough fracture*), giving rise to the characteristic pain of fractured ribs.

5 Cardiovascular effects: patients with Cushing's syndrome often have *hypertension*. This is due to an increase in the peripheral resistance, due to potentiation of the catecholamines. There is also an increase in the cardiac output, due to a direct effect of glucocorticoids on the strength of cardiac muscle contraction. Another factor which leads to high blood pressure is *retention of sodium and water*, as a result of the weak mineralocorticoid action of cortisol.

6 Electrolyte disturbances: there is *sodium retention together with potassium loss*. The wasting of muscle coupled with potassium depletion results in muscle weakness, which is a common feature of Cushing's syndrome.

7 Mental symptoms: about 60% of patients develop mental symptoms, varying from mild depression to frank psychosis, and they may present initially to the psychiatrist.

8 Anti-inflammatory responses: patients with Cushing's syndrome have poor wound-healing, e.g. after surgery, and are more liable to develop infection.

9 Features of excessive production of androgens are seen in secondary Cushing's syndrome, because adrenal androgens are under ACTH control, e.g. *amenorrhoea* and *hirsutism* in the female. The affected female may grow a beard and moustache. Acne is a common feature of excessive androgen activity. Male patients may become impotent.

Excessive aldosterone production

1 **Primary hyperaldosteronism (Conn's syndrome)** is usually due to a secreting tumour affecting the zona glomerulosa cells of the adrenal cortex. Its main features are persistent *hypertension, headache, hypokalaemia, alkalaemia* and severe *muscle weakness*. The increased plasma pH leads to decreased Ca^{2+}, which may cause latent or overt *tetany*. Oedema is uncommon. There is increased aldosterone excretion in urine.

2 Excessive aldosterone production can also occur in disturbances of the renin–angiotensin system, as in congestive heart failure, liver cirrhosis, nephrosis and toxaemia of pregnancy. This is known as secondary hyperaldosteronism.

Adrenocortical insufficiency (Addison's disease). This may be *secondary* to deficiency of ACTH production by

Table 9.12 Defects of corticosteroid synthesis due to congenital enzyme deficiencies (also refer to Fig. 9.27).

Enzyme	Hormonal changes	Clinical abnormalities
17α-Hydroxylase	Failure of cortisol and sex hormone formation. Excess ACTH. High levels of corticosterone	Congenital pseudohermaphroditism in a genetic male
3β-Hydroxysteroid dehydrogenase	Gluco- and mineralocorticoid deficiency. Excess DHEA	DHEA has a weak virilizing effect. Hypospadias
21β-Hydroxylase (commonest defect)	This enzyme deficiency is usually not absolute. Some gluco- and mineralocorticoids are synthesized. Excess androgens and ACTH	Virilizing hyperplasia of adrenal cortex (adrenogenital syndrome in females). Sodium loss
11β-Hydroxylase	Excess deoxycorticosterone and 11-deoxycorticosterone. Excess ACTH	Virilizing hyperplasia of adrenal cortex. Sodium retention and hypertension

the pituitary hypothalamic axis, or it may be *primary*, due to destruction of the adrenal gland by an infection, such as tuberculosis, or due to an autoimmune process. In the primary type there is a high level of plasma ACTH, due to the absence of inhibitory feedback from adrenal steroids. The main features of Addison's disease are:

1 *Hypovolaemia* and *hypotension*, due to loss of sodium and water as a result of absence of aldosterone. Diminished sensitivity to catecholamines and reduced cardiac work, due to decreased glucocorticoids, also lead to lowering of blood pressure.

2 *Hypoglycaemia*, due to loss of the hyperglycaemic action of cortisol and to increased sensitivity to insulin.

3 *Hyperpigmentation*, seen mainly in mucous membranes of the mouth, pressure points, such as the elbows, old scars and areas which are normally pigmented, such as the nipples, axillae and skin creases. Hyperpigmentation, due to excessive production of ACTH and *melanocyte-stimulating hormone*, is a feature in the primary form of the disease. Pigmentation is not seen in the secondary type because of lack of ACTH production.

4 Loss of appetite, vomiting, wasting and weakness. These symptoms are probably due to the water and electrolyte disturbances and to the hypoglycaemia.

All the above symptoms and signs may be suddenly exaggerated, leading to shock or even death, if the patient is subjected to stress or infection. The condition is referred to as adrenal or *Addisonian crisis*, and calls for immediate attention.

Adrenogenital syndrome. Abnormal secretion of adrenal androgens, especially DHEA, occurs in adrenal adenoma or in cases of congenital deficiency of an enzyme responsible for steroid hormone synthesis. The excess androgens result in precocious puberty in a male child or virilization in a female child or female adult. In a male adult, the effects are masked by normal male characteristics. Table 9.12 gives a summary of the clinical manifestations of enzyme deficiencies. These congenital deficiencies are rare; the most common is 21β-hydroxylase deficiency, which leads to one type of virilizing hyperplasia of the adrenal cortex.

Failure of fetal androgen synthesis or androgen excess during pregnancy causes abnormal development of the external genitalia (pseudohermaphroditism), i.e. ambiguous external genitalia different from genetic sex (see Chapter 14).

The adrenal medulla

Since the adrenal medulla represents a modified sympathetic ganglion, its function closely resembles that of the sympathetic nervous system. Its hormones, as in the case of postganglionic adrenergic neurons, are catecholamines. The only difference is that the adrenal medulla produces **adrenaline** (epinephrine) from noradrenaline (norepinephrine). The ratio of secreted adrenaline to noradrenaline is about 4 : 1. This is because the adrenal medullary cells have the enzyme system responsible for *N*-**methylation** (phenylethanolamine-*N*-transferase, PNMT), which converts noradrenaline into adrenaline. The synthesis of this enzyme requires a high concentration of glucocorticoids, which is supplied through the arterial blood from the adrenal cortex (see Fig. 9.26). Therefore atrophy

Tyrosine

Tyrosine hydroxylase

Dihydroxy-
phenylalanine
(DOPA)

DOPA decarboxylase

Dopamine

Dopamine
β-hydroxylase

Noradrenaline

Phenylethanolamine
N-methyltransferase
(PNMT)

Adrenaline

Negative feedback

Fig. 9.30 Catecholamine biosynthesis.

of the adrenal cortex also leads to a decrease in adrenaline synthesis.

The gland is stimulated by a nervous mechanism as part of the sympathetic nervous system. The medullary cells are supplied by **preganglionic cholinergic sympathetic fibres**. Stressful stimuli, such as hypoglycaemia, hypotension, haemorrhage, infection, exercise, fear, anxiety and emotion, are the main stimuli for the release of catecholamines. This is reflected in the widespread effects of catecholamines in the body. Figure 9.30 shows catecholamine synthesis.

Actions of catecholamines

The effects of catecholamines are determined by adrener-gic receptors situated in the target organs. There are two receptors for catecholamine responses: alpha (α) and beta (β). Alpha receptors mainly exhibit excitatory functions, such as contraction of smooth muscle, a notable example of which is vasoconstriction. Beta receptors can be sub-divided into β_1 and β_2 receptors. Beta-1 receptors are found in the heart. Their stimulation accelerates the heart and increases its force of contraction (i.e. chronotropic and inotropic effects) and produces coronary dilatation. Beta-2 receptors are found in bronchial muscle and in other tissues. Their stimulation leads to inhibition of smooth muscles, e.g. vasodilatation and intestinal relaxation.

Noradrenaline acts almost entirely on α receptors and has minor effects on β receptors, except in the heart, while adrenaline acts on both α and β receptors—hence it may cause smooth-muscle contraction in some sites and relaxation in others. Several drugs may be used to block selectively α or β receptors. For example, *propranolol* and *practolol* are β-blockers, while *ergotamine, phentolamine* and *phenoxybenzamine* are α-blockers. *Atenolol* is a selective β_1-blocker and is therefore used in ischaemic heart disease. A β_2-receptor agonist (*salbutamol*) is used in the treatment of bronchial asthma, without producing the unwanted effects of adrenaline on other receptors.

The main function of catecholamines is to prepare the body for an emergency situation—known as the fight-or-flight reaction. Emergency and stressful situations, such as *pain, hypoglycaemia, hypotension, emotional stress* and *muscular exercise*, bring about the release of the hormones of the adrenal medulla. For this reason, the effects of catecholamines are varied and complex:

1 *Metabolic effects.* The general metabolic rate and oxygen consumption are significantly increased by catecholamines, in a similar manner to that of a sympathetic stimulation. Metabolic rate may go up to 100% above normal. This is known as the calorigenic effect of catecholamines:

(a) *Carbohydrate metabolism.* Catecholamines and, in particular, adrenaline, which is about 10 times more active than noradrenaline, are glycogenolytic. They activate glycogen phosphorylase b to the active form a. In the liver, glycogen is ultimately converted to glucose via a cascade of reactions. In muscle, glycogen will only be converted to lactic acid because of very low or absent activity of glucose-6-phosphatase.

(b) *Fat metabolism.* Adrenaline stimulates lipolysis in adipose tissue, releasing FFAs and glycerol. FFAs provide an important fuel to the active muscle. Adrenaline has a direct α-receptor *inhibitory action* on the release of insulin by the B cells of the pancreas.

The consequences of these effects of adrenaline are to

provide FFAs, which are the main fuel for muscles, and to raise the blood sugar and decrease the uptake of glucose by muscles by inhibiting the secretion of insulin. This will make glucose more available for the central nervous system, which explains its usefulness in response to hypoglycaemia.

2 *Cardiovascular effects.* Both chronotropic and inotropic effects on the heart are stimulated by catecholamines; the heart accelerates and contracts more forcibly. Most of the blood-vessels are constricted. The exceptions are vessels of the skeletal muscles, which are dilated by adrenaline through stimulation of β_2 receptors. Thus adrenaline increases skeletal muscle blood flow. Coronary vessels are also dilated by both adrenaline and noradrenaline.

3 *Effects on gastrointestinal and urinary tracts.* Both adrenaline and noradrenaline lead to relaxation of gut musculature and contraction of sphincters. Similar effects occur in the urinary bladder. The detrusor muscle of the bladder relaxes and the internal sphincter constricts.

4 *Effects on respiration.* Both adrenaline and noradrenaline increase pulmonary ventilation by increasing the rate and depth of breathing and by bronchiolar dilatation. However, if there is considerable rise of blood pressure, inhibitory impulses from the carotid and aortic baroreceptors may lead to cessation of breathing (adrenaline apnoea).

Abnormal catecholamine secretion

Phaeochromocytoma is a tumour of the chromaffin tissue of the adrenal medulla which secretes adrenaline and noradrenaline. The patients usually present with episodes of hypertension. When diagnosed, this type of hypertension is curable.

The gastrointestinal hormones

The gastrointestinal tract contains cells which belong to the APUD system (amine precursor uptake and decarboxylation). These cells originate from the embryonic neural crest. APUD cells are widely scattered in the body, especially in the central and peripheral nervous system. Several gastrointestinal hormones are well known for their effects on motility and secretions of the gastrointestinal tract. In the nervous system they act as neuropeptide cotransmitters and parahormones.

Chemically, these hormones are polypeptides, which can be grouped into two main groups. Those in one group are similar in structure to **gastrin**, such as CCK, and those in the other group are similar to **secretin**, such as glucagon, GIP and VIP. In general, gastrointestinal hormones are found with different lengths of the polypeptide chain (macroheterogeneity) and they may also have some minor differences in the amino acid constitution of the chain (microheterogeneity).

The secretion and effects of these hormones are discussed in Chapter 8. Abnormalities of gastrointestinal hormones are rare, the best known being excess of gastrin and VIP due to tumours (gastrinoma and vipoma, respectively). The effects of these hypersecreting tumours are also discussed in Chapter 8.

Prostaglandins, thromboxanes, prostacyclin and leucotrienes

Prostaglandins are considered as local hormones which are produced under a variety of physiological conditions in almost all tissues of the body. They are closely related to **thromboxanes** and **leucotrienes** because they are all synthesized from essential fatty acids. These local hormones have a short half-life and are rapidly inactivated in all tissues, especially the lung and the liver.

The prostaglandins received this name because they were first discovered in the seminal fluid and were thought to be produced by the prostate. Seminal prostaglandins are actually produced by the seminal vesicles. They are synthesized from unsaturated fatty acids, which are incorporated in cell membranes and can be released by the action of an enzyme (phospholipase A_2). Figure 9.31 gives an outline of the synthesis of the above local hormones. The leucotrienes shown in this diagram are aminolipids because they incorporate amino acids in their molecular structure. Thromboxane A_2 is synthesized by the platelets and prostacyclin is synthesized in blood-vessel walls.

Release and effects

Prostaglandins
Prostaglandins are found in many tissues but the regulation of their release is not certain. Their effects are as widespread as the tissues in which they are formed. They have been identified in the hypothalamus and may play a role in the regulation of the pituitary gland by hypothalamic hormones. In the stomach they inhibit gastric acid secretion and may play a role in the prevention of gastric ulceration. They have well-known effects in female reproduction. In very small doses they can induce abortion or labour. They may also play a role in the menstrual cycle by causing luteolysis towards the end of a normal cycle. In the kidney they stimulate renin secretion.

Prostaglandins appear in inflammation and may play a role in the signs and symptoms of inflammation, and their effect in the hypothalamus may produce fever.

Thromboxanes
Thromboxane A_2 is synthesized by the blood platelets. Its release at the site of injury promotes blood clotting by

Phospholipids
in cell membranes

Arachidonic
acid

Cyclo-oxygenase   Lipoxygenase

Cyclic endoperoxides   Hydroxyacids
(PG G2)

Prostaglandins (e.g.   Thromboxane
PGE$_2$, PGF$_2$ and
others)   Prostacyclin   Leucotrienes

Fig. 9.31 Synthesis of prostaglandins, prostacyclin, thromboxane and leucotrienes.

causing vasoconstriction and platelet aggregation. Thromboxane B$_2$ is a breakdown product of thromboxane A$_2$.

Prostacyclin

Prostacyclin is produced by endothelial cells and vascular smooth muscle. It has the opposite effects to thromboxane A$_2$. It causes vasodilatation and inhibits platelet aggregation.

Leucotrienes

Leucotrienes are released in response to allergens acting on most cells. Their effects are those observed in allergic reactions, namely bronchoconstriction, as in asthma, and vascular permeability, as in skin and epithelial membrane allergies. They accumulate in inflamed joints, as in rheumatoid arthritis. Leucotrienes cause high concentrations of eosinophils and neutrophils in inflamed tissues.

Applied physiology

Although knowledge of the physiology of prostaglandins is rather elementary, they have already proved their value in clinical practice. The following are some clinical applications based on knowledge of the biosynthesis and the effects of prostaglandins:

1 *Cortisol* and other steroids inhibit the release of arachidonic acid from cell membrane phospholipids. Thus, as anti-inflammatory agents, steroids have a broad inhibitory action on the synthesis of prostaglandins, thromboxane, prostacyclin and leucotrienes. Therefore, they are used in severe inflammatory conditions.

2 *Aspirin* in small doses (about 300 mg/day) inhibits thromboxane synthesis but not prostacyclin synthesis. It blocks cyclo-oxygenase in platelets but not in vessel walls. This results in a decrease in platelet aggregation and a decrease in the risk of intravascular clotting—hence its use in patients with coronary heart disease.

3 *Indomethacin* (indometacin) is a more selective, non-steroidal, anti-inflammatory drug. It inhibits cyclo-oxygenase but not lipoxygenase and therefore it spares the leucotriene synthesis pathway.

4 *PGE$_2$* is used to induce abortion so as to terminate pregnancy when a valid indication is established.

5 Pain during the menstrual period (dysmenorrhoea) has been found to be due to increased concentrations of prostaglandins in the uterus. Inhibitors of prostaglandin synthesis have been found useful in treatment of dysmenorrhoea.

6 *Prostacyclin*, which has a short half-life (3 min), is used as an inhibitor of platelet aggregation in procedures such as renal dialysis and cardiopulmonary bypass operations.

7 Prostaglandins are believed to increase gastric mucosal resistance to acid. Analogues of prostaglandins may prove useful in the treatment of peptic ulcers.

Further reading

1 Guyton, A.C. & Hall, J.E. (1996) Endocrinology and reproduction. In: *Textbook of Medical Physiology*, 9th edn, pp. 925–1003. Saunders, Philadelphia.

2 Ganong, W.F. (1999) Endocrine functions of the pancreas and regulation of carbohydrate metabolism. In: *Review of Medical Physiology*, 19th edn, 318–339. Appleton & Lange, Stamford, Connecticut.

3 Sherwood, L. (1997) The peripheral endocrine glands. In: *Human Physiology: From Cells to Systems*, 3rd edn, pp. 654–699. Wadsworth, Belmont, California.

10 / The Urinary System

Introduction

The kidneys play a major role in the control of the constancy of the internal environment. The blood flowing in the kidneys is first filtered (**glomerular filtration**) so that all the blood constituents, except blood cells and plasma proteins, go into the microtubular system. In these tubules, modifications of the filtrate take place so that useful substances, including most of the filtered water, are quickly reabsorbed (**tubular reabsorption**) back into the blood. Unwanted substances that escape filtration are actively secreted into the tubular lumen (**tubular secretion**). The final concentration of electrolytes and other constituents of urine is adjusted according to the requirements of the regulation of the extracellular fluid composition. Glomerular filtration, tubular reabsorption and tubular secretion are

rightly described as **renal mechanisms** that allow the kidney to undertake its various homoeostatic functions.

Several hormones (especially antidiuretic hormone (ADH) and aldosterone) act on the kidney to enable it to adjust the final composition of urine in response to changes in the internal environment.

The nephron

Figure 10.1 gives the gross anatomy of the kidney, showing the cortex, medulla and renal calyces.

Nephrons are the functioning units of the kidney (Fig. 10.2). There are about 1 million nephrons in each kidney. The **glomerulus** (200 μm in diameter) is a tuft of capillaries covered by a fibrous tissue capsule (**Bowman's capsule**). The renal tubular system starts at the glomerulus. The capillaries receive their blood supply from the **afferent arteriole** and the blood leaves the glomerulus through the **efferent arteriole**.

The function of the glomerulus is filtration, which occurs across the **capillary endothelial layer**, the tubular epithelium and the **basal membrane** which separates them. The capillary endothelium has **pores** about 100 μm in diameter and the tubular epithelium (also called the **podocyte layer**) has slits 25 nm in width. The basal membrane is made of mucopolysaccharide and has no visible pores.

Functionally, this triple-filtering membrane allows particles about 8 nm in diameter or those of molecular weight about 60 000, such as inulin, to pass. Due to the large number of nephrons, the total surface area of the membrane

Fig. 10.1 Major structural features of the kidney.

Fig. 10.2 Diagrammatic representation of the nephron.

used for filtration has been estimated to be about 0.4 m² for each kidney.

The glomerular filtrate flows first into the **proximal convoluted tubules**. These are about 15 mm long and 5 μm in diameter. They are lined by a single layer of epithelial cells with a well-defined **luminal brush border**. The main function of the proximal tubule is the *reabsorption* of useful substances, including sodium and water.

From the proximal tubules the filtrate passes into the **descending limb** of the **loop of Henle**, which varies between 2 and 14 mm in length. The loop is about 15 μm in diameter and is lined with flat epithelial cells. In humans, only 15% of the nephrons have long loops descending into

the renal pyramids; these are referred to as *juxtamedullary nephrons*, which play a major role in the urine concentration mechanism. The rest (85%) are called *cortical nephrons*. The ascending limb of the loop is about 12 mm in length, the more distal part of which becomes thicker as it joins the distal convoluted tubule. In this place it comes close to the afferent arteriole of the glomerulus and forms the **juxtaglomerular apparatus**, which plays an important role in the regulation of the **renin–angiotensin–aldosterone system**.

The **distal convoluted tubules** are about 5 mm in length and they are lined with microvilli but have no brush border. The distal tubules join the **collecting ducts**, which are

Afferent arteriole
(100 mmHg)

Bowman's
capsule
(18 mmHg)

Interlobular
artery

Glomerular
capillaries
(60 mmHg)

Interlobular
vein

Efferent arteriole
(18 mmHg)

Arcuate artery
(100 mmHg)

Peritubular
capillaries
(12 mmHg)

Arcuate vein
(8 mmHg)

Interlobar
artery

Interlobar
vein
(8 mmHg)

Vasa recta

Fig. 10.3 The blood supply to the
different parts of the kidney.

Renal papilla

about 20 mm in length. These are lined by cuboidal epithelial cells with no brush border. The collecting ducts open at the renal papillae into the minor calyces of the renal pelvis. Each collecting duct serves about 4000 nephrons. The total length of one nephron is about 45–65 mm.

Renal circulation

The special features of the renal circulation deserve an early description. These special characteristics are essential for the nephrons to perform their various functions.

Blood reaches the kidneys through the renal arteries, which are short and come directly from the abdominal aorta. The **renal arteries** divide into several **interlobar arteries**, which give rise to the **arcuate arteries** (Fig. 10.3). These cross the border between the cortex and the medulla of the kidney. From the arcuate arteries many branches radiate into the renal cortex, the **interlobular arteries**. The afferent arterioles arise at right angles from the interlobular arteries and end in the glomeruli.

Thus, blood from the aorta has a short distance to flow until it reaches the glomeruli. The blood pressure in the **afferent arteriole** is about **100 mmHg**, which is about the same as the mean pressure in the aorta. This leads to a high glomerular capillary pressure, about **60 mmHg** in humans. Capillary pressure elsewhere in the systemic circulation is 15–30 mmHg. Thus, glomerular capillaries can only filter fluid and *never allow reabsorption*.

The **efferent arterioles** have a blood pressure of about **18 mmHg**. They also offer high resistance to blood flow and this results in a further fall of blood pressure distal to the efferent arterioles. The efferent arterioles end in the **peritubular capillary plexuses** surrounding the proximal and distal convoluted tubules. In addition, some straight capillaries (**vasa recta**) descend into the renal medulla and drain the interstitial fluid around the loops of Henle. All these capillaries finally drain into venules, which join the **interlobular veins**, which eventually lead to the renal vein. The peritubular capillaries and the vasa recta have a low blood pressure, about **10–13 mmHg**, which is much lower than the colloid osmotic pressure of plasma proteins (25 mmHg). This allows *only the absorption* of fluid and no further filtration. It is worth noting that most of the renal blood supply goes to the renal cortex, where the glomeruli are situated; the medulla receives only **1–2%** of the renal blood flow.

The kidneys receive 20–25% of the cardiac output, approximately 1–1.5 litres/min in a 70 kg man. The total renal capillary surface area is about 12 m^2, i.e. about the same as the total surface of the renal tubules. The kidney is therefore a highly vascular organ, equipped to **filter** blood as well as to **reabsorb** and **secrete** various constituents by means of exchange across the capillary membranes and the tubular surfaces.

Measurement of renal blood flow

The renal blood flow can be measured using the **Fick principle**. The blood flow to an organ can be calculated from the amount of a substance taken up by the organ and the difference in concentration of the substance between arteries and veins supplying that organ:

$$\text{Blood flow} = \frac{\text{Amount of substance taken up}}{\text{Arterial concentration}}$$
$$\text{– venous concentration}$$

A substance which is removed by the kidney can therefore be used. Para-amino hippuric acid (PAH) is used for measurement of the renal blood flow. PAH is filtered through the glomerulus and it is actively secreted in the renal tubules, so that blood loses 90% of PAH in one passage through the kidney.

Renal blood flow can be calculated as follows:

$$\frac{\text{Amount of PAH removed by the kidney}}{\text{Arterial concentration – venous concentration}}$$

The amount removed by the kidney can be calculated by taking a sample of urine over a known period of time—say, 15 minutes. Thus, urine volume × urine PAH concentration = the amount of PAH removed ($U_v \times U_{PAH}$).

There is no need to take an arterial and a venous blood sample because PAH is about 100% removed by the kidney and it is not removed by any other organ in the body. Therefore, a mixed venous blood sample taken soon after PAH administration is representative of the renal artery blood; and, since the removal by the kidney is almost complete, we can assume that the renal vein concentration of PAH is zero. Thus, the arteriovenous difference can be represented by the PAH concentration in a mixed venous blood sample:

Renal plasma flow (RPF)
$$= \frac{\text{Urine volume} \times \text{urine PAH concentration}}{\text{Plasma PAH concentration}}$$

Example:

    Urine volume (U_v) = 1 ml/min
    Urine PAH concentration (U_{PAH}) = 13 mg/ml
    Plasma PAH concentration (P_{PAH}) = 0.02 mg/ml

Substituting in the above formula:

$$\text{RPF} = \frac{U_V \times U_{PAH}}{P_{PAH}}$$
$$= \frac{1 \times 3}{0.02} = 650 \text{ ml/min}$$

This is known as the effective renal **plasma flow**, i.e. blood flow through those parts of the kidney that effectively remove PAH from the bloodstream, i.e. renal tubules. This is to differentiate it from other parts of the kidney, e.g. renal capsules and perirenal fat, which receive 10% of the renal blood flow and do not transport PAH. Therefore, only 90% of the PAH is cleared by the kidney and the actual renal plasma flow is:

$$\frac{650 \times 100}{90} = 721 \text{ ml/min}$$

To calculate the renal blood flow, we use the ratio of plasma to whole blood. The packed-cell volume (PCV) is about 45%. Therefore, if plasma constitutes 55% of the blood volume, blood flow can be calculated as follows:

$$\text{Blood flow} = \text{Renal plasma flow} \times \frac{100}{55}$$
$$= \frac{721 \times 100}{55} = 1309 \text{ ml/min}$$

Glomerular function

The main function of the glomeruli is **filtration**. This is the first of the renal mechanisms that enables the kidney to carry out its functions. It is a passive physical process and does not require energy. The glomerular capillaries are about 50 times more permeable than the capillaries in skeletal muscle. They allow substances up to 60 000 molecular weight or 8 nm in diameter to pass. Albumin, which has a molecular weight of 69 000, passes with difficulty. Only minute amounts of albumin normally appear in the glomerular filtrate. The filtrate, therefore, is described as an *ultrafiltrate*, because it consists of all plasma constituents of small molecular size, e.g. crystalloids, but not plasma proteins or blood cells.

The mechanism of glomerular filtration

Glomerular filtration depends upon three main variables:
1 Glomerular capillary pressure (hydrostatic pressure).
2 Intracapsular pressure.
3 Plasma protein osmotic pressure.

Hydrostatic pressure of the glomerular capillaries

As indicated previously, the glomerular capillary pressure is about 60 mmHg, which is twice as much as capillary pressure in skeletal muscles. The force of this **hydrostatic pressure** tends to help filtration of fluid through the capillary wall, the basement membrane and the glomerular tubular epithelium into Bowman's space.

Intracapsular pressure

Bowman's capsule restricts the size of the glomerulus. The filtrate formed within Bowman's capsule exerts a pressure opposite to that of the capillary hydrostatic pressure. **Intracapsular pressure**, i.e. the pressure of fluid within Bowman's space, is usually about 18 mmHg.

Colloid osmotic pressure of plasma proteins

Plasma protein osmotic pressure acts in the opposite direction to the capillary hydrostatic pressure. It tends to retain fluid in the capillaries. Plasma **colloid osmotic pressure** is about 25 mmHg. Thus:

Net filtration pressure = 60 − (18 + 25)
= 17 mmHg

This is a sizeable pressure gradient in favour of filtration. It guarantees a continuous flow of filtrate, which amounts to about 125 ml/min. This is the normal **glomerular filtration rate (GFR)** in a 70 kg man.

Measurement of the glomerular filtration rate (GFR)

A suitable substance which is filtered freely in the glomeruli is selected and its rate of excretion in urine is measured. From this the rate of filtration of fluid through the glomeruli can be calculated, as will be explained. The substance to be used should have the following characteristics:
1 It should be filtered freely in the glomeruli and neither reabsorbed nor secreted by the tubules. This ensures that all of the amount which appears in urine has come through filtration.
2 It should be stable, i.e. not metabolized or stored in the body. This ensures that the total amount administered stays in the circulation and is available for filtration in the kidney.
3 It should not bind to plasma proteins, which are not filtered at the glomerulus.

4 It should not alter the rate of filtration or glomerular function.
5 It should not be toxic.

A substance which satisfies the above characteristics is **inulin**, a polymer of fructose which has a molecular weight of 5200 daltons.

Procedure

1 An intravenous loading dose of **inulin** is given, which is followed by an intravenous infusion of inulin to maintain the plasma level constant.
2 A timed urine sample is taken, say for 15 or 20 minutes.
3 A blood sample is collected about halfway during the collection of the urine sample.

The quantity of inulin excreted in urine (Q_u) will be the same as that which is filtered (Q_F). And, as inulin is freely filtered, its concentration in the glomerular filtrate (C_F) should be the same as that in plasma (C_p). The volume of the glomerular filtrate per minute (GFR) can therefore be calculated as follows:

$$Q_u = Q_F$$
$$Q_u = u_{in} \times u_v$$
$$Q_F = GFR \times C_p$$
$$GFR = \frac{U_{in} \times U_v}{C_p}$$

where U_{in} is the concentration of inulin in urine and U_v is the urine vol/min.

Example

$$U_{in} = 21 \text{ mg/ml}$$
$$U_v = 1.5 \text{ ml/min}$$
$$C_p = 0.26 \text{ mg/ml}$$
$$GFR = \frac{21 \times 1.5}{0.26} = 127 \text{ ml/min}$$

The GFR is about 125 ml/min for a 70 kg man. The GFR is about 7.5 litres/hour and 180 litres/day. Normally, only about 1–2 litres of urine are passed per day. This means that about 98% of the water is reabsorbed in the renal tubules.

Creatinine is a substance which is produced in the human body from skeletal muscles. It is freely filtered in the glomeruli but is secreted by the tubules to a slight extent. Using the above formula for creatinine, values of GFR closely resemble those for inulin. It is therefore the method of choice for assessing glomerular function in hospitals. Since some creatinine is secreted by the renal tubules, this makes the quantity excreted in urine (Q_u) slightly higher than that filtered (Q_F). However, some chromogenic substances in plasma give the same colour as creatinine and this overestimates the concentration of creatinine in plasma. These sources of error cancel each other and therefore the calculated GFR approximates that obtained when using inulin.

Control of the GFR

The following factors control the GFR:

1 *Capillary hydrostatic pressure*. This is the most important factor in the control of the GFR. When the hydrostatic pressure changes from as little as 75 mmHg to as high as 180 mmHg, the GFR hardly changes. This is called **autoregulation** of the glomerular filtration rate. Over the same pressure range, the renal blood flow also remains unchanged. It is important to maintain a GFR which is not too slow or too fast. If too slow, the glomerular filtrate will flow slowly along the renal tubules; most of its constituents will be reabsorbed and in this way the kidney will fail to excrete the unwanted waste products. On the other hand, if the flow of the filtrate is too fast, the time will not be enough to enable the tubular cells to reabsorb the vital constituents of the glomerular filtrate.

Two feedback mechanisms are believed to be responsible for the autoregulation of the GFR. These are: (i) an afferent arteriolar vasodilator feedback mechanism; and (ii) an efferent arteriolar vasoconstrictor feedback mechanism.

The renal blood-vessels constrict in response to an increased blood flow and dilate when the blood flow is reduced. This change of the vascular resistance maintains the intrarenal vascular blood pressure almost constant in spite of changes in the systemic blood pressure. Autoregulation is a **local myogenic response** of the vascular smooth muscle to the distending force of blood flow. The combination of these two feedback mechanisms is called **tubuloglomerular feedback**. These intrinsic regulatory mechanisms are controlled by the juxtaglomerular apparatus (Fig. 10.4). The juxtaglomerular cells secrete an enzyme called **renin**, which splits a decapeptide (**angiotensin I**) from a plasma protein (α_2-globulin) called **angiotensinogen**. Angiotensin I loses two amino acids in the presence of a converting enzyme to become an octapeptide, **angiotensin II**, which is a potent vasoconstrictor, and also causes the secretion of aldosterone from the adrenal cortex.

The juxtaglomerular cells secrete renin and therefore activate the renin–angiotensin system in response to a high rate of flow in the distal tubule or to a low sodium concentration in the distal tubular fluid. This is possible because the macula densa cells of the distal tubules come in close contact with efferent arterioles. Activating the renin–angiotensin system results in the generation of angiotensin II, which produces constriction of the **afferent**

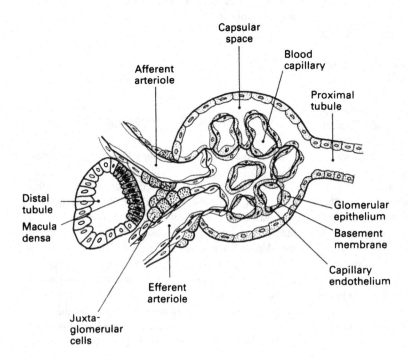

Fig. 10.4 The glomerulus and the juxtaglomerular apparatus.

arterioles, lowers the hydrostatic pressure in the glomerular capillaries and consequently lowers the GFR.

Small amounts of angiotensin II produce constriction of the **efferent arterioles**. This results in a rise in the glomerular capillary hydrostatic pressure and an increase in the GFR. However, as the rate of flow in the glomerular capillaries becomes slower, the rise in the concentration of plasma proteins in the capillaries tends to limit filtration. The net result is also to lower GFR.

In conclusion, the *intrinsic regulation of renal blood flow* makes it possible for the rate of filtration in the glomeruli to be regulated by the rate of flow of the tubular fluid and the degree of concentration of the tubular fluid, so that optimum levels of filtration are achieved. If too much or too little glomerular filtrate is formed, this may result in serious changes in fluid, urea and electrolyte excretion.

2 *Capillary permeability.* The permeability of the glomerular capillary is estimated to be 50 times more than that of muscle capillaries. However, it is the permeability of the pores in the glomerular filtration barrier that finally determines the size of the molecules filtered. Molecules with diameters less than 4 nm are filtered freely, while others with diameters more than 8 nm are not. Besides, the walls of these pores are *negatively charged* due to a predominance of **sialoproteins**. Therefore, molecules which carry a negative charge, such as albumin (molecular diameter = 7 nm), will be repelled and will not pass through these pores. Kidney disease may cause loss of these negative charges, and then albumin will appear in urine (albuminuria).

3 *Renal blood flow.* This is increased on lying down, during physical exercise and in pregnancy. Minor, but significant, increases of the GFR occur in these conditions.

In cases of severe haemorrhage, a reduction in systemic blood pressure and renal blood flow may result in a serious reduction of GFR, which may lead to a complete failure of urine formation (anuria).

Present at the bifurcations of the glomerular capillaries are the contractile **mesangial cells**. When these contract the result will be reduction of both blood flow and the size of the filtration area of the capillary bed and also a reduction of glomerular filtration rate. Mesangial cells contract in response to angiotensin II, vasopressin, noradrenaline (norepinephrine), and thromboxane A_2 (TXA_2) and relax in response to dopamine, prostaglandin E_2 (PGE_2) and cyclic adenosine monophosphate (cAMP).

4 *Plasma albumin concentration.* This increases in patients with dehydration, thus leading to a reduction of GFR. Patients with low plasma albumin (hypoalbuminaemia), due to loss of albumin in urine or liver disease, usually have a high GFR.

5 *Pressure in Bowman's capsule.* This may become abnormally high in cases of intrarenal oedema or haemorrhage due to trauma to the kidney. Increased *renal intracapsular pressure* may also result from a tumour of the kidney. Pressure in the renal tubular system may also rise in cases of obstruction of urine flow in the renal pelvis (hydronephrosis), e.g. as a result of ureteric calculi or fibrosis due to bilharzia.

6 *The number of functioning glomeruli.* This may be reduced due to disease, thus decreasing the rate of glomerular filtration. This may be due to inflammatory or parasitic disease, such as bilharzia of the urinary tract (*Schistosoma haematobium*).

Renal clearance

The term clearance is defined as the volume of plasma completely cleared of a substance by the kidneys per unit time. Most substances are partly cleared; therefore clearance is not a true volume. The concept of clearance originated from the old observation that the function of the kidney is to clear urea and other waste products from the blood. An example is the volume of blood or plasma which is *completely cleared* of urea per minute. This is blood *urea clearance*, which is a measure of the ability of the kidney to remove urea from the blood and to deliver it in urine. In the case of PAH, clearance is used to measure renal plasma flow, as PAH is both filtered and secreted and the blood is almost completely cleared of PAH while passing once through the kidney. It is therefore a true volume in the case of PAH:

$$\text{PAH clearance} = \frac{U_{\text{PAH}} \times U_{\text{v}}}{P_{\text{PAH}}}$$

This formula can be used to calculate the clearance of any other substance which the kidney handles through filtration, reabsorption or secretion. Since substances are filtered and then reabsorbed, the value of clearance becomes a *theoretical volume*, because the blood is not completely cleared of them, e.g. clearance of urea or creatinine. However, the clearance of these substances, as measured under normal conditions, can be used as an index of normal kidney function. Measurement of their clearance in kidney disease is useful for the assessment of renal function.

The normal clearance of **creatinine** is about 125 ml/min. Creatinine is therefore similar to inulin in its clearance. A substance which has a clearance less than 125 ml/min is therefore reabsorbed in the renal tubules. Conversely, a substance which has a clearance more than 125 ml/min must be added to the filtrate, i.e. secreted as it passes through the renal tubules.

The clearance of urea is about 60 ml/min. This indicates that some of the urea which is filtered is reabsorbed in the tubules. The clearance of glucose is zero. All the glucose in the filtrate is reabsorbed in the tubules, so that none appears in urine.

Functions of the renal tubules

The glomerular filtrate is changed both in volume and composition during its passage through the renal tubules. Useful substances such as **glucose**, **amino acids** and **vitamins** are reabsorbed completely. Most of the water is reabsorbed, so that urine volume is much less than the volume of the glomerular filtrate. **Sodium, potassium** and **chloride** are partly reabsorbed, according to the requirements of the maintenance of the constancy of the composition of the internal environment (homoeostasis). On the other hand, the pH of the filtrate, which is initially similar to that of plasma (pH 7.4), becomes more acidic due to the addition of **hydrogen ions** by tubular cells.

The two functions of the renal tubules are therefore **reabsorption** and **secretion**.

Tubular reabsorption

Reabsorption of substances by the renal tubules is either **passive** or **active**. Passive reabsorption depends on the concentration and/or electrochemical gradient. Active reabsorption, on the other hand, is the transport of substances against concentration or electrical gradients. This requires the expenditure of energy or specialized transport systems (**carriers**) in the tubular cells.

Glucose reabsorption

Glucose is reabsorbed rapidly and completely from the early portions of the proximal convoluted tubule by a specialized **cotransport carriers** (sodium–glucose transporter 2, SGLT2), which simultaneously transfer Na^+ from the tubular lumen. No energy is directly used to operate the cotransport carriers, but it depends on the Na^+ concentration gradient created by Na^+-K^+ATPase. The downhill movement of Na^+ into the cell carries glucose with it and drops it into the cell, i.e. glucose gets a 'free ride' at the expense of the energy used to transport Na^+ out of the cell into the basolateral space which maintains the intracellular low concentration of Na^+ (already detailed earlier). This mechanism for glucose transport is called **secondary active transport** i.e. secondary to active transport of Na^+. Once inside the tubular cells, glucose is transported down a concentration gradient by GLUT2 across the basolateral membrane into the interstitial fluid.

Fig. 10.5 Renal handling of glucose. The maximum amount reabsorbed per minute is known as the transport maximum (Tm). Also note that glucose starts to appear in urine (excreted) when the blood glucose level reaches about 180 mg/100 ml.

For substances which require a specific transport system, the tubules have a maximum capacity for reabsorption, called the **transport maximum (Tm)**. For glucose it is about 300 mg/min. Usually the amount filtered per minute is much less than this. For example, if the plasma glucose is 100 mg/100 ml and the GFR is 125 ml/min, the filtered glucose load per minute is only 125 mg/min. However, in cases of diabetes mellitus, the blood glucose is high and the filtered glucose load may exceed the Tm, i.e. more than 300 mg of glucose pass in the filtrate per minute. As a result, the excess glucose appears in urine (**glucosuria**). Phloridzin blocks the source of energy for glucose reabsorption and therefore greatly reduces Tm for glucose. Thus, administration of this substance will result in glucosuria.

Figure 10.5 illustrates the Tm for glucose. It shows that, when the blood glucose rises above 180 mg/100 ml, the tubular maximum is exceeded and glucose appears in urine. The level of glucose in the blood above which it appears in urine is called the renal threshold for glucose. In this case it is 180 mg/100 ml.

Other substances which have a Tm are phosphate, sulphate, urate, lactate, amine acids and proteins.

Protein reabsorption

Small amounts of albumin (30–50 mg/day) escape in the glomerular filtrate. This is reabsorbed in the proximal convoluted tubules. **Albuminuria** may occur in those renal diseases which cause an increase in glomerular capillary permeability. Standing for a long time may give rise to

Lumen   Proximal tubular cell   Blood

Fig. 10.6 Mechanisms of water and electrolyte reabsorption in the proximal tubules. The wheel indicates active transport. Broken arrows indicate diffusion.

Fig. 10.7 Reabsorption of phosphate.

albuminuria, probably due to increased pressure in the renal vein.

Sodium and water reabsorption

Renal transport of Na^+ and water is closely linked. About 70–75% of the filtered water and sodium is reabsorbed in the proximal convoluted tubules. The absorption of sodium is an active process, which takes place against an electrochemical gradient. Anions and water follow Na^+ passively. This reabsorptive process occurs as follows.

The driving force for Na^+ reabsorption from the lumen of the tubule into the proximal convoluted tubular cell is generated by a favourable electrochemical gradient for Na^+. A low intracellular fluid concentration of Na^+ is maintained by the action of a Na^+, K^+ adenosine triphosphatase (ATPase) carrier (pump) located on the **basolateral side** of the cell (Fig. 10.6). As this pump transports Na^+ out of the tubular cell into the interstitial space, it keeps the intracellular concentration of Na^+ concentration low, while it simultaneously builds up Na^+ concentration in the *lateral intercellular space*. Na^+ diffuses down a concentration gradient from the lateral intercellular spaces into the surrounding interstitial fluid and finally into the peritubular capillary blood. Thus, net transport (reabsorption) of Na^+ from the tubular lumen into the blood occurs after energy expenditure which has been estimated to constitute 80% of the total energy used by the kidney. It is also important to note that the entry of Na^+ into the tubular cell is accompanied by a number of *secondary transport processes*, including the reabsorption of Cl^-, amino acids, glucose and bicarbonate and the secretion of H^+. Water also follows Na^+

passively by osmosis. K^+ tends to leak out of the cell, due to concentration gradient.

Sodium and water are also reabsorbed in the distal tubules and the collecting ducts under the effect of the hormones **aldosterone** and **ADH**, respectively. This enables the kidney to maintain homoeostasis by regulating the excretion of Na^+ and water in urine.

Urea reabsorption

Urea is highly diffusible through the renal tubules. When Na^+ and water are reabsorbed in the proximal tubules, urea concentration in the tubular lumen rises. This leads to **passive diffusion** of about 50% of the filtered urea from the tubules to the peritubular capillaries. As the filtrate passes down the descending limb of the loop of Henle, it loses water and regains urea from the surrounding, more concentrated medullary interstitium. The fluid keeps its urea until it reaches the collecting duct. Here, as water is reabsorbed under the effect of ADH, urea concentration rises and, as a result, 40–60% of it diffuses back to the medullary interstitium and the rest is lost in urine.

Reabsorption of uric acid

Up to 90% of the filtered uric acid is reabsorbed. However, uric acid can also be **actively secreted**, so that its clearance can exceed that of inulin.

Reabsorption of Ca²⁺ and phosphate

Both Ca^{2+} and phosphate are reabsorbed actively, mainly in the proximal convoluted tubule. The tubular cell has a low **Tm for phosphate** (Fig. 10.7) and therefore about one-third of the filtered phosphate is excreted in urine, where it acts as a main buffer system. Reabsorption of both Ca^{2+} and phosphate is under the control of **parathyroid hormone** (PTH), which reduces the Tm for phosphate in the proximal tubules; as a result, the excretion of phosphate is increased, with a simultaneous increase in Ca^{2+} reabsorption in the distal tubules.

Phosphate reabsorption is also related to glucose re-absorption. It is possible that their transport mechanisms compete for a common source of energy. Phloridzin, which blocks glucose reabsorption, increases the reabsorption of phosphate.

Tubular secretion

The most important substances secreted by the renal tubules are K^+, H^+, organic anions and cations. Tubular secretion refers to the transport of substances from peritubular blood, interstitium or tubular cells into the tubular lumen. Tubular secretion should, therefore, be viewed as a supplement to glomerular filtration, since it removes from peritubular blood those substances which escaped total elimination by filtration at the glomerulus. A substance whose clearance is more than that of inulin must have been secreted as well as filtered.

Like reabsorption, secretion may be:
1 *Passive*, e.g. NH_3, the drugs quinidine and salicylic acid.
2 *Active—Tm-limited*, e.g. creatinine, glucuronides, PAH, penicillin, chlorothiazide and diodrast. K^+ and H^+ are actively secreted by the tubular cells into the lumen by a mechanism which does not seem to be Tm-limited.

Potassium secretion

Almost 90% of the filtered K^+ is reabsorbed actively from the proximal convoluted tubule (see Fig. 10.6) and the ascending limb of the loop of Henle. However, it is the rate of K^+ secretion in the distal convoluted tubule which determines the rate of K^+ excretion in urine, and this is under the control of the hormone **aldosterone**.

The secretion of K^+ in the distal tubules is reciprocally associated with the absorption of Na^+, so that, when Na^+ reabsorption increases, K^+ secretion increases.

Hydrogen ion secretion

The excretion of K^+ in urine is inversely proportional to H^+ excretion. There is active secretion of H^+ from the renal tubules, which tends to correct acid accumulation in the plasma. The mechanism of H^+ secretion will be detailed below in the section on renal acid–base regulation.

The excretion of water

Body fluid regulation depends largely on the role of the kidney in regulating water excretion. When there is a shortage of water in the body, the kidney secretes a smaller volume of more concentrated urine. When there is an abundance of water, a larger volume of more dilute urine is secreted.

Reabsorption of water takes place in the proximal tubule, the loop of Henle, the distal tubule and the collecting ducts. *In the proximal tubules* water moves passively, following the active transport of Na^+. Micropuncture technique, which enables sampling of tubular fluid, has shown that, in the first 70% of the length of the proximal tubule, the tubular fluid is isosmotic with the plasma. The concentration of inulin at this point, however, rises to about four times that in the glomerular filtrate. This indicates that 75% of the water and other osmotically active solutes have left the proximal tubule for the peritubular blood.

In the loop of Henle about 5% of the filtrate is reabsorbed. By the time fluid reaches the distal convoluted tubules, 80% of the filtrate has been reabsorbed. Water leaves the descending limb of the loop because the osmotic pressure in the surrounding medullary interstitial fluid is much higher than that in the lumen. There is a gradual increase in osmotic pressure from normal near the renal cortex (about 300 mosmol/litre) to about four times the normal in the interstitial fluid in the renal papillae (about 1200 mosmol/litre) (Fig. 10.8). However, as both Na^+ and Cl^- ions also leave the ascending limb of the loop of Henle, the fluid which reaches the distal tubules is **hypotonic**.

Further reabsorption of water takes place in the *collecting ducts*, where the final volume of urine is determined. This is controlled by **aldosterone** and **antidiuretic hormone** (ADH). ADH acts on the V_2 receptor on the peritubular side of the collecting-duct cell. The binding of ADH to the receptor activates the enzyme adenyl cyclase, which in turn catalyses the formation of cyclic AMP. Cyclic AMP is the second messenger, which increases the permeability of the collecting duct to water.

ADH secretion is controlled by the osmotic pressure of the extracellular fluid. When there is reduction of body water (dehydration), the osmolarity of the extracellular fluid rises; this leads to ADH release and therefore more water is reabsorbed in the collecting ducts. When there is a drop in the osmolarity of the extracellular fluid, e.g. after drinking large amounts of water, ADH release is inhibited. This leads to a reduction in the reabsorption of water in the collecting ducts and therefore a large volume of dilute urine is formed.

ADH release is also controlled by blood volume. When there is a fall in circulating blood volume, a reflex mechanism is activated by volume receptors, which results in

Fig. 10.8 Relative osmotic pressure differences in the various parts of the kidney.

an increase in ADH secretion. Thus, conservation of body water is achieved.

The function of the distal tubules and the collecting ducts is the final adjustment of sodium and water excretion. In the absence of ADH, the collecting ducts are impermeable to water. The action of ADH is to increase the permeability of the collecting ducts to water, due to the presence of V_2 receptors. The osmolarity of the interstitial fluid in the renal medulla is high. Therefore, water immediately passes out of the tubules and is reabsorbed into the circulation.

Mechanism of concentration of urine

The loops of Henle of the juxtamedullary nephrons play a key role in the concentration of urine, because they are responsible for the creation and maintenance of the *high*

osmotic pressure in the *interstitial fluid of the renal medulla.*

The **descending limb** of the loop of Henle is **permeable to water** and this leads to loss of water to the more concentrated medullary interstitium. This leads to the gradual concentration of fluid passing down the descending limb. This fluid becomes **hypertonic** as it descends. Some Na^+ and Cl^- go into the descending limb, adding further to the rise in their concentration. In the thick portion of the **ascending limb** of the loop, Cl^- is actively pumped out of the tubule and Na^+ follows passively. This leads to the tubular fluid becoming **hypotonic** by the time it reaches the distal convoluted tubule.

The result of this difference in concentration of the fluid in the descending limb and the ascending limb is a similar change in the concentration of the interstitial fluid surrounding the loop. The osmotic pressure becomes progressively higher towards the tips of the renal papillae.

This process of concentration is known as the *counter-current mechanism* for the concentration of urine.

In summary, the following are the main characteristics of the counter-current mechanism:

1 Water leaves the descending limb and, as a result, the filtrate becomes *hypertonic*.

2 In the ascending limb, which is impermeable to water, Cl ions are actively transported and Na ions follow passively into the interstitial fluid, from where they can re-enter the descending limb.

3 Thus, there is a recirculation of solute between the ascending limb and the descending limb of the loop of Henle, which behaves as a counter-current multiplier system.

4 Fluid becomes *hypotonic* as it approaches the distal convoluted tubule.

5 Since the interstitial fluid in the renal medulla equilibrates with the fluid in the descending limb of the loop of Henle, its concentration increases towards the renal papillae, where it has four times the plasma osmolarity (about 1200 mosmol/litre).

6 Active reabsorption of Na^+ from the collecting ducts and the diffusion of urea into the medullary interstitial fluid leads to further hyperosmolarity.

7 The blood supply of the medulla is poor in comparison with that of the cortex. This reduces the possibility of washing out the concentrated ions in the medullary interstitium and therefore helps to maintain the gradient of hyperosmolarity of the renal medulla.

The **vasa recta** are capillary loops descending from the cortex into the medulla. These loops have a role similar to that of the loops of Henle. Thus, in the descending capillaries water escapes into the interstitial fluid while Na^+ and

Lumen   Interstitial
                                                    fluid

Fig. 10.9 Possible mechanisms of action of aldosterone.

Renal electrolyte regulation

Regulation of sodium reabsorption

There is **active reabsorption** of Na^+ in the proximal tubules up to about 75% of the Na^+ in the filtrate. Further reabsorption occurs in the loop of Henle. Only about 10% reaches the distal tubules.

In the distal tubules and the collecting ducts, fine regulation of sodium reabsorption occurs under the influence of **aldosterone**, according to the needs of homoeostasis. In the absence of this hormone, most of the remaining sodium is lost in urine. When aldosterone is secreted in large amounts, almost all the sodium is reabsorbed.

The kidneys reabsorb quite a large amount of sodium each day. The amount which passes in the filtrate is about 625 g/day. The transport of Na^+ in the distal tubules is an active process, which occurs against a concentration gradient from the tubular cell to the peritubular fluid. This net movement of Na^+ creates a negative electrical potential inside the tubular cell, which tends to draw sodium into the cell from the tubular lumen (see Fig. 10.9).

The active Na^+ transport also results in pumping K^+ into the cell. Sodium transport, however, is greater than that of potassium. This explains the negative intracellular potential. Aldosterone acts by means of stimulating the synthesis of the messenger ribonucleic acid (mRNA) responsible for the synthesis of protein carriers necessary for the transport of sodium.

Aldosterone secretion is regulated by means of the sodium level in the extracellular fluid. Low sodium levels stimulate the secretion of **renin** from the juxtaglomerular cells (JG cells). Renin acts on a circulating α_2-globulin (angiotensinogen) and splits from it a decapeptide, **angiotensin I** (Fig. 10.10). This, in turn, becomes converted to an octapeptide, **angiotensin II**, under the influence of a converting enzyme, which comes mainly from the lung. Further breakdown by means of angiotensinases gives rise to **angiotensin III**. Both angiotensin II and angiotensin III are powerful vasoconstrictors and stimulators of the secretion of aldosterone by the adrenal cortex.

The regulation of aldosterone, therefore, enables the kidney to respond to changes in the extracellular Na^+ and K^+ concentration. This is a major mechanism for the maintenance of the constancy of electrolyte concentrations in the internal environment.

Atrial natriuretic hormone is a peptide hormone released from the atria of the heart when the extracellular fluid volume is greater than normal, probably as a result of increased atrial stretch. It promotes glomerular filtration and inhibits tubular reabsorption of Na^+, leading

urea enter. This leads to an increase in the osmolarity of the blood as it descends. In the ascending capillaries, water is reabsorbed and very quickly removed towards the cortex, as the capillaries rejoin the cortical circulation. In this way the vasa recta operate as passive **countercurrent exchangers** and prevent rapid loss of solutes from the medullary interstitial fluid and consequent loss of its hyperosmolarity. The vasa recta remove any water which is reabsorbed from the distal tubules and the collecting ducts. In addition, and since they are the only blood supply to the medulla, they also transport oxygen and nutrients to it and remove carbon dioxide and waste products.

Sodium is actively reabsorbed in the distal tubules and the collecting ducts under the influence of the hormone **aldosterone**. This is achieved against a high electrical gradient of about -120 mV in the tubular lumen, compared with peritubular fluid (Fig. 10.9). This leads to further concentration of the interstitial fluid in the renal medulla. Normally, about 15% of the filtrate is reabsorbed in the distal tubules by isosmotic reabsorption and a further 4% is reabsorbed in the collecting ducts.

Urine entering the renal pelvis may be hypotonic or hypertonic with respect to plasma. At the beginning of the collecting duct, urine is usually isosmotic, and the presence or absence of ADH determines whether further concentration occurs. In the absence of ADH, the absorption of Na^+ and other solutes is more than the absorption of water and therefore hypotonic urine is formed. In the presence of ADH, the absorption of water is accelerated and hypertonic urine is formed.

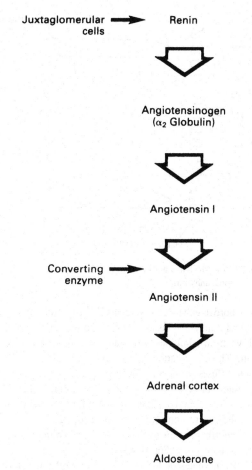

Fig. 10.10 Control of secretion of aldosterone by the renin–angiotensin system.

to increased urinary loss of Na⁺ (*natriuresis*) and water (*diuresis*). This reduces both extracellular and plasma volumes towards normal.

Regulation of potassium excretion

In the proximal tubules and the loop of Henle, potassium moves in the same direction as sodium, i.e. both Na⁺ and K⁺ are reabsorbed. About 65% of K⁺ is reabsorbed in the proximal tubules and 25% in the loop of Henle, which leaves about 10% or less in the distal tubules and the collecting ducts.

In the distal tubules and the collecting ducts, there is a reciprocal relationship between Na⁺ and K⁺. K⁺ is **actively transported** from the peritubular fluid into the tubular cells, from where K⁺ diffuses passively into the tubular lumen, due to concentration gradient. The amount of K⁺

secreted is directly related to aldosterone secretion and to sodium reabsorption.

A small increase of serum K⁺ directly stimulates the adrenal cortex to release aldosterone and thus K⁺ secretion is enhanced. In the absence of aldosterone, K⁺ secretion stops and reabsorption occurs. This shows that K⁺ reabsorption is taking place all the time but it is usually masked by the normally greater amounts secreted.

Hypokalaemia (low serum K⁺) usually results in **alkalosis**. This is because the lack of K⁺ results in excess H⁺ secretion instead, indicating that the same carrier system is involved.

Adequate K⁺ secretion is necessary to safeguard against hyperkalaemia, which is a serious consequence of tubular damage, as in renal failure. Hyperkalaemia can cause cardiac arrhythmia, fibrillation and death. Normally, K⁺ cannot be totally reabsorbed, as in the case of sodium. In potassium deficiency a minimum of 7–12 mmol is lost per day. Regular dietary intake should be ensured; otherwise, hypokalaemia results. Normally urinary K⁺ loss closely indicates K⁺ intake.

The excretion of urea

The level of blood urea is a good indicator of renal function. Normally, it is 4–6 mmol/litre (30 mg/100 ml). In renal disease, it may increase to 40 mmol/litre (200 mg/100 ml) or more.

The excretion of urea depends upon its concentration in both the blood and the GFR. These two factors determine how much urea passes in the filtrate. Normally, 40–60% of this is excreted. Major changes in the GFR greatly influence urea excretion.

Reduction of the GFR due to renal disease or to reduced renal blood flow leads to a reduction in the amount of urea excreted. Two mechanisms are responsible for this. First, the low GFR leads to less urea being filtered. Second, the low GFR results in a slow flow rate of the filtrate in the renal tubules, and more reabsorption of urea. The ultimate result is reduced excretion of urea.

When the GFR is increased, tubular flow is more rapid. This not only increases the amount of urea filtered, but also reduces the amount reabsorbed. Most of the urea filtered is therefore excreted. The significance of these observations on urea excretion is to emphasize the importance of maintaining a good GFR when renal function is decreased.

Urea clearance (normally about 60–70 ml/min) is assisted by the counter-current mechanism involving the collecting duct and the ascending limb of the loop of Henle. Urea leaves the collecting duct and enters the ascending limb and the medullary interstitium because of its concentration gradient. The hypertonicity of the medullary interstitium is due to both sodium ions and urea. This is the basic urine concentrating mechanism, which ultimately enables the maximum reabsorption of water and the excretion of a concentrated urine.

Renal acid–base regulation

The pH of urine produced by the kidneys varies from 4 to 8 according to the requirements of the internal environment, where the pH should be constant at 7.4. This is achieved by the ability of the renal tubules to secrete acid and reabsorb bicarbonate.

The kidney, however, is not the only organ responsible for acid–base regulation. **The lungs** are important for the removal of CO_2 from the blood. Indeed, larger quantities of acid are removed by the lungs than the kidneys can handle. **Blood buffers** tend to minimize changes in pH, while the lungs and kidneys excrete excess acid formed during metabolism. A comprehensive account of acid–base regulation is presented in Chapter 11.

Role of the renal tubules

In the proximal tubules, reabsorption of about 85% of the **filtered bicarbonate** ions takes place. Further reabsorption of bicarbonate occurs in the distal tubules and the collecting ducts. Normally, almost all the bicarbonate in the filtrate is reabsorbed. This is purely a *conservation* process. H^+ is **secreted** in the proximal tubule in exchange for Na^+ which enters the tubular cells along a concentration gradient created by Na^+–K^+ATPase. The distal tubules and the collecting ducts also secrete hydrogen ions (less so in the distal tubules than in the collecting ducts) through an ATP-driven proton pump.

A fall of urine pH to 6 can be achieved by reabsorption of bicarbonate only. Any further fall in pH requires the active secretion of H^+.

Bicarbonate

Mechanism of bicarbonate reabsorption

Most of the bicarbonate is reabsorbed together with Na^+ in the proximal tubules. Sodium in the tubular lumen is present in the form of:

1 $NaHCO_3$.
2 Disodium monohydrogen phosphate (Na_2HPO_4).
3 NaCl and other monovalent salts.

Filtered bicarbonate cannot be reabsorbed directly because the lumenal tubular cell membrane is impermeable to HCO_3^-. It has to combine first with H^+ to form carbonic acid. The presence of **carbonic anhydrase (CA)** in the

Fig. 10.11 Mechanism of absorption of bicarbonate. CA, carbonic anhydrase.

brush border enhances conversion of carbonic acid into CO_2 and water. CO_2 instantly diffuses back into the tubular cell, where it combines with water to form carbonic acid again. The dissociation of carbonic acid gives HCO_3^-, which diffuses through the basolateral membrane. The H^+ is secreted actively into the tubular lumen (Fig. 10.11).

It has been found that there is no Tm for bicarbonate, but when the plasma concentration rises above 26–28 mmol/l, e.g. when there is an expansion of ECF volume, HCO_3^- appears in the urine (Fig. 10.13).

Under normal conditions (GFR = 125 ml/min), up to 3 mmol/min of bicarbonate is filtered and almost all of that bicarbonate is reabsorbed. Any increase in filtered bicarbonate results in bicarbonate appearing in urine.

Formation of 'new' bicarbonate

In the formation of **'new' bicarbonate**, HCO_3^- ions which are formed within the tubular cells (hence the term 'new') are added to the blood. The dissociation of intracellular carbonic acid gives HCO_3^-, which is reabsorbed, and H^+ is secreted into the tubular lumen. This hydrogen ion is picked up by either phosphate or ammonium buffers, rather than being used for the absorption of filtered HCO_3^- (Fig. 10.12).

All of these reactions have four features in common:

1 Na^+ and bicarbonate are reabsorbed into the peritubular capillaries.
2 Carbonic anhydrase is needed to facilitate formation of carbonic acid in the tubular cells.
3 For every HCO^- absorbed one H^+ is secreted into the tubular lumen.

Fig. 10.12 Formation of HCO_3^- and excretion of H^+ through (a) monobasic phosphate; and (b) NH_4^+ formation. Both act as buffers which combine with H^+ in urine.

Hydrogen ions

Excretion of hydrogen ions

The rate of formation of H^+ by the tubular cells is directly related to the concentration of CO_2 in the extracellular fluid. The more CO_2 is formed, the more of it passes into the tubular cell and the more H^+ is secreted (see Fig. 10.12).

The excretion of H^+ by tubular cells, as seen from the above account, is achieved by means of their acceptance in urine by several buffers:

1 They may combine with HCO_3^- in the filtrate, facilitating the reabsorption of filtered HCO_3^- (Fig. 10.11).

2 They may be conjugated with **dibasic phosphate**, giving monobasic phosphate ions ($H_2PO_4^-$). Since phosphate is all

Fig. 10.13 The effect of increased bicarbonate in the filterate (as in expansion of ECF volume) on tubular reabsorption. (Based on Valtin, H. (1983) *Renal Function* 2nd Edn. Little, Brown.)

filtered, its quantity is limited and therefore in acidosis it will readily be utilized as a buffer.

3 H^+ may combine with **NH_3**, formed by the renal tubular cells, to form NH_4^+, which combines with Cl^- to form NH_4Cl. This salt is excreted in urine. In the latter two processes, for each H^+ secreted by the tubular cells, a 'new' bicarbonate ion is added to the bloodstream.

The excretion of hydrogen ions is achieved in exhange for Na^+ (i.e. **H^+–cation exchange**). There is evidence to suggest that K^+ competes with H^+ for exchange with Na^+. In **hyponatraemia**, more Na^+ reabsorption takes place in exchange for K^+. This leaves little K^+ to exchange with H^+, which leads to acidosis. In **hypokalaemia**, more K^+ is reabsorbed and therefore more H^+ is secreted, which leads to alkalosis. **Hyperkalaemia**, on the other hand, results in more K^+ excretion and retention of H^+, with the secretion of alkaline urine, leading to acidosis.

Secretion of ammonia

Ammonia is formed in the renal tubular cells from **glutamine**, which is broken down by the enzyme glutaminase to glutamic acid and ammonia. NH_3 is secreted into the lumen. H^+, secreted by the tubular cells into the lumen, combines with NH_3 to give NH_4^+. About two-thirds of the H^+ secreted by the renal tubules is excreted in this form.

NH_4^+ is an important urine buffer, because it forms a weak acid and therefore can take large quantities of H^+ with little change in pH. The rate of production of NH_3 is proportional to the rate of H^+ formation in the renal tubular cells. The more acidic the urine, the more NH_3 is produced.

Unlike the phosphate buffer, NH_3 is produced by tubular cells and therefore the kidney can increase its NH_3 production up to 50 times when there is excessive need for excretion of H^+.

Urine acidity

Secretion of H^+ can take place until its concentration in the tubular lumen is 900 times that in the extracellular fluid. This is the maximum transport gradient for H^+ and corresponds to a urine pH of 4.5 (limiting pH). The buffers in urine determine whether this pH is reached quickly or not. If the H^+ secreted forms strong acids, urine pH falls quickly, but, if weak acids are formed, then the fall of urine pH is slower and more H^+ can be excreted.

The **titratable acidity** of urine can be measured by adding a strong base to urine until the pH 7.4 (normal pH of plasma) is reached. This will measure the acid excretion by the kidney. It is usually 20 to 40 mequiv of H^+ per day. It should be emphasized, however, that the titratable acidity does not include H^+ which is excreted as bicarbonate or in combination with ammonia.

Micturition

In the adult, passing urine is a voluntary act. However, there are underlying **reflex mechanisms**, which deserve special description for the understanding of disturbances of micturition. The urinary bladder receives innervation from the parasympathetic outflow of the sacral nerves and also a sympathetic supply from the **hypogastric nerves**. These nerves are distributed to the **detrusor muscle** of the bladder as well as the **internal sphincter**. The **external sphincter** receives a somatic nerve supply from the **pudendal nerves**.

Anatomical and functional considerations

Urine travels down the ureters by means of peristaltic waves, which are initiated by a rise of pressure in the renal pelvis. These waves occur at the rate of one every 10 s and travel down the ureter at the rate of 3 cm/s.

The ureters enter the lower part of the bladder at the base of the trigone. They pass obliquely into the muscle coat of the bladder, forming a valve-like arrangement, which makes it difficult for urine to pass back into the ureters, even when the pressure in the bladder rises.

When the bladder is empty, its internal pressure (intravesical pressure) is about zero. When up to 100 ml of urine is collected in the bladder, the pressure rises rapidly to about 10 cm H_2O. Additional collection of urine up to 300 ml produces no further rise in the pressure (Fig. 10.14).

Fig. 10.14 Pressure changes in the urinary bladder.

This is due to **relaxation** of the bladder. When about 350–400 ml of urine has collected, the intravesical pressure rises rapidly. This stimulates stretch receptors in the wall of the bladder and the micturition reflex is initiated. The reflex causes the bladder to contract and empty its contents. This emptying reflex has its **afferent pathway** in the parasympathetic sacral nerves. There are also parasympathetic **efferent nerves**, which come from the same sacral segments (S2, 3 and 4). These nerves trigger the contraction of the detrusor muscle of the body of the urinary bladder and **relaxation** of the **internal sphincter**. Urine distends the posterior urethra and triggers an inhibitory reflex that relaxes the external sphincter.

This basic reflex arrangement can be modified in two ways:
1 Voluntary control.
2 Sympathetic modification.

Voluntary control of micturition
Reflex contraction of the detrusor muscle results in repetitive contraction of the detrusor muscle. If the time and situation are not appropriate for passing urine, there is voluntary suppression of the reflex. The reflex becomes inhibited for a few minutes up to 1 hour. Further stretch of the bladder will initiate another series of contractions that are more frequent and more powerful.

There seem to be inhibitory and facilitatory centres in the brain stem and in the cerebral cortex. Afferents to these higher centres possibly travel in the lateral spinothalamic tracts of the spinal cord. The efferents from higher centres travel deep to the lateral corticospinal tracts.

These higher centres exert their influence as follows:

1 They send impulses which keep the micturition reflex inhibited except when there is a desire to pass urine.
2 They can inhibit reflex micturition even when it has already started. This happens when the time and place are not suitable.
3 Voluntary control of the external sphincter can check emptying of the bladder.
4 Higher centres facilitate the micturition reflex and relax the external sphincter when it is convenient to empty the bladder.

Role of the sympathetic nerves in micturition
Sympathetic stimulation results in relaxation of the detrusor muscle and contraction of the internal sphincter. This occurs in conditions of 'fight or flight' to prevent incontinence of urine. The sympathetic nerves have no role in the control of normal micturition.

Disturbances of micturition
Damage to the spinal cord above the sacral segments results in the abolition of the voluntary control of micturition and **automatic emptying** occurs every time the threshold for the micturition reflex is reached. This occurs in patients with paraplegia. However, some paraplegic patients empty the bladder when the time is convenient and initiate the reflex by stimulating the upper thigh or the skin near the genital organs. During **spinal shock**, which immediately follows damage to the spinal cord, the micturition reflex is abolished. The bladder fills up and **overflow incontinence** occurs. In a few days to a few weeks, the shock state passes and the reflex returns.

Damage to the afferent pathway from the bladder results in loss of the reflex. The bladder tends to overfill and overflow occurs (**autonomous bladder**). It eventually becomes atonic.

Endocrine functions of the kidney
The kidney produces several substances, some of which may not strictly be labelled as hormones. These are renin, erythropoietin and vitamin D_3 (1,25-dihydroxycholecalciferol). These substances either act locally or are responsible for the production of other hormonal agents.

Renin
Renin is produced by the **juxtaglomerular cells** (see Fig. 10.4) in response to a variety of stimuli, e.g. renal ischaemia, as in low blood volume, low extracellular fluid (ECF) volume, low serum Na^+, high serum K^+ concentration, and others as will be explained later. Renin release is the first step in the activation of the renin–angiotensin

system, which results in the production of angiotensin II. The actions of angiotensin II can be summarized as follows:

1 It produces arteriolar constriction, resulting in an increase of both systolic and diastolic blood pressure. It is four times as potent as noradrenaline (norepinephrine). It is not useful therapeutically in cases of sodium depletion because angiotensin II receptors will be already occupied with endogenously produced angiotensin II. Its physiological role in the regulation of arterial blood pressure is mainly through the maintenance of Na^+ concentration rather than of vascular tone.

2 Angiotensin II increases the production and secretion of aldosterone by the adrenal cortex. This response tends to correct low ECF volume and blood pressure through sodium conservation.

3 Angiotensin II modulates sympathetic activity by means of a facilitating effect on catecholamine synthesis and release.

4 Angiotensin II participates in the regulation of water intake by a direct action on the hypothalamus, stimulating the sensation of thirst.

Angiotensin III is formed from angiotensin II by the action of an aminopeptidase. It has much less pressor activity than angiotensin II, but it retains all its stimulating action on aldosterone secretion. It has been suggested that both angiotensin I and angiotensin II can be converted to angiotensin III in the adrenal cortex, but the physiological significance of this mechanism is still uncertain.

Regulation of renin secretion

Renin is released in conditions of low blood pressure, hypovolaemia and Na^+ depletion:

1 Low arterial blood pressure stimulates intrarenal baroreceptors residing in the afferent arterioles.

2 Low sodium and chloride ions at the region of the macula densa.

3 **Prostaglandins** stimulate renin release by direct action on JG cells. Also, the stimuli mentioned in 1 and 2 above may be mediated through the release of prostaglandins in the renal cortex.

4 Plasma concentration of K^+ and the release of renin are inversely related. This may also be associated with the rate of delivery of Na^+ and Cl^- ions at the level of the macula densa.

5 **Angiotensin II** inhibits the release of renin, probably through a feedback mechanism on the JG cells.

6 **Vasopressin** inhibits the secretion of renin.

7 Increased sympathetic discharge leads to the release of renin, both by the action of circulating catecholamines and through the sympathetic nerves to the kidney. This is a β-adrenergic receptor mechanism.

It appears that there are close interrelationships between the above mechanisms involving hypotension, hypovolaemia and Na^+ depletion. It is possible that more than one mechanism may be working at any one time.

Erythropoietin

It is now established that **erythropoietin** is produced by peritubular interstitial cells in the renal cortex and outer medulla. It is released when the kidney is exposed to hypoxia. The physiological role of erythropoietin is to stimulate the bone marrow stem cells to promote erythropoiesis.

The kidneys produce erythropoietin as long as renal tissues are not getting adequate oxygen supply, as in acclimatization to *high altitude*. The half-life of erythropoietin is about 5 hours. If large amounts of erythropoietin are produced, polycythaemia follows. Low levels of erythropoietin are found in severe renal damage, which accounts for the anaemia associated with kidney disease; this is the basis for the therapeutic use of erythropoietin, produced commercially by gene technology, instead of blood transfusion in the treatment of anaemia of renal failure.

Vitamin D_3

Vitamin D is synthesized in the skin or taken in food in an inactive form. It is hydroxylated in the liver at the C_{25} position to give **25-hydroxycholecalciferol (calcidiol)**, which is the major form of vitamin D in the blood. However, this form does not seem to act on the gut, kidney or bone.

Calcidiol is hydroxylated at the C_1 position by a specific kidney enzyme to give **1,25-dihydroxycholecalciferol (calcitriol)**. This is the active form, which acts on:

1 The gut to regulate calcium and phosphate absorption.

2 The kidney to regulate calcium and phosphate excretion.

3 Bone to regulate Ca^{2+} mobilization and exchange with serum calcium.

All of these actions are achieved together with parathyroid hormone. Low serum calcium stimulates parathyroid hormone (PTH) release, which, in turn, increases the conversion of 25-dihydroxycholecalciferol into 1,25-dihydroxycholecalciferol in the kidney. However, low serum phosphorus (P) does not require the mediation of PTH for the conversion of vitamin D into the physiologically active form. The significance of the difference in the two mechanisms lies in the fact that low Ca and low P do not usually occur at one and the same time. The stimulus is usually low Ca or low P. In case of low Ca, the released PTH mobilizes both Ca and P from the bones. PTH will enhance the loss of the excess P in urine. In the case of low P, 1,25-dihydroxycholecalciferol will increase without the release of PTH. Both Ca and P will be mobilized from bone by 1,25-dihydrocholecalciferol and, in this case, excess Ca is lost in urine, due to the absence of PTH, and hypophosphataemia is corrected.

Prostaglandins

Prostaglandins are a group of 20-carbon unsaturated fatty acids. They are rapidly metabolized, particularly by the lungs. They have a short half-life (minutes), which makes them act as local hormones, either within the cells in which they are formed or on the organ in which they are released.

Renal prostaglandin E (PGE) is released in response to renal ischaemia due to sympathetic stimulation, catecholamine release or angiotensin II. It may be involved in the regulation of renal blood flow in these conditions.

PGE_2 and PGI_2 have a vasodilator effect and lead to increased renal blood flow on intrarenal infusion. PGA_2 and PGE_2, on the other hand, have a vasoconstrictor effect. Renal prostaglandins may also modify the action of ADH by reducing the sensitivity of renal tubular cells to the effect of ADH.

Further reading

1 Ganong, W.F. (1999) Section VIII. Formation and excretion of urine. In: *Review of Medical Physiology*, 19th edn., pp. 641–677. Appleton & Lange, Stamford, Connecticut.
2 Lote, C.J. (1994) *Principles of Renal Physiology*, 3rd edn. Chapman & Hall, London.

11 / Regulation of Blood pH

Objectives

On completion of the study of this section, the student should be able to:

1 Define the major clinical classifications of acid–base disturbances.

2 Describe the roles of blood buffers in order to interpret laboratory findings.

3 Explain the respiratory and renal mechanisms concerned with acid–base regulation so as to diagnose and manage the underlying causes of acid–base disturbances.

4 Identify and explain the main responses to acid–base disturbances so as to interpret clinical and laboratory findings.

5 On reviewing clinical information and laboratory data, differentiate between the various types of acidoses and alkaloses.

6 Explain the main relationships between body electrolytes and acid–base disturbances.

Introduction

Acid–base disturbances are one of the most worrying clinical problems to the physician, mainly because of the subtle nature of the physiological changes which lead to them. Furthermore, acid–base imbalance usually indicates a serious disturbance of physiological control mechanisms.

The constancy of the pH in the blood and the extracellular fluids is one of the important characteristics of the internal environment. The normal H^+ concentration in the plasma and extracellular fluid is 0.00004 mequiv/litre (40 nmol/litre). The term pH is the negative log of 0.00004, which is 7.4, i.e. it is slightly alkaline. The cells of the body function within the normal range of 7.35–7.45 (36–44 nmol/litre). Minor deviations outside this range cause serious effects in almost all body functions. Death usually occurs if the pH falls below 7.0 or rises to 7.8.

Every 24 hours, metabolic processes result in the production of about 12 000 to 20 000 mmol of carbon dioxide (CO_2) (**volatile acid**). Other acids, such as sulphuric and phosphoric acids, are given the name non-volatile or **fixed acids**. It is evident that the body has to deal with these acids continuously. In clinical practice there are many conditions which lead to disturbances of the blood pH. The following section explains the physiological mechanisms responsible for the maintenance of the blood pH and the major clinical abnormalities.

Mechanisms of acid–base regulation

Any deviation from the normal pH is counteracted by the mechanisms which tend to stabilize the pH at 7.4. There are three mechanisms which deal with the maintenance and regulation of blood pH, namely the *blood buffers*, the *respiratory mechanisms* (i.e. pulmonary ventilation) and the *renal mechanisms*. The following account gives the main features of these mechanisms, with the objective of integrating the knowledge already gained in studying the blood, the respiratory system and renal physiology.

The blood buffers

The blood buffers are the first line of defence which prevents deviation of the blood pH. They act within minutes. Acids are produced during metabolic activity. CO_2, leading to the formation of carbonic acid, is the main acid product. Other acids, such as lactic acid and keto acids (acetoacetic acid and β-hydroxybutyric acid), are produced under conditions of metabolic stress. Lactic acid accumulates in the muscles and the extracellular fluid when inadequate supplies of O_2 are delivered to muscle, as in severe muscular exercise. The keto acids accumulate when there is increased catabolism of fat with lack of insulin, as in diabetes mellitus.

Thus, the normal metabolism is continuously producing H^+, which is taken up by the blood buffers. There are several buffer systems in the blood. The major ones are the *bicarbonate–carbonic acid* buffer system and *haemoglobin*. The first is extracellular (in the plasma) and the second is intracellular (in the red cells). Other buffers are the plasma proteins and intracellular phosphate.

The bicarbonate–carbonic acid buffer is the main ECF buffer system for H^+ arising from sources other than H_2CO_3. Its extreme effectiveness is due to the fact that CO_2 (and therefore H_2CO_3) is rapidly regulated by the respiratory response. Furthermore, HCO_3^- is regulated by the kidneys. As this buffer pair is found in a relatively high concentration in the ECF, it is a useful first line of defence against any addition of H^+. In fact, the bicarbonate–carbonic acid buffer system determines the pH of the blood and extracellular fluid. According to the *Henderson–Hasselbalch equation*, the dissociation constant of carbonic acid (pK) and the ratio of HCO_3^-/H_2CO_3 determine the blood pH:

$$pH = pK + \log \frac{salt}{acid}$$

pK for carbonic acid = 6.1

$$\log \frac{HCO_3^-}{H_2CO_3} = \log \frac{20}{1} = 1.3$$
$$pH = 6.1 + 1.3 = 7.4$$

This buffer system is closely monitored by the reflexes of the respiratory system to maintain the bicarbonate–carbonic acid ratio at 20/1.

Haemoglobin is also an important blood buffer for a different reason. It is present in high amounts, i.e. 14 g/100 ml. There is about 700 g of haemoglobin (Hb) in the blood of an adult person. This is the reason for its high *buffering capacity*. It is estimated that Hb is responsible for 70% of the buffering power of the blood. Haemoglobin buffers H^+ generated in the tissues as a result of CO_2 production, i.e. it buffers the blood until it unloads CO_2 in the lungs. Both oxygenated and reduced Hb are present partly in the form of anions and therefore act as bases. The combination of Hb with H^+ sets free an equivalent amount of bicarbonate according to the following reaction:

Fig.11.1 Diagrammatic representation illustrating the combination of haemoglobin with CO_2. Note the formation of bicarbonate due to carbonic anhydrase (CA) in the red cell. Efflux of bicarbonate is associated with entry of Cl^-, the chloride shift.

$$H^+ + HCO_3^- + KHb \rightleftharpoons HHb + K^+ + HCO_3^-$$

Carbonic anhydrase is found inside the red cells and K^+ ions are the main intracellular cation. Therefore, this reaction can only take place in the red cells. The resulting bicarbonate ions diffuse to the plasma and they are replaced by chloride ions, which enter the cell (chloride shift). Figure 11.1 illustrates this effect during the process of CO_2 carriage from the tissues. As reduced haemoglobin is a weaker acid than oxygenated haemoglobin, its buffering capacity is greater in the tissues. In the lung HbO_2 releases H^+, which combines with HCO_3^- to form H_2CO_3, which gives off CO_2 to the alveolar air. Note that in this process the H^+ is incorporated in the water molecules.

Proteins act mainly as intracellular buffers. They are useful buffers because they have both acidic and basic groups. Intracellular proteins are the most important buffer in the intracellular fluid (ICF) because of their high concentration. However, the plasma proteins play a limited role in the blood.

The *phosphate buffer* system, due to its concentration, has an important role in the ICF. The phosphate buffer consists of acid phosphate ($H_2PO_4^-$), which can donate H^+, and basic phosphate (HPO_4^{2-}), which can accept H^+, as follows:

$$Na_2PO_4 + H^+ \rightleftharpoons NaH_2PO_4 + Na^+$$

Phosphate filtered in the urine plays an important role as a urinary buffer which takes up secreted H^+ in the urine and therefore stabilizes the pH in the tubular fluid, allowing

Table 11.1 A summary of functions of extracellular (ECF) and intracellular (ICF) buffers.

Buffer system	Site of action	Main function
H_2CO_3/HCO_3^-	ECF	Buffers non-carbonic acid H^+ in blood and interstitial fluid
Haemoglobin	Blood	Main buffer against carbonic acid especially in venous blood
Protein	ICF, ECF	Main intracellular buffer
Phosphate	ICF	Also buffers secreted H^+ in urine

more H^+ to be secreted. The functions of the various buffer systems are given in Table 11.1.

In conclusion it must be emphasized that the buffer systems only prevent larger fluctuations of pH by combining with excess H^+ or giving off H^+ as required. The ultimate removal of excess acidity must take place either through the lungs as CO_2 or by the kidneys.

The respiratory mechanisms

The main advantage of the contribution of the respiratory system in acid–base regulation is its quick response. The partial pressure of CO_2 (Pco_2) and H^+ have a potent stimulatory effect on ventilation (see Chapter 6). Increased depth and rate of ventilation wash out CO_2 and therefore decrease H^+ arising from H_2CO_3. When the H^+ falls, ventilation is decreased, leading to accumulation of CO_2 and H_2CO_3 and therefore H^+ rises towards normal levels. This mechanism is useful when excess CO_2 is produced, as in exercise, and in H^+ accumulation from non-H_2CO_3 sources. However, the response of the respiratory system can only compensate this H^+ excess by up to 75%. Final correction is brought about by the kidney.

The renal mechanisms

The kidney represents the third line of defence after blood buffers and the respiratory system. It has a key role in excretion of H^+ and control of plasma bicarbonate.

Food and other ingested substances are sources of non-volatile acids (i.e. other than carbonic acid). Sulphur-containing amino acids result in the production of sulphuric acid. Phosphorus from proteins and phospholipids results in phosphoric acid production. If calcium chloride is ingested, most of the calcium is not absorbed in the gut and gets excreted in the faeces, but the chloride is absorbed as hydrochloric acid. Ingestion of ammonium chloride salt

gives rise to urea and hydrochloric acid. Furthermore, large amounts of keto acids accumulate in uncontrolled diabetes mellitus, because of inability to complete the oxidation of these acids to carbon dioxide and water. During severe muscular exercise and in hypoxic conditions, accumulation of lactic acid can also lead to acidaemia.

The kidney excretes 100–150 mmol of non-volatile acid per day. This is the main reason for the acidosis which accompanies uraemic states due to renal failure. In acidosis, the renal excretion of acid may increase to 500 mmol/day. The kidney can excrete acid against a concentration gradient so that the urine pH can go down to pH 4 (compared with plasma pH 7.4). Eventually, the bicarbonate–carbonic acid ratio is returned to normal.

Three main renal mechanisms are responsible for the regulation of acid–base balance: (i) bicarbonate is reabsorbed almost completely from the filtrate; (ii) active secretion of H^+ by the renal tubules; and (iii) the synthesis of ammonia by the renal tubular cells.

The reabsorption of bicarbonate and formation of new bicarbonate

The kidney adjusts bicarbonate in two ways: reabsorption of filtered bicarbonate and formation of new bicarbonate in association with H^+ secretion.

About 85% of filtered bicarbonate is reabsorbed in the proximal tubules. At the same time, water and electrolytes are reabsorbed. Because the volume of the filtrate is greatly decreased, there is little change in bicarbonate concentration or pH in the filtrate. Reabsorption of filtered bicarbonate in the proximal tubule is associated with secretion of hydrogen ions. CO_2 is formed by carbonic anhydrase in the brush border and it re-enters the tubular cell (Fig. 11.2a). The reaction results in the reabsorption of bicarbonate with equimolar secretion of H^+ in the urine.

Formation of *new bicarbonate* takes place during the process of H^+ secretion. In the tubular cell, carbonic anhydrase forms carbonic acid from CO_2 and intracellular water:

$$CO_2 + H_2O \rightleftharpoons H^+ + HCO_3^-$$

The hydrogen ions are secreted into the tubular lumen, mainly in exchange for Na^+. The bicarbonate is reabsorbed, together with sodium. This tends to restore the bicarbonate level or to raise it above normal values in case of excess H^+ secretion by the renal tubules (Fig. 11.2a,b).

Secretion of H^+ by the renal tubules

Excess non-volatile acids can only be excreted by the kidney. This is why acidosis is one of the main features

Fig. 11.2 (a) Reabsorption of bicarbonate. In the proximal tubules the filtered bicarbonate is reabsorbed in association with H^+ secretion. In this case, carbonic anhydrase present in the brush border results in CO_2 formation. Reabsorbed CO_2 is used again to form H_2CO_3 in the cell. (b) Excretion of titratable acid. Titratable acid secretion in association with monobasic phosphate in the renal tubules. (c) Excretion of H^+ with NH_3 formed in the distal tubular cell. Both (b) and (c) result in the formation of new bicarbonate, which is returned to the ECF.

of renal failure. The mechanisms for the hydrogen ion secretion and formation of new bicarbonate are summarized in Fig. 11.2b, c.

Ammonia synthesis

Ammonia synthesis accounts for the major part of hydrogen ion secretion, especially that coming from non-volatile acids (Fig. 11.2c). The rate of synthesis of ammonia from **glutamine** is directly proportional to the plasma pH. In this respect, the renal tubular cells are acting as chemoreceptors. Their rate of formation of NH_3 will therefore be adjusted according to the need to excrete H^+. Being a weak acid, NH_3 has a high buffering capacity. Therefore, large amounts of H^+ can be excreted in the urine in this form with little fall of urine pH. The importance of NH_3 synthesis lies not only to its response to a fall in pH but also in its great capacity, as it continues to buffer the urine after exhaustion of all filtered phosphate.

It appears from the above account that the final adjustment of blood pH is slowly, but completely, achieved by the renal mechanisms. In particular, the kidney is the only organ which is able to excrete non-volatile acids, by virtue of its ability to synthesize ammonia and its ability to secrete H^+ actively.

Disturbances of acid–base balance

There are many clinical conditions which disturb the acid–base balance. The result is a state of **acidaemia** or **alkalaemia**, which signifies the change in pH of the blood. More commonly, the terms acidosis and alkalosis are used to signify the generalized nature of the disturbance, which affects the whole of the internal environment. Acid–base imbalance is usually a complication of diseases affecting the systems which regulate the production or excretion of H^+. The disturbances should be viewed as occurring in phases:

1 The primary disturbance is either respiratory or metabolic.

2 The immediate compensation is by the bicarbonate/carbonic acid buffer system.

3 Respiratory and renal compensatory mechanisms are involved.

The clinical classification of such disturbances is as follows.

Metabolic acidosis

This term includes all types of acidosis of non-respiratory origin, i.e. the primary defect is not excess CO_2 in the blood. The problem lies in accumulation of non-carbonic acid H^+ in the extracellular fluid (ECF), or it may be due to excessive loss of HCO_3^-. The following is a review of the main causes of metabolic acidosis:

1 *Diabetes mellitus* results in excessive utilization of fatty acids with decreased utilization of glucose in the absence of normal insulin secretion or its effectiveness. This leads to accumulation of keto acids. Polyuria of diabetes results in dehydration and excessive loss of Na^+. This aggravates the acidosis.

2 *Severe diarrhoea* results in loss of intestinal contents. Pancreatic juice and bile contain large amounts of HCO_3^-. Normally this HCO_3^- is reabsorbed. Severe reduction in the alkali reserve results in a decrease in the buffering power of the blood and therefore high plasma $[H^+]$.

3 *Uraemia* results from renal failure, which leads to the inability of the kidneys to secrete the normal amounts of fixed acids. Also the kidneys fail to reabsorb the HCO_3^- normally filtered into the tubular fluid.

4 *Severe exercise* leads to anaerobic metabolism, which results in the production of large amounts of lactic acid. This acidosis is short-lived, because lactic acid is removed during recovery.

Metabolic alkalosis

Metabolic alkalosis occurs in conditions where there is excessive *ingestion of bicarbonate*, as in the treatment of gastric hyperacidity, heartburn and peptic ulcer. Metabolic alkalosis also occurs as a result of excessive *vomiting*, such as in patients with high gastro-intestinal obstruction (e.g. due to pyloric stenosis). The same thing happens after removal of large amounts of gastric secretions through a stomach tube (gastric suction). Loss of gastric juice, which contains appreciable amounts of hydrochloric acid, leads to metabolic alkalosis due to several mechanisms.

With persistent vomiting, K^+ is also lost in the vomitus and in the kidney. As extracellular K^+ falls, more K^+ will leak out of cells. This is replaced by H^+ entering the cells.

Table 11.2 Examples to illustrate the bicarbonate–carbonic acid ratios in the various types of acid–base disturbances.

	HCO_3/CO_2 (mmol/l plasma)	Ratio in plasma	pH
Normal	26/1.30	20/1	7.4
Metabolic disturbances			
Acidosis	13/1.30	10/1	7.1
Alkalosis	52/1.30	40/1	7.7
Respiratory disturbances			
Acidosis	26/2.60	10/1	7.1
Alkalosis	26/0.65	40/1	7.7

The net effect is extracellular alkalosis and intracellular acidosis.

In metabolic alkalosis, the bicarbonate fraction is high, with little change in carbonic acid.

In most of the above causes of metabolic alkalosis, there is a deficit of chloride ions—hence the term **hypochloraemic alkalosis**. The anion which replaces chloride in the extracellular fluid to maintain the electrochemical balance is bicarbonate.

Respiratory acidosis

Respiratory acidosis occurs in disease processes which interfere with normal respiratory functions, such as congestive heart failure, pneumonia and asthma, or in depression of the respiratory centre by drugs, such as morphine and barbiturates. Therefore, respiratory acidosis is due to accumulation of CO_2 in the blood.

In respiratory acidosis, carbonic acid is high relative to bicarbonate.

Respiratory alkalosis

Respiratory alkalosis occurs after hyperventilation, as in hysteria, high altitude and hepatic failure. It is due to excessive washing out of CO_2 from alveolar air, which leads to a low $P\text{co}_2$ in arterial blood.

In respiratory alkalosis, the carbonic acid fraction is low, with little change in the bicarbonate level.

Table 11.2 gives illustrative examples of the bicarbonate–carbonic acid changes which may be encountered in cases of simple clinical acid–base disturbances of the four types above.

In conclusion, it appears from Table 11.2 that, in metabolic acid–base disturbances, it is the bicarbonate which is disturbed, with little change in carbonic acid. In respiratory abnormalities, the main disturbance lies with the

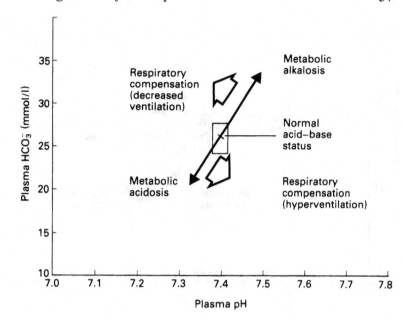

Fig.11.3 The graph shows the relationship between plasma bicarbonate and plasma pH in metabolic acid–base disturbances. The arrows indicate the directions of change due to respiratory compensation.

carbonic acid. However, this simple state of affairs is soon changed by responses aimed at correction of the blood pH.

Responses to acid–base disturbances

Both acidosis and alkalosis have a profound effect on the central nervous system (CNS). Acidosis depresses the CNS, leading to disorientation and coma. Alkalosis causes hyperexcitability of the nervous system, leading to tetany involving peripheral nerves and muscles, and in the CNS it causes extreme nervousness and convulsions.

The immediate response to any deviation of the hydrogen ion concentration in the extracellular fluid is to readjust the pH by means of the blood buffer systems. As was mentioned above, this is a temporary reaction. Adjustments have to be made by means of respiratory and renal mechanisms.

The respiratory response to change in pH

In respiratory acid–base disturbances, the respiratory response is simply to readjust the carbonic acid fraction by increasing or decreasing ventilation and, by so doing, attempt to achieve the normal bicarbonate–carbonic acid ratio of 20/1.

In the case of metabolic acid–base disturbances, however, the respiratory system cannot deal with excess non-volatile acids or get rid of excess bicarbonate. It can only readjust the carbonic acid level. This is achieved

through the effect of H^+ on peripheral chemoreceptors. The increased ventilation does not compensate the acidity completely because when H^+ starts to fall and CO_2 is washed out, the effect of these stimuli weakens and the hyperventilation stops. Conversely, in metabolic alkalosis the compensatory suppression of ventilation results in a higher P_{CO_2} and therefore a higher carbonic acid level (Fig. 11.3).

The renal response to acid–base disturbances

The kidney helps to restore normal pH by adjusting the bicarbonate fraction and therefore works to restore equilibrium according to the Henderson–Hasselbalch relationships. HCO_3^- can only be absorbed when it reacts with H^+ in the lumen of the tubules. Therefore, alkalosis will result in decreased bicarbonate reabsorption due to lack of H^+ in the tubular lumen. Consequently, excess bicarbonate will be excreted. This decreases the bicarbonate level and helps to lower the plasma pH. In acidosis filtered bicarbonate decreases and H^+ secretion increases. The H^+ is excreted in combination with other urine buffers (such as phosphate and ammonium ions). For each H^+ secreted, there is a *new bicarbonate* ion formed. This restores the alkali reserve and gets rid of excess H^+. These changes help to increase the plasma pH (Fig. 11.4).

Intracellular pH

In metabolic and respiratory acid–base disturbances, the cell pH remains relatively constant. The intracellular pH

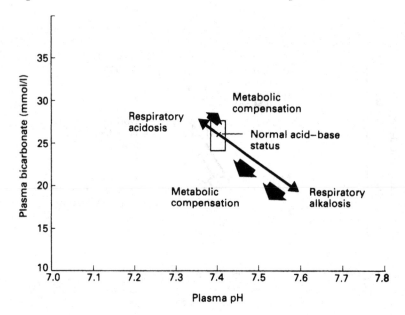

Fig.11.4 The graph shows the relationship between plasma bicarbonate and plasma pH in the case of respiratory abnormalities of acid–base balance. The arrows indicate renal (metabolic) compensation.

differs from one type of cell to another. It is generally lower than that in the extracellular fluid (e.g. 6.9 in muscle, 7.3 in renal tubule cells). It is maintained by active transport of H^+ to the extracellular fluid or the absorption of bicarbonate ions.

In respiratory abnormalities, the pH of the intracellular fluid is rapidly affected by the changes in extracellular pH. This is due to the high permeability of the cell membrane to CO_2.

In metabolic abnormalities, the abnormality of the extracellular fluid may not affect the intracellular pH. Change will take place rather slowly because of the relative impermeability of the cell membrane to H^+ and bicarbonate. For example, if bicarbonate is administered, it depresses respiration, leading to accumulation of CO_2. The CO_2 rapidly crosses the cell membrane, causing intracellular acidosis. As HCO_3^- cannot cross the cell membrane, there will be extracellular alkalosis but intracellular acidosis.

In alkalosis due to vomiting, loss of Na^+ and K^+ leads to exit of intracellular K^+, to be replaced by H^+ from extracellular fluids. This aggravates the extracellular alkalosis and causes intracellular acidosis.

Assessment of acid–base balance

The presence of acidosis or alkalosis can be assessed by direct measurement of blood pH, using appropriate pH meters. To determine the type of acidosis or alkalosis, the status of the bicarbonate–carbonic acid buffer system has to be measured.

Blood pH and Pco_2 are readily and accurately measurable in the laboratory, using suitable equipment. The Henderson–Hasselbalch equation is used to calculate the actual bicarbonate concentration:

$$pH = 6.1 + \log \frac{[HCO_3^-]}{[H_2CO_3]}$$

First, Pco_2 is used to calculate $[H_2CO_3]$. The CO_2 dissolved in plasma depends on the Pco_2 and its solubility coefficient (0.03). Therefore, $[H_2CO_3]$ can be represented in the formula as follows:

$$pH = 6.1 + \log \frac{[HCO_3^-]}{0.03 \times Pco_2}$$

Thus, measurement of pH and Pco_2 will enable us to calculate the bicarbonate concentration. By an analysis of pH, bicarbonate, carbonic acid and Pco_2, the status of the acid–base balance in any clinical situation can be assessed.

In some laboratories **standard bicarbonate** can be estimated. This is what the bicarbonate should be when respiratory compensation is eliminated. The sample of blood is equilibrated with Pco_2 at 40 mmHg when Hb is fully oxygenated. Standard bicarbonate is determined using a special nomogram (the Siggaard–Andersen curve nomogram). The standard bicarbonate reveals the true state of the alkali reserve and therefore the degree of acidosis or alkalosis. The same nomogram can also be used to determine

buffer base and **base excess**. Buffer base represents the total amount of blood buffers (namely, Hb, protein and HCO_3^-). Base excess gives an estimation of the amount of acid or base which can be given to restore the pH to normal. It is used as a guide to therapy. More information on these computed indices can be found in reference works on clinical chemistry.

The following are some examples of the assessment of the acid–base balance.

Metabolic acidosis

In metabolic acidosis the bicarbonate is much reduced but the Pco_2 is within normal limits. If hyperventilation occurs, then Pco_2 will also be decreased and the pH moves towards normal (compensated metabolic acidosis); renal mechanisms contribute to the compensation by retaining HCO_3^-.

To differentiate between different types of metabolic acidosis, the **anion gap** is calculated. It is the difference between the sum of anions and the sum of cations in the extracellular fluid. It is determined by measuring Na^+ and K^+, which account for 95% of the cations, and Cl^- and bicarbonate, which account for 86% of the anions. As the total anions and cations should be equal, the anion gap is mainly accounted for by unmeasured anions, such as protein, phosphate, sulphate and organic acids.

$$\text{Anion gap} = ([Na^+] + [K^+]) - ([Cl^-] + [HCO_3^-])$$

The normal value of the anion gap is 10–16 mmol/litre, with an average of 12 mmol/litre. In metabolic acidosis the presence of acid will change the concentrations of HCO_3^- and Cl^-. The change in the anion gap indicates the type of acidosis. In metabolic acidosis due to keto acids or lactic acid, the anion gap is increased. The bicarbonate becomes used up for buffering and is replaced by fixed acids. Thus, the anion gap provides an indirect estimate of unmeasured anions such as SO_4^{2-}, HPO_4^{2-}, and other organic acids. In diarrhoea or renal acidosis, the lost bicarbonate becomes replaced by Cl^- and the anion gap remains normal. This type is known as hyperchloraemic acidosis, to differentiate it from the first type, in which the anion gap is increased and Cl^- concentration is normal, i.e. normochloraemic.

The anion gap is not increased in metabolic acidosis due to carbonic anhydrase inhibitors or ingestion of NH_4Cl. Thus, the estimation of the anion gap provides a useful laboratory test for the evaluation of patients with acidosis.

Metabolic alkalosis

In the case of metabolic alkalosis, there is a high pH and

Table 11.3 Illustrative examples of plasma bicarbonate–carbonic acid values in cases of partially compensated acid–base disturbances.

	HCO_3/CO_2 (mmol/l plasma)	Ratio in plasma	pH
Normal	26/1.3	20/1	7.40
Partially compensated acidosis			
Metabolic acidosis	13/0.8	16.2/1	7.31
Respiratory acidosis	46/2.6	17.7/1	7.35
Partially compensated alkalosis			
Metabolic alkalosis	39/1.5	26/1	7.51
Respiratory alkalosis	22/0.8	27.5/1	7.54

a high bicarbonate level, with little change in the carbonic acid level. Carbonic acid may be slightly elevated (to satisfy the Henderson–Hasselbalch relationship). When the respiratory suppression takes place in response to the low H^+ concentration, the Pco_2 rises to high levels. This compensation is rather limited due to the O_2 demand, which soon stimulates respiration. In the kidneys not all the bicarbonate filtered is reabsorbed, which contributes to decreasing the HCO_3^- level. Therefore, in compensated metabolic alkalosis, both the Pco_2 and bicarbonate are found to be elevated. This should be differentiated from compensated respiratory acidosis (discussed below) by knowledge of the clinical history and of the previous condition of the acid–base balance (Table 11.3).

Respiratory acidosis

In respiratory acidosis the Pco_2 is high. An attempt will be made to approximate the bicarbonate–carbonic acid ratio to normal, as CO_2 is the source of plasma bicarbonate. This will result in a slight elevation of the bicarbonate fraction, but the pH will still be low. In prolonged respiratory acidosis, renal mechanisms will retain bicarbonate further and this leads to correction of the pH, but both the bicarbonate and the carbonic acid will be high, i.e. compensated respiratory acidosis (see Table 11.3).

Respiratory alkalosis

In the case of respiratory alkalosis, the Pco_2 is low because of the underlying hyperventilation. Due to the Henderson–Hasselbalch relationship, the bicarbonate also falls slightly. However, in chronic respiratory alkalosis, renal compensation sets in, with increased excretion of bicarbonate. Both the bicarbonate and carbonic acid will be low.

Table 11.3 gives examples of possible values obtained in compensated acid–base disturbances. Complete compensation is rather unlikely and the values given in Table 11.3 are illustrative of situations which may be encountered in clinical practice.

The electrolytes in acid–base imbalance

General considerations

There are several situations where Cl^-, Na^+ and K^+ disturbances may result in abnormalities of the acid–base balance. There are also situations where a primary acid–base disturbance may lead to abnormal serum electrolytes. These abnormalities may be explained by the relationship of the bicarbonate ion with Cl^- on the one hand and that of H^+ with body cations (Na^+ and K^+) on the other. Such relationships lead to disturbances in two ways: (i) exchange of similar ions across the cell membrane, i.e. between the ICF and ECF; and (ii) exchange in the renal tubules. The following account gives explanations of these relationships.

Exchange across the cell membrane

1 Bicarbonate has a reciprocal relationship with Cl^-, e.g. the chloride shift during bicarbonate synthesis. In chloride deficiency, bicarbonate ions take its place and therefore HCO_3^- in the extracellular fluid increases.

2 H^+ and K^+ have a reciprocal relationship in the ICF, i.e. K^+ tends to leave the cells when the intracellular H^+ rises, as in acidosis. This leads to hyperkalaemia.

Exchange in the renal tubules

1 The secretion of H^+ is achieved in exchange for Na^+ or K^+ ions. In the case of lack of Na^+ and K^+ in the tubular fluid, H^+ excretion will be curtailed. Therefore, correction of the Na^+ deficit in acidosis is one of the important measures which enable the kidney to excrete acid.

2 Reabsorption of Na^+ in the distal tubules takes place in exchange for K^+ and H^+ secretion, e.g. in hypersecretion of mineralocorticoids excessive K^+ and H^+ will be lost in exchange for Na^+, leading to metabolic alkalosis and hypokalaemia.

3 H^+ and K^+ seem to compete for the same carrier mechanism in the distal tubules. In the case of excessive K^+ in the tubular fluid, as in hyperkalaemia, H^+ secretion will be curtailed (acidosis). In hypokalaemia, H^+ secretion is enhanced (alkalosis).

Alkalosis, whether metabolic or respiratory in origin, results in increased excretion of K^+ in the urine. This is possibly due to increased entry of K^+ in the distal tubules to replace intracellular H^+. The lack of H^+ secretion will result in greater excretion of K^+, which would otherwise be reabsorbed in exchange for H^+ secretion: hence the association of alkalosis with hypokalaemia.

Acidosis, especially if it develops rapidly, results in decreased K^+ excretion and hyperkalaemia. This is probably due to high H^+ content of cells, including the renal tubular cells, which tends to decrease the secretion rate of K^+.

On the other hand, excessive ingestion of K^+ may lead to acidosis. The K^+ will enter the renal tubular cells and cause a net increase in secretion of potassium in the urine. This will tend to curtail H^+ excretion and therefore lead to acidosis.

Examples of electrolyte disturbances

Diabetic acidosis

1 Diabetics with ketoacidosis are usually sodium-deficient. This is brought about in several ways:

(a) The polyuria results in excessive loss of water and sodium, as a result of shrinking of the extracellular fluid volume (dehydration).

(b) The NH_4^+ mechanism for secretion of excess H^+ fails to cope and therefore Na^+ gets excreted with fixed acid in the urine. Thus, acidosis makes the Na^+ deficit worse.

(c) On the other hand, the sodium deficiency curtails the excretion of H^+ in the distal tubules and the collecting ducts. The H^+ ions tend to stay in the extracellular fluid in the place of Na^+ and therefore the acidosis is made worse.

It appears from the above that there is a vicious circle in diabetic acidosis involving Na^+ and H^+. One of the key measures in the management of this condition is to give intravenous NaCl. The correction of the sodium deficit enables the kidney to secrete H^+. Insulin therapy also helps to correct acidosis by oxidation of keto acids. If the pH falls to 6.9, bicarbonate administration is recommended.

2 Potassium abnormalities are also observed in diabetic acidosis. Severe acidosis is usually associated with entry of H^+ and net exit of K^+ from cells. This leads to hyperkalaemia. Another cause for hyperkalaemia is a decrease in renal excretion of K^+. Potassium is believed to enter the tubular cells due to the electrochemical gradient between the interstitial fluid and the intracellular fluid. In acidosis this is curtailed by excessive entry of H^+ into the tubular cell, which leads to less K^+ secretion. However, diabetics are usually K^+-deficient, because of tissue destruction and catabolism of protein. Therefore, the hyperkalaemia does not reflect the true picture of potassium balance. On treatment with insulin and glucose, K^+ ions quickly enter into cells and may therefore precipitate hypokalaemia.

Chronic renal failure

Renal failure (uraemia) is characterized by high blood urea, associated with metabolic acidosis. This is due to failure of the renal mechanisms to excrete adequate amounts of H^+. There is also an accumulation of toxic products of metabolism, particularly those resulting from a breakdown of amino acids and nucleic acids. Uraemic subjects tend to have low intracellular potassium, probably due to toxic interference with the Na^+–K^+ pump. The extracellular potassium is usually normal or high. Insulin normally augments the entry of potassium into the intracellular compartment. In uraemia there is a resistance to the actions of insulin and this probably adds to the possibility of developing hyperkalaemia.

In general, severe acidosis is associated with hyperkalaemia. A simple explanation is generalized K^+ efflux of intracellular potassium in exchange for H^+. This can be corrected by giving bicarbonate and limiting K^+ intake in the diet or in drugs containing potassium.

Patients with uraemia have a slightly expanded extracellular fluid volume, with Na^+ retention. Therefore, it is useful to restrict Na^+ intake. Renal function in these patients may become rapidly worse if they lose fluid by vomiting or diarrhoea. In this case, correcting the fluid and Na^+ loss has to be done cautiously in order not to exceed the required amount, which might result in overloading the circulation and heart failure.

In cases of renal insufficiency, hypokalaemia can be induced by vomiting or diuretic therapy. This is due to the inability of the kidney to conserve K^+ efficiently in case of excessive losses.

Abnormalities of corticosteroids

In Cushing's syndrome there is excessive secretion of cortisol, which exerts some mineralocorticoid activity. There is Na^+ reabsorption and K^+ excretion. This leads to hypokalaemia. Less K^+ will be available in the tubular cells and more H^+ will take their place, leading to excessive secretion of H^+ and reabsorption of HCO_3^-. This is probably the main explanation of the alkalosis which occurs in hyperactivity of the adrenal cortex.

In corticosteroid deficiency, Addison's disease, there is excessive loss of Na^+ in the urine, from failure of reabsorption in the distal tubules due to aldosterone deficiency. There is also potassium retention, less secretion of H^+, and acidosis.

Loss of chloride

There is an inverse relationship between chloride and bicarbonate ion concentrations in the extracellular fluid.

Hypochloraemia is associated with high plasma bicarbonate levels. Alkalosis sets in, but the exact mechanism is not fully understood. In hypochloraemia there is a high content of bicarbonate in the glomerular filtrate. This is known to result in increased reabsorption of bicarbonate. Conversely, low plasma bicarbonate in hyperchloraemia leads to less bicarbonate reabsorption, giving rise to acidosis. Restriction of salt intake is one of the methods used in the management of renal acidosis.

The effects of diuretic therapy

Diuretics that work by their inhibition of carbonic anhydrase, such as acetazolamide (Diamox), result in failure of the renal tubules to make HCO_3^-. This leads to decreased H^+ secretion and decreased HCO_3^- absorption. Therefore, acidosis sets in, with increased sodium and potassium losses.

Other diuretics (non-carbonic anhydrase inhibitors) result in the excretion of a large volume of urine. The kidney works very hard and rapid absorption of Na^+ takes place. Na^+ reabsorption is associated with H^+ and K^+ secretion. Therefore, alkalosis sets in, with associated hypokalaemia.

Summary

1 The normal blood pH depends on a constant bicarbonate –carbonic acid ratio of 20/1. The normal levels in plasma are 24–28 mmol/litre for bicarbonate and 1.2–1.4 mmol/litre for carbonic acid. The pH of blood is predicted by the Henderson–Hasselbalch equation, using bicarbonate–carbonic acid as its buffer system.

2 The constancy of the pH is challenged all the time by constant production of acid during metabolism. The main acid is CO_2 (volatile acid), which can be excreted by the lungs. Other acids, such as sulphuric acid, phosphoric acid, keto acids and lactic acid (non-volatile or fixed) are excreted by the kidneys.

3 There are two main buffers which safeguard the pH of the blood against rapid change:

    (a) The bicarbonate in the plasma neutralizes any excess acid production. The bicarbonate buffer is especially valuable because it converts H^+ from any source to carbonic acid, which can be excreted as CO_2 in the lungs.

    (b) Hb in the red cells neutralizes the excess H^+ associated with CO_2 carriage from tisues to the lungs.

Thus, the blood buffers are the first line of defence. They prevent rapid changes in pH. The buffers, however, have a temporary effect and cannot deal with long-term changes.

4 The respiratory system eliminates or retains CO_2 by readjustment of alveolar ventilation. Therefore, it only adjusts the carbonic acid. The respiratory response takes

Fig. 11.5 Summary diagram of acid–base regulation.

Table 11.4 Causes and effects of acid–base disturbances.

pH Disturbance	Causes	HCO_3	P_{CO_2}
Metabolic acidosis	Diabetic ketosis Renal failure Diarrhoea Ingestion of NH_4Cl	Low	Normal or low in respiratory compensation
Metabolic alkalosis	Ingestion of bicarbonate Excessive vomiting Excessive loss of K^+	High	Normal or high in respiratory compensation
Respiratory acidosis	Lung disease Airway obstruction Oedema of the lung Depression of respiratory centre (e.g. barbiturate poisoning)	Normal or high in renal compensation	High
Respiratory alkalosis	Hyperventilation (e.g. hysteria, high altitude, ventilators)	Normal or low in renal compensation	Low

seconds or minutes and is incomplete in cases of bicarbonate (or metabolic) disturbances.

5 The main long-term defence is the kidney. This is achieved by reabsorption of bicarbonate and the secretion of H^+. Both mechanisms are closely linked so that, with the secretion of H^+, an equivalent amount of bicarbonate is reabsorbed. Thus, the kidney can only readjust the bicarbonate level (alkali reserve), which usually falls in acidosis as a result of the buffering action of bicarbonate. Thus, the renal mechanisms bring about the final adjustment. This is

slow but complete. It may take several days for the kidney to compensate for respiratory acidosis.

Figure 11.5 summarizes acid–base regulation.

6 Disturbances of acid–base balance are clinically classified into four types: acidosis or alkalosis, each of which may be either metabolic or respiratory in origin. Table 11.4 summarizes the main causes of these disturbances and their laboratory findings.

7 Acid–base disturbances encountered in clinical practice are usually due to failure of one of the mechanisms.

The other mechanisms will attempt to compensate, e.g. in compensated metabolic acidosis, the P_{CO_2} will be low due to hyperventilation, and, in compensated metabolic alkalosis, the P_{CO_2} may be slightly elevated due to respiratory adjustments. Different types of metabolic acidosis also lead to changes in the normal value of the anion gap.

8 Acid–base disturbances are usually associated with electrolyte abnormalities. This is because of exchange between the bicarbonate and Cl^- ions, on the one hand, and between H^+ and both Na^+ and K^+, on the other. The exchange takes place at two sites: (i) between extracellular and intracellular fluid, e.g. the chloride shift in association with bicarbonate and the exit of K^+ from cells in exchange with H^+ in acidosis; and (ii) exchange in tubular reabsorption and secretion, e.g. Na^+ reabsorption in exchange for H^+ and K^+ secretion, H^+ secretion in exchange for Na^+ and K^+, and K^+ loss in cases of low H^+ secretion in the urine. Therefore, changes in H^+ secretion rates are reflected in electrolyte disturbances. Conversely, the availability of electrolytes in tubular fluid affects the rate of secretion of H^+.

Further reading

1 Brenner, B.M. & Rector, F.C., Jr (eds) (1996) *The Kidney*, 5th edn, pp. 929–998. Saunders, Philadelphia.
2 Guyton, A.C. & Hall, J.E. (1996) Regulation of acid–base balance. In: *Textbook of Medical Physiology*, 9th edn, pp. 385–403. Saunders, Philadelphia.

12 / The Skin and Regulation of Body Temperature

Introduction

The skin has several important functions in homoeostatic regulatory mechanisms. In addition to its protective role, the skin has a vital role in the regulation of body temperature. By adjusting the blood flow in the skin, the body can adjust the amount of heat lost to the environment. In hot climates the sweat glands secrete sweat so as to cool the skin by means of evaporation. The amount of sweat varies greatly with heat exposure. Large amounts of fluids and electrolytes can be lost through the skin during sweating. This may lead to disturbances of fluid and electrolyte balance.

Anatomical considerations

The skin is one of the largest organs of the body. In a 70 kg man, its total weight is about 4 kg and its surface area about 1.8 m². The skin has a superficial layer, the **epidermis**, and a deep layer, the dermis.

The epidermis consists of several layers of cells. That lying deepest is the **basal layer** of cells. Next to these are

Objectives

On completion of the study of this section, the student should be able to:

1 Describe the microscopic anatomy of the skin and appreciate its functional significance.

2 Acquire knowledge of the major physiological functions of the skin so as to explain abnormalities due to injury or diseases of the skin, e.g. burns, infections and loss of sensations.

3 Explain the passive and active mechanisms involved in the maintenance of thermal balance in order to interpret clinical abnormalities of temperature regulation.

4 Become acquainted with the various disorders of thermal balance so as to differentiate between them for the purpose of clinical management.

5 Become aware of the social and cultural aspects of thermal regulation in order to give appropriate advice to patients and the community.

the keratinocytes, which are responsible for the continuous regeneration of the more superficial layers (Fig. 12.1). The **granular cells** are next. These are flat cells that have lost their nuclei and contain **keratin granules**. As new cells are formed, the granular cells move towards the surface and form the horny layer, which consists of dead cornified cells. It is estimated that the horny layer is entirely shed every 3 weeks.

The **dermis** consists of dense collagen fibres, which give the skin its elasticity.

The skin has several **appendages**: the **hair follicles, nails, sweat glands** and **sebaceous glands**. There are two types of sweat glands. The *eccrine* glands are responsible for sweating associated with the regulation of body temperature. These are present all over the body. The secretory tubules of these glands are coiled up and lie deep in the dermis. Their ducts open on the surface of the skin. These glands are supplied by sympathetic fibres, which stimulate sweating by releasing acetylcholine. The other type of sweat glands are called *apocrine* glands, which are only found in the parts of the body with hair follicles, e.g. the axillae and pubis. Their ducts open into the hair sheath. These glands become active after puberty. Their secretion is not necessarily stimulated by heat. Decomposition of their secretion by bacteria results in the unpleasant smell of the axillae in some adults.

Horny layer

Granular cell layer

Keratinocytes

Basal layer

Epidermis

Epidermal papilla

Dermis

Fig. 12.1 Vertical section through the epidermis showing the layers of cells. (Reproduced from Borysenko, M. & Beringer, T. (1989) *Functional Histology*, 3rd edn. With permission from Little Brown & Co., Boston.) Students are advised to consult their histology textbook for the study of the dermis and skin appendages.

Blood supply of the skin

The skin has a rich supply of blood-vessels. The amounts of blood which flow in various parts of the skin may vary greatly, e.g. the face and scalp have one of the richest supplies. Wounds of the scalp and face tend to bleed more profusely.

The skin is supplied by small arteries which penetrate from the subcutaneous tissues. They supply the capillary beds just below the epidermis. The blood from these capillaries drains into a rich venous plexus just below the dermis. An interesting feature of the venous plexus is that it is connected by **arteriovenous shunts** with the deeper arteries in the subcutaneous tissues. Opening or closing these shunts can greatly influence the flow rate of blood through the skin. No blood-vessels penetrate into the epidermis, which gets its nutrients through the tissue fluid. The constriction or dilatation of the arterioles determines the amount of blood flow in the skin. Normally, vasomotor tone through sympathetic α receptors keeps the arterioles in a state of moderate balanced constriction. Decreasing the vasomotor tone will result in dilatation, while an increase will result in constriction.

The lymphatic drainage of the skin takes place via rich lymphatic capillaries in the dermis. These start in the tips of the papillae and collect to form larger vessels, which run into the subcutaneous fat with the larger blood-vessels. Minor or temporary blockage of superficial lymph drainage due to infection or injury causes localized lymphatic oedema around the site of infection or injury. More serious lymphatic blockage occurs in cases of cancer involving lymph nodes and in parasitic infestation with a worm,

Wucheraria bancrofti, which causes massive swelling of distal parts, e.g. the legs and the scrotum, giving rise to the disease known as elephantiasis.

Functions of the skin

Protective role

The cornified layer of the skin is almost waterproof. It allows the body to keep its water even when the air is very dry. Conversely, it does not allow water to go in during swimming in fresh water or to go out if the body is immersed in salt water. The cornified layer also protects the underlying soft tissues from invasion by microorganisms, by chemical substances and by rough objects. When the horny layer is lost, as in cases of burns, evaporation takes place 10–20 times faster from the underlying tissues. This is particularly serious in hot, dry climates. When large areas of skin are burnt, the evaporative water loss can be enormous, which can lead to serious dehydration.

In addition to its function as a physical barrier to microorganisms, the skin has chemical and **immunological roles**. The intact skin and mucous membranes have a number of secretions which are known to be germicidal, e.g. fatty acids from sebaceous glands and propionic acid produced by normal skin flora. Scattered within the stratum germinativum (**Malpighi's** layer) are found **Langerhans cells**. These are clear cells found among the **keratinocytes**. They seem to act as a trap for **exogenous antigens** which penetrate the cornified layer. They bind the antigen and migrate to the lymph nodes, where they sensitize lymphocytes. Specifically sensitized lymphocytes then migrate to the epidermis to attack the antigens trapped by the cells of Langerhans. Langerhans cells have also been found in other surface epithelium exposed to exogenous antigens, such as the gastrointestinal, respiratory and genitourinary systems.

The skin pigment, melanin, which is present in the basal layer of the dermis, protects the skin against injury by **ultraviolet light**. The greater the amount of pigment, the less the amount of light that penetrates the epidermis. Exposure to the sun stimulates pigment formation and also leads to thickening of the horny layer. Both of these effects decrease the penetration of ultraviolet light and carcinogenic solar radiation (wavelengths less than 320 nm). It is not surprising, therefore, that individuals with congenital lack of pigment (albinos) are prone to develop skin cancer.

Sensory functions

There are numerous nerve endings in the skin which serve the functions of pain, touch and hot and cold sensation. There are also specialized skin receptors for pressure, vibration, stretch and hair movement. These sensations provide the individual with information about the immediate environment. Conscious or reflex responses will take place, depending upon the nature of the stimulus. In this respect, these sensations can also be considered to play a protective role.

Synthesis of vitamin D

Vitamin D_3 (cholecalciferol) can be synthesized in the skin from **7-dehydrocholesterol** (Fig. 12.2). This indicates that this substance can also be looked upon as a hormone synthesized by the skin, which travels in the blood and acts on distant organs. As seen in the sequence of synthesis, both the liver and the kidney are essential for converting vitamin D_3 into its active form, 1,25-dihydroxycholecalciferol. The conversion of vitamin D_3 to the active form by the kidney depends on parathyroid hormone and plasma calcium and phosphate levels.

Regulation of heat loss

The skin temperature under normal conditions is several degrees cooler than the core body temperature (Table 12.1). It appears from these figures that the skin and subcutaneous tissues, shell temperature, varies with the external or ambient temperature, while the core temperature remains relatively constant. Therefore, in hot weather, the skin acts as a cooling organ for the body. Blood flowing through the skin loses heat to the skin, which, in turn, loses it to the environment. At a comfortable ambient temperature, which is usually between 23 and 30°C, the skin blood flow is

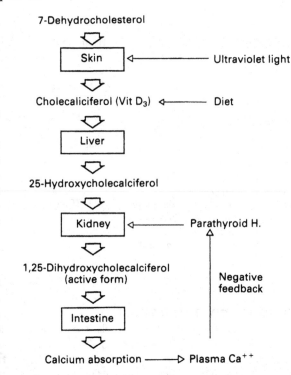

Fig. 12.2 Vitamin D synthesis and regulation of its activation by parathyroid hormone.

Table 12.1 Variations of skin and core temperatures (°C) in a subject exposed to various ambient temperatures.*

| Ambient temperature | Skin | | | | Rectum |
	Foot	Hand	Trunk	Head	
23	24.8	29.5	32.8	34.0	36.4
25	29.0	31.5	33.2	34.5	36.6
27	30.5	33.2	33.5	34.2	36.6
29	32.6	33.5	34.0	34.6	36.8
32	33.5	34.0	34.4	34.8	36.9
34	33.8	34.5	34.6	35.0	37.0

* Approximate temperatures after Dubois, F.F. (1933) *Journal of Nutrition* **15**, 477.

about 20 ml/min/100 g. This constitutes about 4% of the cardiac output. The regulation of heat loss through the skin is achieved in two ways:

1 *Regulation of blood flow in the skin.* This is achieved by adjusting sympathetic vasomotor tone to skin blood-vessels. In hot environments the vasomotor tone is decreased and this leads to vasodilatation and a consequent increase in blood flow. In extremely hot environments, the blood flow to the skin can increase up to 3 litres/min (i.e. 60% of cardiac output). This means that the cardiac output has to be increased to maintain adequate flow to other organs.

In cold environments vasomotor tone is increased and this leads to decreasing the blood flow to the skin, which may fall to 2 ml/min/100 g in extremely cold climates.

2 *Sweating*. When the skin temperature or the core temperature rises, reflex sweating is stimulated. This leads to secretion of sweat on the surface of the skin. When water evaporates, it takes its latent heat of vaporization from the skin and therefore the skin temperature drops to normal or below normal levels. This is a vital mechanism for heat loss in extremely hot environments or when the body is producing large amounts of heat (as in muscular exercise, hard physical labour and fever). Failure of sweating under such conditions leads to a rapid rise of body temperature, which may lead to coma and death (heatstroke).

Thermal balance

The contributions of the skin to heat loss are under active physiological control. However, the body can lose or gain heat from the environment by passive heat transfer mechanisms, i.e. radiation, convection and conduction, and also by the evaporation of water from the surface.

Homothermic, or warm-blooded, animals (e.g. mammals and birds) maintain their body temperature within a narrow range. This is achieved by regulatory mechanisms which adjust the thermal balance. **Poikilothermic** animals, such as fish and reptiles, are referred to as cold-blooded animals because they allow their body temperature to change with that of the environment. Camels are homothermic but they can allow their body temperature to change within a wider range than that of other mammals. This mechanism helps the camel to cool during the night and therefore not to lose water in cooling during the day. It can also allow its temperature to rise to higher levels than is compatible with normal body functions in other mammals.

Thermal balance depends on factors which cause the body to gain or lose heat. Table 12.2 gives the various mechanisms which contribute to thermal balance. Thermal balance can be expressed by the following equation when

Table 12.2 The components of heat gain and heat loss.

Heat gain	Heat loss
Metabolic heat production (M)	Evaporation (E)
Radiation (R)	Radiation
Conduction $\left.\right\}(C)$	Conduction
Convection	Convection

there is no change in body temperature, as in homothermic animals (see Table 12.2 for explanation):

$$M - E \pm R \pm C = 0$$

In fevers or in hypothermia, the thermal balance can be either positive (excess of heat gain) or negative (excess of heat loss). The thermal balance equation does not come to zero:

$$M - E \pm R \pm C = S$$

where S = change in heat store due to change in body temperature, which can be either positive or negative.

Now let us consider the various factors which contribute to thermal balance. Each of the mechanisms in Table 12.2 will be explained.

Heat loss

Radiation

Hot objects emit infrared heat rays (electromagnetic waves) through the air. When the body is surrounded by cooler objects, radiation will result in heat loss. If, however, the surroundings are hotter than the body, radiant heat will travel from the environment to the body. This will result in heat gain. Therefore, the contribution of radiation to heat balance can be either positive (gain) or negative (loss), i.e. $\pm R$ in the thermal balance equation. At a comfortable room temperature, about 60% of heat loss occurs by radiation.

Conduction

Heat transmission by conduction takes place between objects in direct contact with each other. Thus, clothes, chairs and beds will exchange heat with the body. Therefore, the contribution of conduction can be either positive or negative depending on the temperature of the object in contact with the skin. However, the amount of heat exchanged by conduction is very small, except when the temperature difference is high and the surface of the skin in contact is extensive, e.g. cold sponging on large areas of body surface in the treatment of fevers or heatstroke. Heat gain by conduction can be increased by the use of an electric blanket and heat loss by the use of cooling beds and jackets, as in the management of heatstroke.

Conduction of heat to the air in contact with the skin also takes place. But this loss is assisted by movement of the heated air in immediate contact with the skin, to be replaced by cooler air by *convection*. Hot air rises, creating convection currents. Similarly, conduction between the skin and fluid can take place, e.g. when the body is immersed in cool water. Convection currents also move the water in contact with the body, to be replaced by cooler water. If immersed in warm water, the body can gain heat very quickly by conduction.

Convection

It is clear from the above that convection takes place in air and water. Convection currents move the layers of air or water in contact with the body, to be replaced by other molecules with a different temperature. In a cool room, about 10% of the heat loss occurs by conduction and convection. This method of heat loss can be greatly increased by air movement, e.g. the use of fans.

Evaporation

Evaporation of water takes place from the body surface in contact with air, i.e. the lungs and the skin. About 500–600 ml of water is lost every day in this way. This is referred to as inevitable water loss, which occurs irrespective of body temperature or environmental conditions. Evaporation from the skin takes place even in cool environments, due to simple diffusion and evaporation of water from the skin. This is also known as **insensible perspiration**, to differentiate it from sweating, which is an active secretory process. Sweating greatly increases the evaporative heat loss. At comfortable temperatures, the inevitable water loss from skin and lungs accounts for about 30% of the heat loss, and this is relatively constant. Evaporation is clearly associated only with heat loss and therefore its contribution to the heat balance is always negative ($-E$) in the thermal balance equation. The evaporation of 1 ml of water from the skin or lungs results in losing 0.58 kcal of heat.

Sweating

There are about 2.5×10^6 sweat glands in an adult person. However, the number of functioning glands varies with acclimatization. People who live and work in hot environments tend to have more active sweat glands. Persons living in cold environments and who do not perform hard physical labour tend to have a minimum number of active sweat glands. Even in these people, the number of active glands can be increased in a few days during acclimatization to heat and can therefore achieve maximum rates of sweating very quickly.

Thermal sweating is controlled by the hypothalamic heat-regulating centres. Stimulation of central thermoreceptors by the blood temperature leads to activation of the sympathetic nerves to the sweat glands. It is also possible to produce reflex sweating by stimulation of heat receptors in the skin. Quadriplegic patients can sweat reflexly on the trunk and limbs. This indicates that there are centres in the spinal cord capable of producing reflex sweating.

Sweat is a dilute fluid similar to extracellular fluid. For practical purposes, it is a dilute solution of sodium chloride. It has a specific gravity of 1.002–1.003. The concentration of NaCl in sweat varies between 50 and 100 mmol/litre. It is found that, with acclimatization, the concentration of NaCl decreases and therefore sweat is produced without severe losses of NaCl.

Heat gain

Metabolic heat gain

Under basal conditions almost all the energy produced appears as heat. If measured by O_2 consumption, this is about 1 kcal/kg/hour. As the body is composed mostly of water, its specific heat is almost 1. This means that, if there were no heat loss, the body temperature would rise by 1°C every hour at basal conditions. It is clear, therefore, that the body must lose heat all the time, especially when the metabolic rate is high, e.g. during physical work or exercise.

Fevers cause an increase in metabolism of about 10% or more. In children this can cause a rapid rise in body temperature, leading to convulsions. Sweating during an attack of fever is a good sign and helps to cool the body.

Metabolic heat gain can be increased by means of **shivering** and **non-shivering thermogenesis**. The mechanisms responsible for body temperature regulation are described in the following section.

Mechanisms of body temperature regulation

The core temperature of the body remains relatively constant in homothermic animals in spite of the wide variations in heat production and the changes in environmental temperature. In humans, we can measure the core body temperature by inserting a clinical thermometer into the rectum. Alternatively, the mouth temperature is taken as indicative of the core temperature, provided the thermometer is kept in the mouth for 1–2 minutes to equilibrate. The body temperature has a physiological diurnal rhythm. It is highest in the afternoon and lowest in the early hours of the morning (Fig. 12.3). This is an example of circadian rhythm. The changes in core body temperature, however, stay within a range of 1–2°C throughout the day.

The maintenance of a constant body temperature depends on regulation mechanisms, mainly mediated through the hypothalamus, where thermal regulatory centres have been identified. In the **anterior hypothalamus**, the preoptic

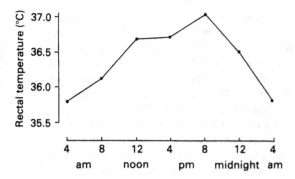

Fig. 12.3 Diurnal circadian rhythm of core body temperature.

nuclei are sensitive to changes in core body temperature. These centres are mainly associated with responses to heat exposure. Parts of the **posterior hypothalamus** are associated with the body responses to cold exposure. Sensory inputs to these regulatory centres come from two main thermal receptors:

1 *Central thermoreceptors.* Receptors sensitive to core body temperature changes have been identified in the anterior hypothalamus. They are responsible for monitoring the temperature of the blood flowing through the hypothalamus. Central thermoreceptors are also found in other parts of the central nervous system, e.g. the spinal cord.

2 *Receptors in the skin.* Nerve endings in the skin that are specialized in detection of heat or cold sensations detect changes in the temperature of the immediate environment in contact with the body.

Neural mechanisms

Lesions in the anterior hypothalamus result in elevation of body temperature. It seems that these centres are constantly keeping the temperature of the body down, i.e. lowering the heat production. The absence of this effect results in fever and the body temperature can only be brought down by cooling the skin artificially. The barbiturate drugs have been found to bring down body temperature in cases of fever caused by central lesions.

On the other hand, lesions of the posterior hypothalamus result in a lower body temperature or hypothermia. This is particularly severe in cold environments, where the body temperature can fall to fatal levels unless artificial warming is introduced. Neural mechanisms which control heat production depend on integrated signals from both **central** and **peripheral thermoreceptors**. Impulses from the skin receptors alone or from central receptors alone do not seem to have an effect. The details of central neural mechanisms responsible for integration of thermal regulatory responses

are not fully understood. However, the following responses have been amply described.

Effects of exposure to heat

The first response to heat exposure is vasodilatation of skin vessels. This is mediated by skin temperature receptors and carried in the spinothalamic tracts to the thalamus. Impulses are relayed to the hypothalamic nuclei and from there to the vasomotor centres in the medulla. Heat exposure causes an inhibition of vasomotor tone to skin vessels, which results in vasodilatation. However, it has recently been reported that there is an **active vasodilator (AVD) system** which can increase skin blood flow to 60% of the cardiac output, i.e. about eight times that at comfortable ambient temperatures. As this system does not depend on α_1, α_2-receptors or on cholinergic receptors, putative mediators have been suggested, such as vasoactive intestinal peptide (VIP) and substance P. Upon vasodilatation, increased blood flow takes place and consequently heat loss by radiation increases. Conduction and convection also increase, but these are responsible for smaller amounts of heat loss. Vasodilatation alone can take care of regulating thermal balance as long as the environmental temperature is 30°C or less and as long as heat production is kept at basal or resting levels.

If the rate of heat production is high (e.g. muscular activity) or the environmental temperature is higher than 30°C, then the core body temperature may start to rise. An increase of core body temperature of a fraction of 1°C results in stimulation of sweating. The **set point** for thermal regulation is around 37°C. It may be a fraction of a degree above or below. Figure 12.4 shows the initiation of sweating in a subject exposed to heat in relation to core body temperature. The sweat glands are controlled by the hypothalamic heat-regulating centres, which send impulses via the cholinergic sympathetic supply to the sweat glands.

Effects of exposure to cold

Vasoconstriction of the skin is the first response to cold. This results in a reduction of heat loss by radiation, convection and conduction. On further exposure, other responses take place.

Shivering. Heat gain can be increased during exposure to cold by increasing the tension of the skeletal muscles at first. Then reflex shivering occurs. The mechanisms of shivering depend on the somatic nerves and cannot occur in muscles deprived of voluntary function (various types of paralysis). Both central and peripheral temperature receptors can initiate shivering. Figure 12.5 shows a

Fig. 12.4 Stimulation of sweating in a subject, showing initiation and increase in sweat rate in relation to core body temperature. (Based on data by Benzinger, T.H. (1959) *Physiological Reviews* **49**, 671.)

diagrammatic representation of the neural mechanisms involved in thermal regulation.

The posterior hypothalamus initiates the shivering response via the midbrain and extrapyramidal nuclei, and the impulses descend in the tecto- and vestibulospinal tracts to the anterior horn cells. This tonic discharge to the anterior horn cells leads to oscillations in the stretch reflex (see Chapter 16) with short-lived contractions and relaxations in all skeletal muscles of the body. Shivering may cause up to a fivefold increase in the resting heat-production level. Shivering starts at a critical skin temperature of 27°C in a nude person but this can be greatly lowered on wearing suitable clothes.

The **rigors** of fever (e.g. malaria) are due to intense cutaneous vasoconstriction with a rapid fall in skin temperature, giving the sensation of cold. Shivering can be induced by cold receptors in the skin even if the core temperature is high. The core and skin temperatures sensed by the receptors seem to be integrated at the level of the hypothalamus. Thus, we find that the thresholds for sweating and for shivering vary with various combinations of skin and core temperatures (Fig. 12.6).

Non-shivering thermogenesis. In the newborn child there is a special type of fat, known as brown fat, which is found around the neck and shoulders. Brown fat disappears after the first 6 months. It is also found in animals that live in cold climates. Brown fat is richly supplied with sympathetic nerves and blood-vessels. Stimulation of these nerves releases noradrenaline (norepinephrine), which results in increased metabolism of the brown fat cells and consequently increases heat production. Vasodilatation in brown fat helps to increase the distribution of heat throughout the body.

Hormonal and chemical mechanisms

Adrenergic stimulation results in the release of adrenaline in the circulation. This has a profound calorigenic effect,

Fig. 12.5 Diagrammatic representation of the pathways of thermal regulation.

(a)

(b)

Fig. 12.6 The variation in thresholds of (a) sweating and
(b) shivering, with various combinations of skin and core body
temperature. (Adapted from Benzinger, T.H. (1959) *Physiological
Reviews* **49**, 671.)

through uncoupling of oxidative phosphorylation (i.e.
oxidation of nutrients releasing heat energy without synthesis of adenosine triphosphate (ATP)). It is fast-acting
but lasts for only a short time. It accounts for the sensation of heat which accompanies anxiety and stress. Sympathetic stimulation is lower during fasting and higher
after feeding. In response to cold, sympathetic stimulation is responsible for the non-shivering thermogenesis
described above.

Thyroid function increases slowly on prolonged exposure to cold environments. It is considered one of the mechanisms for cold adaptation, resulting in increased basal
metabolic rate (BMR). In laboratory animals thyroid-
stimulating hormone (TSH) is stimulated by exposure to
cold; this mechanism is uncertain in humans.

Adaptation

Long-term exposure to hot or cold climates causes a variety
of adaptive changes in thermal regulatory functions. In
essence, these changes lead to more efficient maintenance
of thermal balance under extremes of environmental conditions. Persons who move from one environment to another
also adapt themselves by means of choice of clothes and by
behavioural patterns suited to the new environment.

Acclimatization to heat

On moving from a temperate to a tropical region, an individual experiences discomfort at first but soon becomes
'used to it'. This is due to acclimatization. One of the main
features of acclimatization to heat is a marked increase in
the rate of sweating. This adaptive change leads to more
efficient cooling, a smaller rise in body temperature, a
smaller rise in pulse rate and therefore less discomfort. The
stimulus for heat acclimatization is the rise in body temperature. The more frequently the body temperature rises, the
greater the activity of the sweat glands.

Sweat is similar to extracellular fluid (ECF). However
Na^+ and Cl^- can be reabsorbed in the ducts of the sweat
glands. The concentration of NaCl depends on the rate of
sweating. In well-acclimatized individuals the amount of
sweat is less and the concentration of NaCl is low, due to
increased secretion of aldosterone. An acclimatized person loses less than 5 g NaCl/day, while an unacclimatized
individual may lose up to 30 g/day.

The salt balance also affects the amount of salt in
the sweat. Experiments on Sudanese and British medical
students revealed that the salt intake was 13 g/day in Cambridge and only about half that amount in Khartoum. This
indicates that the salt balance can be maintained on much
lower salt intakes than those seen in temperate climates.

Acclimatization to heat also includes a lower heart rate at
rest, a lowering of the threshold for sweating and a decrease
in the amount of sweat required for cooling compared
with unacclimatized subjects. In hot, dry climates the
sweating mechanism is the main acclimatization mechanism. However, in hot, humid climates, when evaporative
heat loss is low, convection becomes more important. A
higher skin temperature is achieved by a dramatic increase
in skin blood flow. Under these conditions an efficient

cardiovascular response is the main adaptation mechanism, which requires an increase in cardiac output, effective skin vasodilatation and increased circulatory volume. This requires more fitness than acclimatization in hot, dry conditions.

During heat acclimatization, there is an increase in blood volume. This safeguards against circulatory insufficiency on exposure to heat.

Behavioural adaptation includes avoiding the heat by staying in the shade and by working and moving about at a slower pace. The choice of appropriate clothes plays an important part in maintaining a thermal balance.

Acclimatization to cold

There is evidence that, in animals exposed to cold, thyroid gland activity increases by means of an increase in hypothalamic thyrotrophin-releasing hormone (TRH). In humans, such evidence is not available. There is evidence, however, that the metabolism increases in individuals exposed to cold. Increased metabolism is partly explained by increased sensitivity to the calorigenic effect of catecholamines. There is also an increase in corticotrophin-releasing hormone (CRH), which stimulates adenocorticotrophic hormone (ACTH) release and consequently the production of cortisol. Animals also increase their heat production through non-shivering thermogenesis by increasing the amount of brown fat.

Behavioural factors include avoiding cold surroundings, wearing warm clothes, consuming hot drinks and using indoor heating.

Abnormalities of thermal regulation

Disturbances due to heat

Disturbances of temperature regulation can be caused by excessive exposure to hot environments at work or in cars or by direct exposure to the hot sun. Muscular work under such conditions increases the metabolic heat production. This results in a heat load beyond the capacity of heat-losing mechanisms. When the Muslim pilgrimage to Mecca (hajj) occurs in the summer, large numbers of people are exposed to extremely hot environments by walking long distances in the open sun. Hundreds of cases of thermal, fluid and electrolyte disturbances due to heat are brought to the health units for urgent attention. This has necessitated giving appropriate medical advice and the establishment of a special service for cases suffering from various forms of heat exposure.

Exposure to high heat loads causes a variety of heat imbalance syndromes. These can be broadly classified as heatstroke and heat exhaustion.

Heatstroke (heat hyperpyrexia)

Heatstroke may be brought about by a primary failure of sweating or by an inadequate sweating response. The patient usually, but not always, has hot, dry skin. The nature of the primary failure is not fully understood. It may be explained by damage to hypothalamic sweating centres by the rapid rise in body temperature. Post-mortem studies of cases dying of heatstroke have shown evidence of central nervous system damage. In experimental animals, heat stress produces brain oedema and decreased cerebral blood flow (CBF). **H$_2$-receptor** blockers have been found to decrease the oedema and improve CBF, suggesting a role for **histamine** release in the pathogenesis of heatstroke. It is also known that certain **pyrogens** (e.g. in malaria) can produce failure of sweating. This produces hyperpyrexia, associated with cutaneous vasoconstriction and shivering (rigors), making things worse.

Insufficiency of the sweating response occurs in some cases of heatstroke, i.e. heat loss is inadequate for balancing the heat gain. Such insufficiency of sweating occurs when the skin does not have adequate numbers of active sweat glands (e.g. lack of acclimatization or damage by prickly heat rash). In some cases, insufficiency of sweating can result from fatigue of the sweat glands, e.g. after prolonged sweating in hot, humid environments.

Heat exhaustion

Heat exhaustion can be caused by: (i) circulatory deficiency; (ii) dehydration; and (iii) salt deficiency. In most instances, there is a combination of two or more factors.

The predominant feature is salt depletion. The patient feels giddy with a headache and may faint. Nausea and vomiting are common features. There is a low blood pressure and a high pulse rate and the skin is cold and clammy. Heat exhaustion occurs in unacclimatized people who undertake physical effort in a hot environment, often with little water and salt intake. Some patients may proceed to develop **exertional heatstroke (EHS)** as a complication.

Heat syncope. This presents with weakness and fainting without a rise in body temperature or with failure of sweating and predisposes to heat exhaustion. It is brought about by exposure or working in hot environments, usually in unacclimatized individuals or persons with poor physical fitness. The blood pressure is low and the pulse may be slow (vasovagal effect). The skin is moist and cold. The fainting is caused by pooling of blood in the skeletal muscles and the skin, particularly in the lower limbs, due to failure of adjustment of the circulation.

Dehydration. This is usually caused by insufficient water intake to compensate for evaporative water losses. Infants in the tropics are particularly prone to develop this condition. Normal food and salt intake replaces the salt loss but not the fluid deficit. There is a decrease in blood and ECF volume and an increase in ECF osmotic pressure. The pulse rate is high and is closely related to the degree of dehydration. Death occurs as a result of cell damage brought about by abnormally high osmotic pressure and heatstroke. It is of particular importance to be aware of this in the management of dehydrated children in the tropics. High salt or sugar intake without adequate hydration can be fatal.

Salt deficiency. Salt-deficiency heat exhaustion is due to excessive loss of chloride after profuse sweating, accompanied by water intake without salt replacement. Fatigue and dizziness develop, together with muscle cramps. These are painful muscle spasms of limbs and abdominal muscles. Salt depletion and heat exhaustion occur in unacclimatized individuals or workers in hot environments, e.g. boilers, bakeries, the iron industry and mining in the tropics.

The salt-deficiency syndrome presents itself more often without muscle cramps. The osmotic pressure of ECF is low, which results in movement of water to the intracellular compartment. This affects muscle fibres. The kidneys continue to secrete urine. Salt conservation by the kidney is accompanied by an increase in urea reabsorption; hence there is usually a rise in blood urea.

Prevention and treatment of this condition depend on adequate salt intake.

Disturbances due to cold

Hypothermia

Hypothermia is clinically defined as a drop of body temperature to 35°C or less. Exposure to cold affects old people and babies more often than it does other age-groups. It is generally easier to raise the body temperature than to lower it. This is due to the efficiency of shivering. Therefore, the dangers of hypothermia in the general public are much less than heatstroke when extremes of climatic conditions prevail.

The elderly and newborn babies are particularly prone to suffer from cold exposure. In the elderly, there is evidence that the sensation of cold develops less readily than in young adults. There is also an impairment of the shivering response and a disturbance of vasomotor responses, suggesting deterioration in autonomic functions. On the other hand, newborn babies do not have a shivering response but they can produce heat from brown fat, as described before.

However, it is important to remember that, even at normal room temperatures in the tropics, a newborn or a premature infant can lose enough heat overnight to develop fetal hypothermia.

Swimmers can remain in cold water for 10–20 hours without developing hypothermia. This is achieved in two ways: (i) a well-developed layer of subcutaneous fat, which acts as an efficient insulator; and (ii) a high rate of heat production due to muscular work. However, if fatigue sets in, the swimmer becomes slower and can rapidly lose heat.

Hypothermia causes mental confusion and visual hallucinations. First there is skeletal muscle weakness. When the body temperature falls to 33°C or below, shivering stops, and consciousness becomes affected at 32°C. At 30°C the patient becomes completely unconscious. When rewarmed, patients usually recover completely.

Cold injury

Freezing of the extremities (e.g. fingers and toes) occurs at temperatures appreciably below zero. This is due to the high salt content of cell water. When freezing occurs for more than a few minutes, permanent damage to tissues occurs. This is known as frostbite. Vasomotor control of the extremities fails because nerve conduction stops when the temperature of the limbs drops to 9°C or less. Vasodilatation occurs with painful hyperaemia and loss of sensation.

Fever

Fevers are characterized by an elevation of core body temperature by 1–4°C due to infection. The increase in temperature may be fast or slow, depending on the nature of the infective organism. The fever of malaria, brucellosis and typhus (relapsing fever) is intermittent, with rapid rises of body temperature and periods of remission. Fevers caused by typhoid, enteric fevers, pneumonia and tuberculosis tend to be maintained at a continuous plateau.

During the course of an attack of fever, the temperature seems to be regulated, only it becomes maintained at a higher level than normal. It is believed that the regulatory centres are reset at a higher level. The mechanism of this resetting of the hypothalamic 'thermostat' is not understood. If the rise of temperature is rapid, a sensation of cold or chill is experienced by the patient. Actual shivering or rigors may occur. **Chills** and **rigors** are probably produced by skin cold receptors, due to vasoconstriction and cooling of the skin. On the other hand, blood coming from the periphery is relatively cooler than the temperature at which the hypothalamic 'thermostat' has been reset. Both peripheral and central thermoreceptors contribute to the rigors.

Inflammation
endotoxins
other pyrogenic
stimuli

Monocytes
macrophages
Kupffer cells

Interleukin-1
(endogenous pyrogen)

Preoptic
area of
hypothalamus

(Role of prostaglandins
uncertain)
Increased set-point

Fever

Fig. 12.7 The mechanism and pathogenesis of fever.

The mechanism of production of the fever response to infection has been attributed to substances called **pyrogens**, which act on the hypothalamus. Such substances are of two types:

1 Exogenous pyrogens are lipopolysaccharides of large molecular weight (several million). They are part of the cell membrane of pathogenic microorganisms. If injected into animals, exogenous pyrogens produce fever after a delay of up to 1 hour.

2 The endogenous pyrogen (EP), also known as interleukin I, is a protein molecule of about 14 000 daltons. It is produced by leucocytes, macrophages and hepatic Kupffer cells in response to bacterial endotoxins and products of tissue damage. EP acts on the preoptic area of the hypothalamus to produce resetting of the thermostat at a higher level, leading to fever (Fig. 12.7). It has such a powerful effect that an injection of a few nanograms in animals produces fever in 2–3 minutes.

Prostaglandin E₁ has been found to produce fever under experimental conditions. Aspirin blocks prostaglandin synthesis but does not inhibit fever produced by its administration. It is therefore believed that the antipyretic effect of aspirin is due to its inhibitory action on prostaglandin synthesis.

Summary

Effects of exposure to heat

Mechanisms which increase heat loss
1 Cutaneous vasodilatation—increased blood flow to the skin.
2 Increased heart rate—increased cardiac output.
3 Sweating.
4 Increased respiration (panting in animals).
5 Behavioural changes—selection of suitable clothes and assuming a stretched-out, relaxed posture to increase surface area used for heat loss.

Mechanisms which decrease heat production
1 Decreased appetite, decreased specific dynamic action of food (SDA).
2 Decreased sympathetic discharge.
3 Decreased thyroid function and BMR in the long term.
4 Decreased muscular activity (behavioural adaptation).

Effects of exposure to cold

Mechanisms which decrease heat loss
1 Cutaneous vasoconstriction—decreased skin blood flow.
2 Assuming a curled-up position to decrease the surface area exposed to cold.
3 Hair erection (horripilation) in hairy animals.

Mechanisms which increase heat production
1 Increased appetite (increased SDA).
2 Shivering.
3 Increased voluntary muscular activity (behavioural adaptation).
4 Increased secretion of catecholamines.
5 Increased thyroid function as a slow and long-term mechanism.

Further reading

1 Sherwood, L. (1997) *Human Physiology*, 3rd edn, pp. 607–617. Wadsworth, Belmont, California.
2 Guyton, A.C. & Hall, J.E. (1996) Body temperature, temperature regulation and fever. In: *Textbook of Medical Physiology*, 9th edn, pp. 911–922. Saunders, Philadelphia.
3 Ganong, F.G. (1999) Temperature regulation. In: *Review of Medical Physiology*, 18th edn, pp. 234–239. Appleton & Lange, Stamford, Connecticut.

13 / Exercise and Work Physiology

Objectives

On completion of the study of this chapter, the student should be able to:

1 Understand the physiology of muscle contraction kinetics so as to differentiate between different types of muscular exercise.

2 Identify the sources of energy and control of metabolism during exercise.

3 Describe and explain the cardiovascular and respiratory adjustments which take place during muscular exercise.

4 Understand the homoeostatic mechanisms invoked during different grades of muscular work.

5 Explain the effects of training on muscles and the supporting systems.

6 Become aware of the basis and uses of various exercise tests in clinical practice.

Introduction

Exercise physiology is concerned with the description and explanation of the changes that occur in the human body during single or repeated bouts of muscular exercise. The chemical and physical changes which take place during muscular exercise trigger numerous responses in almost all systems of the body, to respond to the increased demands on energy and oxygen and to deal with the increased production of heat and waste products.

Exercise tests are used in clinical medicine to assess the condition of patients with cardiac, vascular or lung diseases for the purpose of diagnosis and follow-up of their treatment.

Skeletal muscle

Skeletal muscle in the human body comprises more than 40% of the total body-weight. Since it is the organ needed for work, the student requires a good knowledge of its physiology. The mechanism of skeletal muscle contraction has been dealt with in Chapter 3.

There are two types of skeletal muscles: red and white. **Red muscles** usually have a large blood flow, numerous mitochondria and a high concentration of oxidative enzymes. The speed of contraction and relaxation of red muscles is slow. Red muscles are therefore suitable for *aerobic work* of moderate intensity and long duration. **White muscles,** on the other hand, contain a highly developed anaerobic enzyme system and therefore they are more suitable to perform *anaerobic work* of high intensity and short duration. However, it was found that the colour of a muscle was not necessarily a good indication of its physiological or metabolic characteristics. A better way of distinguishing between different fibre types is by making a section of a muscle and measuring the activity of oxidative enzymes by histochemical techniques. According to the sensitivity of myosin adenosine triphosphatase (ATPase) to extremes of pH, muscle is classified into at least three types of fibre: I, IIA and IIB. However, type IIA fibres are not found in appreciable amounts in humans.

Type I fibres contain high activities of enzymes of the Krebs' cycle, of free fatty acid (FFA) oxidation and of the electron-transfer chain. They also show a high content of triacylglycerols and low glycolytic capacity. Type I fibres are referred to as *slow twitch* since the time course of the maximal twitch is longer. They are also known as fatigue-resistant, a feature that depends on their capacity for FFA oxidation.

Type IIA fibres have high oxidative and glycolytic capacities with an intermediate content of triacylglycerols, whereas type IIB fibres have low oxidative and high glycolytic capacities and a low content of triacylglycerols. Type II fibres are known as *fast-twitch* fibres, type IIA fibres as fast twitch–oxidative and type IIB fast twitch–glycolytic. Therefore, red muscles contain a large number of type I fibres and white muscles a large number of type II fibres. Although it is recognized that a whole range exists

Table 13.1 Characteristics of fast- and slow-twitch muscle fibres.

Characteristics greater in fast-twitch fibres
Myosin ATPase activity
Anaerobic glycogen and glucose metabolism
Recruitment during maximal exercise of short duration

Characteristics greater in slow-twitch fibres
Activities of enzymes of the Krebs cycle and electron-
    transfer system
Activities of enzymes for fatty acid catabolism
Number of mitochondria per muscle cell
Recruitment during submaximal exercise
Number of capillaries in the muscle

between characteristically fast and slow muscle fibres, some characteristics of fast- and slow-twitch muscle fibres are shown in Table 13.1.

All muscle fibres receiving one motor nerve belong to one type. A motor neuron, together with all the muscle fibres it innervates, constitute one motor unit. The number of muscle fibres supplied by a single motor neuron is largely related to the complexity of the movement subserved. For example, the temporalis muscle, which performs only gross movements, has about 1000 fibres supplied by one neuron. On the other hand, the eye muscles, which carry out more complex movements, have around five muscle fibres innervated by one motor neuron. Muscle contraction is graded, since, as the strength of stimulation is progressively increased from threshold onwards, more and more tension is developed by single twitches (contractions). This is due to a gradual recruitment of more motor units. Ultimately, when all motor units are recruited, the maximum tension possible by separate twitches is reached. Further increase in muscle tension is possible only if the frequency of stimulation is increased, so that contractions add up and get fused (summation and tetanus; see Chapter 3).

Types of skeletal muscle contractions

There are two types of muscle contractions:

1 *Isometric contractions*. These are also called static contractions. In this type of contraction there is no change in the length of the muscle and therefore no external work is done.

2 *Isotonic contractions*. The muscle shortens to produce a given force with constant tension. The force produced in a given movement is not really constant throughout the whole range of movement. Therefore, isotonic contractions are better referred to as *isokinetic*. During isokinetic contractions the length of the muscle may be decreased and

the work is called positive (concentric) or the length may increase and the work is called negative (eccentric). The amount of work done is the product of distance times force.

The tension developed by a muscle is related to its initial length. This applies for a single fibre as well as for the whole muscle because the muscle fibres are arranged in parallel. The length at which a muscle produces maximum tension is called the resting length. Usually this is the length of the muscle in the resting state. If this length is decreased or increased, the tension developed is less. This is due to the fact that in both cases formation of cross-bridges between actin and myosin will be less efficient (see Chapter 3).

Energy sources during exercise

Adenosine triphosphate (ATP) is a high-energy compound formed inside skeletal muscle cells. In combination with adenosine diphosphate (ADP), ATP functions as a system to transfer chemical energy derived from the breakdown of metabolic fuels (e.g. carbohydrates and fats) under aerobic and anaerobic conditions. The concentration of ATP in muscle is only 5–7 μmol/g fresh muscle, which will be depleted in less than 1 second during intense muscular activity and therefore requires regeneration from ADP. The ATP/ADP system couples the cellular oxidative reactions with the contractile process which is entirely dependent on it.

The basic fuels that can supply substrates for oxidation by muscle are glucose transported from the liver via the blood, locally stored glycogen and FFA removed from the blood or, to a lesser extent, derived from triacylglycerol depots within the muscle. When oxidative energy production is insufficient, muscle makes use of anaerobic metabolism to obtain energy.

The stimulation of the myofibrillar ATPase by Ca^{2+}, which initiates the process of muscular contraction, leads to a decrease in the concentrations of ATP and an increase in those of ADP, phosphate and protons; the latter changes favour ATP synthesis. This occurs when oxidative energy production is insufficient to cover the expenditure, as in the early stages of exercise, before readjustment of the blood supply to satisfy oxygen requirements. During short periods of high-intensity exercise, regeneration of ATP is essentially anaerobic, and for this there are two metabolic pathways. The first is from phosphocreatine, which, in the presence of creatine kinase, can directly rephosphorylate ADP to ATP:

$$\text{Phosphocreatine} + \text{ADP} \leftrightarrow \text{ATP} + \text{creatine}$$

The second route is from glycogen and/or glucose, with the formation of lactate.

Energy sources

Fig. 13.1 Sources of energy for working muscles.

In prolonged heavy work, oxygen supplies may also be insufficient. In such conditions glycogen is used for energy production, leading to formation of lactate. The accumulation of lactate decreases muscle activity and decreases utilization of fat to obtain energy. However, when oxygen supplies are sufficient, more fats are used for energy. The increase in circulating fat-mobilizing hormones during exercise is important for the breakdown of triacylglycerols to FFAs, which are then oxidized.

FFAs may provide up to 65% of the energy requirements during exercise, thus sparing glycogen and blood glucose. In aerobic conditions, ADP is phosphorylated to form ATP during oxidative phosphorylation by the mitochondria.

The energy sources and metabolic pathways are given in Figs 13.1 and 13.2, respectively.

The metabolic rate

The metabolic rate is the rate of energy expenditure. Energy expenditure at complete physical and mental rest is known as the basal metabolic rate (BMR). This has been dealt with in Chapter 7.

For practical purposes, energy expenditure during exercise is measured by indirect calorimetry, i.e. calculated from the rate of oxygen consumption. This is because more than 95% of the energy produced is derived from reactions of oxygen with different energy substrates. The rates of energy expenditure at different exercise or workloads are given in Chapter 7 (see Table 7.9).

Physiological responses to exercise

Cardiovascular responses
The changes that occur in the cardiovascular system during exercise are directed to increase the amount of oxygen delivered to the working skeletal muscles to meet the increased consumption. The cardiac output is increased and consequently the blood flow to the working muscles. In

Fig. 13.2 Pathways of energy metabolism during muscular exercise. Acetyl-CoA, Acetyl coenzyme A.

addition to that, the ability of the muscles to extract oxygen from the blood also increases.

Cardiac output

Cardiac output (COP) is the product of stroke volume and heart rate. At rest it is approximately equal to 5 litres/min in a young adult.

During exercise there is a significant increase in the COP. This depends on the intensity of exercise and also on the state of training of the individual. A COP of 40 litres has been reported in an athletic individual during maximal activity. Sedentary young individuals can attain a COP of 20 litres with maximal activity. The increase in COP during exercise is attained by an increase in both heart rate and stroke volume.

Heart rate

Even before the beginning of exercise there is a considerable increase in heart rate. This is due to the effect of higher centres of the brain on the sympathetic nervous system in anticipation (expectation) of exercise. The increase in circulating catecholamines also contributes to the increase in heart rate at this stage.

When exercise starts, there is a progressive rise in heart rate. The increase in heart rate during exercise is explained by several mechanisms:

1 Receptors in joints and muscle spindles are stimulated by movement. Impulses are then transmitted from these receptors to centres in the spinal cord and then to the cardiac centres in the medulla. This results in an increase in the sympathetic discharge and a decrease in the vagal tone to the heart.

2 Catecholamines are released from the adrenal medulla due to increased sympathetic activity.

3 There is an increase in sinus rhythm due to stretch of the sinoatrial node by the increased volume of blood returning to the right atrium. The increased blood temperature also stimulates the sinoatrial node to produce a faster rhythm.

4 Muscular work results in formation of substances, such as lactic acid, which diffuse from muscle into the blood, thus decreasing the blood pH. This stimulates the peripheral chemoreceptors, which, in turn, send impulses to the cardiac centres in the medulla.

5 Stretch receptors in the lungs also send impulses to the cardiomotor centre to increase the heart rate. This occurs as a result of inhibition of the nucleus ambiguus, which is the origin of the cardiac vagal fibres.

The maximum heart rate attained during exercise varies with age. Younger individuals can attain higher heart rates than older individuals. At the age of 20 years, the maximum heart rate is approximately 210/min (beats per minute). This decreases to about 170/min at the age of 60 years. The maximum heart rate at a particular age can be derived from the following equation:

$$\text{maximum heart rate} = 210 - (0.65 \times \text{age in years})$$

Stroke volume

The stroke volume is the amount of blood pumped by each ventricle per beat. At rest it is approximately 70 ml. During exercise stroke volume may increase up to two-fold. Increased sympathetic discharge and catecholamines released from the adrenal medulla increase the force of contraction of the heart muscle, thus increasing the stroke volume. Another factor that causes a rise in stroke volume is the increased venous return, which increases the stretch of ventricular muscle fibres (Starling's law; see Chapter 5). The increase in stroke volume during exercise is greater if the exercise is performed in the supine position (e.g. swimming) compared with the erect posture. This is due to increased venous return in the former position, as a result of decreased gravitational effect.

Blood circulation

Changes in the diameter of arteries and veins occur during exercise. On the arterial side, as a result of increased sympathetic discharge, there is vasoconstriction of arterioles supplying visceral structures. However, both the adrenaline secreted by the adrenal medulla and the sympathetic cholinergic nerves supplying skeletal muscle vessels cause dilatation of these vessels. An important contribution to vasodilatation in working muscle is due to the build-up of vasodilator metabolites. Therefore, skeletal muscle receives most of the cardiac output (Table 13.2). On the venous side during exercise, there is a decrease in the volume of blood contained in the veins. This is brought about by two mechanisms, namely: (i) the working muscles compress the deep veins (muscle pump); and (ii) sympathetic venoconstriction, leading to an increased venous return.

Visceral blood flow. From the above discussion, it is seen that the blood flow to the splanchnic area and kidneys is decreased during exercise. A significant reduction of the blood flow to these areas occurs when exercise of about 30% of the individual's maximum capacity is performed.

Coronary blood flow. The coronary arteries dilate as a result of low partial pressure of O_2 (P_{O_2}), increased P_{CO_2} and increased adenosine, lactic acid and H^+ ion concentrations. All these metabolites accumulate as a result of muscular

Table 13.2 Cardiac output distribution at rest and during heavy muscular exercise.

	Rest (%)	Heavy exercise (%)
Cardiac output	5 litres/min	25 litres/min
Skin	5	*
Muscle	15	80
Liver and gastrointestinal tract	20	3.5
Kidneys	20	2.5
Heart	4.5	4.5
Brain	15	3.5
Adipose tissue	10	1
Bone	3.5	0.5

* Skin blood flow depends on the ambient temperature and status of core body-temperature regulation.

exercise. Dilatation of the coronary arteries increases the amount of oxygen transported to the cardiac muscle, which depends almost completely on aerobic metabolism.

Skin blood flow. The heat produced during exercise is lost mainly through the skin by the various physical processes (radiation, convection, evaporation). This results from dilatation of skin blood-vessels, which transfers heat from the body core to the shell.

Cerebral blood flow. This is not usually affected by moderate exercise. Autoregulation of the cerebral circulation safeguards against major fluctuations due to redistribution of the cardiac output and changes in blood pressure.

Arterial blood pressure

Blood pressure is the product of cardiac output and peripheral resistance. The cardiac output increases during exercise, leading to a rise in systolic blood pressure. However, diastolic blood pressure, which depends on peripheral resistance, remains constant. This is due to the fact that, although there is constriction of some vascular beds, there is also dilatation of other vascular beds.

Arteriovenous (a-v) O_2 difference

In addition to the adjustments in cardiac output and local blood flow in the various tissues, the working muscle extracts more O_2 from the blood. In exercise the O_2 extraction rises, but rather slowly compared with the increase in the cardiac output. Maximal extraction of the order of 13–16 ml O_2/100 ml of blood has been reported. This is

about three times the resting a-v O_2 difference (5–6 ml O_2/100 ml).

Summary of cardiovascular responses

1 Oxygen consumption increases as a result of an increase in cardiac output and extraction of oxygen by skeletal muscle.

2 An increase in cardiac output is achieved by an increase in both heart rate and stroke volume.

3 The skeletal muscles receive most of the cardiac output due to arteriolar dilatation in response to increased metabolic products. Arterioles in viscera constrict, allowing the shift of most of the cardiac output to skeletal muscles.

4 Systolic blood pressure (BP) rises but diastolic BP remains constant.

Respiratory responses

Pulmonary ventilation increases in response to exercise so that it provides the necessary gas exchange. At rest pulmonary ventilation is about 6 litres/min and the amount of oxygen consumed by all tissues is about 250 ml/min. When oxygen consumption increases to 3000 ml/min during exercise, ventilation increases to 80–100 litres/min. Athletes can attain pulmonary ventilation of 150–200 litres/min with maximal physical effort.

During physical work of low intensity, ventilation is increased mainly by an increase in tidal volume. But with heavy physical work the frequency of ventilation (respiratory rate) also increases.

The mechanisms by which pulmonary ventilation increases during exercise are not fully understood. There are only slight changes in Po_2, Pco_2 and pH. These are not sufficient to explain the great change in pulmonary ventilation. The arterial blood pH remains constant during light and moderate exercise. During heavy exercise the pH falls and ventilation is further stimulated by the increased H^+ concentration. However, it is clear that none of the above mechanisms can account for the marked increase in pulmonary ventilation during moderate and light exercise.

Other stimuli have been suggested, such as psychic stimuli and impulses from receptors situated in muscles and joints. These stimuli are probably responsible for the rapid rise in pulmonary ventilation during the first few seconds of exercise.

Other contributing factors include a possible increase in the sensitivity of the chemoreceptors to small changes in Pco_2 and Po_2 and an increased response to the increase in core body temperature during exercise. Another theory holds that radiation of impulses from the cerebral cortex or hypothalamus may be responsible for stimulation of the

Fig. 13.3 Graphic representation of the changes in ventilation during moderate exercise plotted against time. (Adapted from Rhoades, R.A. & Pflanzer, R.G. (1989) Physiology of exercise. In: *Human Physiology*, pp. 841–853. Saunders College Publications, Orlando, Florida.)

respiratory centre, thus serving as a link between central neural mechanisms and working muscle. None of the theories so far proposed is completely satisfactory.

Figure 13.3 shows the changes in ventilation during moderate steady-state exercise. At the beginning of exercise (stage I) there is a sharp rise in ventilation. This is due to neural control mechanisms. In stage II there is a slower rise in ventilation and at stage III the steady state is reached. The slower rise in stages II and III is due to humoral stimuli.

Metabolic and hormonal changes

The plasma levels of most of the hormones are affected by exercise. A brief account of the response of various hormones to exercise is presented in this section:

1 *Antidiuretic hormone (ADH)*. There is increased secretion of ADH in response to exercise for the purpose of conserving body water. This effect is particularly noticed when an individual performs exercise in a dehydrated state.

2 *Growth hormone (GH)*. There is increased secretion of GH during exercise in the postabsorptive state. This serves the purpose of mobilizing fatty acids from adipose tissue to be used as a source of energy. GH takes about 1 hour to produce its fat-mobilizing action, so it is particularly important in prolonged exercise.

3 *Thyroid-stimulating hormone (TSH)*. An increased plasma level of TSH is noticed even before exercise begins, i.e. in anticipation of exercise.

4 *Cortisol*. An increase in cortisol secretion occurs, particularly in severe exercise, and may be due to an increase in adrenocorticotrophic hormone (ACTH) secretion. The expected stress of strenuous exercise may be the factor responsible for stimulation of cortisol secretion.

5 *Catecholamines*. A rise in plasma levels of catecholamines occurs at an exercise intensity of about 60% of maximum. The increased plasma adrenaline causes mobilization of fatty acids and also increases blood glucose level.

6 *Insulin*. Plasma insulin level decreases significantly after exercise. Two mechanisms are involved in this, namely, decreased secretion by the pancreas and increased uptake by skeletal muscles. In view of the antipolytic and antiglycogenolytic actions of insulin, this decrease creates favourable conditions for more FFA mobilization and glycogenolysis.

7 *Glucagon*. There is no change in plasma concentration of glucagon in exercise that lasts up to half an hour, but its level increases three times in prolonged exercise lasting about 1 1/2 hours.

It can be seen from the above discussion that during prolonged exercise, glucose production is increased, as a result of increased secretion of catecholamines, glucagon and cortisol, while insulin levels fall. Following a period of exercise, muscle glycogen is restored from dietary sources under the influence of insulin or from hepatic gluconeogenesis. In skeletal muscle the importance of FFA oxidation is to spare the glycogen stores to some extent, although it does not completely replace glucose as an energy source. FFAs provide energy at a rate of about 6 kcal/min. The rest of the energy must come from glucose. During moderate exercise this presents no problem but, when work intensity increases acutely, the release of FFAs can supply only about 65% of an individual's maximum capacity. So, in very severe exercise, glycogen stores set the limit for the capacity to undertake prolonged exercise.

The contribution of the different fuel supplies to the total energy output by the muscle will vary with both the intensity and the duration of the exercise and will be further influenced by the fitness of the individual, the nutritional status both before and during exercise, the level of anxiety and even the environment. Morphological differences between individuals in their muscle fibre make-up may also affect their use of the different fuels available during standard exercise.

Summary of the metabolic and hormonal responses

1 The blood level of the following hormones increases: ADH, growth hormone, TSH, cortisol, catecholamines and glucagon, causing an increase in blood glucose.

2 The insulin level decreases.

3 After exercise, muscle glycogen is restored by insulin.

4 FFAs play a glucose-sparing role.

Blood responses

Intense exercise causes leucocytosis. The white blood cell (WBC) count increases up to 25 000/mm^3. Haemoconcentration may partly explain this rise, but more important is the washing of WBCs from their storage areas in bone marrow, spleen, liver and lungs. In addition to this, there is increased secretion of interleukin-I due to increased activity of macrophages.

Steady-state exercise

Oxygen consumption rises gradually during the first 2–3 minutes of exercise. There is a similar response of the heart rate, cardiac output and pulmonary ventilation. Then a state is reached when all these parameters remain constant up to the end of exercise. This is called steady-state exercise. During the steady state the oxygen requirements of the tissues equal the oxygen uptake.

This explains the phenomenon of second wind, in which respiration becomes much easier and the athlete can continue in the performance of the exercise without increased breathlessness. The rate of lactic acid removal equals the rate of its production and O_2 consumption is matched by its supply. This is due to adequate cardiovascular and respiratory adjustments.

At the end of exercise, oxygen uptake declines gradually until it reaches the resting level. More oxygen is required to repay what is called the *oxygen debt*, which is defined as the oxygen uptake during the recovery period after exercise in excess of the oxygen uptake at rest (Fig. 13.4). This excess oxygen is mainly used for removal of lactic acid, to restore ATP and myoglobin oxygenation in skeletal muscle and to satisfy the increased metabolic demands of the heart and respiratory muscles during the recovery period. The term *oxygen deficit* is defined as the difference between the theoretical oxygen requirement of a given physical activity and the oxygen actually used during exercise.

Exercise testing

In this section, a brief description of the various methods used for the assessment of physical fitness is presented. Special emphasis is given to the use of exercise testing for clinical purposes.

Two types of exercise tests are in current use: (i) tests of maximal capacity; and (ii) submaximal tests.

Tests of maximal capacity

The aim of tests of maximal capacity is to determine the maximum ability of the individual to perform muscular work. This can be measured directly or indirectly. In the direct method, the maximum oxygen uptake (max. Vo_2) is measured. Max. Vo_2 is defined as the highest oxygen uptake an individual can attain, breathing air at sea level. When estimated under standardized conditions, max. Vo_2 measures the capacity of the cardiovascular system to transport oxygen to the working muscles and the ability of the muscles to consume oxygen. Max. Vo_2 is a very reproducible characteristic of the individual (Fig. 13.5).

Submaximal tests

There are many types of submaximal tests. Those described below are the ones that are most frequently used.

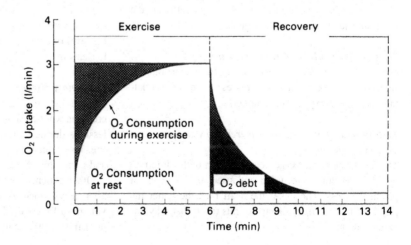

Fig. 13.4 Oxygen consumption during exercise and recovery, showing the oxygen debt.

Fig. 13.5 The relationship between oxygen consumption and the heart rate at three workloads. The extrapolated broken line is extended up to a heart rate of 185/min (the maximum heart rate) and the O_2 consumption of 3.3 litres/min is taken as the maximum Vo_2.

Tests in which both heart rate and oxygen consumption are measured

Tests measuring both heart rate and oxygen consumption are based upon the following principles:

1 The relationship between heart rate and oxygen consumption is linear throughout all workloads, including the maximum levels of work.

2 All subjects within the same age-group show a similar maximum heart rate.

The subject performs progressive workloads but is not taken to the max. Vo_2. Max. Vo_2 is predicted from the relationship between heart rate and Vo_2 by extrapolation to the maximum heart rate for his/her age (see Fig. 13.5).

Tests in which only heart rate is measured

Max. Vo_2 is predicted mathematically from heart rates at submaximal workloads by using regression equations relating heart rate to oxygen consumption.

Tests in which heart rate is measured at a standard oxygen consumption

The heart rate at an oxygen consumption of 1.0 litre/min or 1.5 litres/min is recorded and used as the index of physical fitness. The lower the heart rate, the better the physical fitness. The advantage of this test is that it avoids extrapolation.

Performance-scoring tests

In performance-scoring tests the score of physical fitness is the heart rate at a certain submaximal workload, i.e. the amount of work done at a specified heart rate is the index of physical fitness.

In other tests, the heart rate obtained after exercise (during recovery) is used to obtain the physical fitness score. The Harvard step test has been used extensively to assess manual and factory workers. It consists of the subject stepping up and down a stool until he/she is exhausted. The score is then calculated as follows:

$$score = \frac{duration\ of\ exercise}{2\ (P_1 + P_2 + P_3)}$$

where P_1, P_2 and P_3 are the pulse rates at: 1–1.5, 2–2.5 and 4–4.5 min, respectively. The higher the score, the more physically fit the individual is considered.

The use of exercise tests in clinical practice

It appears from the above that exercise can test the cardiorespiratory capacity to transport oxygen to the working muscles. This fact is made use of in disease conditions related to the respiratory and cardiovascular systems.

Cardiovascular disease

Exercise testing is used to confirm diagnosis and assess the severity of ischaemic heart disease (electrocardiogram (ECG) stress test). ECG changes are related to the level of exercise (walking at different speeds and inclinations on a treadmill). Particular notice is given to various arrhythmias and inversion of the T wave. The Bruce exercise test protocol is used for this purpose. In addition, the test is used to screen the population in order to identify those who are at risk of developing ischaemic heart disease or sudden death.

Exercise testing is also used to assess the severity of arterial disease in the leg. A treadmill walking test will identify the level of exercise that brings claudication (leg pain due to ischaemia).

Pulmonary disease

Patients with restrictive lung disease show a marked decrease in work capacity. Some patients complain of breathlessness during performance of heavy work in their daily life. To establish a diagnosis, an exercise test is carried out and symptoms of bronchospasm are looked for.

Other patients complain of breathlessness that persists after heavy work. To confirm that, the forced expiratory volume in 1 second (FEV_1) or peak expiratory flow is measured after 6–20 minutes of exercise.

Table 13.3 Some uses of exercise tests.

Cardiovascular system
Prediction of heart disease and surveys of
  cardiorespiratory fitness
Assessment of ischaemic heart disease for diagnosis
  and follow-up
Follow-up on drug therapy, e.g. in hypertensive patients
In rehabilitation, to restore patients' confidence after
  myocardial infarction
Assessment of peripheral vascular disease, e.g.
  intermittent claudication

Respiratory system
Assessment of exercise tolerance
Investigation of dyspnoea or hypoxia
Investigation of alveolar ventilation

Muscles
Assessment of muscle disorders

A summary of the uses of exercise tests is given in
Table 13.3.

Further reading

1 McArdle, W.D., Katch, F.I. & Katch, V.L. (1996) *Exercise Physiology: Energy, Nutrition and Human Performance*, 7th edn. Williams & Wilkins, Baltimore.
2 Guyton, A.C. (1997) Sports physiology. In: *Textbook of Medical Physiology*, 9th edn, pp. 1059–1069. Saunders, Philadelphia.
3 Noble, B.J. (1986) *Physiology of Exercise and Sport*. Mosby College Publishers, St Louis.

14 / Physiology of Human Reproduction

Objectives

Upon completion of the study of this chapter, the student should:

1 Understand the neural and hormonal mechanisms concerned with the control of various reproductive functions.

2 Describe and explain the changes which occur at puberty and adolescence to be able to diagnose defects of sexual maturation.

3 Describe and explain the cyclic changes in the human ovary and uterus so as to recognize abnormalities of the menstrual cycle.

4 Understand the neural and hormonal mechanisms which control the sexual act so to be able to recognize deviations from the normal.

5 Become aware of some common abnormalities of reproductive functions so as to pursue further study of their underlying pathology and management.

Introduction

There are similarities as well as differences in male and female reproductive functions. Both are controlled by neural and hormonal mechanisms and both produce *gametes* containing one-half of a set of chromosomes. This chapter is concerned with the functions of the reproductive system in males and females. A knowledge of the anatomy of the reproductive organs is essential.

Reproductive functions in the male consist of: (i) **spermatogenesis**, i.e. production of sperms; and (ii) deposition of sperm in the reproductive tract of the female. On the other hand, the reproductive functions in females are far more involved: (i) **oogenesis** or production of ova; (ii) reception and transport of sperm and ovum to achieve **fertilization**; (iii) **gestation** or pregnancy, which includes the formation and functions of the **placenta**; (iv) **parturition** or giving birth; and (v) **lactation** or breast-feeding. The last three of these functions will be discussed in Chapter 15.

Hormonal control of reproduction

The hormonal control of reproduction in males and females is determined by the interaction of three glands: the **hypothalamus**, the **anterior pituitary** and the gonads—the **ovaries** in females and the **testes** in males.

The gonads secrete the sex steroid hormones—**oestrogen** and **progesterone** in females, and **testosterone** in males. These are the main hormones responsible for the sexual characteristics and regulation of reproductive function of males and females. The interrelationship between the hypothalamic–pituitary–gonadal system can be summarized as follows.

The hypothalamus secretes a decapeptide hormone, known as **gonadotrophin-releasing hormone (GnRH)**. GnRH reaches the anterior pituitary along the hypothalamic pituitary portal vessels. It acts on the anterior pituitary

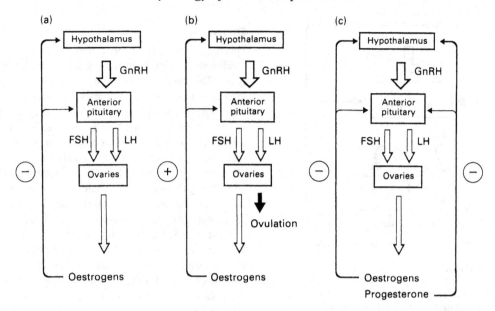

Fig. 14.1 Feedback effects of oestrogens and progesterone on the hypothalamic–pituitary axis. (a) Negative feedback in the proliferative phase. (b) Positive feedback in the preovulatory phase. (c) Negative feedback in the luteal phase.

to increase the synthesis, storage and secretion of the gonadotrophins: **luteinizing hormone (LH)** and **follicle-stimulating hormone (FSH)**. The gonadotrophins are normally secreted in a pulsatile manner every 60–120 min. Both FSH and LH act directly on the gonads to stimulate sex steroid hormone secretion (see Chapter 9). Other endocrine glands are also required for normal reproductive function, e.g. the thyroid and adrenal cortex. Higher cerebral centres have important influences on the normal development and functions of the hypothalamic–pituitary axis. Therefore, factors such as nervous stress and social or mental disorders can affect normal maturity and functions of the reproductive organs.

The differences between females and males do not only lie in the type of sex steroid hormones secreted, but also in the pattern of secretion of hypothalamic–pituitary gonadotrophins and the relationship between the gonads and the hypothalamic–pituitary system.

Female sex hormone regulation

During the female's reproductive life, gonadotrophins are secreted in a cyclic pattern and they regulate the menstrual cycle. In males gonadotrophins have no such pattern.

Another important feature is the effect of sex hormones on the anterior pituitary gonadotrophin secretion, known as the feedback mechanism, which controls pituitary gonadotrophin hormone secretion. FSH acts on the Graafian

follicles, promoting their growth and maturation until at least one ovum is produced. The maturing follicles produce *oestrogens*. On the other hand, LH maintains the *corpus luteum*, formed after ovulation, which secretes *progesterone*.

High oestrogen levels suppress the hypothalamic–pituitary unit by inhibiting FSH secretion (negative feedback) (Fig. 14.1), while having little effect on LH secretion except at mid-cycle, when the high level of oestrogen induces the LH surge (*positive feedback*). Also, progesterone feedback at mid-cycle enhances the LH surge (positive feedback). In the luteal phase, the high level of progesterone acts with oestrogen to inhibit gonadotrophin secretion (negative feedback).

Male sex hormone regulation

In males testosterone from the Leydig cells of the testes is the main sex hormone. It has a negative feedback on pituitary gonadotrophins, thus inhibiting both FSH and LH. However, testosterone has a specific negative feedback effect on LH-secreting cells in the anterior pituitary. Therefore its effect in suppressing the gonadotrophins is stronger on LH inhibition. **Inhibin** produced by Sertoli cells in the testes, is responsible for the feedback regulation of the pituitary FSH hormone (Fig. 14.2). The roles of these hormones in the control of reproductive function are discussed later in this chapter.

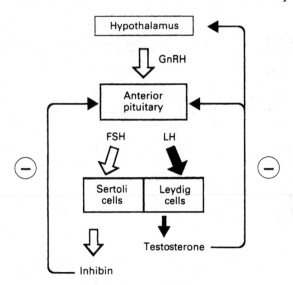

Fig. 14.2 Feedback by testicular hormones testosterone and inhibin to the hypothalamus and the anterior pituitary.

Puberty

Puberty is the period of maturation which follows childhood. At puberty many physiological changes take place. The most important are acceleration of somatic growth, development of secondary sexual characteristics and attainment of reproductive capacity. They are mainly due to increased secretion of the sex steroid hormones, testosterone in males and oestrogens in females. The changes at puberty occur over a period of 2–4 years, usually between the ages of 11 and 15 in boys and between 9 and 13 in girls (Fig. 14.3). **Adolescence** is another term which refers to the period between childhood and maturity; it usually extends between the ages of 10 and 19.

The exact mechanisms which initiate gonadal function at puberty are not known. But during childhood it seems that the pituitary is very sensitive to the normally detectable very low levels of sex steroid hormones, testosterone (in males) and oestrogens (in females). There is evidence that the pineal gland, which releases the hormone **melatonin**, may be involved in prepubertal inhibition of hypothalamic gonadotrophin-releasing hormone (GnRH) secretion. With the onset of puberty the hypothalamic–

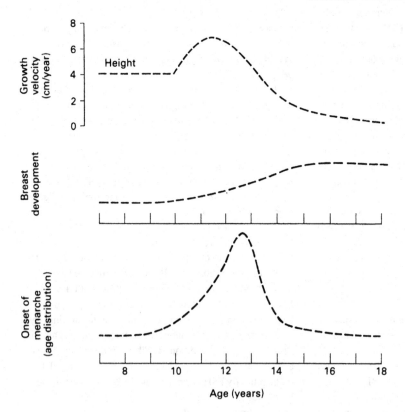

Fig. 14.3 Diagram showing timing of some of the main changes of puberty in females.

pituitary system starts to mature; it seems to become less sensitive to the inhibitory effect of gonadal steroids. The pulsatile secretions of GnRH start to appear and consequently gonadotrophins are secreted by the anterior pituitary, which, in turn, stimulate secretion of the sex steroids by the gonads. The mechanism of hypothalamic maturation is not fully understood, but it is also related to higher centres in the nervous system, which control the pulsatile secretion of the hypothalamic GnRH. Many factors affect the onset of puberty, including psychological, social, nutritional and environmental factors.

Various changes, somatic and sexual, occur at puberty. It is important to recognize these features in order to be able to diagnose abnormalities.

The adolescent growth spurt

In childhood the growth curve normally runs steeply during the first 2 years and then becomes less rapid until puberty starts, when it suddenly becomes steep again. This acceleration of growth is termed the adolescent or *puberty spurt*. In girls the peak is around 12 years of age; in boys it is about 2 years later. It does not begin at the same time in all parts of the body, e.g. the trunk reaches its maximal growth rate about 6 months after the legs.

Development of secondary sex characteristics

In males secondary sex characteristics depend on testosterone secretion. They consist of the following: (i) *male body configuration*, i.e. broad shoulders and development of skeletal muscles; (ii) *hair growth* on the face and chest; (iii) the voice becomes deep (low pitch) due to growth of the larynx and elongation and thickening of the vocal cords (in females the voice remains high-pitched due to lack of laryngeal growth); (iv) thickening of the skin; and (v) the hairline begins to recede, widening the forehead; this may proceed to the development of male baldness in those who are genetically predisposed.

In females the secondary sex characteristics are due to secretion of oestrogens. They consist of: (i) the *development of breasts*; and (ii) the deposition of *body fat* in certain parts, resulting in the characteristic rounded female figure. Other features of female puberty, such as the *growth spurt*, the growth of *axillary* and pubic hair and the development of the libido are due to increased *adrenal androgens* (mainly *dehydroepiandrosterone* (DHEA)) at puberty.

Development of the reproductive organs

There is genital growth in both sexes. The genitalia increase in size and start to show functional manifestations.

In females the vulva takes an adult appearance, with growth of both labia majora and labia minora. The vagina becomes rugose and takes a mature histological appearance, as the thickness of its lining epithelium increases. The vaginal discharge (made of vascular transudation, cervical discharge and desquamated epithelial lining) becomes acidic (pH 4.5), as it contains lactic acid. The acid comes from the breakdown of glycogen present in the vaginal epithelium by *Döderlein's bacilli*, which invade the vagina at puberty and become normal inhabitants. The increased thickness of the vaginal epithelium and the low pH of its secretions are protective mechanisms against ascending infection.

The uterus

In childhood the cervix is about twice the length of the uterine body. During puberty the body of the uterus grows so that it increases to about twice the length of the cervix. Its muscle fibres also increase in bulk. The cervical glands secrete a mucoid secretion. The lining of the uterus, the endometrium, proliferates under the effect of oestrogens and subsequently responds to progesterone. These cycles are responsible for the onset of menstruation (menarche).

Attainment of reproductive capacity

In females signs of maturation of the ovaries start with menstruation but attainment of reproductive capacity is complete when ovulation actually starts. *In males* the production of sperm (spermatogenesis) is essential for attainment of reproductive capacity.

Menarche and ovulation

The word menarche is defined as the age at which the first menstruation takes place. This usually occurs when the hypothalamic–pituitary–ovarian axis matures sufficiently for the ovary to secrete some oestrogen, so as to induce endometrial development followed by some bleeding.

However, menarche does not mean fertility, since it can take 1–2 years before oogenesis and ovulation occur. During this time, cycles are often anovulatory (see ovulation and regulation of menstruation).

Spermatogenesis

Spermatogenesis means the formation of the male germ cells or mature sperm. As with oogenesis in females, spermatogenesis in males is a sign of reproductive maturity. It takes about 74 days to form a mature sperm from a primitive germ cell (Fig. 14.4). The formation of sperm takes place in three phases (Table 14.1).

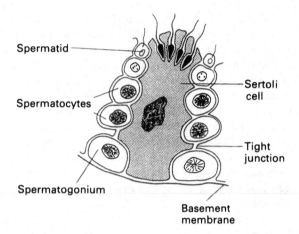

Fig. 14.4 Diagram of a cross-section in a seminiferous tubule showing the phases of sperm maturation. Note the close proximity of the Sertoli cells in relation to the developing spermatocytes.

The first phase. The primitive germ cells (**spermatogonia**) replicate by **mitotic division** and produce several generations of **primary spermatocytes**.

The second phase. The primary spermatocytes undergo a **meiotic** or **reduction division** so that each will form two haploid **secondary spermatocytes** (each having 23 chromosomes). These cells remain at rest for some time, during which the 23 chromosomes replicate, resulting in 23 double-strand chromosomes. A second maturation division occurs, resulting in four haploid **spermatids** arising from

every primary spermatocyte. It has been estimated that 16 spermatids are formed from one spermatogonium. Spermatids have 23 single-strand chromosomes each and no further division takes place after this stage.

The third phase. The spermatids develop into spermatozoa. During sperm maturation the four spermatids remain attached to each other by cytoplasmic bridges. These bridges enable sharing of products between X-bearing and Y-bearing sperms. X chromosomes have the genes needed for cell products essential for sperm maturation. In the absence of such cytoplasmic bridges, Y-bearing sperms cannot mature.

The mature sperm will have shed most of its cytosol, which is not needed for fertilization. The **head** of the sperm consists mainly of the nucleus. The tip of the head acquires an **acrosome** layer, which contains enzymes necessary for penetration of the ovum. The **midpiece** of the sperm contains mitochondria, which generate the energy needed for **tail** motility.

Throughout the stages of maturation, spermatozoa remain in close proximity to **Sertoli cells** and are surrounded by their cytoplasm. These are large cells which span the distance from the basement membrane of the seminiferous tubule to its lumen. Neighbouring Sertoli cells are attached to each other by **tight junctions**, which temporarily separate to allow passage of the spermatocytes towards the lumen of the tubuli.

The composition of fluid in the tubular lumen is different from that of plasma. It has high concentrations of K^+,

Table 14.1 Summary of the stages of spermatogenesis.

Stages	Cell development	Chromosomes
Mitotic division	*Spermatogonium* gives rise to two spermatogonia	46
	One remains to maintain the germ-cell continuity	46
	The other daughter cell migrates towards the lumen of the seminiferous tubule and divides *mitotically* to give rise to four *primary spermatocytes*	46
Meiotic division	Primary spermatocytes divide *meiotically* to give rise to secondary spermatocytes	23
	These replicate their chromosomes before division	23 (double)
	They have a second haploid division giving rise to four *spermatids*	23 (single)
Maturation	Spermatids shed cytosol Spermatids develop head, acrosome, midpiece and tail	23 (single)

Table 14.2 Summary of the functions of the Sertoli cells.

Blood–testes barrier: the tight junctions maintain critical composition of tubular fluid for sperm maturation and prevent antigenic material produced during sperm maturation from reaching the blood
Secrete fluid for carrying sperm into the epididymis
Provide nutrients for maturing sperm
Produce androgen-binding protein (ABP), which maintains the high androgen level needed for continued sperm production
Phagocytic function for cytosol extruded from maturing sperm; phagocytosis of debris of sperm which do not mature
Secrete *inhibin*, a hormone which acts by negative feedback to inhibit FSH secretion from the anterior pituitary

Table 14.3 Summary of the functions of the male reproductive system.

Testes	Germ cell: sperm production Sertoli cell: sperm maturation and production of *inhibin*. Production of ABP Leydig cell: Secretes testosterone
Epididymis	Receives sperm and Sertoli cell secretion under pressure Sperms are stored, mature and gain motility in epididymis Concentration of sperm by absorbing fluid
Vas deferens	Carries semen from epidiymis to the ejaculatory ducts (within the *prostate*), which empty into the urethra Stores concentrated sperm until ejaculation
Seminal vesicles	Secrete the larger part of seminal fluid with *fructose* for sperm nourishment after ejaculation Secrete prostaglandins Secrete fibrinogen for seminal clotting
Prostate	Secretion provides alkaline medium for sperm; helps neutralize vaginal secretions Produces clotting enzymes, which initiate seminal coagulation in vagina soon after ejaculation
Bulbourethral glands	Produce mucus during sexual arousal for lubrication during intercourse

glutamic acid, aspartic acid and inositol, as well as high levels of androgens and oestrogens. On the other hand, it has low levels of glucose and protein. This is explained by the presence of a **blood–testes barrier**, which prevents free exchange. It is believed that the barrier is due to tight junctions between the Sertoli cells near the basal lamina of the seminiferous tubules (Table 14.2). This barrier may serve the purpose of preventing harmful substances (e.g. drugs) in the blood from reaching the lumen. Conversely, it prevents products formed during cell division, which may be antigenic, from reaching the bloodstream and causing an autoimmune reaction.

Endocrine control of spermatogenesis. The hormones responsible for spermatogenesis are **testosterone** and two anterior pituitary hormones, **LH** and **FSH**. LH and FSH are under control of spontaneous pulses of GnRH from the hypothalamus, which occur every 2–3 hours, causing a similar pulsatile pattern of pituitary gonadotrophin secretion. The role of anterior pituitary hormones in males is as important as in females. LH acts mainly on the Leydig cells of the testes to stimulate the production of testosterone, the main androgen responsible for the development and maintenance of secondary sexual characteristics and normal sexual activity in males. The target of FSH is mainly the Sertoli cells of the seminiferous tubules of the testes. In response to both testosterone and FSH, the Sertoli cells produce a high-affinity **androgen-binding protein (ABP)**, which maintains the high androgen content within the seminiferous tubules, an essential factor for normal spermatogenesis. Testosterone is essential for the germ-cell divisions resulting in the spermatids, while FSH acts on the Sertoli cells for completion of the subsequent

stages resulting in the maturation of the sperm. The Sertoli cells also secrete **inhibin**, which controls FSH release by negative feedback.

The functions of the male reproductive system are summarized in Table 14.3.

The menstrual cycle

The menstrual cycle is a term used to describe the monthly cycle of physiological events which prepare the female for pregnancy. The cycle ends in menstruation if pregnancy does not occur. The duration of an average normal menstrual cycle is 28 days from the onset of one menses (period) to the next, with a range of 21–35 days.

The ovarian cycle

Each month a few primordial follicles start to grow in response to the rising level of pituitary follicle-stimulating

Fig. 14.5 Schematic representation of the ovulatory cycle showing the pituitary hormones and ovarian hormone secretion levels during the phases of the ovarian cycle.

hormone (FSH) (Fig. 14.5). Most will undergo atresia, while usually only one 'leading' follicle will continue development to be able to respond to LH and thereby progress to ovulation. The functional and morphological changes which occur in the ovaries and ovarian follicles during the menstrual cycle may be divided into three stages:

1 Follicular development.
2 The ovulatory process.
3 The luteal phase.

Follicular development

Follicular development involves changes in the three components of the primordial follicles: the oocyte, the granulosa cells and the theca cell layers.

The **granulosa cells** proliferate to form several layers, with fluid spaces appearing between cells. These spaces eventually join to form a single fluid-filled space or antrum. The granulosa cells respond to FSH by synthesizing oestrogen hormone.

The **oocyte** enlarges and becomes surrounded by a **zona pellucida**, a mucopolysaccharide layer and some layers of granulosa cells, known as the **cumulus oophorus**.

The **theca cells** differentiate into a well-vascularized theca interna and less vascularized theca externa. The theca cells respond to LH by synthesizing androgens, which normally pass to the granulosa cells to be transformed into progesterone.

During the follicular phase, the rising level of oestrogens exerts a negative feedback on FSH secretion, causing it to decline. The further increase in oestrogen level towards mid-cycle, together with the increased sensitivity of the pituitary to GnRH, exerts a positive feedback on LH and FSH secretion, causing a dramatic mid-cycle peak of LH, which begins the second phase (or ovulation).

The ovulatory process

The ovulatory process usually occurs about 24–36 hours following the LH peak, between the 12th and 15th days of a 28-day cycle. This LH surge is produced only when one follicle has matured and is secreting large amounts of oestrogen. The oestrogen triggers the LH secretion through a positive feedback mechanism. LH causes ovulation by production of prostaglandins, which induce vascular changes, causing the ovum to swell rapidly. Enzymatic digestion of the follicular wall leads to rupture and the ovum is shed. Thus the mid-cycle surge of LH terminates the follicular phase and marks the beginning of the luteal phase.

The luteal phase

After ovulation LH acts on the follicular cells, which differentiate into luteal cells, and the **corpus luteum** is formed (luteinization). The corpus luteum secretes both oestrogen and progesterone. As the levels of these two hormones increase, they inhibit the secretion of gonadotrophins by a negative feedback. If no pregnancy takes place, the corpus luteum gradually reaches the end of its life and oestrogen and progesterone levels decline. This removes the negative feedback effect from the pituitary, allowing the premenstrual rise of FSH to stimulate the maturation of more follicles for the next cycle.

The uterine cycle

The most important target for oestrogen and progesterone is the uterus. In response to the ovarian hormones, both myometrial and endometrial tissues undergo important changes in anticipation of pregnancy.

The myometrium

Oestrogen increases the uterine blood flow. Oestrogen increases and progesterone decreases myometrial activity. This effect is important, as it ensures minimum uterine muscular activity at mid-cycle and in the early luteal phase, in case of early implantation.

Endometrial changes

Within 48 hours after the period of menstruation, the surface of the endometrium is covered by epithelial outgrowth from the remnants of glands in the basal part of the endometrium. Subsequent changes in the endometrium, in response to the ovarian hormones, can usually be described under three phases: **proliferative phase**, **secretory phase** and **menstrual phase**.

The proliferative phase. This phase starts from the end of menstruation and lasts until the time of ovulation. The glands first appear tubular, lined by low columnar cells with centrally placed nuclei. Gradually, they become long and increasingly convoluted. The stromal cells increase in number and become more oedematous. The blood supply of the endometrium also grows. The basal layer is supplied by straight arteries and the superficial part is supplied by the spiral arteries.

During this period the endometrium grows from approximately 0.5 mm to 5 mm in height, a 10-fold increase. This is due to new tissue growth and to stromal expansion.

The secretory phase. This phase occupies the time from ovulation until menstruation. During this phase, progesterone is the dominant hormone and corresponds to the luteal phase of the ovary. Under the influence of progesterone, endometrial growth ceases and functional changes begin to prepare the tissues for implantation. The glands commence secretory activity, with subnuclear vacuoles appearing. They discharge their contents into the lumen of the glands. The secretion consists mainly of glycogen, sugars, amino acids, mucus and enzymes, such as alkaline phosphatase. The arteries become more prominent and increasingly coiled as they continue to grow, while the endometrium height remains relatively static.

Further changes in the late luteal phase depend on whether implantation has taken place or not:

1 *Implantation.* If pregnancy occurs, the early embryo secretes human chorionic gonadotrophin (hCG), a hormone which maintains the corpus luteum, and therefore the secretion of oestrogen and progesterone continues. Further changes in the endometrium will mainly involve the stromal cells, which differentiate into three layers: a superficial, cellular, compact layer, the **stratum compactum**; an oedematous, less cellular layer underneath, known as the **stratum spongiosum**; and a basal layer of endometrium surrounding the straight arteries, known as the **stratum basalis**. This last layer does not show much change.

2 *Non-implantation.* In the absence of implantation and chorionic gonadotrophin support, the corpus luteum declines and consequently both oestrogen and progesterone levels fall. This results in a reduction in endometrial tissue height and more coiling of the spiral arteries, with secondary stasis, ischaemia and eventual blanching of the endometrium. Local release of prostaglandins induces waves of rhythmic contractions in the spiral arteries.

Menstruation. Interstitial haemorrhages occur as a result of the breakdown of superficial arteries and capillaries. Eventually, the non-viable tissues are extruded into the uterine cavity and contribute to the menstrual flow. This process continues until all the layers, except the deep layer of the endometrium, are shed.

The menstrual flow stops in 5–7 days due to vasoconstriction of the spiral arteries and the formation of thrombin–platelet plugs. Resumption of oestrogen secretion by the new crop of developing follicles induces healing and new tissue growth.

Menstrual blood does not normally coagulate unless it is very profuse. Normally the small amounts of blood that collect in the uterus do form clots but these are immediately acted upon by fibrinolytic enzymes secreted by the damaged endometrial cells. Menstrual blood has a large number of leucocytes, which are important for defence of the raw surface of the endometrium against infection.

Changes in the cervix during the menstrual cycle

During the proliferative phase, the mucus secreted by the cervical epithelium is thin and alkaline. This facilitates entry of sperm. After ovulation, under the effect of progesterone, the mucus becomes thick and difficult to penetrate by bacteria or by sperm.

Cyclic changes in the vagina

During the proliferative phase, the vaginal epithelium becomes *cornified* under the effect of oestrogens. This is protection against abrasion during sexual intercourse before ovulation. After ovulation, progesterone increases vaginal secretions. There is proliferation of the epithelium and infiltration by leucocytes.

The sex hormones

The sex hormones are the hormones which are directly responsible for sexual differentiation and function in males and females. They are mainly produced in the gonads, i.e. the testes in males and the ovaries in females, but the adrenal glands also produce minimal amounts of sex steroid hormones in both sexes, which might have an important function before puberty and in females after the menopause.

The steroid hormones are clearly related to each other. Their main precursor is cholesterol, and they are easily converted from one to the other in the appropriate tissues, which possess the required enzymes (Fig. 14.6).

Steroid hormones are secreted in the blood and transported to the target organs bound to serum proteins. At the target organ cells, specific receptor proteins take up the steroid hormones, because their affinity to the hormones is usually much higher than that of the carrier protein. They act by entering the cell, where they become bound to a cytoplasmic protein receptor. The steroid–protein complex becomes attached to the nucleus and stimulates ribonucleic acid (RNA) synthesis, which directs protein synthesis and therefore regulates cell functions.

Oestrogens

The main natural oestrogens found in the circulation are: 17β-oestradiol, oestriol and oestrone. Oestradiol is the most active compound. It is bound to plasma proteins (60% to albumin and 37% to globulin). Oestrogens are C_{18} steroids, mainly produced by the granulosa cells in the ovaries. In pregnancy, the placenta produces a large amount of oestrogen, mainly oestriol. Oestrogens are mainly meta-

Fig. 14.6 Biosynthesis of ovarian steroids.

bolized in the liver by conjugation with glucuronic acid, and most of the conjugate (65%) is excreted in the urine.

Actions of oestrogens

Ovarian oestrogens, which begin to be secreted at puberty, are responsible for the changes that take place at that period. The target tissues include the genitalia, the uterus, the breasts and certain parts of the subcutaneous fat layers. In the breast, they promote the growth of the duct system and slight pigmentation of the areola. General growth is promoted by their anabolic action. However, they cause the epiphyses to close and therefore limit skeletal growth.

During the menstrual cycle oestrogens are responsible for proliferation of the endometrium. Oestrogens also induce the growth of uterine muscle and increase the blood flow in the uterus. The myometrium becomes more sensitive to the effect of oxytocin and its electrical activity becomes more frequent.

Cyclic oestrogen secretion results in regulation of gonadotrophic hormone release, as previously described (see Fig. 14.1). This effect has made it possible to use oestrogens in combination with progesterone as oral contraceptives for inhibition of hypothalamic and pituitary hormones and thus suppression of ovulation. Progesterone seems to potentiate the inhibitory effect of oestrogens on LH secretion.

Undesirable or adverse effects of oestrogens are seen with artificially administered oestrogens (e.g. oral contraceptives). Therefore, oestrogen administration should only be given under medical supervision. The following are common examples of these unwanted effects:

1 Water and salt retention.

2 Effects on blood clotting factors. Oestrogens increase the risk of thrombosis and thromboembolism through changes in platelet adhesiveness and increased synthesis of clotting factors.

3 Biochemical disturbances. Oestrogens increase the level of circulating plasma globulins, which bind iron, cortisol and thyroxine, leading to raised plasma levels of these substances. Like other steroids, oestrogen also disturbs carbohydrate metabolism and may result in a decreased tolerance to glucose.

A summary of the effects of oestrogens is given in Table 14.4.

Progesterone

Natural progesterone is mainly synthesized in the corpus luteum by the theca lutein cells of the follicle. During pregnancy the placenta produces a large amount of progesterone. Progesterone is a C_{21} steroid. It is also found in secreting tissues as an intermediary product in hormone synthesis. In the plasma it is bound to serum proteins (50% to albumin and 45% to transcortin). Progesterone is metabolized in the liver, converted to pregnanediol and conjugated to glucuronic acid, which eventually appears in the urine, where it can be measured in clinical investigation of pregnancy and the menstrual cycle.

Actions

The main action of progesterone is to induce secretory changes in the oestrogen-primed endometrium during the luteal phase of the menstrual cycle. These changes are

Table 14.4 Summary of the effects of oestrogens.

At puberty	Growth of female reproductive system
	Secondary sex characteristics
	Growth of duct system of the breast
On reproduction	Growth of ovarian follicles
	Proliferation of endometrium
	Increased motility of uterine tubes
	Growth of uterine muscle
	Increased uterine blood flow
	Regulation of gonadotrophins
	Sensitizes uterine muscle to oxytocin
	Lactation
Other effects	Protein-anabolic
	Increased formation of adrenal androgens
	Water retention
	Platelet adhesion—in large doses thrombosis
	Lower cholesterol
	Decreased glucose tolerance

necessary for implantation. Secretory changes also take place in the fallopian tubes. These changes provide the necessary nutrition for the fertilized ovum.

Progesterone exerts an antioestrogen effect on the endometrium by decreasing the oestrogen receptors and by increasing the rate of conversion of 17β-oestradiol to oestrogens with weaker physiological effects. Progesterone also exerts antioestrogen effects on the myometrium, making it less excitable and less sensitive to oxytocin. This is reflected in less electrical activity and a higher resting membrane potential.

In breast development, progesterone exerts its effect on the alveolar tissue and lobules, which grow in size during adolescence and subsequently during pregnancy.

During pregnancy progesterone plays an important role in the maintenance of pregnancy, as it inhibits uterine muscle activity (relaxing effect). Also, together with oestrogens, it prepares the mammary glands for lactation. It exerts a thermogenic effect, which is partially responsible for the raised basal metabolic rate (BMR) of pregnancy. It also seems to stimulate the respiratory centre, causing hyperventilation and thus lowering arterial partial pressure of CO_2 (Pco_2).

A summary of the effects of progesterone is given in Table 14.5.

Testosterone

Testosterone is mainly synthesized in the testes by the Leydig cells, which account for about 20% of the testicular

Table 14.5 Summary of the effects of progesterone.

Progestational effects on endometrium
Decreases excitability of myometrium and decreases its
  oestrogen receptors
Cyclic changes in cervix and vagina
Maintenance of pregnancy
Increases conversion of oestradiol to less active
  oestrogens
Development of breast alveoli
Prepares breast for action by prolactin
Stimulates secretions in fallopian tubes for nutrition of
  fertilized ovum

Table 14.6 Summary of the effects of testosterone.

In the fetus	Differentiation of male genital tract
	Differentiation of male external
	genitalia through DHT
	Descent of testes
At puberty	Growth and maturation of male
	reproductive system
	Development sex drive (libido)
	Secondary sexual characteristics
On reproduction	Spermatogenesis
	Libido
	Maintenance of male genital tract
	Feedback regulation of
	gonadotrophins
Other effects	Protein anabolic effect
	Bone growth at puberty
	Closure of epiphyses

mass in adults. The adrenal glands also produce some testosterone, as well as other androgens (see Chapter 9). In females some testosterone is produced by the ovarian stroma cells. Testosterone is a C_{19} steroid which is transported in the plasma bound to albumin (40%), to a β-globulin (40%) and to other proteins (17%). It acts by binding to tissues which contain 5α-reductase and is converted to dihydrotestosterone (DHT). Most of the physiological effects of testosterone are due to DHT. It is metabolized in the liver and conjugated to glucuronic acid and sulphate. Excretion takes place in the urine and bile.

Actions

Testosterone and other androgens develop and maintain the male primary and secondary sex characteristics, already described in the section on puberty. Together with FSH, testosterone is required for spermatogenesis. Androgens also have a protein anabolic effect, which is evident during the growth spurt of puberty, and, like oestrogen, testosterone causes the epiphyses to close. Normal levels of testosterone secretion are also necessary for the sex drive in the male.

A summary of the effects of testosterone is given in Table 14.6.

The menopause

Menopause is a term which describes the last period or the final cessation of menstruation. It usually occurs in the late 40s to early 50s. However, women's reproductive abilities usually decline over 2–3 years before the menopause. This period is known as the climacteric.

Physiology of the menopause

At birth the ovary contains all the germ cells that have the potential to mature into ova during a woman's reproductive life. After puberty, during each menstrual cycle, a number of follicles attempt to mature but only one reaches maturity and becomes shed at ovulation; the others degenerate to form atresic follicles. Gradually, as the woman approaches the menopause, the ovaries become depleted of oocytes and become increasingly small, until they consist mainly of fibrous tissue with no follicles.

As a consequence of ovarian ageing at the menopause, circulating oestrogens fall to very low levels. As a result of the diminished negative feedback effect of ovarian oestrogens and progesterone on the hypothalamus and the anterior pituitary, large amounts of FSH and LH are produced (up to 10 times the levels in premenopausal women). These hormones appear in blood and in urine. Measurement of gonadotrophins can be used to confirm the onset of the climacteric or menopause (Fig. 14.7).

The fall in oestrogen production causes various local and systemic effects, known as the symptoms and signs of the menopause. When severe, these manifestations are considered abnormal and require treatment. The important changes are described below.

Symptoms and signs of the menopause

Vasomotor symptoms

Vasomotor symptoms present as a sensation of warmth, which occurs on the trunk and spreads to the face. These are known as hot flushes and are usually accompanied by sweating and palpitations; they occur mainly at night. The exact cause is unknown, but it is suggested that a hypothalamic disturbance leads to the vasomotor responses associated with a burst of LH secretion. The attacks of hot flushes can be stopped by oestrogen therapy. Similar attacks have been reported in men and women after removal of the

Fig. 14.7 The pituitary–ovarian axis at the menopause.

gonads and continue after removal of the pituitary. Therefore, the hypothalamic origin of the hot flushes, as well as the LH bursts, has been postulated.

Emotional and psychological problems
The subject's attitude towards the menopause, as well as that of her husband and family, determines the extent and severity of emotional and psychological symptoms.

Skeleton
The lack of oestrogens results in increased bone resorption, associated with increased calcium and hydroxyproline excretion. Collagen is lost from other sites of the body as well as bone, namely skin and joints. It is the loss of collagen and elasticity that contributes to the overall ageing appearance. Loss of bone, particularly from the vertebrae, causes a reduction in height, with forward bending and kyphosis in extreme cases. There is an increased incidence of fractures, particularly of the neck of the femur and the distal end of the radius. Ligaments lose their elasticity, and loss of collagen leads to degenerative changes in the joints, leading to osteoarthritis.

Cardiovascular problems
Atherosclerotic changes gradually occur, due to a progressive increase in the plasma concentration of cholesterol, triacylglycerols and low- and very-low-density lipoproteins, so that the mortality rate from ischaemic heart disease comes to equal that of men.

Changes in the oestrogen target organs in the urogenital tract
The oestrogen target organs in the urogenital tract are the uterus and its appendages, the cervix, the vagina, the vulva, the urethra and the bladder. The uterus shrinks as the myometrium becomes converted to fibrous tissues. The cervix and vaginal epithelium undergo atrophic changes, resulting in thinning and dryness. The pH rises to about 7.2, compared with 4.5 in the productive years, because of the absence of glycogen for Döderlein's bacilli to convert to lactic acid. This produces susceptibility to infection and atrophic vaginitis. The latter may be a cause of postmenopausal bleeding, which requires urgent investigation.

The external genitalia decrease in size and there is loss of pubic hair. The transitional epithelium of the bladder trigone undergoes atrophy. The urethra, which arises from the same ectoderm as the vaginal vestibule, also undergoes some atrophic changes.

Coitus (the sex act)
Sexual intercourse, or coitus, is the means of propagation of the species in all mammals. In humans, unlike other species, the act of coitus can take place at any time during the menstrual cycle, whether or not reproduction is possible. The stages of physiological response to sexual stimulation are similar in males and females, namely: excitement, plateau, orgasm and resolution.

The male sex act
The physiological responses during the *excitement phase* include penile *erection* and congestion of the testes. Erection is due to a spinal reflex triggered by stimulation of the penis or other parts of the genital tract. It is usually enhanced by visual, olfactory, auditory and psychic stimuli. The reflex causes arteriolar vasodilatation, which increases the blood flow into the penis, leading to engorgement, and it becomes hard due to the presence of strong fibrous sheaths surrounding the erectile tissue. The penis enlarges in both length and girth. Vasodilatation is due to parasympathetic nerve stimulation. The vasodilator transmitter in these nerves is believed to be **nitric oxide (NO)** and not acetylecholine. The turgidity of the penis compresses the veins and therefore mechanically decreases venous outflow, thus maintaining the erection, which soon achieves penetration into the vagina. Normally arterioles receive only sympathetic nerve fibres and vasodilatation is produced by inhibition of sympathetic flow. In the penis stimulation of parasympathetic vasodilator fibres and inhibition of the sympathetic result in a rapid increase in blood flow, which achieves an erection within a few seconds. It is well

known that sympathetic vasoconstriction before or during the sex act can destroy an erection. Undue anxiety about sex is a common cause of failure of erection (**impotence**).

During the *plateau phase*, due to massage of the penis within the vagina, the turgidity of the penis increases. There is an increase in the heart rate, blood pressure and respiratory rate.

Orgasm is reached at the peak of sexual stimulation and results in **ejaculation**, which is also due to a spinal reflex. It is brought about by sympathetic nerves, which cause the *emission* and *expulsion* of semen. *Emission* is due to contraction in sequence of the prostate, the ejaculatory duct and the seminal vesicles. This causes emission of semen into the urethra. The internal sphincter of the urinary bladder remains closed to prevent semen from passing into the bladder. *Expulsion* is triggered by arrival of semen in the urethra. There is a second reflex, which causes skeletal muscle at the base of the penis (namely, the bulbospongiosus and bulbocavernosus) to contract rhythmically at 0.8 s intervals. These contractions compress the urethra and cause the semen to be expelled into the vagina. This final phase of ejaculation is associated with the feeling of sexual satisfaction and release known as orgasm.

Ejaculation is essentially a spinal reflex but higher centres are also involved. Therefore, emotional and psychological factors can affect the threshold of ejaculation, which explains delayed or premature ejaculation.

The *resolution phase* of the male sex act is associated with relaxation, during which there is decreased blood flow into the penis due to sympathetic vasoconstriction. There is a variable refractory period before another sexual excitation and erection can be produced.

Semen

Sixty per cent of the seminal fluid comes from the seminal vesicles. The rest consists of secretions of the prostate, the vas deferens and the mucous glands of the urethra. About 3–5 ml are ejaculated each time. The pH of semen is alkaline (pH 7.5), unlike that of the vagina. The vas deferens secretes fibrinogen, which causes the semen to coagulate, and the prostatic secretion contains fibrinotrypsin, which causes the clot to dissolve in about 20 minutes. Male fertility depends on a sperm count of about 100 million/ml, on sperm motility and on the absence of a high percentage of abnormal forms. A count of less than 20 million sperm/ml usually indicates infertility.

The female sex act

Initiation of the *excitement phase* is due to physical or psychological stimuli. Touching the clitoris and the skin surrounding the vulva is particularly exciting. The physiological responses during this phase result in vasodilatation of the vagina and external genitalia by parasympathetic vasodilator fibres. This leads to swelling of the labia and erection of the clitoris. The vasodilatation also leads to diffusion of fluid into the vagina. The fluid exudate is one of the early signs of sexual arousal. It serves to lubricate the vagina during intercourse. Lubrication is also served by mucus secretion from the mucous glands at the vulva and secretion from the male. Vasodilatation of the skin leads to a flush, which appears in most women. Vascular congestion of the breasts also occurs during this phase, resulting in erection of the nipples.

The *plateau phase* is characterized by an increase in the responses started during the excitement phase. Further vasodilatation of the lower vagina makes it more tight, which increases the sensation for the male. Systemic responses, such as an increase in blood pressure and respiratory rate, also occur. The cervix is lifted by the uterus, thus increasing the length of the vagina and making space for deposition of the ejaculated semen. Continued penile stimulation during this phase results in *orgasm*, which consists of rhythmic contractions of the pelvic muscles but most intensely in the musculature of the lower third of the vagina. The rate of contractions is the same as that in males. After the orgasm, if intercourse continues, the stimulation only diminishes to the plateau level and another orgasm may be experienced. There is no emission as in males and, unlike males, repeated orgasms can be experienced during one sex act. During the *resolution phase* the vascular responses diminish and the female experiences a great feeling of physical relaxation.

Fertilization

Fertilization is the process of penetration of the oocyte by the spermatozoon. It marks the beginning of the formation of the embryo. Fertilization normally occurs soon after ovulation, for the ovum remains viable for only about 8 hours.

After deposition of sperms in the upper vagina, they penetrate the mucus of the cervical canal into the uterus and reach the outer third of the fallopian tube, where fertilization usually takes place. The cervical canal acts as a reservoir for sperm for about 24–48 hours. Fertilization can occur as long as 72 hours after intercourse. Sperms reach the fallopian tubes 5–10 minutes after ejaculation. They proceed by flagellar motion at about 5–6 cm/min, which is not enough to explain their rapid ascent. It is believed that uterine contractions and antiperistaltic movement of the fallopian tubes help their progress. The ovum, on the other hand, is helped to descend down the tube by the action of cilia, which beat in the opposite direction, i.e.

towards the uterus. Of about half a billion sperm deposited, only 1000–3000 reach the fallopian tubes.

The spermatozoa have to undergo a number of physiological changes during their course in the female genital tract before they are able to penetrate the oocyte, i.e. capacitation and the acrosome reaction.

Capacitation

Sperms are not capable of fertilization immediately after ejaculation. They develop this capacity after a few hours in the female genital tract. This process is known as capacitation. It is probably due to changes in the plasma membranes induced by enzymes located in the acrosome region of the sperm. These changes usually occur as the sperms traverse the cervical canal. Capacitation under artificial conditions was one of the problems of *in vitro* fertilization.

Acrosome reaction

Sperms undergo structural changes, which end by loss of the acrosomal cap (the two layers of the outer acrosomal membranes), leaving the inner acrosomal membrane and the nucleus exposed. These changes usually occur in the ampulla of the fallopian tube, where the oocyte is found soon after ovulation. A large number of sperms attach themselves to the outer layer of the ovum. The acrosome enzymes from this large number are needed for breaking down the outer layers. The acrosome reaction results in the release of the enzyme **acrosin**, which is required for penetration of the zona pellucida.

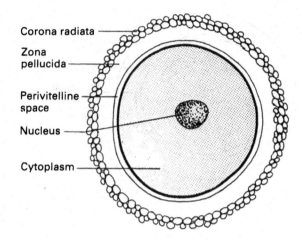

Fig. 14.8 The oocyte and its surrounding layers.

Oocyte penetration

The sperm has to penetrate through several layers of the oocyte, with the aid of the enzymes hyaluronidase and protease. The outermost layer penetrated is the corona radiata (Fig. 14.8). The sperm becomes attached to the second layer or the zona pellucida. Dispersion of the corona radiata is achieved by means of acrosomal enzymes. Sperms attach to the zona pellucida at receptor sites which are species-specific (i.e. sperms of different species cannot attach to ova of another). The sperm reaches the perivitelline space between the zona pellucida and oocyte (Fig. 14.9). Eventually, only one sperm penetrates, activating the oocyte and

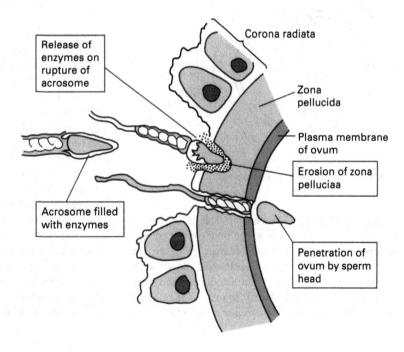

Fig. 14.9 Diagrammatic representation of sperm showing release of acrosome enzymes and penetration of layers surrounding the ovum to achieve fertilization.

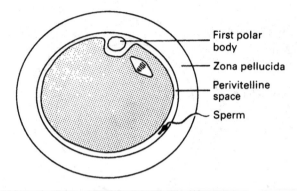

First polar body

Zona pellucida

Perivitelline space

Sperm

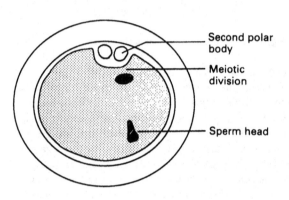

Second polar body

Meiotic division

Sperm head

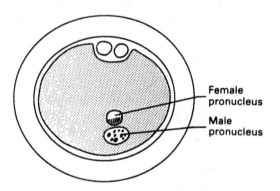

Female pronucleus

Male pronucleus

Fig. 14.10 Fertilization of the human ovum.

blocking further sperm penetration. This is believed to be due to the release of a substance from cortical granules surrounding the ovum. This substance permeates the perivitelline space and the zona pellucida, and it inactivates the remaining sperms. On penetration of one sperm head, the membrane potential of the ovum is reduced and this is followed by changes in membrane structure, which provide further protection against penetration by more sperm (polyspermy).

When the oocyte is activated, it undergoes meiotic division and discards 23 chromosomes as the second polar body, having lost nuclear material as the first polar body in early ovum formation (Fig. 14.10). These chromosomes form the pronucleus from the ovum, which fuses with the pronucleus from the sperm, and the cell is ready to divide with 46 chromosomes. Mitotic division starts immediately and results in the formation of the blastocyst.

Infertility can result from damage to the tubes, e.g. infection, causing their blockage and/or loss of their function in providing the ideal environment for fertilization and early development of the blastocyst.

Abnormalities of human reproduction

Knowing the mechanisms, the signs and the symptoms of normal changes in reproductive life is important in order to diagnose and treat various pathological states. Some of the abnormalities of human reproduction have already been mentioned. The following are some examples of reproductive disorders.

Abnormalities of puberty

Delayed puberty could occur due to disturbance of gonadal hormone production, because of familial delay of maturation, disease states affecting the hypothalamic–pituitary–ovarian axis or congenital abnormalities.

Chromosomal abnormalities

Chromosomal abnormalities result in impairment of development of the reproductive system and hormonal abnormalities. During the formation of the ovum or sperm, the pair of sex chromosomes may fail to separate (non-disjunction) during meiosis. In the case of ova, the result is an ovum with either two X chromosomes or none. If such ova are fertilized, the result is one of the following possible combinations: XO, YO, XXY or XXX. In the XO combination the individual has female internal and external genitalia and suffers from what is known as *ovarian dysgenesis* or **Turner's syndrome**. The ovaries are rudimentary or absent. Such patients fail to develop at puberty and they are short and sterile. A fetus with a YO combination is usually aborted and is probably incompatible with life. The XXY combination is the most common of the sex chromosome abnormalities. The individual develops normal male genitalia. There is adequate testosterone secretion at puberty but the seminiferous tubules are not normal. This is known as

Klinefelter's syndrome or *seminiferous tubular dysgenesis*. Individuals with this condition have a high incidence of mental retardation. When XXX and XYY combinations occur, the first is referred to as the superfemale and is not associated with any particular abnormalities and the second is usually a tall male with severe acne and possibly some aggressive tendencies.

Abnormalities of genital tract differentiation

The external genitalia of both male and female tracts develop from the same primitive tissue. The reproductive tracts, however, develop from different embryonic structures. Genetic male and female embryos have two duct systems: **Wolffian ducts** and **Muellerian ducts**. In male embryos the Wolffian ducts develop into the male genital tract and the Muellerian ducts degenerate. In females the opposite takes place. The differentiation of the embryonic ducts depends on two hormones: **testosterone** and **Muellerian inhibiting factor**, both of which are secreted by the fetal testes on being stimulated by hCG released by the placenta. Both hormones are responsible for male genital tract differentiation. In female embryos the absence of these two hormones results in degeneration of the Wolffian ducts and the Muellerian ducts develop into the female genital tract.

Testosterone from the fetal testes is converted into dihydrotestosterone (DHT), which is essential for differentiation of the male external genitalia. Inappropriate sex differentiation can result from hormonal defects, e.g. failure of conversion of testosterone into DHT due to a genetic enzyme deficiency results in failure of differentiation of the external genitalia of a genetically male fetus. On the other hand, a genetic female fetus may have excess dehydroepiandrosterone, which is a male sex hormone from the adrenal cortex. This leads to enlargement of the clitoris and development of male-like external genitalia. If not diagnosed in infancy or early childhood, this child may be brought up as a boy, until the signs of female puberty reveal the true sex.

Infertility

Successful pregnancy requires fertilization of a mature ovum by a sperm and subsequent implantation in a prepared endometrium. This can be disturbed at several stages; male factors are responsible for infertility as much as female factors. In males, abnormal sperm counts or azoospermia can be a permanent cause of infertility. Hyperprolactinaemia has been associated with infertility in men and women. Prolactin appears to be inhibitory to the effects of LH on the ovaries and of FSH on the testes. Tubal patency and normal function are essential for fertilization. However, the commonest cause of infertility in women is failure of ovulation. This should be the first matter to investigate when there are no genital tract abnormalities in the female. Presence of progesterone in the secretory phase of the cycle indicates ovulation and its absence indicates anovular cycles.

Abnormalities of the menstrual cycle

Primary *amenorrhoea*, or failure to menstruate at puberty, is usually due to failure of sexual maturation. Secondary amenorrhoea, or cessation of normal cycles, is most commonly due to pregnancy. In the absence of pregnancy, it may be brought about by an abnormality of the hypothalamic–pituitary axis, ovarian disease or some systemic disease. *Dysmenorrhoea* is the occurrence of pain during menstruation. This is mainly explained by prostaglandins accumulating in the uterus, and can be relieved by inhibitors of prostaglandin synthesis. The term *oligomenorrhoea* refers to little blood flow during menstruation and *menorrhagia* refers to much bleeding with each menstrual period. *Metrorrhagia* refers to abnormal bleeding which occurs between periods. This is often due to ovarian or uterine disease.

Abnormalities of the testes

Undescended testes occur in about 10% of newborn boys, but by the end of the first year most of these complete their descent into the scrotum. When the testes remain in the abdominal cavity, this is called *cryptorchidism*, which may be treated with gonadotrophins or surgically corrected. If left in the abdomen until puberty, spermatogenesis does not occur, due to the higher abdominal temperature, but testosterone is secreted. There is also the possibility of development of malignant testicular tumours.

Male hypogonadism occurs because of chromosomal abnormalities, failure of the hypothalamic–pituitary axis or testicular damage. If it occurs before puberty, the individual usually grows to be tall and thin. This is explained by the observation that their epiphyses remain open longer than normal, due to the absence of testosterone. The genitalia are small, there are no male secondary sex characteristics and the pubic hair is of a female configuration. Such individuals are sterile and the condition is referred to as *eunuchoidism*.

When male hypogonadism occurs after puberty, there is loss of spermatogenesis and gradual loss of libido. Secondary sex characteristics are not lost, as they can be maintained by adrenocortical androgens. The individual eventually becomes impotent and sterile and may develop symptoms similar to those encountered in menopausal women.

15 / Pregnancy and Perinatal Physiology

Objectives

On completion of the study of this section, the student should be able to:

1 Understand the functions of the placenta and appreciate the physiological integration of the fetoplacental unit.

2 Describe the maternal physiological responses to pregnancy in order to deal with the special needs of antenatal care.

3 Understand the physiology of normal childbirth so as to recognize obstetric abnormalities.

4 Describe the control and maintenance of lactation and its advantages so as to encourage breast-feeding.

5 Explain the special functional features of the new-born so as to give appropriate postnatal care to the neonate.

Early physiological changes

The fertilized ovum undergoes a process of rapid cellular multiplication as it travels along the fallopian tube. Eventually, when it reaches the uterine cavity, the blastocyst is formed. The blastocyst acquires its nutrition from the surface secretions of the endometrium. Inadequate supplies of nutrients result in failure of the completion of implantation. The syncytiotrophoblast layer erodes the endometrium by the action of proteolytic enzymes and implantation is completed in 4–5 days after fertilization (7–8 days after ovulation). The chorion and, later, the placenta have important endocrine functions.

Pregnancy is suspected when an otherwise regular period is missed by the mother. As early as the first week after the time of the missed period, i.e. 5–6 weeks after the last period, a hormone known as **human chorionic gonadotrophin (hCG)** can be detected in the maternal blood. Human chorionic gonadotrophin detection is the basis of pregnancy tests. It may be detected in the urine 14 days after conception. A positive pregnancy test is obtained when hCG is detected by an immunological technique. Earlier biological methods using rabbits or toads, which were injected with maternal urine, a positive test giving rise to ovulation in these animals, are no longer used.

In the early stages of pregnancy, the embryo develops rapidly with little growth in size. About the 12th week it is only about 5 cm in length but all the organ systems have started to differentiate. It is during these first 12 weeks that the effects of radiation, teratogenic drugs and some viruses are most likely to produce fetal abnormalities. During the first 12 weeks, the mother may have nausea and vomiting, known as morning sickness. The reason for this is not known. It is possible that cell degradation products, due to the invasion of the endometrium, may have a role in this. Another possible reason may be the high levels of hCG and sex hormones produced by the placenta. In some cases, morning sickness may develop into severe vomiting, which seriously affects the health of the mother and requires medical attention—a condition known as hyperemesis gravidarum.

The placenta

The placenta has two main functions. The first is an endocrine function and the second is the transfer of substances between maternal and fetal blood. Several hormones are produced by the placenta (Fig. 15.1).

Endocrine functions

Human chorionic gonadotrophin (hCG)
Human chorionic gonadotrophin is a glycoprotein

Fig. 15.1 Hormones of the placenta: levels of secretion in the maternal blood throughout pregnancy. hCG, human chorionic gonadotrophin; hPL, human placental lactogen; O, oestrogens; P, progesterone.

Fig. 15.2 Fetoplacental hormone synthesis. Placental progesterone is also used by the fetal adrenal cortex to synthesize glucocorticoids.

hormone with a molecular weight of about 3000 daltons and similar molecular structure to that of pituitary luteinizing hormone (LH). Its main function is to maintain the corpus luteum of pregnancy beyond the period of the menstrual cycle. It stimulates the corpus luteum to secrete large amounts of progesterone and oestrogens. The latter are essential for maintenance of the endometrium and suppression of menstruation. Peak levels of hCG are reached by about the 10th week. Afterwards, it declines and is maintained at a lower level until the end of pregnancy. hCG also causes the fetal testes to produce small amounts of **testosterone**, which stimulate the development of male sex organs and the descent of the testicles into the scrotum.

Progesterone
Progesterone is produced by the corpus luteum in early pregnancy and in much greater amounts by the placenta. From about the 8th week onwards, the production of progesterone is taken over by the placenta. It reaches a peak value at the end of pregnancy, which reaches levels about 10 times those of early pregnancy.

Progesterone increases the endometrial nutrient stores in early pregnancy. These provide the developing embryo with an important source of nourishment. During pregnancy, progesterone prevents uterine contractions by decreasing the contractility of the myometrium. This prevents spontaneous abortion in early pregnancy. Together with oestrogens, progesterone prepares the breasts for lactation.

The effect of progesterone is to develop the duct system of the mammary glands.

Placental progesterone has an important role as a precursor for fetal steroid synthesis. The progesterone of the placenta is converted to dehydroepiandrosterone (DHEA) by the fetal adrenal cortex. The latter is again converted by placental enzymes to oestriol. Thus, the production of placental oestrogens depends on the fetus and the placenta (**fetoplacental unit**). Figure 15.2 shows the interdependence of fetal and placental steroid synthesis.

Oestrogens
The placenta secretes large amounts of oestrogens, mainly in the form of the less potent **oestriol**, in contrast to the ovaries, which produce mainly **oestradiol**. As mentioned above, the precursors for placental oestrogens come from the fetal adrenal. Therefore, the maintenance of placental oestrogens depends on a living fetus. Intrauterine fetal death causes a sharp fall in maternal plasma oestrogen levels.

Placental oestrogens have several functions. They promote the growth and enlargement of the uterus to accommodate the developing embryo and fetus. Oestrogens also promote the growth of the glandular tissues of the breast. By the end of pregnancy, both the duct and the glandular systems of the breast are developed and ready to produce milk. The external genitalia also enlarge and the pelvic ligaments and joints relax. These changes help the passage of the fetus through the pelvis during labour.

Human placental lactogen (hPL)

Human placental lactogen, also known as **human chorionic somatomammotrophin (hCS)**, is a protein hormone with a molecular weight of 3800. It is secreted by the placenta and is first detected in the maternal circulation around the 5th week of pregnancy. Its concentration increases in the maternal blood as pregnancy progresses. It seems to have an effect on the development of the breasts. It also has metabolic actions similar to those of pituitary growth hormone (GH), which normally decreases during pregnancy. hPL is protein-anabolic and favours mobilization of fat from maternal stores, while inhibiting glucose utilization in maternal tissues. This action contributes to the decreased sensitivity to insulin encountered during pregnancy, which helps to spare glucose for the fetus. The fetus uses glucose as its main source of energy.

Transfer functions

Oxygen and carbon dioxide diffuse freely across the placental membrane lining the villi of the placenta. The *intervillous spaces* receive oxygenated maternal blood from the *spiral arteries* of the uterus. Maternal venous blood drains back by means of the *placental sinuses*, which drain into the many tributaries of the uterine veins. Deoxygenated fetal blood comes to the villi by means of branches of the umbilical arteries. At term, the fetus requires about 20 ml of oxygen per minute. As the arteriovenous oxygen difference in the uterine vessels is about 7 ml/dl and the uterine blood flow is about 500 ml/min or more, 35 ml oxygen/min or more can be supplied to the uterus at term. The extra oxygen is used by the uterine and placental tissues.

The fetal arterial partial pressure of O_2 (Po_2) is about 40 mmHg. The fetal venous blood Po_2 is about 20–30 mmHg. The Po_2 in the placental sinuses is about 50 mmHg. Thus, there is only 20–30 mmHg Po_2 difference between the fetal and maternal blood. Several factors favour the diffusion of O_2 across the placental membrane:

1 The surface area of the villi is huge. In a full-size placenta, which weighs about 500 g, the total surface area for exchange is about 14 m^2.

2 Fetal haemoglobin has a higher affinity for O_2 than adult haemoglobin. It can carry up to 30% more oxygen per gram.

3 The fetal haemoglobin concentration is about 50% higher than that in adults.

4 The fetal blood has a higher Pco_2 (48 mmHg) than maternal blood. CO_2 diffuses quickly into the maternal blood and shifts the O_2 dissociation curve to the left (Bohr effect), helping the release of oxygen from the maternal blood. At the same time, fetal blood becomes more alkaline, thus shifting the curve to the right and favouring more O_2 uptake. Therefore, the Bohr effect works both ways in favour of oxygenation of fetal blood more than it does in the adult lung.

Blood flow to the placenta is decreased during uterine contractions, which squeeze the spiral uterine arteries. Muscular exercise also decreases uterine blood flow, due to redistribution of blood. Smoking mothers have various levels of carboxyhaemoglobin in both maternal and fetal blood. This tends to lower the O_2-carrying capacity of the blood in both mother and fetus, leading to hypoxia in the fetus. Heavy smoking is associated with smaller birth weights and greater risk of perinatal death.

The placenta allows a variety of other substances to cross. Generally, small-molecular-weight substances cross the placental membrane more readily. Electrolytes and lipid-soluble substances cross more easily than water-soluble substances. Fetal blood glucose is 20–30% lower than maternal blood glucose concentration. Therefore, glucose diffuses to the fetal blood down a concentration gradient by facilitated diffusion, using a specific carrier. More glucose tends to diffuse to the fetus when the mother has poorly controlled diabetes mellitus. The baby tends to become obese and overgrown. Many drugs, including anaesthetics and analgesics, cross the placental membrane and may affect the fetus. Protein molecules cannot normally pass across the placenta. However, immunoglobulins and some maternal enzymes are able to cross, possibly by pinocytosis.

Minerals are most probably transported by carrier-mediated transport mechanisms. In the case of **iron**, maternal transferrin does not cross the placental barrier but it interacts with placental binding sites. Iron is then transported into the fetus in bound form. There is a marked increase in the efficiency of maternal intestinal absorption of iron and calcium during pregnancy and there are active transport mechanisms for these substances. Even if the mother is anaemic, the fetus usually has normal haemoglobin levels; but fetal iron stores may be deficient. Therefore, the possibility of developing *iron-deficiency anaemia* during infancy is greater.

Amino acids are actively transported across the placental membrane and usually the fetal concentrations of free amino acids are much higher than those in the mother. This favours the process of protein synthesis, especially in the rapid growth stage during the second and third trimesters. The excretion of urea, uric acid and creatinine takes place by diffusion, due to higher concentrations in fetal blood.

Maternal responses to pregnancy

The mother's systems become prepared for the increased workload and nutritional requirements of the fetus. Almost every system is involved so that there is a wide range of physiological changes during pregnancy.

Body fluids

There is marked water retention—nearly 2.5 litres by the middle of pregnancy, of which about 1.5 litres are in the plasma. During this period, growth of the uterus and mammary glands, amniotic fluid and increased blood volume account for most of the water and electrolytes retained. During the latter half of pregnancy, the tissue fluid and blood account for about 6 litres of retained water. This may be due to the oestrogens secreted by the placenta. There is also increased renin production, which leads to an increase in aldosterone release and sodium retention.

The blood

As mentioned above, blood volume increases. This increase is due to an increase in plasma volume, as well as in red blood cell production. The increase in blood volume is rapid during the 3rd month and levels off during the last 3 months of pregnancy at about 1.5 litres. Although there is an increase in total red-cell mass, the packed-cell volume (PCV) is decreased, due to haemodilution, and may normally be as low as 30%. The haemoglobin concentration is similarly lower than normal (11–12 g/dl). However, the cell haemoglobin should be normal unless iron deficiency occurs. These observations emphasize the importance of haemoglobin measurement in antenatal care and the need for adequate iron supplies during pregnancy.

The plasma proteins show an increase in the β-globulin and fibrinogen. Although the total amount of albumin is increased, plasma albumin is found to be lower in concentration, which leads to a fall in plasma osmotic pressure. These changes raise the erythrocyte sedimentation rate (ESR) to high levels during pregnancy, which, at other times, would be considered abnormal.

The circulatory system

Cardiovascular changes prepare the mother for the increased demands of pregnancy. About 500 ml of blood/min pass to the uterus. Early in pregnancy the cardiac output increases to meet this demand. It is estimated that, by the end of the first trimester, the cardiac output increases by about one-third. This is achieved by an increase in both the heart rate and the stroke volume. One of the important changes during pregnancy is the increase in renal blood

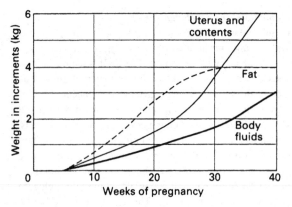

Fig. 15.3 The major components of weight gain during pregnancy. Note the rates of increase of the different components.

flow. This increases by just less than half a litre in early pregnancy and leads to a high glomerular filtration rate (GFR).

The blood flow in the skin is increased. This is useful in the maintenance of body temperature. The increased metabolic heat production leads to vasodilatation and sweating.

The urinary system

There is a rise in GFR due to the high renal blood flow. It increases from a normal level of 110 ml/min to about 150 ml/min in the first 3 months and remains high throughout pregnancy. Renal glucosuria may occur in some mothers if the tubular maximum (Tm) for glucose is exceeded due to the increased GFR. The clearance of urea and uric acid increases and appreciable amounts of amino acids may also appear in the urine. Water-soluble vitamins may also be lost in the urine. In particular, folic acid is lost in appreciable amounts. The possibility of developing megaloblastic anaemia in pregnancy is increased because of higher demands and the renal losses of folic acid.

Changes in body composition

The increase in cell mass due to the growth of the uterus, the breasts and the uterine contents is associated with a net gain in protein. By the end of pregnancy, the net gain in *protein* amounts to about 1 kg. Most of this protein is used for uterine and fetal growth during the third trimester. This is associated with water and electrolyte gain, as part of the tissue fluids and intracellular water. Figure 15.3 shows the rate of change in body-weight during pregnancy, broken down into the major components.

By the end of pregnancy, the pregnant mother stores about 4 kg of *fat*, mainly in subcutaneous adipose tissues. The larger part of this fat is stored during the middle trimester. It provides an energy surplus to be used mainly during the period of lactation. Repeated pregnancies are one of the common causes of obesity.

The pregnant mother gains about 750 mg of iron by the end of pregnancy. The *iron* is used mainly for the mother's haemoglobin during the first and second trimesters and for fetal blood and iron stores during the third trimester. The net gain in *calcium* during pregnancy is about 30 g. This is used mainly for the growth and calcification of the fetal skeleton during the third trimester.

Nutritional requirements during pregnancy

The total weight gain during pregnancy is about 12 kg. The changes in body composition during pregnancy (see Fig. 15.3) serve as a useful guide for the nutritional needs of pregnant mothers. The timing of these changes also gives an indication of the important nutritional needs during the various stages of pregnancy. For more detail on nutritional requirements, see Chapter 7.

Metabolic changes during pregnancy

The metabolic responses during pregnancy can be explained by the changing needs of the pregnant mother and the fetus. The hormonal changes during pregnancy are responsible for these metabolic responses.

Carbohydrate metabolism

Carbohydrate metabolism is characterized by increased glucose utilization during the first few weeks of pregnancy, with increased glycogen storage. This is due to hyperinsulinaemia, probably mediated by high levels of oestrogen and progesterone. In the latter half of pregnancy, hPL, prolactin, cortisol and glucagon are responsible for the appearance of insulin resistance. Latent diabetes may become overt, giving rise to decreased glucose tolerance and glucosuria.

Protein and fat metabolism

Protein metabolism is mainly anabolic. There is a high protein intake, which leads to short-lived increases in plasma amino acid levels. Placental hormones play an important anabolic role. However, protein catabolism is brought about by cortisol and glucagon, which enhance the utilization of amino acids in gluconeogenesis during the latter half of pregnancy.

The above discussion indicates that there are prominent metabolic differences between early and late gestation. Maternal glucose removal from the circulation is increased in early gestation but progressively declines to subnormal levels by term. Basal plasma insulin concentrations are normal early in gestation but rise in late gestation, associated with an increased insulin response to glucose and insulin resistance. Fat storage is greatest in early gestation but almost completely stops in late gestation. All of these observations indicate enhanced maternal ability to store energy in early gestation. We call this the *anabolic phase* of pregnancy; the fetus is small at this stage and requires relatively small amounts of nutrients. However, in the later part of gestation, when fetal growth is much more rapid, there is increased nutrient flow across the placenta to the fetus, i.e. the *catabolic phase*. The insulin resistance experienced by the mother in late gestation helps to maintain glucose concentrations at a higher level than normal and decreases maternal glucose utilization. Therefore, glucose is spared for the fetus. The catabolic phase of pregnancy occurs mainly during the third trimester. During this stage the mother uses an increased amount of fat. In the fed state, the fat is derived from the diet. In the fasting state, increased amounts of fat are mobilized from adipose tissue stores, leading to a state similar to accelerated starvation.

Labour (parturition)

The duration of normal pregnancy is about 40 weeks from the first day of the last menstrual period (38 weeks from conception). Irregular, but usually painless, uterine contractions occur throughout pregnancy. The onset of labour is marked by regular uterine contractions, widely spaced at first and gradually increasing in frequency and strength. During labour, the uterine smooth muscles characteristically contract and retract (shorten). This phenomenon is important as it ensures the gradual descent of the baby as the capacity of the uterine cavity decreases. The initiation of labour is probably due to several factors. Maternal oestrogen increases and progesterone decreases near term. These hormonal changes increase the sensitivity of the uterus to oxytocin. **Oxytocin receptors** on the myometrium and decidua cells increase progressively towards term (Fig. 15.4). Oxytocin stimulates the decidua to produce one of the prostaglandins (**PGF$_{2\alpha}$**). It is found in high concentration in the amniotic fluid and the placenta at term. It has a strong stimulating action on the uterus. However, there is no detectable rise in maternal serum levels of either oxytocin or prostaglandins before labour, but once labour starts their levels increase. Their action in maintaining effective uterine contractions is confirmed, but their role in the initiation of labour is uncertain.

When the time of delivery is near, the cervix, already softened by the action of oestrogens, is gradually taken up and shortened, a process known as cervical effacement.

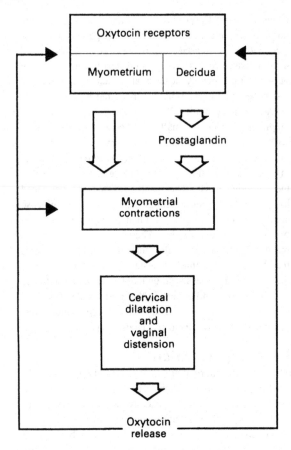

Fig. 15.4 The roles of oxytocin and prostaglandins in parturition.

Once regular contractions are established, the process of cervical dilatation begins, until the cervix is fully dilated. This is called the *first stage of labour*.

The *second stage* begins after full dilatation of the cervix. The advancing head of the fetus causes stretch of the cervix and genital tract. This is a strong stimulus for the release of oxytocin, which acts directly on the myometrium, and the contractions become stronger and more frequent. Oxytocin also acts on the decidua to produce prostaglandins, which enhance the effects of oxytocin on uterine contractions. Drugs which inhibit prostaglandin synthesis delay the progress of labour. During the second stage, the fetal head is pushed slowly through the cervix and vagina until it is born. The strong uterine contractions result in poor circulation to the placenta during this stage; therefore, rapid progress is vital for a safe delivery. When the head is delivered, it is easily followed by the shoulders and the rest of the body. This marks the end of the second stage.

The *third stage* of labour starts after complete delivery of the fetus and ends with complete delivery of the placenta and membranes. Uterine contractions and retractions separate the placenta. Some bleeding normally occurs from the raw surface of the decidua, which helps in completion of placental separation. Further contractions of the uterus and maternal efforts complete delivery of the placenta and membranes. Bleeding is prevented by contraction of uterine muscle and blood clotting, which plug small vessels in the placental bed.

Physiology of lactation

At the onset of puberty, the mammary gland starts to develop and the breast becomes prominent, due to deposition of fat more than glandular tissue. Oestrogen stimulates proliferation of the duct system and progesterone promotes the development of glandular lobules. The presence of normal pituitary function is essential for the effects of the sex hormones. In particular GH, adrenocorticotrophic hormone (ACTH) (and therefore cortisol), thyroid-stimulating hormone (TSH) (and therefore tri-iodothyronine (T_3) and thyroxine (levothyroxine) (T_4) and insulin are required (Fig. 15.5).

Pituitary prolactin increases gradually throughout pregnancy. The placenta secretes human chorionic somatomammotrophin (hCS), which is also known as human placental lactogen (hPL). These hormones, together with oestrogen and progesterone, are important for the development of the lobules and alveolar tissue of the breast in preparation for lactation. However, the main function of prolactin is *milk production*. During pregnancy, very little milk is produced, because of the high levels of placental sex hormones, which inhibit the actions of the lactogenic hormones.

After delivery, the initial breast secretion is known as colostrum. It has a high protein content but almost no fat. It contains antibodies (immunoglobulin A (IgA)), produced by lymphocytes in the mammary gland. The antibodies help to protect the newborn against infections, in particular, those affecting the gastrointestinal tract. Therefore, the baby should be allowed to suckle as soon as possible after delivery. Milk production in appreciable amounts usually takes 2–3 days to start, under the effect of pituitary prolactin. Oxytocin released during suckling stimulates the *milk ejection* reflex. The rapid decrease of oestrogens and progesterone allows the uninhibited production of milk. Similarly, after an abortion, milk production may also start. Suckling is important for continuation of prolactin secretion and also for oxytocin release during breast-feeding. Therefore, breast-feeding should be started

Puberty   Pregnancy   Lactation

Fig. 15.5 The hormones acting on the mammary gland during various physiological conditions. PRL, prolactin.

Puberty	Pregnancy	Lactation
Oestrogens	Oestrogens	Cortisol
Progesterone	Progesterone	PRL
Cortisol	Cortisol	T_3, T_4
T_3, T_4	Insulin	Insulin
Insulin	GH and PRL	
	hPL	

on the first day and carried on regularly thereafter, so as to stimulate and maintain milk production.

During breast-feeding, menstrual cycles usually stop or may become irregular. Even if menstruation occurs during lactation, the cycles occur without ovulation (*anovular cycles*). This is due to an inhibitory effect of prolactin on gonadotrophin-releasing hormone (GnRH) release. Prolactin also decreases the effects of LH and follicle-stimulating hormone (FSH) on the ovaries. Therefore, prolonged breast-feeding is recommended not only for the welfare of the baby and mother, but also for spacing of pregnancies.

Human milk is now recognized as the food most suitable for infant nutrition (see Chapter 7). Mother's milk also contains defensive cells, such as T and B lymphocytes, macrophages and polymorphonuclear white blood cells (WBCs), and antibacterial and antiviral substances (such as IgA, lysozymes and complement components).

The metabolic response to lactation

During lactation, the energy requirements of the mother increase by about 25% above the normal energy needs, so as to provide for milk production (see Chapter 7). The metabolic changes which occur in the mammary gland at the onset of lactation are probably larger than those in any other organ during normal development. For each volume of milk secreted, about 400–500 volumes of blood are circulated through the gland.

A few millilitres of colostrum are usually produced each day throughout pregnancy. Colostrum contains similar concentrations of protein and lactose to milk but almost no fat.

At the peak of lactation, about 1.5 litres of milk may be formed each day. On average, the energy cost of lactation is about 3 MJ/day. Also, some 1–3 g of calcium is used each day; therefore, lactating mothers are advised to take adequate quantities of milk and vitamin D to avoid a negative calcium balance.

Perinatal physiology

A scientific group of the World Health Organization (WHO) defined a mature infant at birth as one who shows functional competence, providing a reasonable safety margin in extrauterine life. This means that a fetus born before completion of 9 months of gestation could be functionally mature. Birth is viewed as an event in a continuing process of development, which marks the beginning of interactions between the newborn and the environment (Fig. 15.6). It is noteworthy that the highest velocity of brain growth occurs in the perinatal period.

During gestation, the fetal organs mature at different rates. An effective circulation is established with placentation, but the lungs and kidneys are not needed for survival until birth. The liver develops gradually and, until birth, some liver functions are still not fully developed. The nervous system and the liver continue to mature after delivery. Kidney function during gestation is required for formation of amniotic fluid. The fetus shows a wide variety of neurological and muscular activities, including breathing movements, which become increasingly vigorous and varied with age. These movements seem to be necessary for the development and maturation of the fetal lungs. For these activities, the circulatory, metabolic, endocrine and

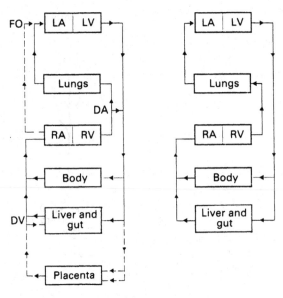

Fig. 15.7 Schematic diagram of fetal and adult circulatory systems. The broken lines indicate the channels which become obliterated after birth. LA and LV denote the left atrium and left ventricle. RA and RV denote the right atrium and right ventricle. FO denotes the foramen ovale, DA the ductus arteriosus and DV the ductus venosus.

Fig. 15.6 Body-weight, crown–feet length and head circumference during the perinatal period and the first year of life. Note the continuity of skeletal growth at birth, while the growth of the head is much faster during the last few weeks of pregnancy. (Based on Gairdner, D. & Pearson, T. (1971) Growth charts. *Arch. Dis. Childh.* **46**, 783.)

nervous support systems must be provided. Three important systems are selected for detailed discussion below.

The fetal circulation

The fetal circulation differs from that of an adult by: (i) low pulmonary blood flow; (ii) high placental flow; and (iii) shunting of blood from the right atrium to the left atrium through the foramen ovale, and from the pulmonary artery to the aorta via the ductus arteriosus. These shunts allow the blood to bypass the fetal lungs (Fig. 15.7).

The placenta receives about 55% of the fetal cardiac output, through the umbilical arteries. **Oxygenated blood** comes back from the placenta through the **umbilical vein**, which joins the portal vein, but it bypasses the liver and goes to the **inferior vena cava** via the **ductus venosus**. On reaching the right atrium, most of this blood flow passes directly through the **foramen ovale** to the left atrium. Minimal mixing occurs with the stream of deoxygenated blood coming through the superior vena cava from the head and neck. This stream passes mainly into the right ventricle. The mixing is kept to a minimum by the position of the left atrium, which lies further posteriorly and to the right than in adults. Also, the crista dividens (the superior margin of the foramen ovale) lies over the entry of the inferior vena cava. The crista dividens directs approximately half of the oxygenated blood from the inferior vena cava directly into the left atrium and the rest goes into the right atrium.

From the left ventricle oxygenated blood is pumped into the aorta, where it is joined by the flow from the main pulmonary artery through the **ductus arteriosus**. The right ventricle pumps about two-thirds of the combined cardiac output. The ductus arteriosus shunts about 90% of the right ventricular output into the aorta and the rest goes to the fetal lungs. It is noteworthy that the ductus arteriosus, which brings mixed blood, joins the aorta beyond the exits of the coronary and carotid arteries, thus permitting a higher O_2 delivery to the heart and the brain. The aortic blood flow is distributed to the various parts of the fetal body, but the main bulk goes to the placenta through the **umbilical arteries**.

Changes at birth

Several cardiocirculatory changes take place at birth. *First*, there is a marked drop in the pulmonary vascular resistance. This is mainly due to the opening up of the **pulmonary arterioles**, no longer compressed by solid lung tissue, and to vasodilatation due to the increased Po_2. The pulmonary artery pressure decreases from 60 to 35 mmHg during the first 8 hours after birth and falls to 25 mmHg by the end of 48 hours. *Second*, the systemic peripheral resistance increases about twofold, due to clamping of the **umbilical arteries** and cessation of the larger flow through the placenta. This increases the pressure in the aorta and consequently in the left ventricle and left atrium. These changes result in a reversal of the pressure difference between the right and left atria and bring about the closure of the valve of the **foramen ovale**. For several weeks, the foramen ovale is kept closed by these haemodynamic forces alone. A rise in right atrial pressure can reopen it and re-establish a right-to-left shunt. This occurs in **hyaline membrane disease (HMD)**, leading to respiratory distress syndrome (RDS) of the newborn. The foramen ovale remains potentially open, but anatomical fusion occurs in 30% of normal adults.

Closure of the **ductus arteriosus** is brought about by contraction of the smooth muscle in the vessel wall. Due to the fall in the pulmonary vascular resistance described above, flow in the ductus arteriosus is reversed at birth. There is also an increase in systemic Po_2, resulting from the establishment of normal ventilation and the closure of the foramen ovale. The Po_2 in the newborn reaches about 50 mmHg above that in the fetus. It is believed that the constriction of the ductus arteriosus is in response to high Po_2. This closure is sufficient to stop the blood flow within a few hours after birth, which is known as physiological closure. Permanent or anatomical closure takes 1–4 months, by infolding of the endothelium and disruption of subintimal layers, followed by fibrosis.

Respiration

In mammals, fetal breathing movements are present from early gestation. In the human fetus, irregular breathing movements have been detected as early as the 11th week of pregnancy. They become increasingly regular after the 5th month, and by 36 weeks of gestation they acquire regular rhythm. However, these breathing movements do not seem to respond to changes in Po_2 and Pco_2, as in

postnatal life. This leads to the hypothesis that the respiratory centre must be under some form of inhibition. Changes which decrease or may even stop the breathing movements include hypoglycaemia, fetal infection, cigarette-smoking during pregnancy and administration of pethidine and barbiturates to the pregnant mother.

During fetal breathing activity, lung liquid flows up the trachea, with continuous small outward spurts of fluid synchronous with fetal breathing activity. At birth, up to 35 ml of fluid drains from the mouth during normal vaginal delivery. The rest is absorbed by the pulmonary lymphatics and capillaries. Fetal adrenaline (epinephrine) and noradrenaline (norepinephrine), which are very high during delivery, stimulate the absorption of lung fluid. The lungs are rapidly cleared of fluid and within 60 minutes a normal functional residual capacity is established in the newborn infant.

About 90% of the epithelial lining of fetal alveoli at birth is made up of type I cells of flat epithelium. Other cells, more round and lying mostly beneath the surface, are type II cells, which produce **surfactants**. Early aeration of the alveoli is important for a layer of surfactant to spread and provide the stability of alveoli, preventing them from total collapse during expiration. Surfactants are complex **lipoproteins** which lower surface tension at the air–liquid interface. The lining of alveoli with surfactants, when the lung is inflated, keeps the pressure constant within all alveoli, irrespective of their diameter. This decreases the work of breathing during inspiration and keeps alveolar patency during expiration.

Aeration of the lungs takes place with the first breath within 60 s of clamping the cord. Various physical stimuli, individually and in combination, can initiate respiration. These include lowering the skin temperature and physical tactile stimuli. Hypoxia, as a result of clamping the cord, is an important factor in initiating the onset of breathing. The response to hypoxia and, particularly, to raised carbon dioxide tension in arterial blood seems to be **chemoreceptor-mediated**. It is abolished in experimental animals by cutting the carotid sinus nerve. At birth, the chemoreceptors become much more sensitive to small changes in arterial blood gas tensions and are important in the postnatal control of respiration. Also, the prenatal inhibition of the respiratory centre is somehow removed. **Sensory inputs** to the central nervous system are also involved in the onset of breathing and, if they are surgically interrupted in animals, the electrical activity of the respiratory centre is greatly reduced.

It seems, therefore, that there is not one single event that initiates the onset of respiration or one single controlling mechanism. The enormous sensory input at birth, the

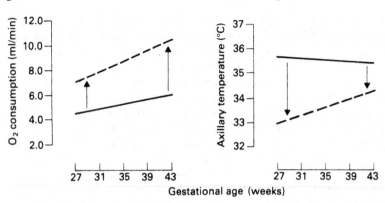

Fig. 15.8 Oxygen consumption and body temperature changes in premature neonates. The solid lines are responses in a thermoneutral environment and the broken lines are responses to a cool environment at 25–36°C. Note that at low gestational age the premature neonate fails to raise O_2 consumption and to maintain body temperature. (Adapted from Heim, T. *et al.* (1981) Homeothermy and its metabolic cost. In: *Scientific Foundations of Paediatrics*, 2nd edn, p. 105. William Heinemann Medical Books, London.)

change in chemoreceptor sensitivity, the hypoxia resulting from cord clamping and the increased activity of the central nervous system—all these factors combine to stimulate the newborn gasp which aerates the lungs.

The kidneys

Fluid, electrolytes and acid–base balance can be easily disturbed in the newborn because of several considerations. *First*, considering the weight of the newborn, the fluid turnover—intake and excretion—is seven times as much as in the adult. *Secondly*, the kidney of the fetus at birth can only concentrate urine up to 1.5 times the osmotic pressure of extracellular fluid, while the adult kidney can concentrate up to four times. The GFR rapidly increases from 20 to 60 ml/min during the first month, compared with 120 ml/min in the adult. Renal tubular function is not fully developed, so that sodium reabsorption and hydrogen ion excretion are poor at birth and develop rapidly during the first month. Therefore, during the first few weeks there is inability to conserve sodium and to excrete acid. *Thirdly*, the metabolic rate of the newborn is twice that of the adult. Consequently, twice as much acid is produced by metabolic processes relative to body-weight. All these factors indicate that fluid and electrolyte loss can rapidly take place in newborn infants and that there is a tendency to develop **acidosis**.

The premature newborn kidneys are even less developed and therefore medical care should include close monitoring of fluid and electrolyte balance, as dehydration or even overhydration can easily occur.

Temperature regulation

The set point for thermal regulation is slightly lower in neonates. Thermal regulatory mechanisms are not fully developed. However, the neonate can maintain a constant body temperature within a narrow range of ambient temperature. Extremes of heat or cold can rapidly result in drastic changes in core body temperature. Room temperatures less than 20°C can rapidly cause **hypothermia**. It is possible that maturation of hypothalamic thermoregulatory centres and availability of nutrients for peripheral thermogenesis may be among the underlying causes. Other contributory factors include the large surface area in the newborn relative to body mass and limited insulation by a thin layer of subcutaneous fat.

Mechanisms of heat production are mainly by increasing **non-shivering thermogenesis**. This is achieved by adrenergic stimulation of hydrolysis of triacylglycerols in **brown fat** to release heat energy. Brown fat is located at the root of the neck and between the scapulae, along the aorta, in the mediastinum and around the kidneys. It may constitute up to 6% of fetal body-weight. Non-shivering thermogenesis is associated with increased oxygen consumption. Therefore, hypoxic infants have a weaker response to cold. Chronic exposure to cold environments can result in energy loss and therefore poor weight gain early in infancy. Neonates only shiver when the environmental temperature falls to 15°C or less. The premature neonate, in particular, is less capable of maintaining body temperature (Fig. 15.8).

Heat conservation mechanisms, on the other hand, are well developed. Infants curl up and decrease their body surface exposure. Vasoconstriction is well developed in the neonate, but its effectiveness may be decreased by the thin layer of subcutaneous fat.

Heat loss occurs, as in adults, through conduction, convection, radiation and evaporation. Conduction is insignificant, unless the baby is laid, without insulation, on a surface which is too cold or too warm. Convective heat loss is small and is due to air currents surrounding the skin. Radiation heat loss depends on the surroundings, either the room temperature or the walls of an incubator. If an infant is naked, e.g. for the sake of observation in the ward, heat loss by radiation is much greater in an open cot than in an incubator. Evaporative heat loss depends on the presence of liquid on the surface, e.g. amniotic fluid immediately after birth. Air movement also increases the rate of evaporative heat loss. In premature infants, the skin is more permeable to water and therefore more evaporative heat loss takes place.

Neonatal jaundice

During intrauterine life, fetal bilirubin crosses the placenta and is excreted by the liver of the mother. For the first few days, the fetal liver functions poorly, so that conjugation of bilirubin with glucuronic acid does not proceed satisfactorily. This leads to accumulation of bilirubin, giving rise to **physiological hyperbilirubinaemia** and jaundice. Fortunately, this is usually mild; serum bilirubin reaches up to 5 mg/100 ml (normal 1 mg/100 ml) and there is a mild yellow coloration of the sclera and mucous membranes.

A pathological cause of neonatal jaundice is **rhesus (Rh) incompatibility**. The fetus is Rh-positive and the mother is Rh-negative but has had previous exposure to Rh antigens (Rh-positive red blood cells (RBCs)), either from a previous pregnancy or from a blood transfusion. The mother's serum will then have Rh antibodies. *Maternal antibodies* may cross the placenta and, when they reach the fetal circulation, they start to destroy fetal RBCs. This creates a high bilirubin concentration in fetal blood. Fortunately, this condition can now be treated before the child is born.

Further reading

1 Emslie-Smith, D., Paterson, C.R., Scratcherd, T. & Read, N.W. (1988) Pregnancy. In: *BDS Textbook of Physiology*, 11th edn, pp. 336–350. Churchill Livingstone, Edinburgh.
2 Guyton, A.C. & Hall, J.E. (1996) Foetal and neonatal physiology. In: *Textbook of Medical Physiology*, 9th edn, pp. 1033–1056. Saunders, Philadelphia.

16 / The Central Nervous System (Clinical Neurophysiology)

Objectives

On completion of the study of this section, the student should be able to:

1 Describe the structural and functional organization of the central nervous system.

2 Understand the sensory functions of the central nervous system, so as to apply tests for sensory abnormalities.

3 Explain the mechanisms of the sensation of pain, in order to use appropriate measures in its treatment and management.

4 Comprehend the mechanisms of reflexes, so as to explain their roles in the control of motor functions.

5 Understand the voluntary and involuntary motor functions of the central nervous system, so as to test for motor disorders resulting from lesions of the motor pathways.

6 Understand the roles of the cerebellum and vestibular apparatus in the regulation of posture and equilibrium.

7 Understand the higher functions of the brain, so as to explain disturbances of memory, learning, speech and other processes.

8 Explain the relationships and functions of the hypothalamus with emotions, visceral functions and neuroendocrine integration.

Introduction

The vast complexity of body functions controlled by the nervous system is unique. These functions range from the somatic motor and sensory functions to highly integrated functions, such as perception, memory, learning and emotions.

The central nervous system (CNS) consists of the brain and spinal cord. The peripheral nervous system, on the other hand, consists of 43 pairs of nerves which enter and leave the CNS. Afferent (sensory) fibres carry nerve impulses from the periphery to the CNS and efferent (motor) fibres carry impulses from the CNS to effector organs, i.e. muscles and glands.

The nervous system responds to changes in the external and internal environments. Receptors sensitive to various stimuli (e.g. light, sound, touch, blood pressure, muscle tension, etc.) are excited. Nerve impulses carried along afferent fibres to the CNS are processed and integrated before appearing in the efferent fibres to produce appropriate responses in the effector organs (e.g. muscle contraction, glandular secretion). The pathway the impulses follow from receptor to effector is called the *reflex arc* and the action that results is called a *reflex action*. Reflex arcs vary in complexity. They are simple at the level of the spinal cord, but get more complex at the level of the brain stem. The most complex reflex arcs are in the cerebral cortex.

Cells of the nervous system

Neurons

The neuron is the functional unit of the nervous system and the human brain has 10^{11} neurons. These vary in size and shape, but they all basically consist of the cell body (soma), one or more dendrites and only one axon, with synaptic terminals (Fig. 16.1).

The soma contains the nucleus and the cytoplasm contains granules which stain with basic dyes, known as Nissl substance. These are the source of the neuron's protein. Dendrites are tapered branches from the cell body that make contact with other neurons. Both soma and dendrites receive information from synaptic connections with other neurons. They are thus usually considered to be the sensory end of the neuron.

The single axon varies in length (from a few hundred micrometres to more than a metre) and also in diameter. It arises from the part of the soma known as the axon hillock, which is the most excitable part of the neuron. Axons are usually covered by myelin sheaths and their ends branch to form terminals, which make contact with other neurons at synapses.

A synapse consists of: (i) a presynaptic terminal, which contains the synaptic vesicles enclosing a neurotransmitter; (ii) a synaptic cleft, which is a small space (20–30 nm wide) between neurons that the transmitter has to cross to arrive at the postsynaptic neuron; and (iii) the postsynaptic membrane which contains the receptors specific to a particular neurotransmitter.

It is important to note that, by about the 6th month of age, the maximum number of neurons one will ever have is attained, because mature neurons do not multiply. Therefore dead neurons will not be replaced by new ones. In fact, there is progressive loss of neurons from birth onwards, due to the normal ageing process.

Neuroglia

Neuroglia (or supporting cells) are the matrix of the CNS and maintain its structure. There are three types of neuroglia (Fig. 16.2). *Astrocytes* are large and function also to maintain a constant K^+ environment around neurons. This is necessary for the normal functioning of the nerve cell.

Oligodendroglia form and maintain myelin sheaths around axons, similar to the Schwann cells in the periphery. *Microglia* are the macrophages of the CNS which phagocytose tissue debris, thus helping the process of tissue repair.

Electrical signals in the nervous system

Membrane potentials

Resting membrane potential (RMP)

The intracellular fluid has more K^+ and protein and less Na^+ and Cl^- than the extracellular fluid. This unequal distribution of ions between the two sides of the cell membrane causes a difference in electrical potential across it, called the **resting membrane potentials** (for full description of mechanisms, see Chapter 3).

Local potentials

Local (electrotonic) **potentials** arise when the movement of charge responsible for the change in potential is limited to a particular site on the membrane of the neuron. This takes place when the movement of charge is small, and it usually occurs at points of discontinuity, e.g. environment-sensory receptor (i.e. receptor potentials), CNS synapses (excitatory and inhibitory postsynaptic potentials) and nerve–muscle junctions (end-plate potential).

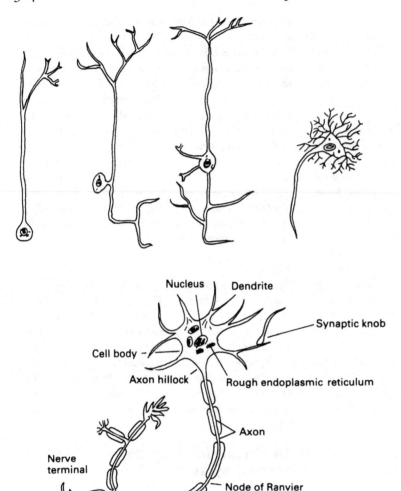

Fig. 16.1 Diagram showing various types of neurons. Below is a motor neuron. (Reproduced with modifications from Bray, J.J., Cragg, P.A., Macknight, A.D.C., Mills, R.G. & Taylor, D.W. (eds) (1989), *Lecture Notes in Physiology*, 2nd edn. Blackwell Scientific Publications, Oxford.)

In local potentials, the change in potential is greatest at the particular site and falls off exponentially with distance. Thus, they are typically restricted to 1 or 2 mm from their point of origin in the cell body or dendrite.

Action potentials

When the movement of charge is large (such as the influx of Na^+ at a sensory nerve terminal), the membrane of the neuron is depolarized to a point called the threshold, beyond which an all-or-nothing response, called an action potential, occurs (see Chapter 3).

Table 16.1 shows the important differences in the characteristics of local and action potentials.

Types and properties of nerve fibres. Nerve fibres are classified into A, B and C fibres (Table 16.2). A fibres have the thickest covering of myelin, followed by B fibres and, finally, C fibres, which are unmyelinated fibres. The more myelin covering the nerve has, the more its thickness, conduction velocity, metabolic activity, excitability (i.e. having lower threshold) and capability of repetitive firing. Type A fibres are subdivided into Aα, Aβ, Aγ and Aδ. Examples of A fibres are spinocerebellar tract fibres and somatic motor fibres. Preganglionic autonomic fibres belong to class B. Examples of C fibres are the slow pain fibres and the postganglionic autonomic motor fibres.

Larger myelinated fibres, because of their higher metabolic activity, are more susceptible to cold, compression and anoxia than smaller fibres. Therefore, these agents block conduction in myelinated fibres before unmyelinated ones. Local anaesthetic drugs, on the other hand, preferentially block unmyelinated fibres: hence their use to block pain sensation from the skin.

The compound action potential. If activity from a whole nerve (with different types of fibres in it) is recorded, we get the summated action potentials of all fibres in the nerve. This is called the compound action potential (AP). If we give stimuli of increasing intensity to the nerve, the compound AP grows in amplitude with increased stimulation strength until it reaches a maximum, when all the fibres are excited. This is because various fibres in the nerve have different thresholds, making the compound AP graded and not obeying the all-or-none law. Its absolute refractory period is the absolute refractory period of the largest fibres. The compound AP may display a number of peaks, each of which represents fibres having similar conduction velocities (Fig. 16.3). The separation of peaks increases as the distance between the stimulating and recording electrodes is increased. Type A fibres usually dominate the record, not necessarily because they are more numerous but because they have the lowest threshold and highest conduction velocity.

Neuronal chemical synapses

The synapse is the site of contact between the axon

Astrocyte

Oligodendroglia   Microglia

Fig. 16.2 Three types of neuroglia. (Reproduced with modifications from Bray, J.J., Cragg, P.A., Macknight, A.D.C., Mills, R.G. & Taylor, D.W. (eds) (1989), *Lecture Notes in Physiology*, 2nd edn. Blackwell Scientific Publications, Oxford.)

Table 16.1 Important differences in the characteristics of local and action potentials.

Action potential	Local potential (electrotonic potential)
Site: at axons	At dendrites and soma (postsynaptic potentials) At sensory receptors (receptor potential) At motor end-plate (end-plate potential)
Permeability: voltage-dependent	Permeability: variable
All-or-none law: response to threshold is complete depolarization	Graded to the strength of the stimulus: non-threshold partial depolarization
Refractory period: summation impossible	No refractory period: summation possible
Propagated potential: not localized	Not propagated: localized
Amplitude: little change with distance	Decremental: maximum amplitude at point of origin, falls rapidly with distance
Conduction: potential change over long distance (range in mm or m) (active spread)	Conduction over short distance (in mm) (passive spread)

Table 16.2 Characteristics of nerve fibres.

	Type of nerve fibre		
	A	B	C
Fibre diameter (μm)	1–20	< 4	0.3–1.5
Conduction velocity (m/s)	5–120	3–15	0.6–2.5
Spike duration of AP (ms)	0.3–0.5	1.2	2.0

AP, action potential.

Divergence

Fig. 16.3 Record of a compound action potential. The letters refer to the type of nerve fibre.

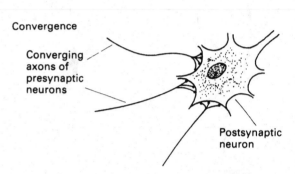

Fig. 16.4 Convergence and divergence.

terminal of one neuron (the *presynaptic neuron*) and another neuron (the *postsynaptic neuron*) across which transmission of nerve impulses occurs. The axon terminal of the presynaptic neuron (i.e. presynaptic fibre) divides into many branches, which end in small swellings, called *synaptic knobs*. These may then synapse either with a dendrite, with the soma or with the axon of the postsynaptic neuron, forming *axodendritic*, *axosomatic* or *axoaxonic synapses*, respectively. Inside the synaptic knob, there are many vesicles which contain a chemical substance, the **neurotransmitter**; there are also many mitochondria, which provide for the synthesis and release of the neurotransmitter.

Axons from many neurons may *converge* on a single neuron postsynaptic (Fig. 16.4) to influence its activity (**convergence**). Some of the converging presynaptic inputs may be excitatory, while others may be inhibitory. The balance between these inputs determines the output of the postsynaptic neuron. Alternatively, the axon of a single neuron may divide and synapse with many postsynaptic neurons, and therefore influences the excitability of many other neurons (Fig. 16.4). This is called **divergence**. It allows the spread of information to different parts of the CNS.

Synaptic transmission

When an action potential arrives at the synaptic knob, it opens voltage-gated Ca^{2+} channels there. As a result, Ca^{2+} influx occurs and causes the release of the neurotransmitter by vesicle fusion and exocytosis at distinct membrane sites, known as active zones (Fig. 16.5). The amount of transmitter released is related to the magnitude of Ca^{2+} influx, so extra amounts of Ca^{2+} are rapidly sequestered and removed from the neuron by an active pump. The neurotransmitter diffuses across the cleft and binds to receptor proteins on the postsynaptic membrane. The neurotransmitter–receptor complex then produces changes in the permeability of the postsynaptic membrane by opening, *chemical-gated* channels for specific ions. As a result these ions are allowed to pass across the membrane, causing a small local change in membrane potential (i.e. synaptic potential). Separate Na^+, K^+ and Cl^- channels are located in the postsynaptic membrane.

A transmitter that opens Na^+ channels increases positive charge inside the cell and so excites the postsynaptic neuron. Such a transmitter is an *excitatory* one. On the other hand, a transmitter that opens K^+ or Cl^- channels or both leads to loss of positive charge from inside the cell. As a result, the neuron is inhibited, due to hyperpolarization.

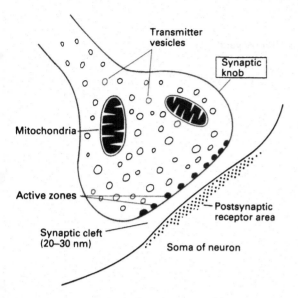

Transmitter
vesicles

Synaptic
knob

Mitochondria

Active zones

Synaptic cleft
(20–30 nm)

Postsynaptic
receptor area

Soma of neuron

Fig. 16.5 Physiological anatomy of a synapse.

Such a transmitter is *inhibitory*. It is believed that, with very few exceptions, each neuron releases only one type of transmitter, and it releases this same transmitter at all of its separate terminals.

However, it has been recently discovered that some neurons may release one or more neuropeptides from their terminals along with the classical small-molecule, rapidly acting neurotransmitter. Neuropeptides are large molecules and their reponses are much slower in onset and more prolonged. In addition, most neuropeptides function more as neuromodulators rather than neurotransmitters—that is, their release is not directed towards opening various ionic channels and the production of postsynaptic potentials, but instead leads to the activation of '*second-messenger*' systems inside the presynaptic or postsynaptic neuron. The activated second messenger brings about long-term changes, which basically alter the effectiveness of synaptic transmission, e.g. long-term increases in the amount of transmitter released or a long-term increase in the number of receptors. Such prolonged changes, which can last from days to years, are thought to be possible mechanisms of the process of memory.

Among the well-known classical, small-molecule, rapidly acting transmitters are **acetylcholine, noradrenaline** (norepinephrine), **adrenaline** (epinephrine), **serotonin, dopamine** and **gamma-aminobutyric acid (GABA)**. Neuropeptides include **endorphins, encephalins, substance P, hypothalamic releasing hormones,**

pituitary peptides, some peptides acting on the gut and brain and peptides from other tissues.

Electrical events during neuronal excitation

The resting membrane potential in most neurons is somewhat less than that found in large peripheral nerve fibres or in muscles, i.e. –65 mV. This makes the neuron more excitable.

Excitatory postsynaptic potential (EPSP).

If the presynaptic neuron is one that secretes an excitatory neurotransmitter, it will increase the permeability of the postsynaptic neurons to Na^+. Na^+ rushes in, due to the large electrochemical gradient across the membrane. The net effect is a localized depolarization of the postsynaptic cell membrane next to the excitatory knob. This increases the excitability of the neuron because part of the negativity of the RMP is neutralized, and it is brought closer to the threshold. The increase in voltage above RMP is called excitatory postsynaptic potential (EPSP).

It is important to note that the duration of the EPSP is much longer than that of an action potential. Also, note that an EPSP has to exceed a certain threshold before it triggers an action potential in the postsynaptic neuron. A single EPSP can never increase the postsynaptic neuronal potential to that level. Instead, the effects of several EPSPs must add up or summate to trigger an action potential.

There are two types of summation (Fig. 16.6):
1 *Temporal summation*. This occurs when successive postsynaptic potentials of an individual synaptic knob develop rapidly enough to summate. Each postsynaptic potential adds up to the previous one before it decays.
2 *Spatial summation*. This occurs when postsynaptic potentials from several knobs over the surface of a neuron summate.

The EPSP is thus not an all-or-none phenomenon but is graded in direct relationship to the intensity of the stimulus. As the excitability of the postsynaptic neuron reaches the threshold value of excitation, an action potential is initiated at the axon hillock. The axon hillock is the most excitable part of the neuron, because it has a much larger number of Na^+ channels than the body of the neuron or its dendrites.

Electrical events in neuronal inhibition

Inhibitory postsynaptic potential (IPSP) or postsynaptic inhibition.

When the presynaptic neuron is one that secretes an inhibitory transmitter, it will increase the permeability of the postsynaptic membrane to K^+ and Cl^-.

Spatial summation

Temporal summation

Fig. 16.6 Above: Spatial summation. Simultaneous stimuli from several presynaptic fibres summate to excite the postsynaptic neuron. Below: Temporal summation. Repetitive stimuli from one source summate to excite the postsynaptic neuron.

K^+ efflux decreases positive charge inside, and Cl^- influx increases negative charge inside. The net effect is an increase in the degree of intracellular negativity—a state of hyperpolarization. This will inhibit the neuron by pushing the membrane potential away from the threshold for excitation. The increased negativity below the normal RMP is known as the *inhibitory postsynaptic potential* (IPSP). Note that another type of inhibition can occur at the level of the presynaptic membrane (see below).

IPSPs can also undergo temporal and spatial summation.

Presynaptic inhibition. In this type, an inhibitory synaptic knob releases a transmitter at the termination of a presynaptic excitatory fibre (Fig. 16.7). The inhibitory transmitter released is mostly gamma-aminobutyric acid (GABA), which opens chloride channels. During simultaneous stimulation of the inhibitory synaptic knob and the presynaptic fibre, the negatively charged chloride ions rush into the presynaptic excitatory fibre, cancelling out a large part of

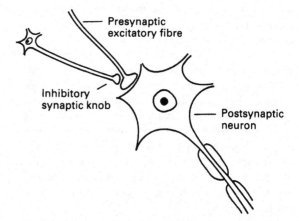

Fig. 16.7 Presynaptic inhibition. The inhibitory synaptic knob secretes a transmitter that depresses the voltage of an action potential at the synaptic membrane of the presynaptic excitatory fibre. The transmitter released from the latter is therefore reduced in amount and the degree of excitation of the postsynaptic neuron is decreased or inhibited.

the excitatory effect produced by the entry of the positively charged sodium ions. As a result, the action potentials reaching the excitatory ending are reduced. The Ca^{2+} influx decreases and therefore the amount of excitatory transmitter released at the synapse is also decreased.

Presynaptic inhibition takes longer to develop than postsynaptic inhibition, but persists longer when it is produced. It occurs in many sensory pathways. The fibres in a particular pathway give rise to collaterals, which inhibit nearby fibres via the interposition of an inhibitory interneuron. Thus lateral spread of excitation is greatly reduced, allowing a finer perception of the sensory pattern. Presynaptic inhibition is also known as **lateral inhibition**.

Properties of synapses

One-way conduction. Impulses conducted through synapses always pass from the pre- to the postsynaptic neuron and never in the reverse direction.

Synaptic fatigue. The number of impulses from the postsynaptic neurons decreases progressively when the presynaptic neuron is repetitively stimulated at a rapid rate. This is mainly due to exhaustion of neurotransmitter stores in synaptic knobs, but also partly due to progressive inactivation of postsynaptic receptors.

Synaptic fatigue can serve as a protective mechanism. A good example is the cessation of an epileptic fit (due to synaptic fatigue), which otherwise would have been fatal.

Post-tetanic facilitation. Repetitive stimulation of an excitatory synapse for a period of time leads to a few moments of synaptic fatigue, followed by a period of increased excitability of the postsynaptic neuron, which might extend from a few seconds to several hours. This is called post-tetanic facilitation and is thought to be due to accumulation of Ca^{2+} in the presynaptic terminals as a result of the repetitive stimulation. The excess Ca^{2+} would eventually lead to increased release of transmitter from knobs.

Post-tetanic facilitation is considered to be one of the mechanisms for short-term memory, in which information is stored as a continuous electrical activity.

Synaptic delay. This is the minimum time required for transmission across one synapse (about 0.5 ms). Most of this time is spent in the release of transmitter.

Uniqueness of central synapses. Although synapses are found both in the CNS and in the autonomic ganglia of the peripheral nervous system, the property of inhibition is unique to central synapses.

Blood pH. Alkalosis greatly enhances neuronal excitability and synaptic transmission, while acidosis decreases synaptic transmission. A rise of blood pH to 7.8 causes convulsions and a fall to 7.0 or below results in coma.

Hypoxia. Synaptic transmission depends on adequate oxygenation. If the blood supply to the brain stops, a subject becomes unconscious within about 5 seconds and may suffer permanent damage to the brain.

Drugs. Some drugs increase the excitability of neurons and enhance synaptic transmission. Caffeine, theophylline and theobromine (found in tea, coffee and cocoa) act by decreasing the threshold for excitation of neurons. Strychnine, on the other hand, acts by inhibiting the action of inhibitory chemical transmitters.

Other drugs decrease the excitability of neurons and thereby decrease synaptic transmission. Anaesthetics act by making neuronal membranes less responsive to excitatory agents.

Functional anatomy of the central nervous system

The CNS comprises the brain lying within the skull and the spinal cord lying within the vertebral column.

Spinal cord

The spinal cord consists of segments, each of which has a pair of nerve roots, on each side (Fig. 16.8). The dorsal roots carry impulses from peripheral receptors into the spinal cord, while the ventral roots carry impulses to the periphery

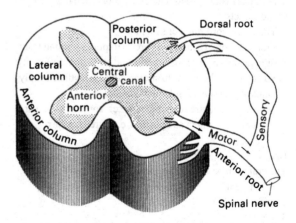

Fig. 16.8 Transverse section of the spinal cord.

(a)

(b)

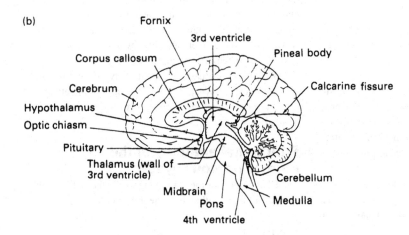

Fig. 16.9 The human brain. (a) Lateral view. (b) View at a midsagittal section. (Reproduced from Bray, J.J., Cragg, P.A., Macknight, A.D.C., Mills, R.G. & Taylor, D.W. (eds) (1989) *Lecture Notes in Physiology*, 2nd edn. Blackwell Scientific Publications, Oxford.)

(i.e. muscles). Grey matter forms the core of the spinal cord and appears like the letter 'H' in cross-section. It contains the cell bodies of neurons. White matter surrounds the grey matter. It is made up of ascending (sensory) and descending (motor) tracts.

The spinal cord functions include:

1 Transmission of sensory (afferent) impulses coming from peripheral receptors to the brain and of motor (efferent) impulses from the brain to motor neurons, which supply effector organs (i.e. muscles and glands).

2 Serving as a centre for some reflexes, some of which are the basis of movement and posture, e.g. stretch reflex.

Brain

The brain can be divided into four subdivisions (Fig. 16.9):

1 Brain stem.
2 Diencephalon.
3 Cerebellum.
4 Cerebrum.

Brain stem

The brain stem consists of the medulla, pons and midbrain.

The medulla forms the upper extension of the spinal cord. It contains motor and sensory nuclei of the throat, mouth and neck, and nuclei for respiratory and cardiovascular control centres. The medulla also contains the nuclei of cranial nerves IX, X, XI and XII.

The pons is continuous with the medulla and also contains control centres for the respiratory and cardiovascular systems. It also contains nuclei of some sensory and motor nerves (i.e. nuclei of cranial nerves V, VI, VII and VIII).

The midbrain is continuous with the pons below and the diencephalon above. It contains nuclei of cranial nerves III and IV which mediate pupillary reflexes and eye movement.

The recticular formation of the brain stem extends from the medulla through the pons to the midbrain. It is composed mainly of ascending and descending tracts and some nuclei. The reticular formation plays an important role in the control of *muscle tone* and in *arousal* or *alerting mechanisms*.

Diencephalon

The diencephalon is composed of the two thalami laterally and the hypothalamus ventrally. Thalamic nuclei are functionally divided into several groups. The most important of these are as follows. One group relays all types of sensation to the sensory cortex except olfaction. Another group relays signals from the cerebellum and basal ganglia to the motor cortex. The third group controls the general level of activity of the whole cerebral cortex and is therefore responsible for the level of consciousness. The hypothalamus is the higher autonomic centre (e.g. control of blood pressure, heart rate and body temperature). It also secretes hormones that control the release of other hormones from the pituitary gland. Being part of the limbic system, the hypothalamus plays a role in the generation of emotions. There are also centres for control of appetite and water intake.

Cerebellum

The cerebellum lies in the posterior aspect of the brain stem and is connected to it by three thick bundles of white matter (cerebellar peduncles), which carry impulses in and out of the cerebellum. It consists of two lateral hemispheres and a central part called the vermis. All parts have the same histological structure—a thin superficial layer of grey matter or cerebellar cortex lies on the outside, enclosing an area of white matter. This latter consists of the fibres that enter and leave the cerebellar cortex. Masses of grey matter, the cerebellar nuclei, are found within the white matter.

The cerebellum is concerned with:

1 Control of rate, range and direction of movement.
2 Control of muscle tone.
3 Control of equilibrium and posture.

Cerebrum

The cerebrum consists of the right and left cerebral hemispheres, connected in the midline by the corpus callosum. The superficial layer of each hemisphere is composed of grey matter—the cerebral cortex. This encloses a larger area of white matter, inside which lie a number of nuclei, known as basal ganglia. These play a very important role in the planning and control of movement.

The cerebral cortex has elevations (gyri) and depressions (sulci), which greatly increase its surface area (see Fig. 16.9).

Each hemisphere is divided into four lobes. The temporal lobe lies on the lateral surface of the hemisphere below the lateral fissure (deep groove) that separates it from the frontal and parietal lobes above. The temporal lobe contains the *primary auditory area*, which is the centre of hearing. The central sulcus forms the borderline between the frontal lobe anteriorly and the parietal lobe posteriorly. The precentral gyrus lies immediately in front of the central sulcus, and this forms the *primary motor area*, which controls muscular movements. The postcentral gyrus lies immediately behind the central sulcus and forms the *primary sensory area*, which perceives sensory information arriving from skin, muscles, joints and the viscera.

The occipital lobe lies most posterior in the cerebral hemisphere. In it is located the *primary visual cortex*, the centre for vision.

The parietal, temporal and occipital lobes meet in the angular gyrus. Just in front of this gyrus is an area of cortex called *Wernicke's area*. This area, often called the general interpretative area, knowing area or gnostic area, plays a crucial role in higher functions of the brain, such as thinking, speech and language. On the undersurface of the medial occipital and temporal lobes is a special area which plays the important role of recognition of faces. Bilateral lesions of this area produce *prosopagnosia*, i.e. inability to recognize people by faces.

The white matter of the cerebral hemisphere constitutes three types of fibres:

1 *Association fibres*. These connect gyri in the same hemisphere.
2 *Projection fibres*. These form the ascending and descending tracts, which carry impulses to and from the hemispheres.
3 *Commissural fibres*. These connect gyri of one hemisphere with corresponding gyri of the other hemisphere. The most important commissure is the *corpus callosum*.

It is of interest to note that splitting of the corpus callosum causes each hemisphere to behave independently of the other—a condition known as split brain. A patient with split brain will identify an object placed on his hand while his eyes are closed but will be unable to identify it as the same object when it is transferred to the other hand.

The sensory system

The sensory system provides us with information about our environment—both the external and the internal environment. All information comes to us through our sense organs, which contain structures called receptors. Receptors are therefore detectors and are also transducers that convert the various forms of energy (light, sound, chemical, mechanical, etc.) they detect into action potentials. When these action potentials reach the brain and enter consciousness, we experience a sensation, e.g. vision, hearing, pain, touch, cold, etc. Every sensation is associated with a feeling that it is pleasant or unpleasant. This emotional component of a sensation is called its affect.

Anatomically, receptors are specialized structures present at the peripheral terminations of afferent fibres. From the receptors to the brain are pathways made up of chains of neurons. These pathways, e.g. visual pathway, pain pathway, etc., make up the sensory system.

Sensory receptors

Classification of receptors
1 *Telereceptors (distance receptors).* These are receptors that detect events at a distance, i.e. rods and cones for light and hair cells of the cochlea for sound.
2 *Exteroceptors.* These are concerned with information about the immediate external environment. They are found in the skin, e.g. touch receptors, temperature receptors.
3 *Interoceptors.* These are concerned with information about the internal environment, e.g. chemoreceptors, osmoreceptors.
4 *Proprioceptors.* These are concerned with information about the position of the body in space. They are found in muscles, tendons and joints.
5 *Nociceptors.* These are pain receptors. They are called nociceptors (from the Latin *nocere*: to injure) because all painful stimuli arise due to injury or damage to tissues.

Properties of receptors
Receptors have the properties of specificity, excitability and adaptation.

Specificity. Each type of receptor is most sensitive to one specific form of energy, which is called its adequate stimulus, and is almost non-responsive to the normal intensities of other forms of energy; e.g. light is the adequate stimulus for the rods and cones of the eyes but they do not respond to heat or cold (Fig. 16.10).

Pain receptors are not stimulated by a blunt object touching the skin, but they discharge as soon as the blunt object is pushed with enough force to damage tissues.

The sensation perceived as a result of stimulation of a receptor is called the *modality* of sensation. Thus, cold, warmth, touch and pain are different modalities of sensation.

Excitability. Different types of receptors are excited in different ways. Some are stimulated by mechanical deformation, others by application or release of a chemical and others by changes of temperature or by electromagnetic radiation. The receptor transforms these various stimuli

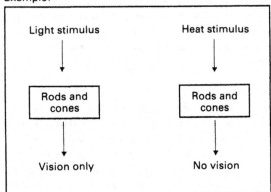

Fig. 16.10 The concept of the adequate stimulus.

into a local electrical change, called the **generator** or **receptor** potential. This is a state of non-propagated partial depolarization. Successive receptor potentials can be summated; and when the threshold value is reached, an action potential (AP) is triggered, then propagated along the sensory nerve from the receptor. The response to receptor stimulation is not a single AP but a volley of action potentials, the frequency of which is directly related to the intensity of the applied stimulus.

Adaptation. When a stimulus of constant strength is continuously applied to a receptor, the frequency of action potentials in the afferent nerve fibre leading from that receptor gradually declines. This phenomenon is called adaptation, and the rate at which it occurs varies in different types of receptors. Some adapt slowly and are known as tonic receptors. These continue to transmit impulses to the brain at a relatively constant rate during continuous

Fig. 16.11 Diagram showing a comparison between the rates of adaptation of receptors.

stimulation, and are therefore useful in detecting changes in the body, which the brain needs to be constantly informed about (Fig. 16.11). Examples of tonic receptors are:

1 Muscle spindle, for information about posture.

2 Joint receptors, for information about the position of different parts of the body.

3 Baroreceptors, for information about arterial blood pressure.

Pain receptors do not adapt at all. This is useful because pain serves as a protective mechanism for the body.

Another group of receptors adapt rapidly. These are known as phasic receptors because, although they show a rapid decline in the magnitude of the receptor potential (and thus a decrease in the frequency of AP along its nerve) with maintained stimulation, they react strongly while a change in the intensity of the stimulus is taking place. They are therefore useful in transmitting information about events which undergo rapid changes, but are of no use in transmitting information about constant events, e.g. touch receptors.

Temperature receptors occupy a position between the above two groups. Thus, they are rated as moderately adapting receptors.

The mechanism of adaptation is specific to the type of receptor. For example, mechanoreceptors, such as Pacinian corpuscles, adapt due to readjustment in their structure when the applied pressure is continued. Other receptors may adapt by the accommodation of the sensory nerve fibre to the receptor potential. It is proposed that accommodation occurs due to gradual inactivation or the **Na+ channels** in the nerve fibre membrane.

Coding of sensory information

Most sensory information aims at causing an awareness of the state of the body and its surroundings. Coding of sensory information enables higher centres to discriminate modality, locality and intensity of different sensory stimuli, although all sensory information is presented to these centres in the form of action potentials similar in all nerve fibres.

Modality

Modality discrimination is made possible by the following:

1 There is a specific stimulus for each receptor—the adequate stimulus.

2 A receptor or its nerve pathway when stimulated gives rise to one type of sensation, regardless of the method of stimulation. This is called the *law of specific nerve energies*. For example, stimulation of a pain receptor or the nerve pathway leading from it will cause a subject to perceive pain whether the stimulus was heat, electric shock or crushing of the tissues.

3 A specific pathway exists for each modality of sensation, i.e. pain pathway, touch pathway, etc.

4 Each nerve fibre in the pathway ends at a specific area in the CNS. The modality perceived is determined by that area, i.e. a subject perceives touch or temperature because their respective pathways end at a specific touch or temperature area in the brain.

Localization

Locality discrimination is explained by the *law of projection*. Conscious perception of a particular sensation is always projected to the locality of the receptor, irrespective of where the sensory pathway (leading from the receptor) is stimulated.

This explains the **phantom limb** phenomenon which occurs after amputation. In someone with an amputated lower limb, squeezing the nerves in the stump causes the patient to report pain in the little toe or ankle, i.e. in parts which have been lost. As the impulses reach the sensory cortex, the sensation is projected to the site of the receptors previously removed with the amputated part. This gives rise to the false interpretation.

Intensity

The increased intensity of stimulus is coded to the brain in two ways (Fig. 16.12): by an increase in the *frequency* of action potentials along the sensory nerve and/or by an increase in the *number of receptors* stimulated.

The somatic sensations

The somatic sensations are those sensations carried from the various parts of the body by somatic nerves.

Strength of stimulus	Weak	Moderate	Strong
Number of receptors(*) stimulated	↓ *	⬇ ***	⬇ *** ****
Frequency of discharge from each receptor	‖‖‖‖‖	‖‖‖‖‖‖‖	‖‖‖‖‖‖‖‖‖‖

Fig. 16.12 Effect of increasing stimulus intensity on receptor excitation.

Classification of somatic sensations

Somatic sensations can be classified into three types:
1 Mechanoreceptive senses, stimulated by mechanical displacement of body tissues.
2 Thermoreceptive senses, stimulated by heat and cold.
3 Pain sense, stimulated by any factor that leads to tissue damage.

Mechanoreceptive senses include touch, pressure, vibration and tickle senses (which are frequently called the tactile senses) and the position sense.

Cutaneous receptors

A large number of tactile receptors have been described. These include free nerve endings, encapsulated nerve endings and expanded-tip tactile receptors, the distribution of which vary in different regions of the body. Free nerve endings are widely distributed in the skin and have been shown to respond to nearly all sensory modalities. The expanded-tip tactile receptors include *Merkel's discs* and *Ruffini endings*. These are relatively slow adapting touch receptors, which, due to this property, enable determination of continuous touch stimuli on the skin. *Meissner's corpuscles* and *Pacinian corpuscles* are encapsulated, rapidly adapting receptors. The former are the receptors for fine touch, i.e. recognition of locality, form and texture of objects touched, while the latter are particularly important for detection of extremely rapidly changing mechanical events, e.g. vibration sense. Another important tactile receptor is the tactile hair and its basal nerve fibre, collectively called the hair end organ. This receptor detects mainly movements of objects on the surface of the body. Pacinian corpuscles and Ruffini endings are also described among receptors found in deeper tissues and joint capsules. There they subserve the sensation of deep pressure and position (i.e. proprioception).

In spite of the large number of types of mechanoreceptors, they transmit their impulses via three types of fibres. Receptors such as Meissner's and Pacinian corpuscles, Merkel's discs, hair end receptors and Ruffini endings transmit impulses via quick-conducting type Aβ fibres. The less specialized free nerve endings transmit via the slower fibres, type Aδ and type C.

Thermoreceptive sensations are discriminated by two types of receptors that detect heat changes, i.e. cold and warmth receptors, and others that detect pain resulting from extremes of temperature. Warmth receptors, and probably cold receptors, are free nerve endings, although specific encapsulated endings for cold sensation have been described. Since cold is not a form of energy, both warmth and cold receptors actually respond to different degrees of warmth. Cold receptors are more densely distributed than warmth receptors. Indeed, there are three to 10 times as many cold receptors as warmth receptors in the skin. They respond to skin temperatures from 10°C to 40°C and probably transmit their impulses via **type C** fibres. Encapsulated cold receptors, however, transmit via type **Aδ** fibres. Warmth receptors respond from 30°C to 45°C and transmit impulses via **type C** fibres. At temperatures below 10°C and above 45°C, tissue damage begins to occur and the sensation experienced is pain, due to stimulation of two subtypes of pain receptors: cold-pain and heat-pain receptors, respectively.

Thermoreceptors are rated as moderately adapting receptors. This happens at skin temperatures between 20°C and 40°C, but no adaptation occurs at skin temperatures below 20°C and above 40°C. It is important to note that thermoreceptors respond vigorously to changes in temperature but they also respond to steady states of temperature.

Pain receptors are all free nerve endings. They are dis-

Fig. 16.13 Schematic diagram of (a) a typical sensory pathway from a receptor in the head region; (b) a typical sensory pathway from a receptor in the trunk region.

tributed in almost every tissue of the body and transmit their impulses in two types of fibres, Aδ and C fibres. The physiological significance of these two types will be discussed later.

To conclude, it can be seen that receptors are classified according to the kind of energy to which they are most specific. Thus, mechanoreceptors respond to mechanical energy, thermoreceptors to heat, and pain receptors to chemicals released as a result of tissue damage. In some cases, specificity can be associated with a particular structure (e.g. Pacinian corpuscle), but more often structures (or receptors) which appear histologically similar show different specificities. Thus free nerve endings that signal itch and tickle sensations are different from those free nerve endings which detect temperature.

Neural basis of sensation

Having described the characteristics and properties of

receptors, we can consider the construction of a typical sensory pathway. Figure 16.13 shows a typical sensory pathway from a receptor in the head region and one from the body to the brain. Lesions can occur at any level in that pathway.

Somatosensory tracts

After entering the spinal cord, sensory fibres follow one of two ascending tracts within the spinal cord:

1 *The dorsal (posterior) column lemniscal tracts.* These subserve the following:

    (a) Touch sensations characterized by sharp localization and high-intensity discrimination (i.e. fine touch).

    (b) Rapidly repetitive sensations, such as the sense of vibration.

    (c) Position sensations.

    (d) Pressure sensations characterized by high-intensity discrimination (i.e. fine pressure).

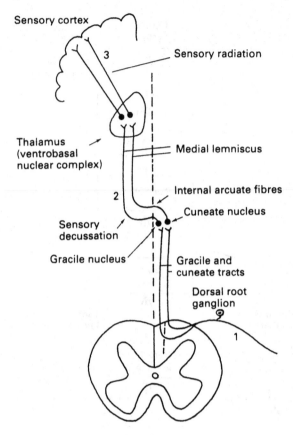

Sensory cortex

3

Sensory radiation

Thalamus
(ventrobasal
nuclear complex)

Medial lemniscus

2

Internal arcuate fibres

Cuneate nucleus

Sensory
decussation

Gracile nucleus

Gracile and
cuneate tracts

Dorsal root
ganglion

1

Fig. 16.14 The dorsal column pathway. (1), (2) and (3) refer to first-, second- and third-order neurons.

2 *The anterolateral tracts (spinothalamic tracts).* These subserve the following:

(a) Pain.

(b) Thermal sensations, including both warm and cold sensations.

(c) Touch sensations characterized by crude localization and poor-intensity discrimination (i.e. crude touch).

(d) Pressure sensations characterized by poor-intensity discrimination (i.e. crude pressure).

(e) Tickle and itch sensations.

(f) Sexual sensations.

Dorsal column lemniscal pathway. The fibres destined for this pathway are mainly large myelinated type $A\beta$ fibres. These are actually the axons of first-order neurons (Fig. 16.14).

The pathway contains three orders of neurons, which are:

1 *First-order neurons.* Afferent fibres enter the spinal cord via the medial portion of the dorsal root. They enter the ipsilateral dorsal column and ascend upwards as the gracile and cuneate tracts to relay, respectively, in the gracile and cuneate nuclei of the medulla.

2 *Second-order neurons.* These are located in the gracile and cuneate nuclei and give rise to axons which cross to the opposite side, forming the sensory decussation. They then pass upwards as the medial lemniscus, which traverses the midbrain to end in the ventrobasal nuclei of the thalamus.

In its pathway through the brain stem, the medial lemniscus is joined by additional fibres from the sensory nuclei of the trigeminal nerve. These fibres carry the same sensations from the head that the dorsal column fibres carry from the body.

3 *Third-order neurons.* These arise from the ventrobasal nuclear complex of the thalamus and pass in the posterior limb of the internal capsule as part of the sensory radiation to the somatosensory cortex.

Anterolateral pathway (spinothalamic pathway). Fibres contributing to this pathway are small, myelinated type $A\delta$ and unmyelinated type C fibres, which enter the spinal cord via the lateral division of the dorsal roots.

The paths of the three orders of neurons are as follows:

1 *First-order neurons.* Afferent fibres, after entering the spinal cord, ascend a few segments before synapsing on the cells of the dorsal horn lamina I, II, III, IV, V and VI (Fig. 16.15).

2 *Second-order neurons.* These are the cells of the dorsal horn and give rise to axons, which cross to the opposite side in front of the central canal (i.e. anterior commissure) and ascend as the spinothalamic tracts through the anterolateral columns of the spinal cord. The fibres then ascend through the brain stem to end in the ventrobasal nuclear complex of the thalamus.

In the anterior commissure of the spinal cord, the temperature fibres are nearest to the central canal. Next to these are the pain fibres, and the furthest from the central canal are the touch fibres. Therefore, in *syringomyelia*, a developmental defect of the central canal, the temperature and pain fibres and damaged and the touch fibres escape. This leads to loss of temperature and pain sensation with preservation of other sensations—a phenomenon known as dissociated anaesthesia or dissociated sensory loss.

3 *Third-order neurons.* These arise from the thalamus and send axons which ascend in the posterior limb of the internal capsule as part of the sensory radiation, to reach the somatosensory area of the cerebral cortex.

It is worth mentioning here that the anterolateral pathway can be divided into two separate pathways: the anterior spinothalamic and the lateral spinothalamic tracts

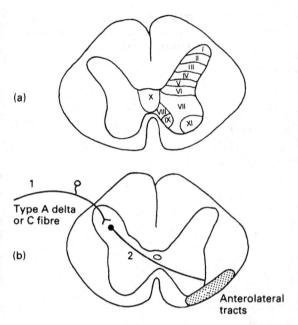

Fig. 16.15 (a) Cross-section of the spinal cord showing the anatomical laminae I to XI of the cord grey matter. (b) Cross-section of the spinal cord showing the first- and second-order neurons in the anterolateral spinothalamic tract. 1, First-order neuron; 2, second-order neuron. (Reproduced from Bray, J.J., Cragg, P.A., Macknight, A.D.C., Mills, R.G. & Taylor, D.W. (eds) (1989) *Lecture Notes in Physiology*, 2nd edn. Blackwell Scientific Publications, Oxford.)

(see Fig. 16.20). While the anterior tract carries crude touch and pressure, itch and tickle, and sexual sensations, the lateral tract transmits pain and temperature sensations.

Table 16.3 shows some major differences in the functional and anatomical characteristics between the two major sensory pathways. One of these is a difference in the spatial orientation of nerve fibres in each. Due to this difference, tumours arising outside the spinal cord (extramedullary tumours) first damage the sacral fibres of the spinothalamic pathway, whereas intramedullary tumours damage the sacral fibres last of all (i.e. sacral-sparing).

Role of the thalamus and the sensory cortex in the appreciation of sensation

All sensory tracts, except the olfactory pathway, synapse in the thalamus on their way to the cerebral cortex. When impulses mediating a given sensation reach the thalamus, the subject becomes crudely aware of the sensation but he/she cannot perceive all of its fine details: e.g. a person will be aware of a change in temperature if he/she contacts a hot object but his/her perception of how hot the object

is, will be less acute. Gradations and spatial and temporal characteristics are appreciated at the level of the sensory cortex and not at the level of the thalamus (Fig. 16.16). Pain and, to a lesser extent, temperature however, seem to be the only sensations that are fully appreciated at the thalamic and probably even at the reticular formation level or even lower. Still, interpretation of the quality and localization of these sensations occurs at the level of the cerebral cortex.

The somatosensory cortex

The somatosensory area is that part of the cerebral cortex to which sensory signals are projected. It comprises two areas, which receive direct afferent fibres from the specific nuclei of the thalamus. Somatosensory area I is the primary sensory area and lies in the postcentral gyrus, and somatosensory area II lies in the wall of the Sylvian fissure (Fig. 16.16).

Somatosensory area I of one cerebral hemisphere is stimulated by impulses arriving from the contralateral side of the body, with the exception of the face, which is bilaterally represented in both hemispheres. The legs are represented on top and the head at the bottom of the gyrus (Fig. 16.16). Moreover, the area of representation of a specific part of the body is related to the density of receptors in the part and not to its size. In humans the lips are represented by the greatest area, followed by the face and thumb, while the entire trunk is represented by a relatively much smaller area (Fig. 16.17). Recordings from somatosensory area I have also shown that it is organized functionally into columns. The cells in a given column are stimulated by afferents from a particular part of the body and all respond to the same sensory modality.

The sensory cortex is concerned with three discriminative faculties:

1 *Spatial recognition*. This includes localization of the site of the stimulus and two-point discrimination. The latter is defined as the ability of a person to perceive two touch stimuli applied simultaneously as two separate points while both eyes are closed. The ability of tactile discrimination varies according to the site. Normally, 2 mm of separation of points can be recognized as two separate stimuli on the fingertips but about 30 mm of separation of points are needed in the back region to perceive two separate stimuli. The acuity of two-point discrimination increases with increase in the number of touch receptors per unit area of skin and with the increase in the width of area of representation in the sensory cortex. The ability of tactile discrimination is lost in dorsal column and parietal cortical (i.e. somatosensory cortex) lesions.

Dorsal column lemniscal pathway	Anterolateral pathway
Is concerned with fine type of transmission (e.g. there is a high degree of spatial orientation of nerve fibres in respect of their origin on the surface of the body)	Is concerned with a cruder type of transmission (e.g. Poor degree of spatial orientation)
Gradations of intensities are acute	Gradations of intensities are far less acute
Responsiveness is not greatly altered by stimuli from other areas of the nervous system	Responsiveness can be greatly altered by stimuli from other areas of the nervous system (i.e. brain and spinal cord analgesic system)
Fibres from the lower parts of the body lie towards the centre, while fibres from higher levels form successive layers laterally	Fibres from the lower parts lie laterally, while those from higher levels form successive layers towards the centre
Receives afferent sensory fibres of the dorsal root, which belong to type Aβ fibres, which ascend directly in the dorsal columns	Receives afferent sensory fibres, which are thin myelinated type Aδ fibres or unmyelinated type C fibres. These travel in Lissauer's tract and relay in the dorsal horn, to give rise to the anterolateral pathway
Has a very fast velocity of transmission (i.e. 30–110 m/s)	Has a relatively slow velocity of transmission (8–40 m/s)
Has great ability to transmit rapidly repetitive sensations (i.e. vibration sense)	Has poor ability to transmit rapidly repetitive sensations
Is limited to transmission of mechanoreceptive sensations only (i.e. fine touch and pressure sense, vibration sense, position sense)	Has the ability to transmit a broad spectrum of modalities (i.e. pain, thermal sensation, crude touch and pressure, itch and tickle sensations, sexual sensations)

Table 16.3 Comparison between the different characteristics of the two major sensory pathways.

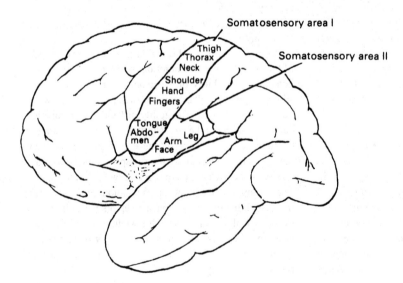

Fig. 16.16 The two somatosensory cortical areas, somatosensory areas I and II. (Reproduced with permission from Guyton, A.C. (1987) *Textbook of Medical Physiology*, 7th edn. Saunders, Philadelphia.)

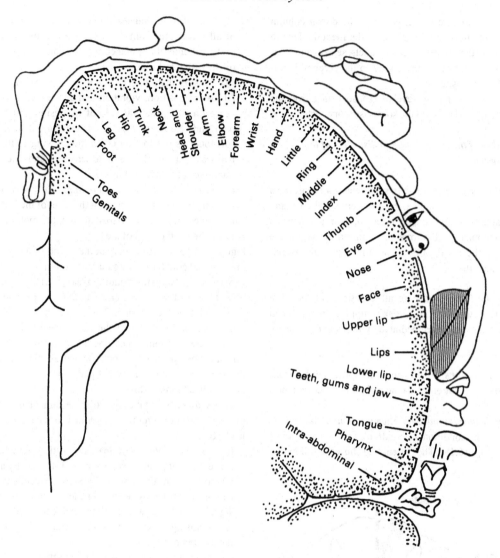

Fig. 16.17 Representation of the different areas of the body in somatosensory area I of the cortex.

2 *Recognition of relative intensities of different stimuli.* An increase in intensity of stimuli is transmitted to the brain in the form of an increase in the number of afferent fibres stimulated and increased frequency of action potentials in these fibres. These two features are perceived as an indication of the strength of the stimulus.

3 *Stereognosis.* This is defined as the ability to recognize objects by touch without the aid of vision. Loss of this ability, called *astereognosis*, occurs due to dorsal column or cortical lesions. In addition to astereognosis, dorsal column lesions cause loss of other sensations carried by the tract. These include other aspects of fine touch (i.e. two-point

discrimination and localization) and proprioceptive and vibration senses. In cortical lesions, however, somatic sensations are not abolished, since some perception is possible at the level of the thalamus, but pure cortical functions, such as localization, tactile discrimination and stereognosis, are lost.

Disordered function of the sensory system
In discussing features that accompany disordered function of the sensory system, it is useful to recall that, at the level of the spinal cord: (i) the spinothalamic pathway is crossed; and (ii) the dorsal column pathway is uncrossed. It is also

of importance to note that crossing of the dorsal column lemniscal system occurs higher up in the medulla. Due to the crossing of the two major sensory tracts, sensory information from one half of the body goes to the cerebral hemisphere of the opposite side.

Lesions can occur at any level of a sensory tract, from the afferent peripheral nerve to the somatosensory cortex.

Localization of the site of lesion in disorders of the sensory system

Lesion of a peripheral nerve. In such a case, all sensations are lost in the area supplied by the nerve. When many peripheral nerves are diffusely affected, as in polyneuritis or polyneuropathy, all forms of common sensation are impaired in the distal parts of the limbs (e.g. glove-and-stocking anaesthesia).

Lesion of the dorsal root. Here, all sensations are lost in the relative dermatome, i.e. area of skin supplied by the dorsal root. The tendon reflexes mediated by fibres in the root are also lost.

Spinal cord lesions. The features in spinal cord lesions depend on the location of damage. The three commonest lesions are:

1 *Brown-Séquard syndrome (hemisection of the spinal cord).* In this condition one-half of the spinal cord is damaged (Fig. 16.18). The patient will show the following:

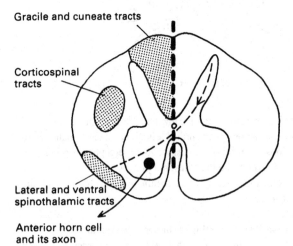

Gracile and cuneate tracts

Corticospinal tracts

Lateral and ventral spinothalamic tracts

Anterior horn cell and its axon

Fig. 16.18 Brown-Séquard syndrome. The pathways (tracts) damaged in Brown-Séquard syndrome are shown by the shaded areas. The thick broken line indicates the limits of the lesion.

(a) Sensory disturbances at the level of the lesion: loss of all sensations from the area supplied by the dorsal roots that enter the spinal cord at the damaged segments on the ipsilateral side.

(b) Sensory disturbances below the level of the lesion: (i) loss of position, vibration and tactile discrimination sense on the ipsilateral side of the lesion; (ii) loss of pain and temperature sense on the contralateral side; (iii) touch is not lost on either side, owing to the dual pathway for touch, i.e. one crossed and the other uncrossed at spinal cord level.

(c) Motor disturbances, including: (i) lower motor neuron lesion manifestations at the level of the lesion on the same side; and (ii) an ipsilateral upper motor neuron lesion below the level of the lesion.

Figure 16.19 gives a summary of the effects of hemisection of the spinal cord (Brown-Séquard syndrome).

2 *Syringomyelia.* In this condition, damage is to the central part of the cord, where the crossing fibres of pain, temperature and touch decussate. This leads to loss of these sensations on both sides of the body at the affected segments. However, fine touch, including tactile discrimination, and position sense are not affected, as they are carried in the dorsal column/lemniscal pathway. Thus, the result is dissociated sensory loss.

3 *Tabes dorsalis.* In tabes dorsalis, the damage is confined to the dorsal root central to the dorsal root ganglion. This leads to:

(a) Loss of tactile discrimination, position and vibration sense. Loss of position sensation leads to sensory ataxia, which is incoordination of voluntary movements. This can be confirmed by testing for the positive Romberg's sign, in which the patient will be unable to stand steadily when closing his eyes. Ataxia also causes the patient to have a stamping gait.

(b) Loss of pain and temperature sensation.

(c) Loss of all reflexes (i.e. superficial, deep and visceral) mediated by fibres in the dorsal root affected. Certain areas are more susceptible to be affected by the disease than others (i.e. cervicothoracic and lumbosacral regions).

Brain stem lesions. At the level of the brain stem, the main sensory tracts have already crossed the midline. Therefore, lesions in this area lead to loss of all sensations on the contralateral side.

Thalamic lesions. Spontaneous pain of a most unpleasant quality, together with exaggerated response to painful stimuli due to facilitation of neurons in the thalamus (i.e.

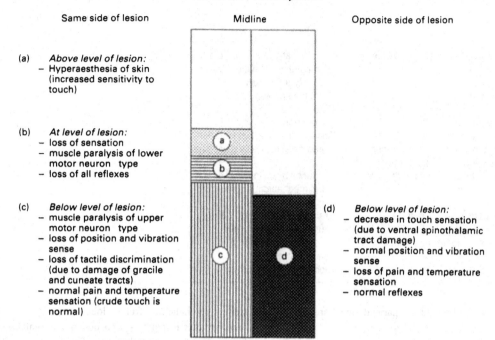

Same side of lesion   Midline   Opposite side of lesion

(a) *Above level of lesion:*
 – Hyperaesthesia of skin (increased sensitivity to touch)

(b) *At level of lesion:*
 – loss of sensation
 – muscle paralysis of lower motor neuron type
 – loss of all reflexes

(c) *Below level of lesion:*
 – muscle paralysis of upper motor neuron type
 – loss of position and vibration sense
 – loss of tactile discrimination (due to damage of gracile and cuneate tracts)
 – normal pain and temperature sensation (crude touch is normal)

(d) *Below level of lesion:*
 – decrease in touch sensation (due to ventral spinothalamic tract damage)
 – normal position and vibration sense
 – loss of pain and temperature sensation
 – normal reflexes

Fig. 16.19 A schematic diagram showing the manifestations of the Brown-Séquard syndrome.

secondary hyperalgesia), is characteristic of this condition. Other sensations are lost on the opposite side of the body.

Cortical lesions. Lesions in the sensory cortex lead to loss of *topognosis* (i.e. ability to localize the site of stimulus), loss of two-point discrimination and astereognosis.

A small area lying posterior to the main sensory area in the cerebral cortex is called the *secondary somatic area.* This area plays an important role in interpreting the meaning of sensations perceived by the main sensory area. Damage to this area may produce a disturbance of the body image and of spatial orientation. The patient may ignore one side of his/her body—a condition called *amorphosynthesis* or sensory inattention.

When lesions occur at the highest cortical level, the condition arising is known as *hysterical sensory loss.* In this condition the sensory loss does not correspond to the anatomical nerve supply of the part. There are sharp lines of demarcation between normal and abnormal areas of sensation. The areas of sensory loss may change in response to suggestions made by the doctor.

The physiology of pain

Pain sensation is produced by stimuli that cause or threaten to cause tissue damage (i.e. noxious stimuli). Sherrington defined pain as 'the physical adjunct of an imperative protective reflex', i.e. pain is the mental component of an urgently operating reflex designed for protection of the body from injury.

Properties of pain sensation

1 All pain receptors are free nerve endings. They are neither encapsulated nor expanded-tip receptors.

2 Pain receptors are the most widely distributed amongst receptors to other modalities.

3 Pain sensation can be produced by various types of stimuli (i.e. mechanical, thermal and chemical): hence the existence of mechanosensitive, thermosensitive and chemosensitive pain receptors.

4 Localization of pain stimuli is less exact than that of other modalities. In fact, pain sensation may originate in one place and be felt in another (i.e. referred pain).

5 Pain receptors adapt very little, if at all. In fact, the sensitivity of pain receptors increases with time (i.e. hyperalgesia).

6 The pain threshold is higher than that of other modalities, i.e. painful stimuli must be strong and noxious. However, pain remains a specific sensation and can never be caused by overstimulation of other receptors.

7 Certain visceral areas are insensitive to pain. These include brain tissue, liver parenchyma and lung alveoli, but the brain blood-vessels and meninges, the liver capsule and

Fast pain	Slow pain
Fast, felt within 0.1 s after stimulation. Mostly felt *during* injury	Slow, felt after 1 s or more after stimulation. Thus, mostly felt shortly *after* injury
Pricking nature	Burning or aching nature
Localized	Diffuse
Short duration	Longer duration
Arises from receptors in superficial tissues and in serosal membranes (pleura, pericardium and peritoneum	Arises from receptors in superficial and deep tissues and viscera.
Produced by mechanical and thermal energy	Produced by all forms of energy, i.e. mechanical, thermal and chemical
Transmitted by type Aδ (fast myelinated) fibres	Transmitted by type C (slow unmyelinated) fibres
Blocked later by local anaesthetics	Blocked earlier by local anaesthetics
Blocked earlier by ischaemia	Blocked later by ischaemia

Table 16.4 Qualities of pain.

bile-ducts and the bronchi and parietal pleura are sensitive to pain.

Effects associated with pain sensation

Besides the distinct sensation of hurt, pain is associated with the following:

1 *Motor reactions.* These may take the form of reflexes which remove part or all the body from the painful stimulus, e.g. the **withdrawal reflex**. Alternatively, they may be in the form of muscle rigidity (stiffness), which is reflex contraction of somatic muscles in response to deep somatic and visceral pain, e.g. **guarding** over an inflamed appendix and neck stiffness in meningitis.

2 *Autonomic reactions.* These vary with the intensity and site of stimulation. Generally, mild pain occurring in superficial tissues stimulates the **posterior hypothalamic nuclei** and results in sympathetic changes, i.e. tachycardia, rise in blood pressure, pupillodilatation, etc. Severe pain in superficial and deep tissues, and organs may stimulate the **anterior hypothalamic nuclei**, leading to parasympathetic changes, i.e. bradycardia and a decrease in blood pressure.

3 *Emotional reactions.* Impulses from pain receptors reach the hypothalamus through thalamohypothalamic pathways. Pain has a built-in unpleasant affect in normal individuals. The reactions are those of anxiety, anguish, crying, depression, etc. Emotional reactions vary widely among people, although the threshold for pain is nearly the same for all individuals.

The different reactions described above originate from different parts of the nervous system (i.e. spinal cord, brain stem, hypothalamus, frontal lobe, etc.). This is clearly demonstrated in patients who undergo frontal lobotomy for treatment of intractable pain. These patients still feel the pain postoperatively, but the emotional reaction is absent.

Qualities of pain (fast and slow pain)

When subjected to a painful stimulus, e.g. a hot object, a person experiences an immediate (fast) pain followed shortly after by delayed (slow) pain. The two pains are of different quality:

1 *Fast pain.* This is also known as first pain or pricking pain. It is an acute sensation which occurs within 0.1 s after application of a painful stimulus. It is usually well localized, the kind of sensation felt when a pin is stuck into the skin or when the skin is cut with a knife. Fast pain is usually superficial and is not felt in most of the deeper tissues. It is transmitted via **type Aδ fibres**.

2 *Slow pain.* This is often known as second pain or burning or aching pain. It is delayed pain whose intensity increases with time and is difficult to endure. It can occur both in the skin and in deeper tissues and organs, e.g. skin burns, toothache and intestinal colic. Slow pain is transmitted via **type C fibres**.

The two qualities reflect not only the dual nature of the input, i.e. Aδ and C nerve fibres, but also the two sets of connections within the spinal cord and brain. Table 16.4 gives a summary of the qualities of pain.

Mechanism of stimulation of pain receptors

Pain receptors are depolarized by threshold stimuli either

directly or through production of chemicals known as pain-producing substances (PPS). Tissue damage causes the release of PPS. The most important of these is *bradykinin*, but *serotonin, histamine, potassium ions, acetylcholine, proteolytic enzymes* and many others also produce pain. Prostaglandins and substance P do not stimulate pain receptors, but they cause pain by lowering the threshold of the receptors.

Ischaemia causes pain possibly through the release of large amounts of metabolites, mainly lactic acid, formed in the process of anaerobic metabolism or through the release of chemicals from cells damaged by hypoxia.

Muscle spasm causes pain by chemicals released from tense muscles becoming ischaemic or possibly by a direct mechanical effect. Thus both chemosensitive and mechanosensitive pain receptors may be responsible for headache or colic.

Types of pain

According to the site of stimulation, pain can be classified into:

1 *Cutaneous pain.* Arising from the skin and subcutaneous tissues.
2 *Deep somatic pain.* Arising from tissues deeper than the skin, e.g. muscles, tendons, joints, ligaments and bones.
3 *Visceral pain.* Arising from the viscera.

Cutaneous pain

When elicited, cutaneous pain occurs in the two phases of fast pricking followed by slow burning pain. In some diseases, e.g. tabes dorsalis, fast fibres are damaged while slow fibres are spared. Therefore, pain is felt after a long latent period. Unlike the other two types, cutaneous pain can be accurately localized due to the large number of receptors. Touch and vision also aid greatly in localizing the site of the pain.

The pathway of cutaneous pain is as follows.

Receptors. These are free nerve endings.

Peripheral nerves. Pain is carried by two types of nerve fibres (Fig. 16.20):
1 Type Aδ fibres: thick rapidly conducting fibres that transmit impulses at the rate of about 20–30 m/s. These carry fast pain.
2 Type C fibres: thin (unmyelinated) slow-conducting fibres that transmit impulses at the rate of about 1 m/s. These carry slow pain.

Spinal cord. Pain fibres ascend a few segments in Lissauer's tract before forming synapses on the neurons of the dorsal horn (Fig. 16.20). Type Aδ fibres terminate mainly in lamina I and lamina V, and type C fibres end in laminae II and III (i.e. *substantia gelatinosa of Rolandi*; see Fig. 16.15).

Type Aδ fibres excite second-order neurons of the *neospinothalamic* tract. Type C fibres excite few interneurons in the dorsal horns which deliver the signals mainly to laminae V–VIII. The last interneurons in the series cross the anterior commissure (along with the fibres of the neospinothalamic tract) and pass upwards in the lateral columns as the *palaeospinothalamic* tract.

It is known that **glutamate** is the neurotransmitter released by type Aδ fibres in the spinal cord and is therefore involved in transmitting fast pain, while **substance P** is the neurotransmitter released by type C fibres and is therefore concerned with the transmission of slow pain. Glutamate is rapidly released and is short-acting compared with substance P, which is released and removed slowly to give a prolonged sensation.

Brain stem and thalamus

1 The neospinothalamic tract. Most of the fibres in this tract pass through the brain stem to terminate mainly in the ventrobasal complex of the thalamus, the somatosensory cortex and other basal regions of the brain. Few fibres end in the reticular formation of the brain stem (Fig. 16.21).
2 The palaeospinothalamic tract. Most of the fibres in the tract terminate diffusely in the reticular formation of the brain stem (Fig. 16.21). Several interneurons then carry the inputs mainly to the intralaminar nuclei of the thalamus. Impulses also pass to the hypothalamus and to adjacent regions of the basal brain. Because the reticular areas of the brain stem and intralaminar nuclei of the thalamus form part of the reticular activating system, impulses arriving there have a strong arousal effect.

It should be emphasized that full perception of pain occurs when the signals enter the reticular formation of the brain stem, thalamus and probably other basal regions.

Cerebral cortex.

The somatosensory cortex plays an important role in **topognosis** i.e. localization. Fast pain is localized better than slow pain because a large proportion of the signals carried in the neospinothalamic tract reach the somatosensory cortex, while a smaller proportion of pain signals in the palaeospinothalamic pathway reach there. Indeed, most of the palaeospinothalamic tract fibres terminate in the reticular formation of the brain stem. Furthermore, the cerebral cortex is also responsible for interpreting the quality of pain.

Sensory cortex

Sensory radiation

③

Thalamus
(ventrobasal
nuclear complex)

Anterior
spinothalamic
tract

Lateral
spinothalamic
tract

②

Substantia gelatinosa
(pain and temperature)

Lissauer's tract

Lateral
column

Dorsal root ganglion

Main sensory
nucleus (crude
touch)

Anterior
column

①

Type C
fibres

Type A delta
fibres

Anterior
column

Fig. 16.20 The anterolateral pathway.
1, 2 and 3 indicate first-, second- and
third-order neurons.

Deep somatic pain

Deep somatic pain is produced by stimulation of pain receptors in deep structures, i.e. muscles, tendons, periosteum of bones, joints and ligaments. Unlike cutaneous pain, it is dull, diffuse, intense and prolonged. The pathway of deep somatic pain is the same as that of cutaneous pain, but the first-order neuron afferents run in sensorimotor nerves. This type of pain is usually associated with autonomic stimulation, e.g. sweating, vomiting and changes in heart rate and blood pressure. Pain from deeper structures can also initiate reflex contractions of nearby muscles, e.g. the

muscle spasm associated with bone fractures. It may show the phenomenon of referral to a distant site, e.g. pain arising in the hip may be referred to the knee.

The adequate stimuli for deep somatic pain include:
1 Mechanical forces, e.g. severe pressure on a bone, traction of a muscle, ligament, etc.
2 Chemicals, e.g. venoms.
3 Ischaemia, e.g. muscle ischaemia.

Ischaemic muscle pain occurs in active muscles when their blood supply becomes inadequate. The intensity of pain is related to the degree of exertion and is due to the

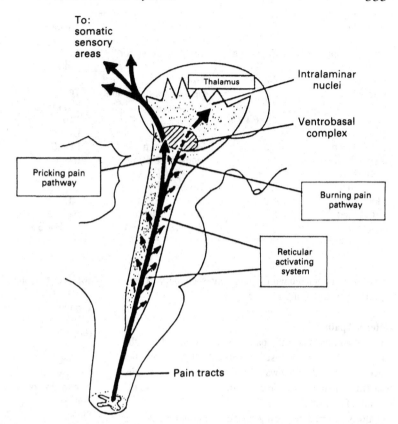

Fig. 16.21 Transmission of pain
signals into the hind-brain, thalamus and
cortex via the 'pricking pain' pathway
and the 'burning pain' pathway.
(Reproduced with permission from
Guyton, A.C. (1987) *Textbook of
Medical Physiology*, 7th edn. Saunders,
Philadelphia.)

liberation and accumulation of a chemical substance
called **Lewis's P factor**, which stimulates pain receptors.
An important clinical example is *angina pectoris* (i.e. angina
of effort). The coronary arteries are narrowed by disease
and the blood supply does not match the needs of cardiac
muscle during exercise. This causes severe chest pain,
which forces the subject to stop.

Visceral pain

Pain receptors in the viscera are sparsely distributed and
therefore severe visceral pain indicates diffuse stimulation
of pain receptors from a wide area of the viscus. Localized
damage does not usually cause severe pain.

The pathway of visceral pain is the same as that of cutaneous and deep somatic pain, but the first-order neuron afferents pass in sympathetic and parasympathetic nerves. The
fibres are type C fibres; thus the pain is of the dull aching
type. When arising from the parietal peritoneum, pleura or
pericardium, the pain is often of the sharp pricking type.
This is because these serous membranes are supplied by
spinal nerves similar to the skin and not by the autonomic
nerves of the viscera.

Pain impulses from the thoracic viscera and lower pelvic
viscera reach the CNS along parasympathetic nerves (i.e.
the vagi and the glossopharyngeal and pelvic nerves), while
those from the rest of the viscera reach the CNS through
sympathetic nerves.

The adequate stimuli for visceral pain include distension of hollow viscera. A good example is the pain we
experience when the urinary bladder is full or when we
overfill our stomachs. Spasm of a viscus is another potent
stimulus, which gives rise to pain when the viscus becomes
ischaemic, e.g. labour pain and intestinal colic. The last,
but not least, stimuli are chemical irritants. Indeed, damage
to the abdominal viscera by leaking HCl acid from a
perforated gastric ulcer gives rise to one of the most severe
pains known to humans.

Visceral pain is characterized by the following:

1 It is poorly localized.
2 It is often referred or radiates to other sites.
3 It is often associated with autonomic disturbances, e.g.
vomiting, sweating, tachycardia.
4 It can be associated with rigidity and tenderness of
nearby skeletal muscles.

Structure	Supply	Structure	Supply
Face and anterior cranium	Trigeminal	Intrathoracic viscera	T1–T4 and vagi
Back of head	C2	Nipple area	T5
Neck	C3	Upper intra-abdominal viscera	T6–T10 and vagi
Diaphragm	C3, C4, C5	Umbilicus	T10
Shoulder area	C4	Groin	L1
Deltoid area	C5	Pelvic viscera	L1–L3
Radial forearm and thumb	C6	Medial side of knee	L3
Index finger	C7	Big toe	L5
Middle finger	C8	Little toe	S1
Little finger	C8	Back of thigh	S2
Inner forearm	T1	Genitosacral area	S3, S4, S5

Table 16.5 Sensory innervation of the body.

5 It may be associated with primary and secondary **hyperalgesia** of the overlying skin (see p. 337).

Referred pain

Visceral and deep somatic pain are often referred, i.e. the pain is not felt in the diseased structure itself, but at another place in the body far away from the site of its origin. Sometimes pain radiates from the diseased structure to the distant referral site.

Pain is referred according to the dermatomal rule, i.e. it is referred to the dermatome (area of skin) supplied by the same dorsal nerve roots as the diseased structure. For example, cardiac pain is referred to the precordium, the inner part of the left arm and the epigastrium. The pain fibres from the cardiac muscle as well as the sensory nerves from these areas pass through the dorsal roots to C3–T5 cord segments.

The sites to which pain from different structures may be referred can be deduced from a knowledge of the segmental and peripheral innervation of the body (Table 16.5).

Table 16.6 shows some important examples of usual sites of referral of pain from some organs.

Mechanism of referred pain

Convergence and facilitation both play a part in the production of referred pain.

Convergence theory. According to this theory, pain fibres from an area of skin and a diseased viscus converge on the same spinothalamic neurons in the dorsal horn (Fig. 16.22). The skin has a richer nerve supply and is more exposed to stimulation than any viscus. Because of this, the somatosensory cortex is more accustomed to

Table 16.6 Important examples of referred pain.

Organ	Site of referral
Heart	Precordium; inner aspect of left arm; epigastrium
Appendix	Umbilicus
Small intestine	Umbilicus
Central part of diaphragm	Tip of shoulder
Pleura	Abdomen
Kidney	Costovertebral angle (loin)
Ureter	Testicle
Trigone of bladder	Tip of penis
Tongue	Ear
Teeth	Head
Hip	Knee
Uterus	Low back radiating to lower abdomen

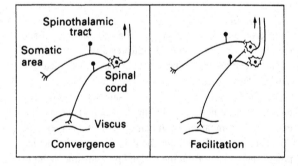

Fig. 16.22 Mechanism of referred pain. The diagrams show the convergence and facilitation theories.

receiving impulses from the skin than from the viscera. So pain impulses carried to the cortex along spinothalamic neurons shared by afferents from the skin and others from the diseased viscus (i.e. convergence) are misinterpreted as coming from the skin. In other words, the cortex will project the sensation to the skin area instead of projecting it to the diseased viscus (i.e. an error of projection).

Facilitation theory. Pain fibres from the skin are always carrying impulses, but these are normally not enough to produce pain, i.e. the spinothalamic neurons on which they converge are only subliminally stimulated (subthreshold stimulation). When the viscus is diseased, many impulses arise from it. These pass through afferents which give collaterals to the spinothalamic neurons receiving pain fibres from the skin (dermatome for that segment). As a result, the spinothalamic neurons' excitability is raised (i.e. they are facilitated) to reach threshold level (see Fig. 16.22). The signals reaching the brain from these neurons are no different from those coming to it from the skin and the sensation is projected to the skin area. The result is pain felt in the skin dermatome and a lowering of its pain threshold. The pain felt in the skin is called **referred pain**, basically an error of projection, and the lowering of its pain threshold is *hyperalgesia* of the skin. It is possible sometimes to abolish mild referred pain by local anaesthesia applied to the dermatome of reference. This confirms that facilitation is responsible for referred pain.

Primary and secondary hyperalgesia

Hyperalgesia is hypersensitivity to pain. In **primary hyperalgesia**, there is increased sensitivity of the pain receptors resulting from release of certain chemicals (e.g. histamine, prostaglandins, etc.) at and around the site of injury. As a result, the threshold for pain is lowered at these sites. An example of primary hyperalgesia is the excessive sensitivity of sunburnt skin to touch. In **secondary hyperalgesia**, the threshold for pain is not changed and may be raised in an area surrounding the injury. However, if a stimulus is strong enough, the pain experienced is far more than it would have been before the injury. Secondary hyperalgesia is due to *facilitation* of sensory transmission within the CNS. Impulses from the injured site facilitate those from a healthy skin area (i.e. area of secondary hyperalgesia). This type can result from injury to the spinal cord or the thalamus.

Muscular rigidity and tenderness associated with visceral and deep somatic pain

The rigidity of nearby skeletal muscle associated with dis-ease of a viscus is distributed regionally and not segmentally, and so its position varies according to the anatomical position of the diseased viscus. The rigidity is most marked when the parietal peritoneum or pleura becomes irritated by the diseased viscus. For example, the rigidity in the right iliac fossa that accompanies acute appendicitis is secondary to irritation of the parietal peritoneum by the inflamed appendix. However, rigidity can occur without involvement of the pleura or peritoneum. The anatomical details of the reflex pathway by which impulses from a diseased viscus initiate skeletal muscle rigidity are still not clear. The spasm protects the underlying inflamed structure from trauma. Indeed, this reflex spasm is sometimes called guarding. Yet, if it continues for long periods, the muscles become ischaemic and chemicals accumulate in them which reduce their pain thresholds. This accounts for the soreness and tenderness of the rigid muscles.

Central inhibition of pain

Several observations have led to the belief that pain transmission and perception are subject to inhibition in the central sensory pathways by ascending and descending impulses. These observations include the following:

1 Stroking the area around the injury or rubbing or shaking it often reduces the pain of injury.

2 The degree to which each person reacts to pain is subject to wide variation.

3 Injuries caused while playing a game or in battle may be completely ignored at the time (stress analgesia). The same injury if inflicted, for example, in surgery without anaesthesia would cause agonizing pain.

4 Irritation of the skin overlying a diseased viscus, for example, with a mustard plaster, relieves pain.

5 Acupuncture has been used for years to prevent or relieve pain.

The *gate control theory* of pain inhibition (proposed by Melzack and Wall) can account for these observations. According to this theory, the dorsal horn of the spinal cord and, in particular, the neurons of the substantia gelatinosa of Rolandi form the 'gate' through which pain impulses must pass in order to reach the brain (Fig. 16.23). The sensation of pain not only is dependent on an input from afferents transmitting pain signals, but also is significantly affected by the input from large myelinated mechano-receptive afferents (type Aβ fibres). Impulses coming along small-diameter (pain) fibres (type C fibres) cause the release of substance P from these fibres and open the gate, while impulses coming along the large-diameter type Aβ fibres close the gate, probably by the process of presynaptic inhibition. Stimulation of the large type Aβ fibres, there-

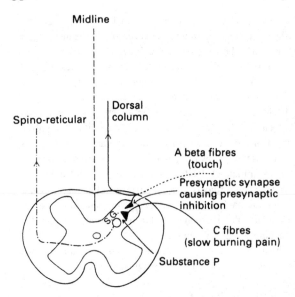

Fig. 16.23 The gate control of pain. Substance P is released from the first-order neuron in the 'slow burning' pain pathway to stimulate the substantia gelatinosa. The presynaptic synapse releases a transmitter which inhibits release of substance P and thus inhibits pain transmission. S.G., substantia gelatinosa.

fore, can reduce or eliminate some types of pain. The common practice of rubbing the skin surface when one is hurt provides a stimulus to the large-diameter fibres. Clinically, the use of cutaneous electrodes over peripheral nerves (transcutaneous stimulation) and the implantation of dorsal column stimulators in treating certain painful conditions have proved to be very successful. Both methods electrically stimulate large-diameter fibres. Also, destruction of these fibres in certain peripheral neuropathies (e.g. herpetic neuralgia) often results in a severe, prolonged, painful state, in which minor stimuli can cause severe unbearable pain. Large-diameter fibres are also presumably stimulated by counterirritants, such as mustard plaster applied to the skin to relieve pain of a diseased viscus, and also by acupuncture, although the latter appears to work mainly by the release of certain transmitters.

The 'gate' is also under the control of higher centres by means of an analgesic system of corticospinal and reticulo-spinal fibres.

The opiate system of the brain

Morphine is a powerful pain-killer (analgesic) found in opium. It acts by combining with receptors in the CNS. Because it seems unlikely that these receptors had been specifically evolved to combine with morphine, a search

was made for morphine-like substances in the brain itself, and two major types of compounds with morphine-like properties (i.e. opioids) have been isolated from the brain, the **encephalins** and the **endorphins**.

The encephalins are a group of naturally occurring peptides found in high concentrations in the periaqueductal grey matter. Their effects are thought to be mediated by acting on **opioid receptors** found in a number of places, including the periphery at sites of injury, the dorsal horn, the periaqueductal grey matter, the hypothalamus and the limbic system. These receptors are originally produced in the dorsal root ganglion but travel peripherally to reside in afferent fibres; there, they are acted upon by **opioids** released from immune cells during inflammatory processes. Opioid receptors from the dorsal root ganglia also migrate centrally, mainly to the dorsal horn region and the rostral brain. Stimulation of the dorsal horn opioid receptors causes presynaptic inhibition of first-order neuron pain afferents and consequently decreases the release of substance P. Stimulation of the periaqueductal grey region activates descending pathways that release **encephalin** at the **raphe magnus** nucleus of the medulla oblongata (Fig. 16.24). The latter projects serotoninergic pathways to interneurons which synapse with the first-order neurons of the pain pathway. These release **encephalins** and pain transmission is inhibited by both pre- and postsynaptic inhibition. Encephalins, like morphine, also influence pain in another way; they modify the emotional state of the individual via their action on the limbic system, thus promoting a sense of well-being.

Endorphins form another group of peptides, which are plentiful in the hypothalamus and pituitary. They also function via interacting with opiate receptors. Indeed, endorphins were found to prevent withdrawal symptoms in opium addicts. Their presence in high concentrations in some women during parturition suggests that these naturally occurring peptides form, in a sense, the body's own analgesic system.

Endogenous opioids are released by a variety of stimulants besides pain. These include various stresses, sexual stimulation, placebos and acupuncture.

The discovery of the transmitters involved in pain sensation has explained some of the various observations we spoke about earlier. Acupuncture acts partly by causing the release of encephalins. This is indicated by the blockage of acupuncture analgesia by naloxone, a drug that competes with morphine and opioids for receptor sites. Endorphins, on the other hand, are secreted together with adrenocorticotrophic hormone (ACTH) from the anterior pituitary in stressful situations. This could explain why injuries are

Fig. 16.24 Mechanism of the role played by descending fibres in determining the threshold of pain. +, Excitation; –, inhibition; PNRG, peripheral nerve root ganglion; 5-HT, 5-hydroxytryptamine.

often painless during playing a game or during a period of fighting.

Methods of treatment

There are many procedures used to alleviate or treat pain. However, they differ in their mode of action and their relative merits. They include the following:

1 Treatment and cure of the cause. This is definitely the best, if possible.

2 Use of analgesics (i.e. pain-killing drugs).

3 Large-fibre stimulation. This can be done by using counterirritants, e.g. hot-water bottles, balms, cold packs and antiphlogistic plasters. Other methods include cutaneous electrodes and the use of dorsal column stimulators.

4 Use of local anaesthetics in minor surgery, e.g. procaine, and general anaesthetics in major surgery, e.g. Pentothal, nitrous oxide, etc.

5 Use of vasodilators in ischaemic pain, e.g. use of nitrites in angina pectoris or increasing blood supply to an ischaemic part, e.g. coronary bypass in angina pectoris.

6 Use of antacids in peptic ulcers and antispasmodics in, for example, intestinal or ureteric colic.

7 Suppression of inflammation by use of steroids.

8 Acupuncture. This works in certain limited circumstances.

9 Electrical stimulation of the periaqueductal grey matter.

10 Surgical denervation (Fig. 16.25) of diseased organs by:

(a) Neurectomy; sympathectomy.

(b) Rhizotomy, i.e. dorsal root sectioning.

(c) Myelotomy, i.e. section of spinothalamic fibres in the anterior commissure.

(d) Anterolateral cordotomy, i.e. sections of pain and temperature fibres in the anterolateral tract of the spinal cord.

(e) Medullary tractotomy.

(f) Mesencephalic tractotomy.

(g) Thalamotomy.

(h) Gyrectomy.

11 Frontal lobotomy. By this procedure abolition of the emotional reaction to pain is achieved. This is a method of last resort for relief of intractable pain in terminal cancer.

12 Psychotherapy, hypnosis and placebos can be used in cases with pain of psychological origin.

The motor system

I Motor functions of the spinal cord and spinal reflexes

Introduction

Sensory information is integrated at all levels of the nervous system and causes different types of motor reflexes:

1 Sensory information integrated in the spinal cord leads to simple spinal reflexes.

2 Sensory information integrated in the brain stem leads to more complicated brain stem reflexes.

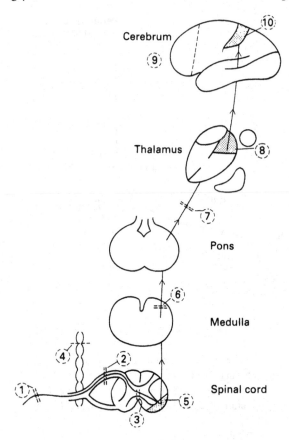

Fig. 16.25 Diagram of the various surgical procedures designed to relieve pain. 1. Neurectomy. 2. Rhizotomy. 3. Myelotomy to section spinothalamic fibres in anterior white commissure. 4. Sympathectomy (for visceral pain). 5. Anterolateral cordotomy. 6. Medullary tractotomy. 7. Mesencephalic tractomy. 8. Thalamotomy. 9. Frontal lobotomy. 10. Gyrectomy.

3 Sensory information integrated in the cerebral cortex initiates the most complicated motor responses and also leads to the perception of sensations.

The reflex arc
The basic unit of integrated neural activity is the reflex arc (Fig. 16.26). It consists of:

1 A sense organ (i.e. the receptor).
2 An afferent neuron.
3 One or more synapses (in the CNS or a sympathetic ganglion).
4 An efferent neuron.
5 An effector.

The simplest reflex arc has a single synapse between the afferent and the efferent neuron. Few of the sensory

impulses that enter the spinal cord pass directly to the anterior horn cells across one synapse to form a *monosynaptic* reflex arc, e.g. the stretch reflex. Reflex arcs in which there are one or more *interneurons* between the afferent and efferent neurons mediate *polysynaptic* reflexes, e.g. the withdrawal reflex. Such reflexes are far more common than monosynaptic ones.

Some of the components of the reflex arc (i.e. the receptor and synapses) have been previously discussed. The rest deserve discussion in some detail.

The afferent neuron
Afferent impulses entering the spinal cord via the posterior root are conducted to two separate destinations. Some end on cells in the grey matter of the spinal cord of the same segment or nearby segments. These cells are either posterior horn cells (e.g. the substantia gelatinosa, or the main sensory nucleus), which form the origin of sensory tracts, or interneurons interposed between the afferent fibre and the efferents, or anterior horn cells, which are actually motor effector neurons. A large number of the afferent impulses, however, ascend to higher levels of the nervous system, i.e. the brain stem, the cerebellum, the thalamus or even the cerebral cortex.

Afferent neurons carry impulses from receptors to the CNS. They can undergo divergence (see Fig. 16.4), thus helping to spread a single stimulus to a wide area of the CNS, or convergence, thus helping the process of spatial summation. At the level of the spinal cord, afferent impulses will lead to facilitatory effects (i.e. raising excitability of neurons, but not enough to fire) or local excitatory effects, or to the induction of spinal cord reflexes.

Interneurons
Interneurons are small, highly excitable cells, which may be excitatory or inhibitory. In the spinal cord they lie in all areas of the cord's grey matter, making connections with one another, and many of them directly synapse with anterior motor neurons.

Interneurons are also arranged to allow convergence and divergence to occur. Their organization also allows the important process of after-discharge. In this process an impulse in an afferent neuron is not merely relayed but causes a prolonged output discharge even after the incoming impulse is over. After-discharge can last from a few milliseconds to as long as many minutes to hours. Two types of circuits formed by interneurons allow the process of after-discharge—parallel and reverberating circuits.

Fig. 16.26 The reflex arc. AP, action potential (all-or-none); EP, motor end-plate potentials (graded); EPSP, IPSP, excitatory and inhibitory postsynaptic potentials (graded); GP, generator potential (graded). Note that at the receptor and at each of the junctions in the arc there is a non-propagated graded response that is proportionate to the magnitude of the stimulus. In the portions of the arc specialized for transmission (afferent and efferent nerve fibres, muscle membrane) the responses are action potentials which are not graded and obey the all-or-none law.

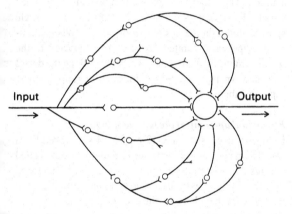

Fig. 16.27 Diagrammatic representation of the parallel after-discharge circuit. (Reproduced with permission from Guyton, A.C. (1987) *Textbook of Medical Physiology*, 7th edn. Saunders, Philadelphia.)

Parallel circuits. In this type, the input impulse reaches the output neuron through different numbers of interneurons which converge on it (Fig. 16.27). As synaptic delay is about 0.5 ms at each synapse, the impulses reach the output neuron one by one after varying periods of delay. Thus, the output neuron continues to discharge for many milliseconds.

Reverberating circuits. These form the most important circuits responsible for after-discharge. They are positive feedback pathways where the output of one neuron feeds back to restimulate itself (i.e. via interneurons) for a long time (Fig. 16.28). The system gets more complex as the number of interneurons increases in the circuit.

The duration of reverberating circuits varies and they only stop as a result of synaptic fatigue or by inhibitory impulses from other parts of the CNS. Examples of important reverberating circuits in the nervous system include the following:

1 During respiration, the inspiratory neurons in the medulla become excited for about 2 s during each respiratory cycle for life by reverberating circuits. These circuits can be stopped by inhibitory impulses from other areas of the CNS, for example, pulmonary vagi stimulation.

2 One theory of wakefulness is that arousal impulses set up within the brain stem continual reverberation to keep wakefulness lasting for up to 18 hours. Sleep sets in when the synapses in the circuit fatigue. This passive theory no longer holds.

The efferent neuron

The efferent neurons are the motor neurons present in the anterior horn of the spinal cord. Their axons leave the spinal cord through the anterior roots to innervate skeletal muscles.

Anterior motor neurons (i.e. anterior horn cells or AHC) are of two types: alpha and gamma motor neurons. The alpha motor neurons are the larger cells, and they give rise to large myelinated type Aα fibres (9–20 μm diameter). Each fibre excites from three to several hundred skeletal muscle fibres. The fibre and the muscle fibres it supplies are collectively called a motor unit. The size of the latter varies according to the type of movements; the more delicate the

Input   Output

Facilitation

Inhibition

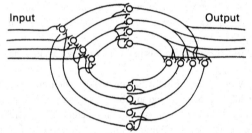

Fig. 16.28 Diagrams of reverberating circuits of increasing complexity. (Reproduced with permission from Guyton, A.C. (1987) *Textbook of Medical Physiology*, 7th edn. Saunders, Philadelphia.)

movement is, the fewer the number of muscle fibres in a single motor unit; e.g. in hand muscles, each motor unit contains around five fibres, while, in the leg muscles, it contains about 100 muscle fibres. Gamma motor neurons are smaller cells, with small axons which are type Aγ fibres (5 μm diameter). They innervate special skeletal muscle fibres, the intrafusal fibres of *muscle spindles*.

In addition to motor neurons, the anterior horn contains large numbers of a special interneuron, located in close association with motor neurons. This is called the **Renshaw cell**. It is an inhibitory cell excited by collaterals from an alpha motor neuron to project back and inhibit the same motor neuron (in a negative feedback fashion) and neighbouring motor neurons (Fig. 16.29). Thus the initial activity

of the motor neuron is soon cut short and is prevented from spreading laterally: this focuses the boundaries of the area stimulated. Renshaw inhibition is also known as *recurrent inhibition*.

Types of reflexes

During examination of the nervous system, three types of reflexes are usually investigated. These are deep reflexes, superficial reflexes and visceral reflexes.

Deep reflexes

Deep reflexes result from stimulation of receptors present in muscles and tendons. They include:
1 The stretch reflex.
2 The Golgi tendon reflex.
3 Postural spinal reflexes.

The stretch reflex (also called the myotatic reflex), is a monosynaptic reflex elicited by applying sudden stretch to a muscle. The response is reflex contraction of the stretched muscle. The receptors for the stretch reflex are the **muscle spindles** found in the fleshy part of muscle. When stimulated, impulses generated in them are conducted to the spinal cord via thick afferents, which enter along the dorsal roots and synapse directly with the anterior motor neurons supplying the same muscle.

Functional anatomy of the muscle spindle

Each spindle consists of 3–12 muscle fibres enclosed in a spindle-shaped connective-tissue capsule. These are called intrafusal fibres, and they are smaller and less developed than the ordinary extrafusal muscle fibres, but they lie in parallel with them because the ends of the spindle capsule are attached either to the muscle tendons or to the sides of the extrafusal fibres. Each intrafusal fibre consists of a central non-contractile area, which is the receptor area, and peripheral contractile parts (Fig. 16.30).

There are two types of intrafusal fibres: (i) nuclear bag fibres, whose central area is dilated with an aggregation of nuclei. Each spindle contains about two nuclear bag fibres; and (ii) nuclear chain fibres, which are smaller than nuclear bag fibres and have one line of nuclei spread in a chain along the receptor area. There are three to nine nuclear chain fibres per spindle.

Innervation of the muscle spindle

Afferent fibres. The receptor area of the intrafusal muscle fibres is supplied by two types of afferent fibres:
1 *Primary (annulospiral) endings.* These are group Ia fibres, which are thick and rapidly conducting (i.e. diameter

Anterior horn cells

Axon to skeletal muscle

Collateral branch

Renshaw cells

Fig. 16.29 Circuit diagram for recurrent inhibition of a motor neuron by a Renshaw cell. (+), stimulation; (–), inhibition.

Dynamic gamma efferent

Static gamma efferent

Group la fibre (primary afferent)

Group II fibre (secondary afferent)

Nuclear bag

Fig. 16.30 The muscle spindle. Note the two types of intrafusal muscle fibres and also the sensory and motor innervation of the muscle spindle.

Nuclear chain

16–17 μm). They encircle the receptor areas of both nuclear bag and unclear chain fibres, and synapse directly with the anterior horn motor neurons that supply the extra-fusal fibres of the same muscle. Thus, the reflex pathway here is monosynaptic. The primary endings discharge most rapidly while the muscle is being stretched and less rapidly during sustained stretch. Therefore they measure mainly the *rate of change* in muscle length and to a lesser extent the absolute muscle length. This response of the primary afferents is called the *dynamic response*. Since nuclear bag fibres are only supplied by primary endings, they are considered responsible for the dynamic response.

2 *Secondary (flower-spray) endings.* These are terminals of smaller myelinated fibres (8 μm diameter). They are group II fibres and they encircle the receptor area of the nuclear chain fibres only. Unlike the first type, these terminate principally on interneurons of the spinal cord, although some fibres terminate directly on the anterior horn cells. The secondary endings discharge at an increased rate throughout the period a muscle is being stretched, in direct proportion to the degree of stretch. Therefore they measure mainly *muscle length*. This response is known as the *static response*. Since nuclear chain fibres are supplied by both primary and secondary endings (see Fig. 16.30), they are considered responsible for the static response. Similarly to the secondary endings, the primary endings also show a static response when a muscle is stretched, but it is much smaller than the dynamic response.

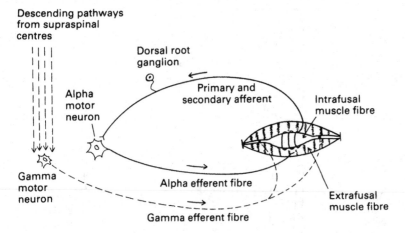

Descending pathways from supraspinal centres

Dorsal root ganglion

Alpha motor neuron

Primary and secondary afferent

Intrafusal muscle fibre

Gamma motor neuron

Alpha efferent fibre

Extrafusal muscle fibre

Gamma efferent fibre

Fig. 16.31 Diagram illustrating the circuit involved in the stretch reflex and the effects of gamma motor neuron stimulation. The dashed lines represent descending pathways bringing impulses from supraspinal centres to the gamma motor neuron and its axons, which supply the peripheral edges of the intrafusal muscle fibres.

Efferent fibres to the muscle spindle. These are axons of the gamma motor neurons, situated in the anterior horn of the spinal cord and the brain stem. They supply the peripheral contractile parts of the intrafusal muscle fibres and are of two functional types (see Fig. 16.30):

1 Dynamic gamma efferents, which end mainly on the nuclear bag fibres (as plate endings).

2 Static gamma efferents, which end mainly on nuclear chain fibres (as trail endings), while some end on nuclear bag fibres.

When gamma motor neurons are stimulated, impulses pass along the gamma efferents to cause contraction of the peripheral contractile parts of the intrafusal fibres. As a result, the receptors in the mid-portion of the intrafusal fibres will be stretched. This, in turn, causes stimulation of the primary and secondary endings encircling the receptor area (see Fig. 16.30). Afferent impulses enter the spinal cord and stimulate alpha motor neurons of the anterior horn, which send impulses along type Aα efferent fibres to ordinary muscle fibres, causing the muscle to contract. (Fig. 16.31)

Function of muscle spindles

The function of the muscle spindle is to keep the CNS informed about muscle length and the rate of change in muscle length. The spindle can be stimulated under two conditions:

1 When the whole muscle is stretched, e.g. by gravity or by tapping a muscle tendon with a hammer during examination of tendon jerks.

2 When the peripheral parts of the intrafusal fibres contract (by gamma efferent discharge) and the central receptor area is stretched. It is worth noting here that a muscle will contract either directly, when alpha motor neurons to extrafusal fibres are stimulated, or indirectly, when gamma motor neuron discharge activates the stretch reflex.

Maximal stimulation of the muscle spindle occurs whenever the muscle is stretched and there is a simultaneous increased rate of discharge of gamma efferents. Minimal or no stimulation occurs when the muscle actively contracts, since the muscle spindles lie in parallel to the extrafusal fibres.

However, there is evidence indicating that, whenever muscles actively contract (i.e. via alpha motor neuron discharge), the gamma motor neurons are simultaneously stimulated, an effect called *'alpha–gamma coactivation'*. This causes the intrafusal fibres to shorten simultaneously with the extrafusal fibres, so that the length of the receptor portion of the muscle spindle, however, does not change. Therefore the muscle spindle maintains its ability to respond to stretch, regardless of muscle length. In this way the muscle spindle can adjust alpha motor neuron discharge throughout a contraction. Coactivation of alpha–gamma motor neurons is the basis of *Jendrassik's* reinforcement manoeuvre, i.e. eliciting a tendon jerk (basically a stretch reflex) while the patient is strongly contracting some other voluntary muscles. An example of this is the hooking of one's fists together while the examiner is eliciting the knee-jerk.

Control of gamma efferent discharge. Gamma motor neuron discharge is controlled by both facilitatory and inhibitory pathways from supraspinal centres (see Fig. 16.31). Facilitatory pathways increase gamma motor neuron discharge, which increases the sensitivity of muscle spindles to stretch; inhibitory pathways do the reverse. Selective simultaneous facilitation of gamma motor neurons supplying some muscles while inhibiting those supplying other muscles leads to variation in the degree of reflex contraction of the different muscles of the body, i.e. *muscle tone*. Such variations in tone are important for the maintenance of posture. Gamma motor neuron discharge is influenced

Action potential in:

Fig. 16.32 Action potentials from muscle spindle afferents. The primary and secondary endings increase their discharge when the muscle is suddenly stretched. Note that the discharge decreases when a constant length is maintained and returns to a basal level when the muscle goes back to its initial length.

by psychic factors, and hyperreflexia of anxious patients is a good example. Noxious cutaneous stimulation also increases gamma efferent discharge to the ipsilateral flexor muscle spindles, but decreases that to extensors. The opposite pattern occurs in the contralateral limb.

Components of the stretch reflex. The stretch reflex can be divided into two separate components, the dynamic and the static stretch reflex.

The dynamic stretch reflex is elicited by sudden rapid stretching of a muscle. The muscle spindle responds by synchronous strong signals transmitted to the spinal cord mainly along the primary endings (Fig. 16.32). Anterior alpha motor neurons respond with a corresponding synchrony, and impulses pass along their axons to cause contraction of all the muscle fibres of the stimulated muscle. This is seen as a jerky movement. As the muscle contracts and the receptor portions of intrafusal fibres becomes relatively lax, discharge from the afferents declines, causing the muscle to relax rapidly. This is the basis of tendon jerks (deep reflexes) examined clinically.

The static stretch reflex is the second component and is elicited by maintained stretch of a muscle. As long as stretch is maintained, impulses enter the spinal cord, mainly along secondary endings, and pass to alpha motor neurons, stimulating them to cause muscle contraction. Because different spindles are subjected to different degrees of stretch, they discharge at different rates. The result is a highly asynchronous discharge bombarding alpha motor neurons, which, in turn, discharge with corresponding asynchrony to the extrafusal fibres. The net result is a sustained contraction of the muscle as long as it is stretched. This forms the basis of *muscle tone.*

Muscle tone. Muscle tone is the static component of the stretch reflex. It is a continuous mild muscular contraction that acts as a background to actual movement. It is present during the wakeful state in all muscles of the body, especially the antigravity muscles. These are mainly the extensors of lower limbs, extensors of the back, muscles of the anterior abdominal wall, flexors of the upper limbs, extensors of the neck and elevators of the mandible. This is why the head falls forward and the mouth opens when one falls asleep. The stimuli for muscle tone are: (i) stretch of muscle fibres naturally found in all skeletal muscles, since normally they tend to be shorter than the distance between their origin and insertion; (ii) gravitational forces tend to flex the lower limbs at the ankles, knees and hip joints, which leads to stretching the extensors of the same limbs; and (iii) reflex muscle contraction (i.e. tone), due to gamma efferent discharge. A low level of gamma efferent discharge is associated with hypotonia (or flaccidity), while a high level of discharge results in hypertonia (or spasticity). Table 16.7 summarizes the functions of muscle tone.

Table 16.7 Summary of the functions of muscle tone.

Muscle tone is responsible for maintaining the erect posture against gravity. The tone of various muscles of the body can be changed in response to postural reflexes so as to maintain suitable body positions at rest and during movement
Muscle tone is enhanced when muscles are relaxed and decreased when muscles are contracted. This averages out contractions and prevents jerkiness of movements
In abdominal muscles muscle tone holds the viscera back and prevents bulging
In abdominal muscles, and especially in the muscles of the lower limbs, muscle tone is important for venous return
Through its contribution to the basal metabolic rate, muscle tone maintains normal body temperature

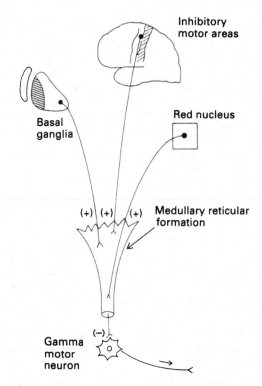

Fig. 16.33 Diagram of the supraspinal centres that facilitate gamma efferent discharge and consequently the stretch reflex: motor area 4 of the cerebral cortex, the dorsolateral part of the pontine reticular formation, the cerebellar cortex neocerebellum and the vestibular nucleus. +, stimulation, –, inhibition.

Fig. 16.34 Diagram of the supraspinal centres which inhibit gamma efferent discharge and consequently the stretch reflex: cortical inhibitory areas, the basal ganglia, the ventromedial part of the medullary reticular formation and the red nucleus. –, inhibition, +, stimulation.

Supraspinal influence on gamma efferent discharge (on the stretch reflex)

The gamma motor neuron discharge to muscle spindles is influenced by facilitatory and inhibitory impulses from higher centres (i.e. supraspinal centres). Through these impulses the sensitivity of the stretch reflex and thus muscle tone can be changed (Figs 16.33, 16.34). These centres include:

1 *Cortical areas.* The primary motor area (motor area 4) is **facilitatory** to gamma motor neurons. Thus selective lesions of motor area 4 or the pyramids in the medulla oblongata cause hypotonia. On the other hand, adjacent cortical areas (i.e. extrapyramidal portions) are normally **inhibitory**, and they exert a predominant effect. Thus lesions of the motor cortex, such as strokes (which damage both facilitatory and inhibitory areas), are characterized by hypertonia (or spasticity).

2 *Basal ganglia.* These are generally **inhibitory**; however, the pathway is indirect. The basal ganglia exert their effect by stimulating a small area in the reticular formation of the brain stem (medullary reticular formation). The latter sends inhibitory impulses to gamma motor neurons via the *lateral reticulospinal tracts*. On the whole, lesions of the basal ganglia cause hypertonia, e.g. *Parkinsonism*.

3 *The brain stem.* Some brain stem centres are **facilitatory**; an important area is the spontaneously active pontine reticular formation, which delivers facilitatory impulses to gamma motor neurons via the *ventral reticulospinal* tracts. The *vestibular nuclei*, particularly the lateral vestibular nucleus, stimulate gamma efferent discharge directly via the *vestibulospinal tracts* and indirectly by sending excitatory signals to the *pontine reticular area*.

The brain stem contains other areas which are **inhibitory**: the **medullary reticular area** has already been mentioned. This part of the reticular formation does not possess inherent activity and is driven by impulses from the **inhibitory** cortical areas, the basal ganglia and also the **red nucleus**.

4 *The cerebellum.* The cerebellar cortex exerts an **inhibitory** influence on the stretch reflex. However, the deep cerebellar nuclei (DCN) are **excitatory**. Cerebellar lesions in humans are usually characterized by *hypotonia* (Fig. 16.35c), because they involve the deep cerebellar nuclei, which exert their excitatory influence through the

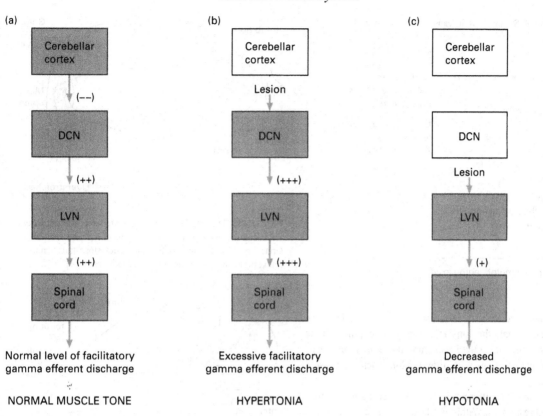

Fig. 16.35 Effects of the cerebellum on gamma efferent discharge (i.e. on muscle tone). The shaded boxes represent functioning areas; the clear boxes represent areas damaged by lesions; DCN, deep cerebellar nuclei; LVN, lateral vestibular nucleus; (+), stimulation; (–), inhibition. For detailed explanation see text.

Table 16.8 Summary of factors that enhance and others which inhibit the stretch reflex.

Enhances the stretch reflex	Inhibits the stretch reflex
Supraspinal centres	Supraspinal centres
Primary motor area (cortical pyramidal area).	Cortical motor areas (cortical extrapyramidal areas)
Vestibular nuclei	Basal ganglia
Pontine reticular formation of the brain stem	Medullary reticular formation of the brain stem
The cerebellum	The red nucleus
Anxiety	Excessive stretch of the muscle
Cutaneous stimulation, especially by noxious stimuli	(which leads to Golgi tendon organ stimulation)
	Muscle contraction

lateral vestibular nuclei and consequently on the gamma motor neurons (Figs 16.33, 16.35a). Selective cortical lesions, however, leave the excitatory effect of the DCN unchecked and lead to *hypertonia* (Fig. 16.35b).

Table 16.8 summarizes factors that enhance and others which inhibit the stretch reflex, and Table 16.9 lists some of the causes of disturbance of muscle tone.

The Golgi tendon reflex (inverse stretch reflex)

If a muscle is subjected to excessive tension either through passive stretch of the tendon or through active muscle contraction, it relaxes, contrary to the response in the stretch reflex. This reflex is known as the inverse stretch reflex to emphasize the opposite response. The receptors are **Golgi tendon organs** located in the tendons of muscles and

Table 16.9 Summary of the causes of disturbance of tone.

Hypotonia	Hypertonia
Neural shock (cerebral or spinal)	Corticospinal lesions (UMNL) after the stage of neural shock
Lower motor neuron lesions	
Cerebellar lesions	Some extrapyramidal lesions, e.g. Parkinsonism
Some extrapyramidal lesions, e.g. chorea	Psychogenic
Interruption of the afferent limb of the stretch reflex (e.g. tabes dorsalis)	
Myopathies	

UMNL, upper motor neuron lesion.

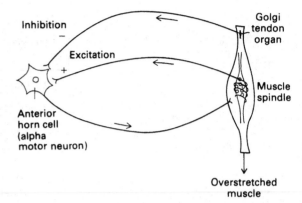

Fig. 16.36 The lengthening reaction. Moderate stretch causes reflex contraction. The receptor is the muscle spindle. Greater stretch increases the tension, the contraction stops and the muscle relaxes. The receptor is the Golgi tendon organ.

connected in series with extrafusal muscle fibres. They are stimulated when the muscle contracts and pulls on its tendons. They detect the *tension* and the *rate of change of* tension that develops within the tendon when the muscle contracts.

It appears that different degrees of muscle stretch cause different responses. Within limits, muscle stretch produces reflex contraction proportional to the degree of stretch (the receptor is the muscle spindle). However, if the muscle is overstretched, muscle contraction is suddenly replaced by relaxation and the muscle lengthens (the receptor is the Golgi tendon organ). This protects muscles against rupture and/or evulsion of their tendons. Such behaviour of a muscle when subjected to different degrees of stretch resembles that of a clasp-knife and is enhanced in hypertonic muscle. This is described by the term 'clasp-knife spasticity' or '*the lengthening reaction*' (Fig. 16.36).

Pathway of the reflex. When these receptors are stimulated, impulses pass to the spinal cord via fast type Aα fibres (group Ib). These produce excitation of inhibitory interneurons, which end on alpha motor neurons supplying the same muscle (Fig. 16.37). As a result, the motor neurons are inhibited and the muscle relaxes.

Tendon jerks: clinical significance
Tendon jerks are examined clinically to test the dynamic component of the stretch reflex. When examined properly, they provide useful information:

1 The presence of a normal tendon jerk indicates that the reflex arc concerned is intact. Except during neural

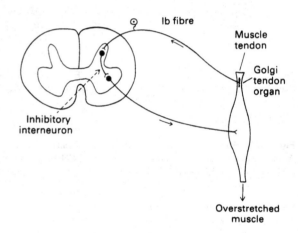

Fig. 16.37 Diagram illustrating the circuit of the tendon reflex.

shock, absence of a tendon jerk almost always means that the reflex arc subserving it has been interrupted, as in poliomyelitis, tabes dorsalis and peripheral neuropathy. In such conditions the static component of the stretch reflex is also affected and the muscles are hypotonic or atonic.
2 Tendon jerks may also be absent, as in lower motor neuron lesions, or decreased when supraspinal facilitatory impulses to the spinal cord are lost, e.g. cerebral or spinal shock.
3 Tendon jerks are generally exaggerated in lesions of the supraspinal inhibitory centres. In such lesions, the static component of the stretch reflex is also enhanced and the muscles show hypertonia. Upper motor neurons exert a net inhibitory effect on the stretch reflex, and therefore upper motor neuron lesions result in exaggeration of

Table 16.10 The spinal centres of the four primary tendon jerks.

Reflex	Spinal centre
Biceps jerk	C5, C6
Triceps jerk	C7, C8
Knee-jerk	L2, L3, L4
Ankle jerk	S1

tendon jerks. However, tendon jerks may also become exaggerated in anxiety states, tetanus, thyrotoxicosis and strychnine poisoning.

4 Abnormal tendon jerks on one side of the body enable determination of the side of the lesion.

5 The level along the longitudinal axis of the body at which tendon jerks are abnormal enables localization of the segmental level of the lesion. Table 16.10 lists the centres in the spinal cord of the four primary tendon jerks.

6 Tendon jerks change characteristically in certain diseases. In cerebellar disease the tendon jerks become *pendular*, and in myxoedema the contraction and relaxation phases of the stretch reflex are prolonged.

Clinical examples. The knee- and ankle jerks in the lower limbs and the biceps and triceps jerks in the upper limbs are the tendon jerks commonly examined. Details of how to elicit these reflexes are important in clinical practice and may be studied in the practical physiology course.

Clonus

This consists of rhythmic regular contractions, which occur when a muscle is subjected to sudden stretch and the stretch is maintained. It is characteristic of states of increased gamma efferent discharge (i.e. hypertonia), as in upper motor neuron lesions. Examples of clonus are ankle clonus and knee clonus. Ankle clonus is elicited by suddenly dorsiflexing the foot at the ankle and maintaining that. This stretches the gastrocnemius muscle and the response is rhythmic plantar flexion at the ankle as long as the stretch is maintained. Knee or patellar clonus is elicited on stretching the quadriceps femoris tendon by pushing the patella down and maintaining that for a while.

The explanation of clonus is as follows. Sudden stretch activates the already hyperactive muscle spindles and the muscle contracts. As the muscle contracts, the muscle spindles stop firing and the muscle relaxes. When the stretch is maintained by the examiner, the muscle spindles discharge again, causing muscle contraction. The cycle continues as long as the stretching force is maintained.

Superficial reflexes

Superficial reflexes result from stimulation of receptors present in the skin. They are clinically important because they aid in localizing lesions.

Superficial abdominal reflexes

When the skin on one side of the abdomen is stroked with a blunt object, the underlying muscles contract. The centres for these reflexes lie in thoracic segments T7 to T12.

Plantar reflex

In healthy adults stimulation of the sole of the foot produces plantar flexion of the toes. The centre for this reflex lies in lumbar segment L5 and sacral segment S1.

Cremasteric reflex

When the skin of the upper and inner aspects of the thigh is stroked, the cremasteric muscle contracts, elevating the testicle on that side. The centre of the reflex lies in lumbar segments L1 and L2.

The flexor reflex (withdrawal reflex)

The flexor reflex is elicited by an injurious and usually painful stimulus to the skin, subcutaneous tissue or muscle. The response is reflex contraction of the flexor muscles, and the part is withdrawn away from the injurious stimulus. Figure 16.38 shows the pathway.

Fig. 16.38 The flexor reflex, the crossed extensor reflex and reciprocal innervation (reciprocal inhibition). (Reproduced with permission from Guyton, A.C. (1987) *Textbook of Medical Physiology*, 7th edn. Saunders, Philadelphia.)

Stimulation of pain receptors in the hand region causes a volley of impulses to travel to the spinal cord via type $A\delta$ or C fibres. These impulses pass via several interneurons before reaching the anterior horn cells supplying the muscles which move the hand away from the injurious stimulus—in this case the flexor muscles. The flexor reflex is a good example of polysynaptic reflexes. Figure 16.38 also shows that excitation of flexors is accompanied by inhibition of extensors, a phenomenon occurring through inhibitory interneurons synapsing with extensor motor neurons. This is known as reciprocal innervation (or reciprocal inhibition). In addition to flexion and withdrawal of the stimulated limb, the figure also shows extension of the opposite limb. This usually occurs when the strength of the stimulus becomes severe enough and is called the crossed extensor response (or reflex), considered by many physiologists to be a part of the withdrawal reflex. The process of reciprocal innervation also occurs in the *crossed extensor reflex*, i.e. flexors are inhibited while extensors are excited. This pushes the entire body away from the injurious agent and supports the body-weight. The circuitry of the withdrawal reflex is also characterized by *after-discharge*, which prolongs the response and so further enhances the protective role of the reflex.

Scratch reflex

The scratch reflex is initiated by the itch-and-tickle sensation caused, for example, by a moving insect on the skin. It results in a to-and-fro scratching movement. The pathway is also endowed with reciprocal innervation and can occur in decerebrate animals.

Visceral reflexes

The clinically important visceral reflexes are those concerned with micturition, defecation and erection.

Micturition reflex

The micturition reflex is basically a spinal reflex, which becomes subject to cortical voluntary control after the first 2–3 years of life.

The urinary bladder is controlled by the autonomic nervous system. Parasympathetic nerves (S2, 3 and 4) cause contraction of the bladder wall and relaxation of the internal sphincter and so encourage emptying, while sympathetic nerves (L1 and 2) relax the bladder wall and contract the internal sphincter, and thus prevent emptying. Somatic supply, via the pudendal nerve (S2, 3 and 4), controls voluntary voiding of urine by contracting the external sphincter of the urethra. Table 16.11 shows the various lesions and states which disturb bladder function.

Table 16.11 Effects of various lesions on bladder function.

Lesion	Defect in bladder function
Damaged parasympathetic nerves (nervi erigentes)	Initially retention, with overflow; later bladder becomes decentralized and functions as an autonomous bladder
Damaged lumbosacral dorsal roots or columns	Patient does not feel bladder sensation but can empty bladder at will
Spinal cord transection above sacral segments	Retention, with overflow initially; later bladder functions as automatic bladder through sacral reflexes
Injury to bladder area in cortical centres	Inability to start or stop micturition at will
Emotional stress	Frequency of micturition due to loss of bladder's ability for adaptation

Defecation reflex

Distension of the rectum results in reflex contraction of its wall and relaxation of the internal anal sphincter, leading to emptying. The reflex is under voluntary control by the external anal sphincter. The nerves involved are the same ones that are involved in the micturition reflex. Neural lesions which disturb bladder function usually also disturb rectal function in much the same way, but consequences are less severe.

Erection reflex

This reflex is initiated by psychic stimuli from the brain and also by physical stimuli from the genitalia. Parasympathetic impulses pass from the sacral spinal cord to the penis, causing dilatation of the penile arteries. Blood accumulates in the corpora cavernosa (erectile tissue of the penis) under great pressure, causing swelling and stiffness of the penis.

General properties of reflexes

Adequate stimulus

Each reflex has a precise stimulus called the adequate stimulus. For example, a painful stimulus to the sole of the foot produces the flexor withdrawal reflex, while deep pressure applied to the same area produces the positive supportive reaction.

Local sign

The pattern of response in a reflex depends on the afferent nerve fibre stimulated. This is called the 'local sign'. A painful stimulus, if applied to the lateral side of the arm, produces flexion and adduction, but, if the same stimulus is applied to the medial aspect, it results in flexion and abduction of the limb.

Irradiation

The extent of the response in a reflex depends on the intensity of the stimulus. The more intense the stimulus is, the greater is the spread of activity in the spinal cord, involving more and more motor neurons (i.e. irradiation of the stimulus). For example, when the sole of the foot is stimulated by a weak painful stimulus, only the big toe is dorsiflexed. A stronger stimulus will cause reflex flexion of the big toe plus the ankle. The strongest stimulus will cause withdrawal of the whole leg by causing reflex flexion of the big toe, ankle, knee and hip. Impulses may also cross to the other side of the spinal cord to cause extension of the other leg (see the crossed extensor reflex).

Summation

In spatial summation, two or more stimuli, through different sensory routes, which by themselves are insufficient to elicit a reflex contraction, may elicit a contraction when given together (see Fig. 16.6).

In temporal summation, two or more stimuli given at different times, which by themselves are insufficient to elicit a reflex contraction, may elicit a contraction if given within a short time of each other (15 ms). Spatial summation seems to be more important than temporal summation in reflex action.

Occlusion

The tension obtained in a certain reflex by strong simultaneous stimulation of two adjacent afferents (i.e. which give rise to the same reflex) is less than the sum of tensions developed by stimulation of each of them separately. This is due to overlap of some of the motor neurons excited by the two afferents.

In Fig. 16.39, the upper diagram shows that strong stimulation of afferent 'a' alone causes four motor neurons to discharge and strong stimulation of afferent 'b' alone also causes four motor neurons to discharge. In total, eight motor neurons discharge when the two afferents are stimulated separately. The discharging motor neurons are said to be in the 'discharge zones' of their afferents. When the two afferents 'a' and 'b' are strongly stimulated simultaneously, the total discharging motor neurons are only six (not eight). This is because there are two neurons common to the

discharge zones of the two afferents. Therefore, *occlusion* occurs, due to overlap of discharge zones.

Summation of subliminal fringes

The tension obtained in a certain reflex by weak (but threshold) stimulation of two adjacent afferents simultaneously is more than the sum of tension developed when each is stimulated separately. Stimulation of each afferent separately causes discharge of some neurons but only facilitates some nearby neurons (i.e. excites them but not enough to discharge). Those facilitated neurons are said to lie in the *subliminal fringe* zone of those discharging. Simultaneous stimulation of the two afferents causes overlapping of the subliminal fringe zones and raises the excitability of the neurons (within the subliminal zones) to discharge.

In the lower part of Fig. 16.39, stimulation of 'a' alone causes two motor neurons to discharge and two to be facilitated. Also, stimulation of 'b' alone causes two motor neurons to discharge and two to be facilitated. In total, four neurons discharge when the two afferents are stimulated separately. When the two afferents are stimulated simultaneously, six neurons (not four) discharge. This is due to overlap of the *subliminal fringe zones*.

Recruitment and after-discharge

If a repetitive stimulus is maintained, the strength of the reflex contraction slowly increases to a final level. The slow build-up is due to gradual activation of more motor neurons (i.e. recruitment) (Fig. 16.40).

The reflex response may continue some time after cessation of the stimulus, due to after-discharge, the main type being reverberating circuit after-discharge.

Reciprocal innervation (or reciprocal inhibition)

Reflex contraction of an agonist muscle is accompanied by inhibition of the antagonist. For example, when the biceps is involved in a stretch reflex, the triceps must relax; otherwise no movement will take place. This is known as *reciprocal inhibition* (Fig. 16.41). The impulses that enter the spinal cord will activate the motor neurons supplying the stimulated muscle and, through an inhibitory interneuron, inhibit the motor neurons supplying the antagonist muscle.

Final common path

Many sensory inputs converge on the motor neuron. Each motor neuron is thus the common efferent path for several reflexes.

Response time

Response time is an indicator of the number of synapses in the reflex arc. Very short response times indicate a smaller

Dorsal
root
ganglion

Stimulation
of 'a' alone
excites 4
neurons

Stimulation
of 'b' alone
excites 4
neurons

Stimulation of 'a' and
'b' simultaneously
excites 6 neurons

Total is 8 neurons discharging

Stimulation of 'a' alone
excites 2 neurons to discharge
and 2 subliminally.
Stimulation of 'b' alone
excites 2 neurons to discharge
and 2 subliminally
Total is 4 neurons discharging

Stimulation of 'a' and
'b' simultaneously
excites 6 neurons

Fig. 16.39 Upper diagram shows
occlusion; lower diagram shows
summation of subliminal fringes.

Fig. 16.40 A diagram showing recruitment and
after-discharge in reflex action.

number of synapses in the reflex path. The knee-jerk, which
has the shortest response time, is a monosynaptic reflex.

Rebound phenomenon

This is the exaggeration of a reflex after a temporary period
of inhibition. For example, a flexor withdrawal reflex in
one limb involves stimulation of flexors and inhibition
of extensors. If this is followed by another reflex which
involves stimulation of extensors of the same limb (such as
the crossed extensor reflex), the extensor response will be
greatly exaggerated.

Rebound is one of the important mechanisms for coordinating the rhythmic to-and-fro movement required in
locomotion (i.e. walking and running).

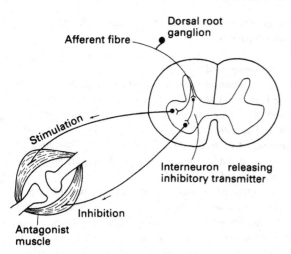

Fig. 16.41 The circuit in reciprocal inhibition. Note the presence of an interneuron releasing an inhibitory transmitter at its junction with the anterior horn cell supplying the antagonistic muscle.

II Motor functions of the brain stem and cerebral cortex

The brain stem

The brain stem is a complex extension of the spinal cord which performs sensory, motor and reflex functions.

Besides containing centres that regulate cardiovascular, respiratory and gastrointestinal functions, the brain stem plays a major role in the control of eye movements, in the support of the body against gravity and also in the control of other complex reflex movements.

The reticular formation of the brain stem

The reticular formation is a large structure occupying the core of the brain stem from the caudal medulla to the rostral midbrain (Fig. 16.42). It consists of areas of diffuse neurons of two types: sensory neurons, which are greater in number and which make multiple connections within the reticular formation itself, and motor neurons, which are larger in size and receive impulses from sensory neurons. Motor neurons give rise to axons, which divide into ascending branches and descending branches. The former pass to the non-specific thalamic nuclei, to the basal ganglia and to the cerebral cortex via the thalamus. This is known as the *reticular activating system*, which plays a major role in the control of brain activity and related phenomena, such as consciousness and alertness. The descending branches, however, pass to the spinal cord to supply the anterior motor neurons. These are the lateral and ventral reticulospinal tracts. A number of nuclei function in association with the reticular formation of the brain stem. These are the *vestibular nuclei*, the *red nucleus* and the *substantia nigra*.

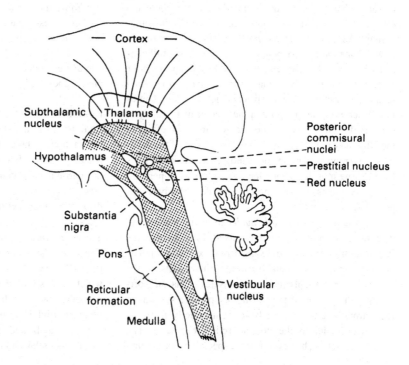

Fig. 16.42 The reticular formation of the brain stem. (Reproduced with permission from Guyton, A.C. (1987) *Textbook of Medical Physiology*, 7th edn. Saunders, Philadelphia.)

Motor functions

Functionally the reticular formation can be divided as follows:

1 The pontine reticular system, often called the facilitatory reticular formation, is located in the dorsolateral part of the pons. It has spontaneous intrinsic activity which is enhanced by impulses from motor area 4 of the cerebral cortex, the vestibular nuclei and the deep cerebellar nuclei, and also from the classical sensory pathways. This area transmits facilitatory impulses to the gamma motor neurons supplying the muscles of the axial parts of the body (i.e. extensors of the lower limbs, and muscles of the vertebral column), which support the body against gravity. Impulses reach the anterior horn cells via the ventral reticulospinal tracts.

2 The medullary reticular system (or inhibitory reticular formation) occupies the ventromedial part of the medulla. Unlike the pontine reticular system, it does not discharge spontaneously, but it is driven by impulses from the inhibitory area of the motor cortex, the basal ganglia and the red nuclei. It transmits inhibitory impulses via the lateral reticulospinal tracts to the gamma motor neurons supplying the same antigravity muscles. This counterbalances the strong excitatory signals from the pontine reticular system so that a state of continuous mild muscle contraction—the normal muscle tone—is maintained under normal conditions. Thus the two systems are antagonistic to each other; but very often situations arise where the effects of one system are required unopposed by the other system. An example is the *positive supportive reaction* in which the *facilitatory pontine system* exercises full control while the inhibitory effects of the *medullary reticular system* is suppressed by signals from higher centres. As a result, antigravity muscles stiffen when the foot comes in contact with the ground and the weight of the body is supported against gravity. In other situations, the effect of the inhibitory medullary system overrides that of the facilitatory pontine system on some antigravity muscles, so as to allow the muscles of one leg (for example) to perform other movements, e.g. kicking a ball, while the body is supported by the other leg.

The role of the *vestibular nuclei* in exciting antigravity muscles cannot be overemphasized. In particular, the lateral vestibular nuclei transmit strong excitatory signals via the lateral and medial vestibulospinal tracts to the motor neurons supplying these muscles. This supports strongly the effects of the facilitatory pontine system. In fact, strong excitatory signals are sent directly from the vestibular nuclei to the pontine reticular system. The vestibular nucleus, however, is more specialized in exciting antigravity muscles in response to impulses from the vestibular apparatus.

Decerebrate rigidity

This condition is seen in animal preparations in which the brain stem has been sectioned at the midbrain level (between the superior and inferior colliculi). Most striking in such an animal is the extreme rigidity in the antigravity muscles. As a result, the animal assumes a characteristic posture—extended limbs, retracted head, arched back, closed jaw and an erect tail.

The effect of supraspinal centres on gamma efferent discharge contributes to the genesis of **decerebrate rigidity**. Normally the cortical inhibitory area, the basal ganglia and the red nuclei (which lie above the level of the section) drive the *medullary reticular formation* to inhibit gamma motor neurons. On the other hand, the *pontine reticular formation* and the *vestibular nuclei* (which lie below the level of the section) excite gamma motor neurons. As shown in Fig. 16.43, the first section interrupted the impulses driving the inhibitory (medullary) reticular formation into activity, leaving the discharge from the facilitatory (pontine) reticular formation and vestibular nuclei unopposed. The result is an excess of excitatory impulses to gamma motor neurons causing rigidity.

Deafferentation of a limb in a decerebrate animal decreases the rigidity (indicating that it is primarily *gamma rigidity*), but does not completely abolish it. This is because the lateral vestibular nucleus sends excitatory impulses via *alpha motor* neurons as well. If, however, another section is made below the level of the vestibular nuclei or the lateral vestibular nucleus is destroyed, rigidity is completely abolished.

Equilibrium and the vestibular apparatus

Equilibrium is maintained by variation in the degree of contraction of the individual antigravity muscles; i.e. if a person begins to fall to one side, the extensor muscles on that particular side contract while those on the opposite side relax. This variation is controlled by signals, mainly from the vestibular apparatus.

The vestibular apparatus

The vestibular apparatus is the sensory organ for equilibrium (Fig. 16.44). It is composed of the bony labyrinth, which consists of a group of bony cavities and canals connected with each other in the temporal bone. The bony labyrinth is formed of the vestibule, three bony semicircular canals and a bony cochlea. This encloses the membranous labyrinth, composed mainly of the cochlear

Fig. 16.43 The genesis of decerebrate rigidity. The top broken line represents the first section at the midbrain level resulting in decerebrate rigidity; the lower broken line represents the second section below the vestibular nuclei which abolished rigidity. (+), Stimulation; (−), inhibition.

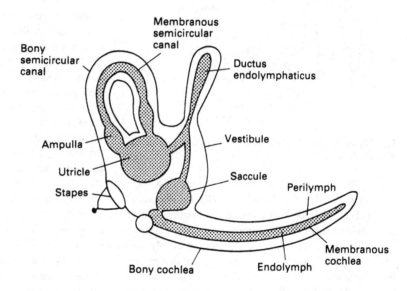

Fig. 16.44 The vestibular apparatus (bony and membranous labyrinths).

duct (membranous cochlea), three membranous semi-circular canals and two chambers: the utricle and saccule (Fig. 16.45). Between the bony and membranous labyrinths is a space filled with fluid, the *perilymph*. Inside the membranous labyrinth there is also fluid, called the *endolymph*. The cochlear duct is the sensory organ for hearing, while the utricle, saccule and semicircular canals contain receptors concerned with the control of equilibrium.

The utricle and saccule. Located on the floor of the utricle and on the wall of the saccule of each membranous labyrinth are small organs called the **maculae** or **otolithic**

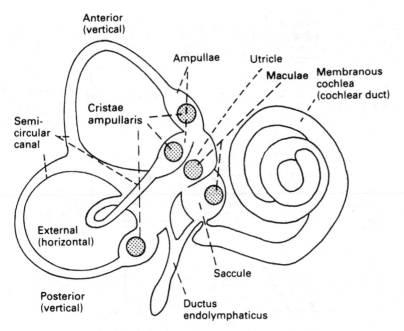

Fig. 16.45 The membranous labyrinth. (Reproduced with permission from Guyton, A.C. (1987) *Textbook of Medical Physiology* 7th edn. Saunders, Philadelphia.)

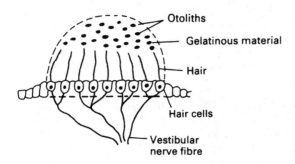

Fig. 16.46 The macula of the saccule and utricle (stimulated by the pull of gravity).

organs (Fig. 16.45). Each macula is formed of a ridge of columnar epithelial cells and hair cells and is covered by a gelatinous layer. Embedded in the gelatinous layer are numerous small calcium carbonate crystals (**otoliths**), which are more dense than the surrounding endolymph. The otoliths lie on top of the hairs or processes that project from the apical ends of hair cells (Fig. 16.46). Because of their weight, otoliths will bend the hairs in the direction of the pull of gravity. A single hair cell has on average about 30–150 small hairs (**stereocilia**) plus one very large cilium called the **kinocilium**. The kinocilium is always located on one side of the cell, and the stereocilia become progressively shorter in an axis away from the kinocilium (Fig. 16.47). Electron microscopy shows that very fine filamentous attachments called *tip links* connect the kinocilium to the nearest longest stereocilium, this to

the next shorter stereocilium and so on up to the other end of the cell. The bases of hair cells synapse with afferent fibres of the vestibular branch of the 8th cranial nerve.

The macula detects deviation of the head from the upright vertical position. Under resting conditions when the head is upright and vertical, the macula generates action potentials at a constant rate in the afferent fibres. Bending the hairs changes the rate of discharge according to the amount and the direction of bending. In a hair cell when the stereocilia bend in the direction of the kinocilium, tip links pull the stereocilia one after the other away from the body of the hair cell. This opens ion channels and the cell is depolarized, i.e. the discharge rate increases in the afferent nerve fibre (Fig. 16.47). Note that, for a given amount of bending, there is only one direction which causes the maximum rate of discharge from that hair cell. When the stereocilia are bent in the opposite direction, i.e. the stereocilia are bent away from the kinocilium, the pulling effect of the tip links on the stereocilia is reduced. This closes the ion channels and the cell is hyperpolarized, i.e. the discharge rate decreases. Again, for this amount of bending, only one direction causes the greatest decrease in discharge rate.

On the surface of each macula, hair cells are orientated in all different directions, so that tilting the head in any direction is signalled. In the upright position with the head vertical, the macula of the utricle lies in the horizontal plane (Fig. 16.48); the hairs pointing upwards. This position allows some cells to signal tilting of the head forwards,

Fig. 16.47 Diagram showing two hair cells of the membranous labyrinth and their mode of stimulation. A tonic level of discharge is recorded from the nerve fibre leading from the hair cell. This level of discharge, however, increases when stereocilia bend towards the kinocilium, and decreases when stereocilia bend away from the kinocilium. (Reproduced from Bray, J.J., Cragg, P.A., Macknight, A.D.C., Mills, R.G. & Taylor, D.W. (eds) *Lecture Notes in Physiology*, 2nd edn. Blackwell Scientific Publications, Oxford.)

Fig. 16.48 Orientation of the maculae in the utricle and saccule.

others to signal tilting backwards and still others to signal lateral tilting of the head on either side. Thus a changing pattern of stimulation is created with each movement, and it is this changing pattern which informs the brain about the orientation of the head in space and in relation to the pull of gravity or the forces of linear acceleration.

In the saccule, the macula lies in a vertical plane with processes of the hair cells pointing laterally (Fig. 16.48). This allows them to operate only when the head is not in the vertical position, e.g. when one is lying down.

Functions of the utricle and saccule. The macula in the utricle (and to a lesser extent in the saccule) plays two important functions:

1 *Detection of a static tilt.* In the upright vertical position, impulses from the right and left utricles balance each other. However, if the body tilts from the precise upright position to one side (e.g. as when the support under one foot gives way), the utricles on the two sides of the head signal a different pattern, informing the brain about the new position of the head in space. In addition to giving the sensation of imbalance, the signals go to the brainstem and the vestibular and cerebellar motor systems, which stimulate the appropriate muscles to restore equilibrium.

2 *Detection of linear acceleration.* Otoliths are also displaced when the body accelerates. Forward thrust, as when a person stands in a bus which suddenly accelerates, causes the otoliths to fall backwards on the hair cell's processes. This creates a sense of malequilibrium (i.e. the person feels he/she is falling backwards), which is corrected by leaning forwards so that the otoliths shift anteriorly. Backward acceleration on the other hand, as when the bus suddenly decelerates, causes the otoliths to fall forwards and the sense of malequilibrium (i.e. the person feels he/she is falling forwards) is corrected by leaning backwards so as to shift the otoliths posteriorly. The utricular maculae detect horizontal acceleration. The saccular maculae respond to vertical acceleration. However, both detect forward and backward acceleration in the horizontal plane.

The semicircular canals. There are three semicircular canals on each side, known as external (horizontal), anterior and posterior (both are vertical), which lie in the three planes of space perpendicular to each other (Fig. 16.49). Each canal opens at both ends into the utricle; one of these ends is dilated to form the **ampulla**, which houses the receptor organ called the **crista ampullaris**. The crista is a ridge of hair cells and supporting cells surmounted by a gelatinous mass, the cupula, which extends across the ampulla, sealing it. Embedded within the cupula are the *stereocilia* and *kinocilia* protruding from the hair cells (Fig. 16.50). Bending of the cupula bends these hairs, and this occurs whenever the endolymph moves along the semicircular canal. The crista is different from the macula in that all hair cells in each crista are orientated in the same direction, i.e. the kinocilium of every hair cell is located on one and the same side of the cell in relation to its orientation on the crista. The kinocilia of the crista in the horizontal canals are located at the edge of the cells towards the utricle, whereas the kinocilia of the cristae in the anterior and posterior canals are located at the edge of the cells towards the canal side.

Semicircular
canals

Anterior —
(vertical)

External
(horizontal)

Posterior —
(vertical)

Left   Right

Fig. 16.49 Planes of the semicircular
canals showing directions of rotation.

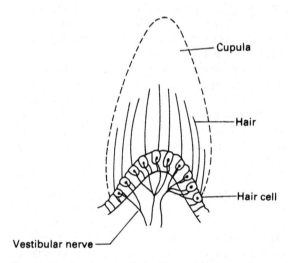

Cupula

Hair

Hair cell

Vestibular nerve —

Fig. 16.50 The crista ampullaris of the semicircular canals
(stimulated by rotation).

The canals are stimulated by rotational movement (i.e.
angular acceleration) of the head, and each canal detects
rotation in its own plane. This causes flow of endolymph in
the canal towards the ampulla on one side of the head, but
flow of endolymph away from the ampulla in the corresponding canal on the other side of the head. Since orientation of hair cells in the crista of one canal is a mirror image
of the orientation of hair cells in the crista of the corresponding canal on the other side of the head, the stereocilia
bend towards the kinocilium (i.e. excitation) in one canal
and away from the kinocilium (i.e. inhibition) in the corresponding canal. The pattern of discharge is reversed if head
rotation occurs in the same plane but in the opposite dir-

ection. In summary, the semicircular canals (SCCs) inform
the CNS of the plane as well as the direction of rotation of
the head.

Signals from the hair cells of the crista ampullaris are
carried along afferent fibres of the vestibular division of the
8th cranial nerve.

Function of the semicircular canals. The cristae of the
semicircular canals detect head rotation in any direction.
This movement is called angular acceleration.

Under resting conditions, the cristae on both sides of the
head transmit a continuous series of impulses, averaging
about 200/s. But when the head suddenly begins to rotate
in any direction, suppose from left to right in the horizontal plane (Fig. 16.51a), the horizontal semicircular canal
moves in the same plane. However, the endolymph inside
it remains stationary for a while, due to inertia. It is as
though the endolymph is flowing in the canal in a direction
opposite to that of the head rotation, i.e. from right to left
(Fig. 16.51a). The cupula is bent by the endolymph and
so are the projecting hairs. Since the kinocilia in the cristae
of the horizontal canals are located on the side of the hair
cells towards the utricle, the frequency of impulses from
the cristae of the right canal is increased, as the stereocilia
are bent towards the kinocilium, while that from the cristae
of the left canal is decreased, because the stereocilia are
bent away from the kinocillium. This unbalanced discharge
from the two sides will give the sensation of rotation to the
right.

With continued rotation, the endolymph will soon rotate
(in the same direction of rotation, i.e. from left to right)
as rapidly as the semicircular canals due to friction inside
the canals, and the cupulae, by virtue of their elasticity,

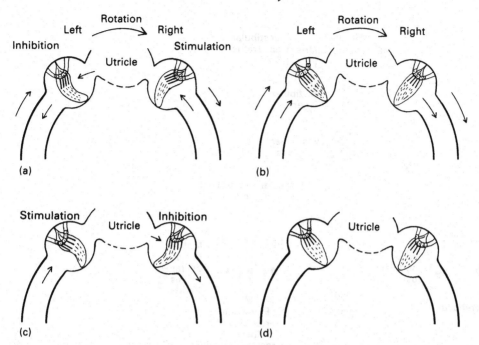

Fig. 16.51 Mode of action of semicircular canals during rotation in the horizontal plane. The right and left horizontal canal ampullae are shown. The arrows drawn inside the canal indicate movement of the endolymph and the arrows outside indicate direction of rotation of the canal. Note the direction of bending of the hairs at the base of the ampulla. See text for explanation of stages (a), (b), (c) and (d).

Fig. 16.52 Response of a hair cell when a semicircular canal is stimulated first by rotation and then by stopping rotation. (Reproduced with permission from Guyton; A.C. (1987) *Textbook of Medical Physiology*, 7th edn. Saunders, Philadelphia.)

return to the resting position (Fig. 16.51b). This causes the discharge from the two sides to decline back to tonic level (i.e. resting level). The equal and balanced discharge from the two sides makes the person unaware of the sensation of rotation, provided that his/her eyes are closed. Figure 16.52

shows the response of one hair cell when the semicircular canal is stimulated at the beginning of rotation and then the decline in the number of impulses to tonic level as rotation continues.

If the rotation suddenly stops, the opposite sequence of events occurs. The canal stops rotating but the endolymph continues to flow for some time due to its momentum in the same direction of rotation (from left to right), bending the cupulae—this time in the opposite direction to when rotation was first started (Fig. 16.51c). Thus, discharge from the left canal crista increases and that from the right decreases. Imbalance in the discharge between the two sides gives the person a false sensation of rotation, this time from the right to the left side. This is known as vertigo. In a few seconds, then, the endolymph stops moving and the cupulae recoil back to the resting position. Discharge will consequently return to tonic level (Figs 16.51d and 16.52) and the false sensation of rotation (vertigo) disappears.

Thus, the semicircular canals detect only the beginning of rotation, end of rotation and changes in the rate of rotation (i.e. angular acceleration). Constant rates of rotation stimulate the semicircular canals for a maximum of 30 seconds, after which the discharge goes down to tonic levels (see Fig. 16.52). However, rotations (i.e. turnings)

Fig. 16.53 Neural connections of the vestibular apparatus.

in everyday life are of short duration, and prolonged periods of rotation at a constant rate are non-physiological. By early detection of rotation or turning, the semicircular canals send impulses to the equilibrium centres to adjust posture accordingly.

Neural connections of the vestibular apparatus

Figure 16.53 shows that fibres from the maculae and cristae ampullaris pass as the vestibular nerve to the medulla to synapse in the ipsilateral vestibular nucleus. From the vestibular nuclei, nerve fibres pass to four main sites:

1 *Cerebellum*. Fibres pass to the flocculonodular lobe and dentate nucleus. Some of the fibres pass directly from the receptors to the cerebellum without synapsing in the vestibular nucleus.

2 *Motor cranial nuclei of cranial nerves 3, 4 and 6.* These supply the extraocular muscles. These fibres are called the medial longitudinal fasciculus. They serve to correct eye movements and so help fixing objects seen in the visual fields when the head is rotating.

3 *Reticular formation.* This in turn sends fibres to the spinal cord (i.e. reticulospinal tracts).

4 *Spinal cord.* The fibres form the vestibulospinal tract.

The impulses from the reticular formation and vestibular nuclei maintain equilibrium by sending impulses that facilitate or inhibit the stretch reflex and thus regulate the tone of various muscles.

Effects of stimulation of the semicircular canals

The semicircular canals can be stimulated in the laboratory or clinic using various methods, including the rotational method, in which a subject is rotated in a rotatory chair at a high speed with the head fixed at certain angles to stimulate a specific semicircular canal. Other methods include the caloric method and the electrical method, about which one will find more details in a physiology practical schedule.

Stimulation of the semicircular canals produces the following effects.

Vertigo. This is the false sensation of spinning with respect to the surroundings that a person feels when rotation is stopped. The sensation is always in the opposite direction to that of the original rotation. The pathway involves impulses that pass from the stimulated semicircular canals to the cerebellum and reticular formation. These then pass to the superior temporal gyrus of the opposite side, via the thalamus.

Nystagmus. This is a series of jerky oscillatory movements of the eye, observed at the beginning and end of rotation. It is a reflex aimed at fixing objects in the visual field during rotation. It has two components:

1 A slow component which is in the direction of flow of the endolymph (vestibulo-ocular reflex). Its pathway involves impulses that travel from the semicircular canals via the medial longitudinal fasciculus to stimulate the 3rd, 4th and 6th cranial nerves, supplying the extraocular muscles.

2 A fast component which is a compensatory flick-back movement when the slow-component movement reaches its limit. The centre for the fast component is in the brain stem, which also sends impulses via the medial longitudinal fasciculus.

By convention, the direction of eye movement in nystagmus is identified by the direction of the fast component. During rotation the fast component is in the same direction as that of rotation and when rotation is stopped it is in the opposite direction to that of rotation.

Stimulation of the semicircular canals may also cause nausea, vomiting, bradycardia, hypotension and sweating. These are autonomic reactions that occur due to stimulation of the autonomic centres in the brain stem by impulses from the vestibular apparatus. It also leads to an increase in muscle tone on the ipsilateral side and a decrease on the opposite side. This is obviously a reflex mechanism to support the body on the side of stimulation.

Other receptors contributing to equilibrium

The maintenance of the upright posture depends on three types of information:

1 Information concerning the position of the body in relation to space. This is signalled by receptors in the *vestibular apparatus*, the maculae being the most important. *Visual and auditory* receptors also contribute. Indeed, visual mechanisms can maintain balance reasonably well in the absence of vestibular function, as long as movements are performed slowly. Vision can also compensate for loss of proprioceptive information. In tabes dorsalis, a late manifestation of syphilis, the patient loses proprioception in the legs. This patient can maintain balance as long as his/her eyes are open, but loses balance and

may fall as soon as the eyes are shut (positive **Rhomberg sign**).

2 Information concerning the position of various parts of the body in relation to each other. This is signalled by *proprioceptors* in muscles, ligaments and joints as follows:

(a) *Neck proprioceptors.* These provide the most important proprioceptive information required for the maintenance of equilibrium. The neck proprioceptors detect the position of the head in relation to the trunk. Tilting the head in any direction (by bending the head on the neck) stimulates neck proprioceptors as well as receptors of the vestibular apparatus. The impulses from the two sources balance each other. However, when the whole body is tilted in relation to gravity (e.g. as when the support under one foot suddenly gives way), the impulses from the vestibular apparatus are unopposed by impulses from the neck muscles. This unbalanced discharge gives the person a sensation of malequilibrium.

(b) *Body proprioceptors.* When we are standing, we sway gently back and forth (and from side to side) throughout the period, making continuous adjustments in *muscle tone*, particularly of the antigravity muscles through the stretch reflex. This is sufficient to hold the body up in exact balance and prevent falling over.

3 Information concerning the direction of support. This is signalled by *cutaneous pressure receptors* located in the parts that support the body. For example, pressure sensations from the soles of the feet provide information about the relative distribution of body-weight on the two feet. This stimulates the positive supportive reaction: the response is reflex extension in the direction of applied pressure (i.e. magnet reaction).

Postural reflexes

The upright posture characteristic of humans is produced, maintained and restored, when upset, by a series of coordinated reflexes called the postural reflexes.

Posture depends on the degree and distribution of muscle tone, and muscle tone depends principally on the stretch reflex. Therefore, the stretch reflex is the basic postural reflex.

The role of the stretch reflex in the maintenance of posture is reinforced and modified by afferent impulses from proprioceptors of the muscles of the neck, trunk and limbs, from the eyes, from the vestibular apparatus and from exteroceptors in the skin. Impulses from these sources, which stream into the central nervous system, are integrated by the coordinated activity of the spinal cord, brain stem, cerebellum, basal ganglia and cerebral cortex. Postural reflexes are divisible into two groups: (i) static reflexes; and (ii) phasic reflexes (*statokinetic reflexes*).

Static reflexes

Static reflexes maintain posture when the body is at rest. They are of two types, stance and righting reflexes.

Stance reflexes. These are static reflexes that keep the body the right way up. They also give attitude. There are three subtypes:
1 Local static reflexes, which are confined to the stimulated limb. By means of these reflexes, a limb which is freely movable at a given moment can be converted at the next moment to a rigid pillar for bearing weight, i.e. *positive supportive reaction or magnet reaction.*
2 Segmental static reflexes are mediated by one segment of the spinal cord for adjusting the position of one limb in relation to movements of the opposite, as in the *crossed extensor reflex.*
3 General static reflexes produce reflex alterations of tone and posture of the trunk and limbs in accordance with the position of the head in space. They are initiated by impulses arising from the neck muscles, when they are known as neck *statotonic reflexes*, and/or from the otolith organs, when they are called *labyrinthine statotonic reflexes.*

Neck statotonic reflexes are studied in decerebrate animals after destroying the labyrinth. They depend on stimulation of the abundant muscle spindles in the neck muscles by changes in the head position. The result is movement involving limbs. For example, turning the head to the right relative to the body causes the right limb to extend and the left limb to flex. Turning to the left produces the opposite effect. Dorsiflexion of the head will extend the forelimbs and flex the hind limbs, while ventroflexion has the opposite effect.

Labyrinthine statotonic reflexes are also studied in the decerebrate animal after elimination of the neck proprioceptors. The receptors are the otolith organs (receptors in equilibratory vestibular apparatus) and the response consists of extension of four limbs on dorsiflexion of the head and flexion on ventroflexion.

Righting reflexes. These are reflexes which come into operation when the upright position is disturbed, as in falling down. The afferent impulses come from the eyes, which mediate the optical righting reflexes, i.e. an animal can appreciate the position of its body with respect to the surroundings by the visual images from the periphery. If the position is disturbed, it is corrected. Afferent impulses also come from the labyrinth, which mediates the labyrinthine righting reflexes. These correct the position of the head if the body is not in the proper position, e.g. an animal held in the air from its pelvis by a sling keeps its head level. The receptors are the otolith organs. The body righting reflexes are mediated by afferent impulses from the trunk muscles, which arise as a result of pressure on one side of the body (e.g. when an animal is laid on its side). The response is reflex correction of the position of the head and body.

Although all the previously mentioned reflexes are functional in humans, the optical righting reflexes are particularly important. They are the reason why a person with sensory ataxia compensates quite well for the deficit with eyes open but tends to fall when they are closed (positive *Romberg's sign*).

Phasic or statokinetic reflexes

These operate to maintain posture when the body is in motion. The afferent impulses originate in the vestibular apparatus, semicircular canals being stimulated during angular acceleration and otoliths (maculae) during linear acceleration. Some examples of phasic reflexes that come into play when the body is displaced in the horizontal plane are the hopping and placing reactions. The *hopping reaction* consists of the hopping movements that keep the limbs in position so as to support the body-weight when a standing animal is pushed laterally. Its sensory input comes from the labyrinths. The *placing reaction* can best be elicited by suspending a blindfold animal in the air. When the animal is moved towards a supporting surface, the feet are placed firmly on the supporting surface as soon as they touch it. Its sensory input comes from touch receptors in the soles of the feet. Both these reflexes are integrated in the cerebral cortex.

Although all postural reactions are reflex in nature, impulses from the various receptors are integrated in the reticular formation of the brain stem and then transmitted to the cerebral cortex. This is responsible for the conscious perception of being equilibrated or not.

Motion sickness

This is a complication of modern travel, i.e. 'travel sickness', and is considered a major problem in space flights. The person in a moving vehicle suffers vertigo, nausea and vomiting and may walk unsteadily. The genesis of motion sickness is attributed to conflicts between inputs from various sensory systems, e.g. conflict between the vestibular apparatus, which tells the person in a moving car that he/she is moving, and the visual field inside the vehicle, which appears stationary. In fact, a passenger feels much better if he/she sits on the front seat or keeps looking out of the side window to watch the moving visual field. The two inputs would then match and cut down the conflict. Motion sickness can be controlled by some tranquillizing medicines.

The motor cortex

Movement is the result of contraction of skeletal muscle fibres. These contract when stimulated by signals arriving along motor nerves. The motor nerves are actually the axons of the anterior motor neurons of the spinal cord or the homologous cranial motor nuclei of the brain stem. Each axon controls a group of muscle fibres, the **motor unit**, the size of which is variable. In the spinal cord, the anterior motor neurons are arranged in groups in an orderly manner. The neurons of the medial group innervate the trunk and proximal muscles which control posture and gross movements, while the neurons of the lateral group innervate the muscles of the most distal parts of the limbs concerned with fine skilled movements.

Motor neurons are influenced by inputs from widespread areas of the CNS—inputs from the same or higher spinal segments and others from supraspinal centres via descending pathways. The **pyramidal system** controls the voluntary skilled movements of the distal parts of the limbs. The **extrapyramidal system** is more concerned with setting the postural background needed for performance of the skilled movements and with subconscious gross movements. Last but not least, the **spinocerebellum** is important for smoothing and coordinating these movements, especially voluntary movements. Because motor neurons are the final path via which all inputs must pass to reach (and influence) skeletal muscle fibres, they are called the **final common path**.

Thus, the performance of normal voluntary movement depends on the integrity of two sets of neurons:
1 *Upper motor neurons.* These consist of the motor neurons originating in the cerebral cortex and the brain stem, which synapse directly or indirectly with the anterior horn cells or with the motor neurons of the cranial nerves. Upper motor neurons are grouped into pyramidal and extrapyramidal systems.
2 *Lower motor neurons.* These include the following cranial motor nuclei and their axons, i.e. motor fibres of the cranial nerves (3rd, 4th, 5th, 6th, 7th, 9th, 10th, 11th and 12th). In the spinal cord they are the anterior horn motor neurons and their axons, i.e. the motor nerves to skeletal muscles (Fig. 16.54).

The upper and lower motor neurons constitute the motor pathways that bring about skeletal muscle contraction. Lesions of the upper or lower motor neurons result in loss of voluntary muscle movement, i.e. **paralysis**.

Fig. 16.54 The upper and lower motor neurons.

Motor areas of the cerebral cortex

The areas in the cerebral cortex from which movement can be evoked by stimulation are (Fig. 16.55): (i) the primary motor area (known also as motor area 4 or MI); (ii) the supplementary motor area (MII); (iii) the premotor area (MIII); and (iv) the parietal lobe (especially the somatosensory area).

1 The primary motor area

The primary motor area, also known as MI or motor area 4, occupies the precentral gyrus (Fig. 16.55) and is highly excitable, due to the presence of the biggest pyramidal cells of the cortex, the *Betz cells*. This area is one of the main regions of origin of the pyramidal tracts. MI of one side controls skeletal muscles of the opposite side of the body, but there still is some cerebral dominance. For example, in right-handed individuals, the left motor cortex may control some muscles on the left side as well. This explains how left-side strokes not only cause paralysis on the right side of the body but may also affect some muscles on the left side.

Representation of the body is unilateral, except for the upper part of the face (i.e. forehead and eyes), which is represented in both cerebral hemispheres. The various parts of the body are represented in an inverted manner, i.e. the feet at the top and the face at the bottom and medially (Fig. 16.56). The area of representation of any part is proportional to the degree of complexity of skilled movement of

(a)

(b)

Fig. 16.55 The motor areas of the cerebral cortex. (a) A lateral view of the cerebral hemisphere showing MI (the primary motor area), MII (the supplementary motor area), MIII (the premotor area). (b) A medial view of the cerebral hemisphere showing parts of MI and MII.

column is arranged into six distinct layers, numbered I to VI from the cortical surface. This horizontal layering reflects the different distribution of various types of cells. Layers I to IV receive input signals from various areas of the nervous system. Layer V contains the pyramidal cells which are the origin of the output fibres from area MI to the spinal cord and brain stem, and layer VI gives rise to fibres that travel to other regions of the cerebral cortex.

Lesions in the primary motor area (MI) lead to flaccid paralysis of the contralateral muscles. The cause of flaccidity is due to loss of the facilitatory effect of MI on gamma motor neurons.

2 The supplementary motor area (MII)

The supplementary motor area is a small area located on the lateral side of the brain in front of area 4 and above the premotor area. It extends on the medial side of the hemisphere down to the cingulate sulcus. This area projects mainly to the motor cortex and appears to be concerned with planning and programming motor sequences. Unlike the primary motor area, lesions here do not cause paralysis but they disturb performance of complex integrated movements.

3 The premotor area (MIII)

The premotor area lies, in front of the primary motor area on the lateral surface of each hemisphere and below the supplementary motor area (see Fig. 16.55). Body representation in this area is also in an inverted manner, and the area contains very few neurons that project nerve fibres directly to the spinal cord. Stimulation of the premotor area produces complex coordinated movements, such as setting the body in a certain posture to perform a specific task. This is achieved by sending signals to brain stem areas that regulate posture and/or to MI to excite multiple groups of muscles. The premotor area receives diffuse sensory input from the posterior parietal cortex. This processed sensory information is considered necessary for the premotor cortex to accomplish its function. Indeed, lesions of the posterior parietal cortex or in MIII lead to **apraxia**. Apraxia is inability to carry out purposeful skilled movements, although the muscles are not paralysed. MIII also contributes fibres to the pyramidal system.

Within the premotor area are located some of the most important specialized motor centres.

Figure 16.56 shows an area that lies immediately above the Sylvian fissure in front of the primary motor area, representing the tongue, lips and larynx. This is known as *Broca's* area or the 'word formation centre', and its stimulation leads to vocalization. Damage in Broca's area, however, does not prevent a person from vocalizing, but it does

that part rather than to its size. Thus, the areas representing muscles of speech (i.e. lips, tongue and vocal cords) and those representing muscles that control hand movement are large. Cortical representation of trunk muscles is noticeably small (Fig. 16.57).

Recently, it has been shown that the neurons in MI are organized so as to represent movements carried by groups of muscles and not by individual muscle contractions. An efferent fibre from MI diverges to contact motor neurons of multiple muscles, and may even contact their far-away synergists. As a result, action potentials along the efferent fibre will spread to cause contraction of all *agonist* muscles and produce a movement. Furthermore, the signals may inhibit the *antagonist* muscles by *reciprocal inhibition*.

The cells in MI are arranged in vertical columns which operate as functional units, each usually stimulating a group of synergistic muscles into action. Each vertical

Fig. 16.56 Representation of the different muscles of the body in the motor cortex and location of other cortical areas responsible for certain types of motor movements.

make his/her vocabulary limited to very few words, a condition known as motor (non-fluent) aphasia.

The voluntary eye movement field is another area that lies immediately above Broca's area and is connected to the occipital visual centres. It controls conjugate eye movements. Damage to this area prevents voluntary movement of the eyes towards different objects.

Above the voluntary eye movement area lies the head rotation area. It controls head rotation. The area has connections with the eye movement area so as to direct the head towards different objects.

The area for hand skills is an important region in the premotor area which lies immediately anterior to the primary motor area for the hands and fingers. A lesion destroying this area leads to *motor apraxia*.

4 The parietal lobe
The relationship between the posterior parietal lobe and the premotor area has already been described. In addition, this part of the cortex contributes about 40% of the fibres that run in the pyramidal tracts.

Connections of the motor cortex

Afferent fibres
The commands to the motor cortex to bring about con-

traction of the exact muscles and cause movements are based on receiving integrated sensory information from the somatic sensory, visual and auditory areas. As the sensory signals arrive, the motor cortex, in association with the basal ganglia and cerebellum, executes its functions. The following are the main inputs:

1 Fibres from nearby cortical areas, i.e. somatosensory areas of the parietal cortex, the prefrontal areas, the visual and auditory areas. Somatosensory information is also delivered by fibres which pass directly from the ventrobasal complex of the thalamus.

2 Fibres from the corresponding motor areas of the cerebral cortex of the other hemisphere.

3 Fibres from the ventrolateral and ventroanterior nuclei of the thalamus. These nuclei receive signals from the cerebellum and basal ganglia.

Also the motor cortex receives diffuse input from the intralaminar nuclei of the thalamus, which control the general level of excitability of the cortex.

Efferent fibres
The primary output of the motor cortex goes to the spinal cord via the corticospinal projection, which passes through the pyramidal tract. Strictly, the pyramidal tract should include solely the fibres which arise from the motor cortex and pass through the medullary pyramids to synapse with

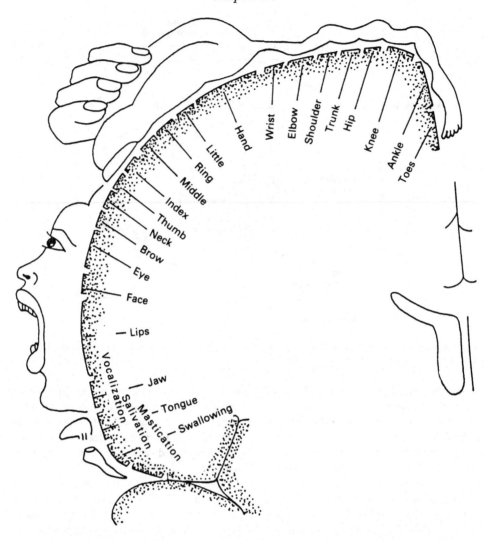

Fig. 16.57 Degree of representation of the different muscles of the body in the motor cortex.

the motor neurons of the brain stem and spinal cord (i.e. *corticobulbar* and *lateral corticospinal tracts*). These fibres are primarily concerned with the control of fine skilled movements. However, the term has been extended to include other fibres of cortical origin which do not pass across the pyramids (i.e. the *anterior corticospinal tracts*) and which are concerned with control of postural movements.

The motor cortex projects to other brain areas (the *basal ganglia*, the *cerebellum* and the *brain stem*), either directly or via collaterals from the corticospinal pathways. Many interactions occur between these areas but the output to the spinal cord is only from the motor cortex or the brain stem (i.e. *reticular formation, vestibular nuclei, red nucleus*). This output passes via the extrapyramidal tracts. It is of interest that, while the fibres of these tracts are rapidly conducting, the pyramidal fibres are comparatively slow-conducting. In fact, at least half of the pyramidal tract fibres are *non-myelinated* and are therefore slow conductors. Thus impulses along the *extrapyramidal projection* that regulate the appropriate postural background reach the cord and consequently muscles much faster than impulses passing along the *pyramidal tracts* to perform fine skilled movements.

The pyramidal and extrapyramidal systems
The motor areas of the cerebral cortex project down to the spinal cord via the pyramidal and extrapyramidal tracts.

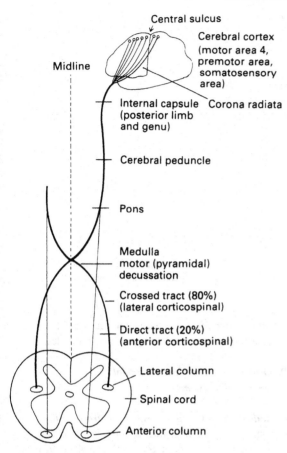

Central sulcus

Cerebral cortex
(motor area 4,
premotor area,
somatosensory
area)

Midline

Internal capsule   Corona radiata
(posterior limb
and genu)

Cerebral peduncle

Pons

Medulla
motor (pyramidal)
decussation

Crossed tract (80%)
(lateral corticospinal)

Direct tract (20%)
(anterior corticospinal)

Lateral column

Spinal cord

Anterior column

Fig. 16.58 The pyramidal (corticospinal) tract to the whole body below the head.

The pyramidal (corticospinal) tract. This consists of approximately one million fibres. Of these, 30% originate from the primary motor area, 30% from the premotor areas and 40% from the somatic sensory areas posterior to the central sulcus. About 3% of the fibres are large myelinated fibres, derived from the large pyramidal Betz cells of the motor cortex. These form monosynaptic connections with the motor neurons of the spinal cord. The rest are fibres from the small pyramidal cells found in many areas of the cerebral cortex.

The fibres from the cortex descend in the *corona radiata* to reach the internal capsule (Fig. 16.58). There they occupy the genu and the anterior two-thirds of the posterior limb and then the fibres descend through the cerebral peduncle of the midbrain and pons. In the medulla 80% of the fibres cross to the opposite side, forming the pyramidal or motor decussation, and descend as the *crossed* or *lateral corticospinal* tracts. Although some of these fibres end monosynaptically on anterior motor neurons (and on

sensory neurons of the dorsal horn), the majority end on interneurons in the intermediate region of the cord grey matter. Whether the connection is direct or via interneurons, the fibres of the lateral corticospinal tract supply the lateral neurons of the anterior horn, which control the fine skilled movements of the distal limb muscles.

The remaining 20% of fibres descend to the spinal cord on the same side, as the direct or anterior corticospinal tract. Some of these fibres cross to the opposite side at the segments, where they synapse with the anterior horn cells, but the rest pass ipsilaterally. The fibres of the anterior corticospinal tract end mainly on interneurons which synapse with motor neurons in the medial part of the anterior horn. These control the axial and proximal muscles of the limbs responsible for posture. Ipsilateral fibres make possible the bilateral innervation of some muscles on both sides of the body which move together (e.g. muscles of the upper face, respiratory and abdominal muscles).

As the corticospinal tracts descend through the brain stem, they give rise to fibres which cross to the opposite side and synapse with cranial motor nuclei supplying the skeletal muscles of the head. These fibres constitute the **corticobulbar tracts** (Fig. 16.59).

Function of the pyramidal system. The lateral corticospinal and corticobulbar tracts are primarily concerned with the execution of complex, fine, skilled, voluntary movements, especially of the fingers, toes and face. They are facilitatory to muscle tone and deep reflexes. This is evidenced by the fact that sectioning of the pyramids (which contain only pyramidal fibres) in monkeys results in hypotonia. Some corticospinal fibres pass directly to the sensory relay nuclei of the dorsal horn. These are probably corticofugal feedback pathways that modulate the intensities of incoming sensory signals.

The extrapyramidal tracts. The extrapyramidal system is made up of all those parts in the central nervous system that are concerned with motor control, other than the pyramidal system and cerebellum. These consist of:
1 Cortical motor areas, especially the premotor area and the parietal cortex.
2 The basal ganglia.
3 The reticular formation, the red nuclei, the tectum of the brain and the vestibular nuclei.

Axons from the cortical areas descend in the corona radiata and internal capsule, intermingled with the pyramidal fibres. In the basal ganglia, these fibres synapse with neurons of the caudata, putamen and globus pallidus. The globus pallidus, being the efferent centre of the basal ganglia, sends impulses to the thalamus, red nucleus,

Cerebral cortex
(Primary and
premotor areas)

Internal
capsule
(genu)

Brain stem

Cranial
nerves
(motor
nuclei)

5
7
9
10
11
12

Corticobulbar
tract

Midline

Fig. 16.59 The corticobulbar
(pyramidal) tract to the head.

substantia nigra, reticular formation, vestibular nucleus and inferior olivary nucleus. The fibres then descend to the spinal cord, to supply the anterior horn cells in the following extrapyramidal tracts:

1 Rubrospinal tract.
2 Reticulospinal tract.
3 Tectospinal tract.
4 Vestibulospinal tract.
5 Olivospinal tract.

Although the *rubrospinal tract* is categorized as extrapyramidal, it is functionally more associated with the corticospinal system in that it forms another pathway (*corticorubrospinal tract*) via which impulses can pass from the motor cortex to the muscles responsible for fine movements. Indeed, the rubrospinal tract lies in the lateral columns of the spinal cord close to the lateral corticospinal tract, and its fibres are distributed in a similar way.

Functions of the extrapyramidal system. This system is concerned with the planning, programming and initiation of movement (operating together with the motor cortex and cerebellum as one unit). It is also responsible for the subconscious gross movements occurring in groups of muscles, such as the associated movements which underlie voluntary actions, e.g. swinging of arms while walking. The extrapyramidal system also provides the necessary postural background for performance of skilled movements by the pyramidal system. Some tracts in this system are facilitatory while others are inhibitory to muscle tone; however, cortical extrapyramidal fibres have a strong

inhibitory effect over gamma motor neurons. Therefore, damage of these areas leads to hypertonia of muscles.

Disordered function of the pyramidal and extrapyramidal systems

Pyramidal lesion (upper motor neuron lesion). In humans, pure pyramidal tract lesions do not occur, but pyramidal fibres are most commonly involved in cerebrovascular accidents (strokes) due to haemorrhage, thrombosis or embolism, as they pass through the internal capsule. In such lesions, many extrapyramidal fibres are damaged too. Thus, clinicians talk of upper motor neuron (UMN) lesions and not of pyramidal lesions.

An upper motor neuron lesion is characterized by the following:

1 *Spastic paralysis or paresis.* There is loss, or more commonly weakness, of voluntary movement on the opposite side of the body (i.e. hemiplegia or hemiparesis) if the lesion is at or above the pyramidal decussation. The effects are widespread, due to damage involving a large number of fibres, and the lesion is characterized by poor recovery. The spasticity is due to the increased muscle tone.

2 *Hypertonia.* Although paralysed, the muscles are hypertonic. On examination, there is stiff resistance to passive movement and at one point the resistance suddenly gives way, just like closing a clasp-knife; thus it is called *clasp-knife spasticity.* Hypertonia is due to loss of the inhibitory effects of the cortical extrapyramidal centres on gamma

motor neurons in the presence of intact facilitatory centres of the brain stem. The latter are released and become over-active in stimulating the spinal motor neurons.

3 *Exaggerated tendon jerks.* These are seen on the affected side, e.g. by the knee- and ankle jerks, and are due to the release of the stretch reflex from cerebral inhibition.

4 *Clonus.* There is occurrence of rhythmic contractions of muscles when they are subjected to sudden sustained stretch, e.g. ankle clonus. This phenomenon is associated with increased gamma efferent discharge.

5 *Loss of superficial reflexes.* The abdominal and cre-masteric reflexes are lost on the paralysed side. This is due to loss of supraspinal facilitation. Examination of the plantar reflex shows a positive **Babinski's sign**. Normally scratching the outer aspect of the sole using a blunt object results in plantar flexion of all toes. When the pyra-midal fibres are damaged, this normal response disappears and is replaced by a primitive reflex, in which there is dorsiflexion of the big toe and fanning of the other four toes. This is described clinically as a positive Babinski's sign.

A positive Babinski's sign is physiological during the first year of life, due to immaturity (i.e. incomplete myelination) of the pyramidal tract. It can also occur in adults, sometimes during deep sleep, anaesthesia or coma, due to the depressed activity of the motor cortex.

6 *Absence of significant muscle-wasting.* This is because, although the muscles cannot be used voluntarily, they can still contract reflexly and the spasticity saves them from disuse atrophy.

Extrapyramidal lesions. Extrapyramidal disease is charac-terized by three features:

1 *Disturbance of voluntary movement.* There is difficulty in initiating voluntary movement (e.g. *akinesia* or *hypo-kinesia* of Parkinsonism). Associated movements are lost (poverty of movements).

2 *Alteration of tone.* Tone may be increased (as in Parkinsonism) or decreased (as in chorea). The hypertonia of extrapyramidal disease is called *rigidity*, to differentiate it from the clasp-knife spasticity of pyramidal disease, e.g. lead-pipe and cog-wheel rigidity of Parkinsonism.

3 *Involuntary movements.* These are four types: tremors, chorea, athetosis and ballismus.

Disordered function of the lower motor neurons

Lower motor neuron lesion (LMN lesion)
A lesion of the lower motor neurons or their axons is char-acterized by the following features:

1 *Flaccid paralysis.* Loss of voluntary movement occurs in the muscles supplied by the affected segments only (e.g. muscles of a limb only) on the same side of the lesion. The flaccidity is due to decreased muscle tone, and recovery is better than in upper motor neuron lesions.

2 *Hypotonia or atonia.* The paralysed muscles show de-crease or loss of tone. This is due to damage of the efferent part of the stretch reflex pathway.

3 *Absent deep reflexes.* This occurs in the muscles supplied by the axons of damaged motor neurons.

4 *Absent superficial reflexes.* Abdominal, cremasteric and plantar reflexes are lost if their reflex arcs are affected by the lesion.

5 *Marked muscle-wasting (atrophy).* The affected muscles show trophic changes due to disuse. These changes are due to the inability of the muscles to contract reflexly or volun-tarily. Intact motor innervation seems to be essential for the well-being of muscles. A denervated muscle shows marked wasting even if it is kept contracting by suitable electrical stimulation.

6 *Presence of fasciculations.* These are visible, spontane-ous contractions of bundles of fibres in the affected muscles (i.e. motor units), due to pathological discharge of spinal motor neurons. Fasciculation continues during the degen-erative process and stops once the nerves have atrophied. Persistent fasciculation in muscle indicates neuropathy.

7 *Changes in the electrical excitability of the affected muscles.* These include appearance of fibrillation potentials, e.g. fine, irregular contractions of individual muscle fibres, which occur due to hypersensitivity to acetylcholine. Other changes include an increase in chronaxie, i.e. the time required to elicit a response by a current twice the rheobasic strength. The rheobase is the minimum strength of current required to elicit a response.

Since the muscles of the upper part of the face (i.e. fore-head and eyes) are represented in both cerebral hemi-spheres, they are bilaterally innervated by the UMNs. On the other hand, the muscles of the lower part of the face (i.e. mouth) are only unilaterally innervated by UMNs. There-fore, in unilateral UMN lesions (supranuclear paralysis), the patient can wrinkle his/her forehead and shut his/her eyes, but cannot show his/her teeth on the affected side; thus it is the lower part of the face which is chiefly affected. In unilateral LMN lesions (infranuclear paralysis) of the 7th cranial nerve (facial nerve), both the upper and lower parts of the face are paralysed.

Internal capsule and spinal cord lesions
Having described the functions of the sensory system and the relevant part of the motor system, it is convenient

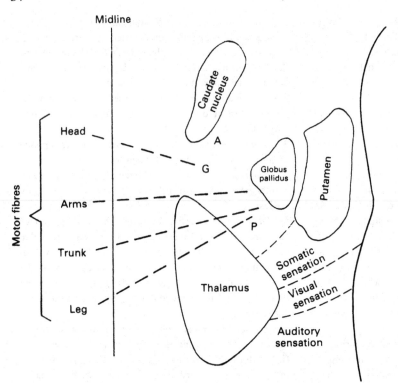

Fig. 16.60 The internal capsule. A, anterior limb; G, genu; P, posterior limb. (Redrawn from (1982) *Samson Wright's Applied Physiology*, 13th edn. With permission from Oxford University Press, Oxford.)

to introduce the reader to examples of disturbances of function that result from damage to the two systems simultaneously.

Effects of a unilateral lesion in the posterior limbs of the internal capsule

The internal capsule is a V-shaped area occupied by a mass of axons lying between the basal ganglia and the thalamus (Fig. 16.60). In transverse section, the angle of the V, called the genu, points medially. This angle is interposed between the anterior and posterior limbs of the internal capsule.

Pyramidal tract fibres occupy the genu and the anterior two-thirds of the posterior limb in an orderly fashion, i.e. the most anterior fibres are concerned with control of the head muscles, followed by those of the arm, trunk and leg muscles. Extrapyramidal fibres are intermingled with the pyramidal fibres. Immediately behind the pyramidal fibres lies the sensory radiation, followed by the optic radiation and, most posteriorly, the auditory radiation.

The posterior limb is a common site for lesions due to haemorrhage or thrombosis in the lenticulostriate artery. Such a lesion is usually unilateral and is characterized by widespread sensory and motor disturbances. These include:

1 Paralysis or paresis of the UMN lesion type on the opposite side of the body (*hemiplegia*). The hypertonia causes the limbs to acquire a specific posture; the upper limb is adducted to the side of the trunk and flexed at the elbow and the forearm is semipronated, with flexion of the wrist and fingers. The lower limb is also adducted but is extended at the knee and ankle.

2 Loss of sensation on the opposite side of the body (*hemianaesthesia*), due to damage of the thalamocortical fibres.

3 Loss of vision in two corresponding halves of the visual fields in both eyes (*homonymous hemianopia*), due to injury of the optic radiation. For example, injury to the left optic radiation causes blindness of the left halves of both retinae. As a result, the patient cannot see objects in the right halves of the visual fields of the two eyes (Fig. 16.61).

4 Hearing may be slightly diminished, but complete deafness does not occur, in spite of damage to the fibres of the auditory radiation. This is because the auditory centre in each cerebral hemisphere receives impulses from the cochleae of the two ears.

Spinal cord lesions

Spinal cord transection may result from fractures of the spine, primary tumours or metastasis from malignant

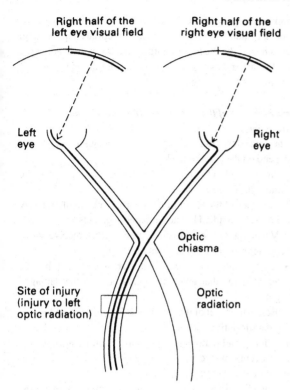

Right half of the
left eye visual field

Right half of the
right eye visual field

Left
eye

Right
eye

Optic
chiasma

Site of injury
(injury to left
optic radiation)

Optic
radiation

Fig. 16.61 Diagram showing site of lesion in the left optic radiation resulting in loss of vision in the right half of the visual field of both eyes (homonymous hemianopia).

tumours. The clinical manifestations are determined by the level and extent of the injury.

Complete transection of the spinal cord

Obviously, the higher the level of the section, the more serious are the consequences. If the transection is in the upper cervical region, immediate death follows, due to paralysis of all respiratory muscles; however, if it occurs in the lower cervical region below the 5th cervical segment, diaphragmatic respiration is still possible, but the patient suffers complete paralysis of all four limbs (i.e. *quadriplegia*). Transection lower down in the thoracic region allows normal respiration but the patient ends up with paralysis of both lower limbs (i.e. *paraplegia*).

When the cord is completely sectioned, the patient passes through definitive stages.

The stage of spinal shock. In the immediate period following transection, there is complete loss of spinal reflex activity below the level of transection. This is known as the *stage of spinal shock* and is thought to occur due to the

sudden withdrawal of facilitatory supraspinal influence (i.e. corticospinal, reticulospinal and vestibulospinal tracts). The stage of spinal shock is characterized by the following manifestations, all of which occur below the level of the lesion:

1 Loss of all sensation (complete anaesthesia) and voluntary movement (complete muscular paralysis), due to section of all sensory and motor tracts, respectively.

2 Loss of all reflexes (superficial, deep and visceral). Absent deep reflexes are manifested in the absence of tendon jerks and the loss of muscle tone, which results in flaccidity. The flaccid muscles lead to a decrease of the efficiency of the muscle pump in the affected part and so venous return is reduced, causing the part to become cold and blue and the body temperature to decrease.

Absent visceral reflexes include the micturition, defecation and erection reflexes. Clinically, the loss of bladder reflexes is the most important. The wall of the urinary bladder becomes paralysed and urine is retained until the pressure in the bladder overcomes the resistance offered by the tone of the sphincters and dribbling occurs. This is known to clinicians as 'retention with overflow'.

3 Loss of vasomotor tone occurs, due to interruption of fibres that connect the vasomotor centres in the medulla oblongata with the lateral horn cells of the spinal cord, which project sympathetic vasoconstrictor impulses to blood-vessels. The resulting relative vasodilatation causes a fall in blood pressure; the higher the level of the section, the lower the blood pressure.

4 Bedsores are seen where the body-weight against the underlying support (i.e. bed) exerts enough pressure on the skin to hinder the circulation. The patient lies in one position for long periods because of the paralysis; moreover, the skin is anaesthetic and the patient lacks the normal protective pain sensation. Bedsores occur particularly over bony prominences, i.e. back, heel and gluteal region. As a result, the skin sloughs off at these points, forming ulcers that heal with difficulty, known as decubitus ulcers.

This stage varies in duration but usually lasts a maximum of 2–6 weeks, after which some reflex activity is recovered.

The stage of recovery of reflex activity. As the stage of spinal shock wanes, reflex spinal activity appears again. The partial recovery may be due to an increase in the natural degree of excitability of the spinal cord neurons below the level of the section, presumably to make up for the loss of supraspinal facilitatory influences. It may also be due to sprouting of fibres from remaining inputs.

Recovery is gradual and includes the following manifestations:

1 Gradual rise of arterial blood pressure towards normal, due to return of activity in the lateral horn cells of the spinal cord (the spinal vasomotor centre). As a result, excitatory impulses are sent to the muscle walls of arterioles and venules. But, since vasomotor control from the medulla is absent, the blood pressure is very labile. The patient develops a sudden fall in blood pressure when made to sit up or stand, because blood pools in the legs and venous return is reduced. This reduction in blood pressure is called orthostatic hypotension, and the patient may faint.

2 Spinal reflexes also return. Flexor reflexes return earlier than extensor ones. A positive Babiniski sign is one of the earliest that appears and, although often described as an 'extensor plantar response', it is actually a physiological flexion. Deep reflexes also recover earlier in flexors. As a result, flexor tone causes the lower limbs to take a position of slight flexion, a state referred to as *paraplegia in flexion*. The return of deep reflexes (i.e. muscle tone) and vasoconstrictor tone in arterioles and venules improves the circulation through the limbs.

3 Visceral reflexes also recover, as evidenced by return of the micturition, defecation and erection reflex. For example, distension of the urinary bladder or rectum causes impulses to travel to the spinal centres, leading to reflex contraction of the bladder or rectal wall and relaxation of the internal sphincters. Consequently, complete emptying usually occurs, but voluntary control over micturition and defecation and the sensation of bladder and rectal fullness are permanently lost.

4 Sexual reflexes, consisting of erection or even ejaculation on genital manipulation, recover.

5 Mass reflex, a state that reflects the heightened excitability of the spinal cord neurons, appears in this stage. A minor painful stimulus to the skin of the lower limbs will not only cause withdrawal of that limb but will evoke many other reflexes through spread of excitation (by irradiation) to many autonomic centres. So the bladder and rectum will also empty, the skin will sweat, the blood pressure will rise, etc.

Since effective regeneration never occurs in the human central nervous system, patients with complete transection never recover fully. Voluntary movements and sensations are permanently lost; however, patients who are rehabilitated and properly managed may enter into a more advanced stage of recovery.

The stage of paraplegia in extension. During this stage the tone in extensor muscles returns gradually to exceed that in the flexors. The lower limbs become extended. Extensor reflexes become exaggerated, as shown by brisk tendon jerks and by the appearance of clonus. The positive

supportive reaction becomes well developed and the patient can stand on his/her feet with appropriate support (e.g. crutches). The flexor withdrawal reflex which appeared in the earlier stage is associated during this stage with the crossed extensor reflex.

Hemisection of the spinal cord (Brown-Séquard syndrome)

The manifestations of the Brown-Séquard syndrome depend on the level of the lesion.

At the level of the lesion, all manifestations occur on the same side. These consist of:

1 Paralysis of the lower motor neuron type, involving only the muscle supplied by the damaged segments.

2 Vasodilatation of the blood-vessels that receive vasoconstrictor fibres from the damaged segments.

3 Loss of all sensations in the areas supplied by the afferent fibres that enter the spinal cord in the damaged segments.

Below the level of the lesion (see Fig. 16.19), the following manifestations occur:

1 Widespread paralysis of the upper motor neuron lesion type occurs on the same side, due to the interruption of pyramidal and extrapyramidal tracts.

2 Vasodilatation also occurs, due to interruption of the pathway of fibres from the medullary vasomotor centres.

3 Sensory loss occurs, due to interruption of the ascending pathways. Crude touch, pain and temperature are lost on the opposite side of the lesion, due to damage of ventral and lateral spinothalamic tracts, respectively, while fine touch, position and vibration sense are lost on the same side, as a result of damage of the gracile and cuneate tracts.

III The cerebral hemispheres: secondary and association areas

Close to each primary area of the cerebral cortex is a **secondary area**. Each secondary sensory area is concerned with analysis and interpretation of information received from the nearby primary sensory area. On the motor side, the secondary motor area works in collaboration with the primary motor area to integrate patterns of movements. The secondary areas shown in Fig. 16.62 are:

1 The secondary somatosensory area.

2 The secondary visual area.

3 The secondary auditory area.

4 The secondary motor area (i.e. premotor and supplementary motor areas).

The **association areas** of the cerebral cortex exert a higher level of processing, analysis and integration of

Fig. 16.62 The secondary and association areas of the cerebral cortex including specific functional areas. B, Broca's area; W, Wernicker's area.

Labels: Primary motor area; Secondary motor area; Supplementary and pre-motor areas; Pre-frontal association area; Limbic association area; Primary auditory area; Secondary auditory area; Primary somatosensory area; Secondary somatosensory area; Parieto-occipito-temporal association area; Secondary visual area; Primary visual area

signals from sensory and motor areas of the cerebral cortex, as well as from subcortical structures. Moreover, each of these areas has its own functional specialities. The association areas of the cerebral cortex are:

1 The *parieto-occipitotemporal association area* is surrounded by the somatosensory, visual and auditory cortices. Information from these areas pools into this association area, which integrates all into a more meaningful, holistic interpretation. In addition, this area houses some of the important speech centres; thus lesions here give rise to many kinds of high-level sensory and motor disturbances. These can be divided into:

(a) **Agnosia**, which is inability to recognize an object, although perception in the particular modality (i.e. tactile, visual or auditory) is intact.

(b) **Apraxia**, which is the inability of a person to perform a skilled, learned purposeful movement when instructed to do so, despite normal muscle power, tone and coordination, full alertness and normal comprehension. The same movement may occur spontaneously.

(c) **Aphasia**, which is the inability of a person to communicate by using language symbols, despite normal articulation and normal visual and auditory perception.

2 The *prefrontal association area* is the anterior pole of the frontal lobe in front of the premotor cortex. Many roles are attributed to this area:

(a) Planning of complex patterns of movements (in association with the motor cortex).

(b) Personality characteristics and social relationships.

(c) Production of deep, more abstract and logically sequenced thoughts, which enable attainment of goals. The area has the capability of holding thoughts long enough to allow memory storage, and therefore facilitate learning.

(d) '**Working memory**': This area has the ability to tie thoughts together in a logical sequence by comparing many bits of new information with appropriate stored knowledge, and be able to instantly recall this information for future planning. This is called the working memory.

Lesions in the prefrontal association area are characterized by changes in personality and behaviour. The patient becomes restless and easily distracted, with labile moods, and yet his/her level of aggressiveness is decreased. There is lack of interest in people and things and inability to weigh consequences of actions beforehand. Social behaviour becomes inappropriate. The patient will use indecent language and may defecate or urinate in the presence of visitors without showing any emotion.

3 The *limbic association area* consists of the anterior and inner portions of the temporal lobe. It forms part of the limbic system; therefore it is primarily concerned with emotions, behaviour and the motivational drive for different tasks, most importantly learning. Lesions in this area may lead to decreased aggression, lack of emotions, hypersexuality (observed in animal experiments) and hyperphagia.

IV Motor functions of the basal ganglia and cerebellum

The power and precision of muscle activity are the product of normal function not only of the cerebral cortical areas, but also of two other essential brain structures, namely the basal ganglia and the cerebellum. These work in close association with the cerebral cortex and corticospinal tracts.

The basal ganglia

Anatomically the motor portions of the basal ganglia

are composed of the caudate nucleus and the putamen, collectively known as the *neostriatum*, and of the *globus pallidus*. The substantia nigra, the subthalamus, part of the thalamus and the reticular formation are functionally related to the basal ganglia.

Connections of the basal ganglia

Functionally important pathways connect the basal ganglia with each other and with other areas of the central nervous system. The main connections are:

1 Pathways from the cerebral cortex to the basal ganglia and back to the cortex. These consist of two circuits, one passing through the putamen and the other through the caudate nucleus.

(a) The putamen circuit (Fig. 16.63a). The putamen circuit originates mainly in the premotor and supplementary motor areas of the motor cortex and in the primary somatic sensory area. The fibres pass to the putamen, then to the internal part of the globus pallidus and next to the ventroanterior and ventrolateral nuclei of the thalamus, from where the fibres finally return to the cerebral cortex, mainly to the primary motor area. A few fibres go to some portions of the premotor and supplemental motor areas. Thus, the putamen receives input mainly from accessory motor areas, concerned with patterns of movement, and sends its output mainly to the primary motor cortex, responsible for the execution of these patterns. Figure 16.63a also shows three other pathways: one passing from the putamen to the globus pallidus, to the subthalamus and then to the motor cortex through the thalamus; another one passing from the putamen to the globus pallidus, next to the substantia nigra, then thalamus and finally to the motor cortex; and the third is a feedback circuit between the subthalamus and the external globus pallidus.

(b) The caudate circuit (Fig. 16.63b). A large proportion of the nerve fibres in this circuit arises from the cortical association areas. These areas are involved in integrating information, new and stored, from various sources into thoughts that can be used to attain goals. From these areas, the fibres pass to the caudate nucleus, next to the internal globus pallidus and then to the ventroanterior and ventrolateral nuclei of the thalamus. From the thalamus, the fibres pass to the prefrontal, premotor and supplementary areas of the cerebral cortex, which are areas concerned with patterns of movement. None of the fibres pass directly to the primary motor area of the cerebral cortex.

2 Pathways from the neostriatum to the substantia nigra and to the globus pallidus release **GABA** (Fig. 16.64); from the substantia nigra to the neostriatum and to the ventrolateral nucleus of the thalamus release **dopamine**; and from the raphe nuclei to the neostriatum release **serotonin**. The neurons in the neostriatum also receive **glutamate-** and **acetylcholine**-releasing fibres from the cerebral cortex. In the basal ganglia, **GABA**, **dopamine** and **serotonin** are inhibitory, whereas acetylcholine and glutamate are excitatory. It seems that the balance between the different transmitters is important for normal function of the basal ganglia. Lesions in one or more of the pathways described lead to a number of clinical syndromes.

3 The main efferent pathway from the basal ganglia is made up of axons from neurons in the internal part of the globus pallidus (Fig. 16.65). Fibres pass from there to the subthalamic nuclei and substantia nigra and then into the reticular formation, which sends impulses via the extrapyramidal tracts to the motor neurons of the spinal cord. Some fibres pass directly from the globus pallidus to the reticular formation.

Functions of the basal ganglia

The most important functions of the basal ganglia include the following:

1 They help the corticospinal system in executing slow sustained movements (i.e. ramp movements), such as writing letters of the alphabet, cutting with scissors, some aspects of vocalization, etc. This is thought to be executed by the *putamen circuit*. Damage to the basal ganglia causes gross abnormality of these patterns, even in the presence of a normally functioning cortical motor system.

2 The *caudate nucleus*, in association with the cortical association areas, plays an important role in the cognitive control of motor activity. Thoughts generated in the association areas are used by the caudate nucleus to help plan patterns of movements in the right sequence and appropriate to every situation that arises. For example, planning the immediate and fast motor response to an approaching danger is altogether different from the patterns of movements planned in response to a friendly stimulus.

The caudate circuit is also responsible for modifying the timing and spatial dimensions of the slow sustained movements executed by the putamen circuit (in collaboration with other areas of the motor system).

3 The basal ganglia are inhibitory to muscle tone throughout the body. This is brought about by sending impulses which activate the inhibitory reticular formation of the brain stem. Therefore, widespread damage of the basal ganglia produces rigidity.

4 The basal ganglia are also responsible for the initiation and regulation of the gross, subconscious, associated

(a)

(b)

Fig. 16.63 (a) The putamen circuit. Inputs to the putamen arise from the premotor, supplementary motor and somatosensory areas (none from the primary motor cortex). Returning signals pass to the primary motor cortex mainly and to portions of the premotor and supplementary motor cortex. EGP, external globus pallidus; IGP, internal globus pallidus; SN, substantia nigra; STh, subthalamus. (b) The caudate circuit. Input signals to the caudate arise from the cortical association areas. Returning signals pass directly to the prefrontal, premotor and supplemental motor areas of the cerebral cortex, with no fibres passing to the primary motor area.

movements of the body (e.g. swinging of the arms while walking, facial expressions).

5 The globus pallidus is responsible for the posture taken by the body to perform a particular voluntary movement (e.g. one assumes a certain posture of trunk and limbs to be able to write).

Clinical syndromes associated with damage to the basal ganglia

Chorea. This is a syndrome which occurs due to degeneration of the *caudate nucleus* mainly, but the putamen may be involved too. It is characterized by spontaneous,

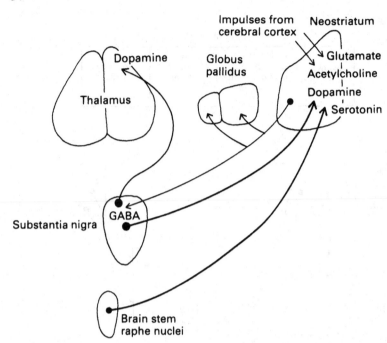

Fig. 16.64 Afferent and efferent pathways of the neostriatum showing several transmitter substances: acetylcholine in corticostriatal endings, GABA in the substantia nigra and globus pallidus, and dopamine and serotonin in the neostriatum.

uncontrolled, flicking movements, which occur one after the other at rest and are increased by muscular activity and emotions. As a result, the normal progression of voluntary movement is interrupted and replaced by distortional movements called dancing movements. These abnormal movements disappear during sleep and are associated with hypotonia and muscle weakness. Examination of the stretch reflexes reveals a *pendular* knee-jerk.

It has been proposed that choreic movements are due to absence of the inhibitory effect of GABA (released by the neostriatum) on the globus pallidus and substantia nigra. Consequently, the globus pallidus and substantia nigra become uninhibited and generate uncontrollable bursts of signals, which cause involuntary movements (see Fig. 16.64).

Athetosis. This occurs due to damage of the lateral portion of the *globus pallidus*. It is characterized by involuntary, slow, writhing movements of the hand, neck, face and tongue or some other part of the body, which occur continuously. The contracting muscles show a high degree of spasm and the movements are increased by emotions or by excessive signals from sensory organs. As a result, voluntary movements in the affected part become impaired or even impossible.

The mechanism behind the succession of abnormal movements is proposed to be due to the interruption of the

feedback circuit between the basal ganglia, thalamus and cerebral cortex which occurs with damage to the globus pallidus. This causes impulses to take unusual routes, leading to abnormal movements.

Ballism. This is a condition which occurs due to lesions in or near the *subthalamic nuclei*. It is characterized by continuous, gross, abrupt contractions of axial and proximal muscles of the extremities, resulting in flailing movements. In most cases, this disorder affects one side of the body (hemiballism). This may be associated with hypotonia and chorea. When the movement occurs in the legs, it is likely to cause the person to fall. In these patients, attempts at performing voluntary movements often cause ballistic movements instead.

Figure 16.63a shows a pathway from the subthalamus to the globus pallidus. The fibres in this pathway generate signals which regulate the output of the globus pallidus (via extrapyramidal pathways) to skeletal muscles. The result is integrated, smooth, progressive movements. Damage to the subthalamic nuclei disrupts this pathway and causes the flailing movements of *ballism*.

Parkinson's disease (paralysis agitans). This is a syndrome that occurs due to widespread degeneration of the *substantia nigra*, which secretes dopamine into the neostriatum and the thalamic nuclei. The causes of degeneration

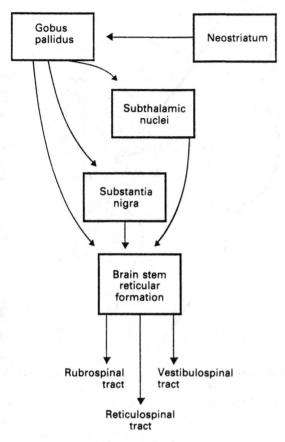

Fig. 16.65 Diagram showing the main efferent pathways from the basal ganglia to the brain stem reticular formation.

are not yet clearly identified, but cerebral atherosclerosis, prolonged treatment with phenothiazines, a tranquillizer that blocks dopamine receptors, and repeated trauma to the head are all implicated. Parkinsonism can also be produced rapidly in humans by 1-methyl-4-phenyl-1,2,5,6-tetrahydropyridine (MPTP) administration. This drug is degraded by monoamine oxidase B in glial cells to l-methyl-4-phenylpyridium (MPP), a strong oxidant which destroys dopaminergic neurons in the substantia nigra. This has led to the hypothesis that an MPTP-like substance probably present in the environment may cause Parkinsonism.

The syndrome is characterized by three principal features: (i) *rigidity* of muscles, either in a widespread area or in isolated areas; (ii) *tremor*; and (iii) *akinesia*. In fact, the name paralysis agitans derives from these manifestations. Paralysis refers to the *akinesia*, manifested as disinclination of the patient to move body parts although the muscles are not paralysed. Agitans, on the other hand, refers to

tremors, which coexist with the akinesia. Different patients show the various manifestations to different degrees, probably due to differences in the distribution of the lesion. Thus one patient may complain of uncontrollable tremor, while another may suffer disabling rigidity and shows no tremors. The mechanism behind the abnormal motor effects is not known, but it is definitely related to the loss of dopamine secretion. Rigidity is different from that seen in decerebration, i.e. spasticity, as here increased motor neuron discharge occurs to both agonist and antagonist muscles. However, flexors are more affected than extensors and proximal more than distal parts, which causes the body to be bent forwards. On examining the patient, passive movement (e.g. flexion of a limb) is met with a plastic, dead-feeling resistance (similar to bending a lead pipe). In patients who also suffer from tremors, this is sometimes interrupted by a series of catches, known as cog-wheel rigidity.

Basically, the flow of information in the basal ganglia is from the cerebral cortex to the neostriatum, thence to the globus pallidus and back to the cortex again via the thalamic nuclei. This feedback pathway is modified by inputs from many sources. One important source is the inhibitory *dopaminergic nigrostriatal pathway*. Parkinson's disease causes loss of this inhibitory input. As a result, the feedback pathway to the cortex becomes overactive and excessive impulses are sent via the corticospinal pathways to both alpha and gamma motor neurons supplying skeletal muscles, causing rigidity.

Tremors are involuntary regular contractions of muscle, which occur at rest (thus the name static tremors), but they may continue during voluntary movements, rendering them clumsy and uncoordinated. These tremors consist of flexion and extension or pronation and supination, usually affecting the distal joints. Pill-rolling movement describes the movement that occurs due to tremors of the thumb and index finger. The *nigrothalamic* pathway shown in Fig. 16.63a is dopaminergic (see also Fig. 16.64). It is thought that, with lack of the inhibitory effects of dopamine, the ventrolateral nucleus of the thalamus is released from inhibition and excessive impulses pass from there to activate the motor cortex (since the *thalamocortical projection* is excitatory). This produces oscillations, which cause the muscle tremors.

Akinesia is the most incapacitating of the motor abnormalities that patients experience. The patient finds the greatest difficulty in initiating voluntary movements, which come out slow and rigid. As a result, movements become scarce (*poverty of movement*) and the patient looks like a statue. Akinesia appears also in the slow monotonous speech, the shuffling gait and the scarcity of blinking. In addition, there is loss of *subconscious associated movements*, such as the natural swinging of the arms during walking, and the facial expression related to emotions and to the content of speech, etc. The combined lack of facial expressions and rigidity give rise to the characteristic '*mask face*'.

The specific disability in akinetic patients is the initiation of voluntary movement, but this can be readily overcome if provoked by a strong enough external stimulus. For example, a patient may find it impossible to start to walk, but a touch on the leg (nowadays dogs are trained to do that) may be enough tactile stimulus to switch on the movement. Also a patient may shuffle heavily across the road, but runs quickly when a speeding car approaches. From the previous description, the problem here appears to be one of self-motivation. Indeed, along with the dopamine deficiency in the basal ganglia of patients with Parkinsonism, the transmitter secretion was also found decreased in some areas of the limbic system. The limbic system is the centre for motivational drives and dopamine is one of the transmitters connected with self-stimulation; its deficiency should therefore explain the lack of psychic drive to move.

On the whole, the basal ganglia are stimulated by acetylcholine and inhibited by dopamine, and balance between them is necessary for normal muscle tone. Thus, treatment of Parkinsonism consists of promoting dopamine activity by levo-dopa (L-Dopa), and reducing acetylcholine activity by anticholinergic drugs. L-Dopa is administered instead because, unlike dopamine, it crosses the blood–brain barrier and is converted by the brain tissue into dopamine. Unfortunately, this is only effective in relieving the rigidity, whereas the effects on tremors are minimal. Stereotaxic destruction of the ventrolateral nucleus of the thalamus was found particularly effective in the attenuation of tremors. Some cases respond to *deprenyl*, a monoamine oxidase inhibitor. This strengthens the view that Parkinson's disease is probably caused by an MPTP-like substance. Transplantation of adrenal medullary tissue or implants of fetal basal ganglia tissue have also been tried as alternative sources of dopamine.

The cerebellum

The cerebellum lies below the occipital lobes of the cerebral hemispheres. It is connected to the brain stem by three cerebellar *peduncles: superior, middle* and *inferior* (Fig. 16.66). Various fibres enter and leave the cerebellum via these peduncles. The cerebellum consists of two **cerebellar hemispheres** connected by the midline **vermis**. Both the vermis and hemispheres show extensive

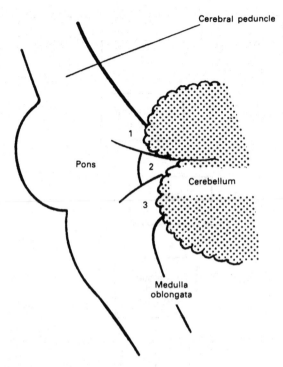

Fig. 16.66 Diagram of the brain stem to show the relationship to the pons and to the superior (1), middle (2) and inferior (3) cerebellar peduncles.

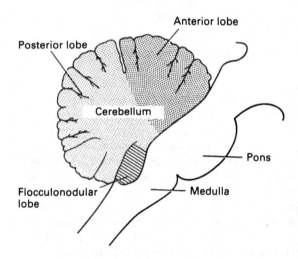

Fig. 16.67 Side-view of cerebellar lobes. (Reproduced with permission from Guyton, A.C. (1987) *Textbook of Medical Physiology*, 7th edn. Saunders, Philadelphia.)

folding and fissuring. Two deep transverse fissures divide the cerebellum into three major parts (Figs 16.67, 16.68): the *flocculonodular lobe*, the *anterior lobe* and the *posterior lobe*.

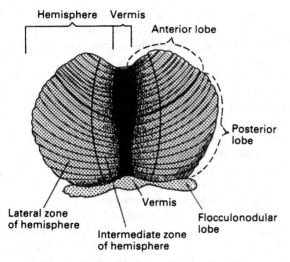

Fig. 16.68 Posteroinferior view of the cerebellum. (Reproduced with permission from Guyton, A.C. (1987) *Textbook of Medical Physiology*, 7th edn. Saunders, Philadelphia.)

Functional divisions of the cerebellum

From the functional point of view, the cerebellum can be organized along the longitudinal axis of the anterior and posterior lobes to give three parts (Fig. 16.68):

1 *The vestibulocerebellum.* This consists of the flocculonodular lobe. Functionally this part is more related to the vestibular system and therefore it is mainly concerned with coordination of various **postural mechanisms** and the maintenance of equilibrium.

2 *The spinocerebellum.* This consists of the vermis and the adjacent medial portions of the anterior and posterior lobes on both sides of the vermis. The spinocerebellum receives vast proprioceptive information from the spinal cord. This information is used in the co-ordination of rapid muscular activities.

3 *The corticocerebellum (pontocerebellum).* This includes the lateral parts of the cerebellar hemispheres (i.e. the lateral zones). The name is derived from the fact that most of the input to this region is from the cerebral cortex. It is also sometimes referred to as the *pontocerebellum* because input fibres from the cerebral cortex go through the pontine nuclei before reaching the cerebellum. The corticocerebellum is one of the higher centres concerned with the planning and programming of movements.

Structure and connections of the cerebellum

Each cerebellar hemisphere is composed of a superficial layer of grey matter, the **cortex**, covering a deeper mass of white matter. **Deep cerebellar nuclei** are embedded in the white matter. These are the *fastigial*, the *interpositus* and the *dentate*. Specific parts of the cerebellar cortex project to specific nuclei: the vermis projects to the fastigial nucleus, the more lateral parts of the spinocerebellum (i.e. the intermediate zones) project to the interpositus and the corticocerebellum (i.e. the lateral zones) projects to the dentate. The vestibulocerebellum is different, however, in that it projects directly to the brain stem.

All afferent fibres to the cerebellum end in the cerebellar cortex. The information they carry flows from the cerebellar cortex to the deep nuclei. These nuclei project in a systematic fashion: the fastigial mainly to the *vestibular nuclei*, the interpositus to the *red nucleus* and the dentate to the *ventrolateral nuclei of the thalamus* and then to the cerebral cortex.

The **cerebellar cortex** shows three distinctive layers of grey matter (Fig. 16.69):

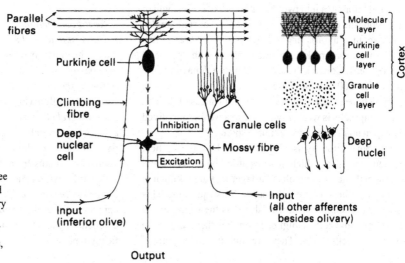

Fig. 16.69 Neuronal connections of the cerebellum. On the right are the three main layers of the cerebellar cortex and on the left the deep nuclei and excitatory inputs. (Reproduced with permission from Guyton, A.C. (1987) *Textbook of Medical Physiology*, 7th edn. Saunders, Philadelphia.)

1 A superficial **molecular** layer containing mainly large numbers of nerve fibres.

2 A middle Purkinje cell layer.

3 A deep granular layer. This layer contains small neurons, 'the granule cells', which appear as granules.

In the cerebellar cortex, afferent fibres synapse directly or indirectly with the large **Purkinje cells**. Purkinje cells have extensive *dendritic* ramifications, which extend into the superficial molecular layer. Their *axons* constitute the only output from the cerebellar cortex, and they discharge continuously at rest at the rate of 50–100 spikes/s. They release GABA at the neurons of the deep cerebellar nuclei, thus inhibiting them. However, the activity of the Purkinje cells is continuously modified by other cerebellar *cortical cells* and *afferent* inputs. Other cortical cells include the *granule* cells, the *basket* cells, the *stellate* cells and the *Golgi* cells. These are all considered as interneurons, as their axons end within the cerebellar cortex.

There are two types of afferent nerve fibres to the cerebellar cortex (i.e. to the Purkinje cells): the **climbing** and **mossy fibres**. Both types are excitatory.

1 *Climbing fibres* originate from the **inferior olive** of the medulla, which receives proprioceptive information from all over the body. After giving collaterals to the deep nuclear cells, each climbing fibre ascends to make up to 10 000 synapses on the dendrites of a Purkinje cell. These synapses release *glutamate*, are strongly excitatory and give rise to a prolonged response, called the '*complex spike*'.

2 *Mossy fibres* enter the cerebellum from a very wide range of sources including the **higher brain**, **brain stem** and **spinal cord**. These fibres also give collaterals to excite the cells of the deep cerebellar nuclei before they enter the cortex, where they synapse with a number of granule cells. Each granule cell axon ascends towards the molecular layer and bifurcates into two thin terminal branches, which run in opposite directions to each other (i.e. at right angles to the mother axon), making the *parallel fibres*. Each parallel fibre may make synaptic contacts with up to 500 Purkinje cells. Conversely, each Purkinje cell may synapse with up to 200 000 of these parallel fibres. Unlike the climbing fibres, the excitatory effect of the mossy fibres on the Purkinje cells is weak, giving rise to a weak, short-lived action potential, known as 'a simple spike'.

The above circuitry is also influenced by the cortical interneurons, all of which are inhibitory. The **basket** and **stellate cells** lie in the molecular layer and are stimulated by parallel fibres to inhibit nearby Purkinje cells. This causes lateral inhibition and so sharpens the signal of the excited Purkinje cells. **Golgi cells**, on the other hand, lie in the granule cells layer. They are stimulated by parallel

fibres and by mossy fibres collaterals to inhibit the granule cells in a negative feedback fashion. This serves to limit the duration of excitation of the cerebellar cortex by the granule cell.

The *efferent output of the cerebellum* consists of the axons of the deep cerebellar nuclei. Like the Purkinje cells, the cells of the deep cerebellar nuclei discharge continuously at rest, but at a higher rate. The cells are directly *stimulated* by climbing and mossy fibres, but are *inhibited* by impulses from the Purkinje cells (see Fig. 16.69). The balance is in favour of excitation, since the output of the deep nuclear cells is always excitatory. The level of this excitation is not fixed but changes appreciably during the execution of movement. It is proposed that the cerebellar circuitry functions mainly by modulating the output of the deep cerebellar nuclei to extracerebellar motor areas. It is via this output that movements initiated elsewhere in the motor system are co-ordinated and brought to precision. This is a gradual process which requires repeating the movement over and over again until perfection is approached; apparently the cerebellar circuitry learns from previous mistakes in motor tasks.

Topographic representation of the body in the cerebellar cortex

There are two separate representations. In the anterior lobe the body is represented upside down, while it is erect in the posterior lobe. The axial portions of the body lie in the vermis (Fig. 16.70), whereas the limbs and facial region lie in the lateral spinocerebellum (i.e. intermediate zone). As the corticocerebellum (i.e. lateral zones) is concerned with the planning and programming of sequential patterns of muscular activity, there is no topographic representation of the body in it.

Afferent connections

1 *Corticopontocerebellar pathway*. This pathway originates in the motor, premotor and somatosensory cortices and then passes via the pontine nuclei and pontocerebellar tract (through the middle cerebellar peduncle) to the opposite corticocerebellum (Fig. 16.71a).

2 *Olivocerebellar tract*. It originates in the inferior olive and passes through the inferior cerebellar peduncle to all parts of the cerebellum. The inferior olive acts as a relay nucleus for inputs from the cerebral cortex, basal ganglia, reticular formation and spinal cord.

3 *Vestibulocerebellar fibres*. These arise in the vestibular apparatus or vestibular nuclei and pass through the inferior cerebellar peduncle to end in the flocculonodular lobe and fastigial nucleus.

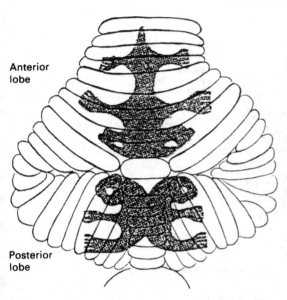

Anterior
lobe

Posterior
lobe

Fig. 16.70 Sensory projection areas of the cerebellar cortex. (Reproduced with permission from Snider, R.S. (1958) *The Cerebellum.* © 1958 by Scientific American, Inc. All rights reserved.)

4 *Reticulocerebellar fibres.* These arise in the reticular formation of the brain stem and pass via the inferior cerebellar peduncle to terminate mainly in the vermis.
5 *Dorsal and ventral spinocerebellar tracts.* The fibres constituting the spinocerebellar tracts are rapidly conducting. The dorsal spinocerebellar tracts transmit signals coming from body proprioceptors, such as muscle spindles, Golgi tendon organs and large tactile receptors of the skin and joints, to the spinocerebellum of the same side through the *inferior cerebellar peduncle* (Fig. 16.72). These signals inform the cerebellum about motor performance in the periphery.

The ventral spinocerebellar tracts also pass ipsilaterally and then through the *superior cerebellar peduncles* to terminate on both sides of the spinocerebellum. These tracts are mainly excited by motor signals arriving at the anterior horn cells of the spinal cord along the corticospinal and rubrospinal tracts. Thus the ventral pathways deliver to the cerebellum a 'copy' of the motor drive to the final common path (i.e. anterior horn cells). Some proprioceptive signals are also transmitted through the dorsal columns of the spinal cord to the *cuneate nuclei* of the medulla and then relayed through to the cerebellum.

Efferent connections
Efferent signals are discharged from the deep cerebellar

nuclei (Fig. 16.71b) to various areas in the CNS along the following pathways:
1 *Three pathways originate in the spinocerebellum* (the intermediate zone) and pass through the *interpositus nucleus*: (i) to the ventroanterior and ventrolateral nuclei of the thalamus to reach the **cerebral cortex**; (ii) to the midline structures of the thalamus and ending in the **basal ganglia**; and (iii) to the red nucleus and reticular formation of the brain stem.
2 *A pathway which originates in the vermis* and then passes through the *fastigial nucleus* into the **reticular formation** of the medulla and pons.
3 *A pathway that originates in the corticocerebellum* and then passes through to the *dentate nucleus* to the ventrolateral and ventroanterior nuclei of the **thalamus** to end in the **cerebral cortex**. Fibres also pass from the *dentate* nucleus to the **red nucleus** and then along the rubrospinal tract to the spinal cord.

Note that each cerebellar hemisphere is connected *ipsilaterally* to the spinal cord but is connected *contralaterally* with the cerebral hemisphere and basal ganglia. The efferent pathways from the cerebral hemisphere and basal ganglia of one side cross to supply the contralateral motor neurons of the brain stem and spinal cord. Because of this *double crossing*, each cerebellar hemisphere controls movements of the ipsilateral muscles.

Table 16.12 gives a summary of the important afferent and efferent connections of the cerebellum. See also Figs 16.71 and 16.72.

Functions of the cerebellum
The cerebellum is vitally important for the correct execution of rapid movements, particularly the finer types of skilled movement. Damage to the cerebellum causes incoordination of movements, making them clumsy and useless. The cerebellum is concerned with equilibrium and has profuse connections with the vestibular system. It is also involved in the learning of motor skills, such as typing, playing the piano, gymnastics, etc. The lateral zone of the cerebellum (*corticocerebellum*), in association with the motor cortex and basal ganglia, is concerned with planning and programming movements.

Function of the cerebellum in voluntary movements. The motor areas of the cerebral cortex on one side are connected to the intermediate zone of the cerebellar hemisphere (**spinocerebellum**) of the opposite side by a closed feedback circuit (*cortico ponto-interpositus-thalamocortical pathway*) (Fig. 16.73).

When impulses are transmitted from the motor cortex via

(a)

Anterior lobe

Superior cerebellar
peduncle

Ventral
spinocerebellar
tract

Cerebropontile tract

Pontocerebellar
tract

Middle cerebellar
peduncle

Vestibulocerebellar tract

Olivocerebellar and
reticulocerebellar tract

Inferior cerebellar peduncle

Posterior
lobe

Flocculonodular
lobe

Ventral spinocerebellar tract

Dorsal spinocerebellar tract

(b)

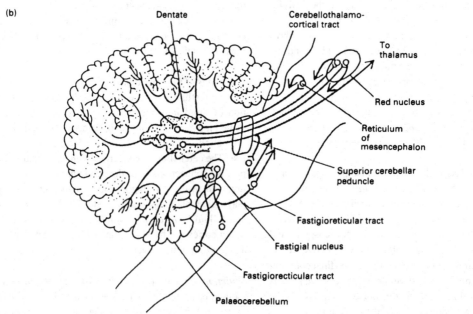

Dentate

Cerebellothalamo-
cortical tract

To
thalamus

Red nucleus

Reticulum
of
mesencephalon

Superior cerebellar
peduncle

Fastigioreticular tract

Fastigial nucleus

Fastigiorecticular tract

Palaeocerebellum

Fig. 16.71 (a) The main afferent tracts to the cerebellum. (b) The main efferent tracts from the cerebellum. (Reproduced with permission from Guyton, A.C. (1987) *Textbook of Medical Physiology*, 7th edn. Saunders, Philadelphia.)

Fig. 16.72 The spinocerebellar tracts.

Table 16.12 Afferent and efferent connections of the cerebellum.

Peduncle	Afferent	Efferent
Superior cerebellar peduncle	Ventral spinocerebellar tract	1 Dentatothalamocortical tract 2 Dentatorubrospinal tract
Middle cerebellar peduncle	Corticopontocerebellar tract	Fibres to reticular formation of pons
Inferior cerebellar peduncle	1 Dorsal spinocerebellar tract 2 Vestibulocerebellar tract 3 Olivocerebellar tract 4 Reticulocerebellar tract	Fibres to reticular formation of medulla

the pyramidal and extrapyramidal tracts to excite muscles, simultaneous impulses pass through the *pontocerebellar* and *olivocerebellar* fibres into the spinocerebellum to inform the cerebellum about the 'intended' motor plan. As the muscles contract, various proprioceptors are stimulated and transmit signals via the *dorsal spinocerebellar* tracts to the cerebellum. In addition, a copy of the motor signals arriving at the anterior horn cells of the spinal cord (from pyramidal and extrapyramidal tracts) is carried by the *ventral spinocerebellar* tracts to the cerebellum. When the muscles contract, signals arrive at the cerebellum via the *dorsal spinocerebellar tracts*.

Having information about the peripheral performance plus information about the intended motor plan, the cere-

bellum now compares the two sets of information. If the comparison is not favourable, the *interpositus nucleus* sends corrective signals via the *ventrolateral nuclei*, mainly back to the motor cortex where the stimulus first originated. The outcome is smooth coordinated movements. Co-ordination is known to improve with training. This learning function of the cerebellum is based on the circuitry of the *inferior olivary complex*. Indeed, selective lesions of the olivary complex greatly diminish the ability to learn certain motor tasks.

Various mechanisms are proposed to explain how the cerebellum adjusts voluntary motor function:

1 *The braking effect of the cerebellum*. It has already been mentioned that the cerebellum acts as a '*comparator*', i.e. it

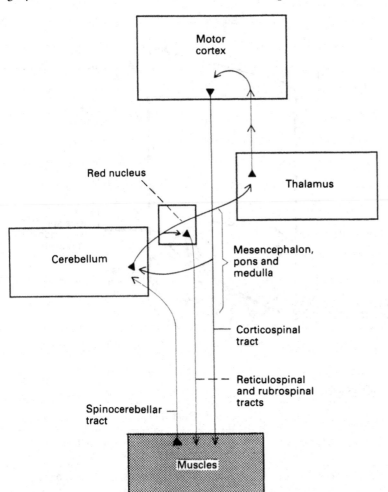

Fig. 16.73 Cerebellar control of voluntary muscular movement. (Reproduced with permission from Guyton, A.C. (1987) *Textbook of Medical Physiology*, 7th edn. Saunders, Philadelphia.)

compares the 'intentions' of higher motor areas and the actual performance. In everyday life, and especially during rapid movements, the motor cortex transmits far more impulses than needed to perform each movement. If the target is not to be surpassed, the cerebellum must act to inhibit the motor cortex appropriately after the muscles have begun to contract. By calculating the difference between the instant position of the limb and the target, the cerebellum will transmit signals related to errors arising to the motor cortex—to inhibit the agonist and excite the antagonist muscles towards the end of movement. Thus the cerebellum can apply '*braking*' impulses to slow down the movement of the limb and stop it at the intended target.

2 *The damping function of the cerebellum.* Voluntary movements performed develop momentum, which, if left unchecked, results in rapid progression and overshooting. The cerebellum dampens the momentum and checks unwanted acceleration. If the cerebellum is damaged, overshooting occurs. The cerebral cortex recognizes the error and sends corrective signals to bring the moving part (e.g. an arm) to the target. However, overshooting occurs again. Repeated overshootings and corrections result in oscillation of the movement before it settles on the target. This is the basis of the *kinetic* or *intention tremor* of cerebellar disease. The tremor becomes especially obvious towards the end of the voluntary movement, when the limb needs the finest control.

3 *The control of ballistic movements by the cerebellum.* Ballistic movements are very fast movements. Their duration is shorter than the time needed for proprioceptive feedback and subsequent modifications before the movement is already over. Examples of such movements are hitting the keys of a typewriter or a piano and the saccadic movements of eyes during reading, etc. These learned movements

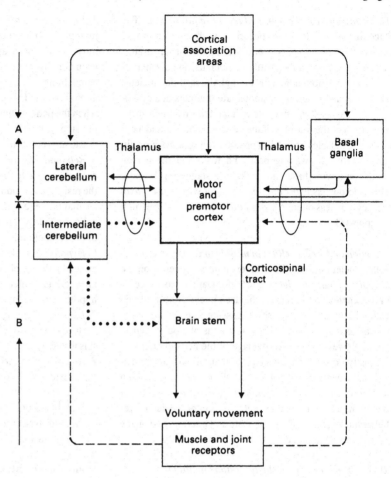

Fig. 16.74 Planning and execution of voluntary movement. A, represents parts concerned with planning voluntary movement; B, represents parts concerned with execution of voluntary movement. Solid lines indicate tracts concerned with motor information, the broken lines indicate sensory information and the dotted lines indicate tracts carrying corrective signals.

develop extra quickly with an extra force at the beginning of the movement but are turned off equally quickly and efficiently to prevent overshoot. At the beginning of movement, afferent impulses enter the cerebellum via the climbing and mossy fibres, where they first excite deep nuclear cells (Fig. 16.69). In response, these cells send strong excitatory signals out to the motor cortex *reinforcing* the onset of the ballistic movement. After a short delay, afferent impulses pass upwards to reach and stimulate the *Purkinje* cells. As a result, inhibitory signals pass back to the motor cortex to apply brakes to the ballistic movement and stop it appropriately. Obviously, the learning mechanisms of the cerebellum are utilized in the performance of such movements.

4 *The planning and timing function of the cerebellum.* Recent studies have shown that electrical activity related to a particular voluntary movement can be detected in the *dentate nuclei* well before the beginning of the movement and while the movement is being executed. The cortico-

cerebellum, in association with other areas, plans movements. Efferent signals encoding this plan are then sent from these areas to the motor areas of the cerebral cortex, where movement is initiated via corticospinal and other pathways (Fig. 16.74).

Another important function of the neocerebellum is its ability to provide appropriate *timing* of each movement. Lesions to this area lead to inability to judge the distance moved by a particular part in a given time. Thus the person is unable to control the beginning of the next movement. The result is failure of the smooth progression of repetitive movement.

Function of the cerebellum in involuntary (postural) movements. The **spinocerebellum** (vermis) coordinates involuntary postural movements initiated in various areas of the motor system (i.e. motor cortex, basal ganglia, brain stem), by acting as a comparator. Corrective signals are sent to the motor area where the motor impulses were first initiated.

The function of the cerebellum in equilibrium. The **flocculonodular lobe** is concerned with equilibrium. It receives profuse inputs from the vestibular apparatus, either directly or via the vestibular nucleus, and discharges back to the vestibular nucleus through the fastigial nucleus. These signals are used for immediate maintenance of balance. Lesions of the flocculonodular lobe result in incoordination of the muscles of the vertebral column and axial body, i.e. muscles utilized in postural reflexes. As a result, there is truncal swaying back and forth and the person stands on a wide base and walks in a staggering fashion. This is known as *trunk ataxia*. A patient with *trunk ataxia* can nevertheless operate his/her limbs normally if the trunk is supported.

Function of the cerebellum in muscle tone. The deep cerebellar nuclei normally have an excitatory influence on the *lateral vestibular nuclei* (Fig. 16.35). Damage to the **cerebellar cortex** would release the deep nuclei from Purkinje cell inhibition. This causes excessive excitation of the lateral vestibular nuclei. The outcome is obviously *hypertonia*. However, selective damage of the cerebellar cortex is mostly *experimental*, because in naturally occurring disease damage usually involves both the **cortex** and the **deep nuclei**. In these patients, *hypotonia* and *hyporeflexia* occur due to the absent normal excitatory effect of the deep cerebellar nuclei (especially the dentate and interpositus) on the lateral vestibular nuclei.

Defects produced by cerebellar lesions in humans (the neocerebellar syndrome)

This is due to damage of the deep cerebellar nuclei as well as the cerebellar cortex. The manifestations occur on the same side of the lesion, i.e. a lesion of the left cerebellar hemisphere produces its effects on the left side of the body, etc.

The manifestations include:

1 *Dysmetria and ataxia.* Dysmetria is the inability of the person to judge properly ahead of time the range of his/her movements. Therefore, the movements usually overshoot their intended mark, i.e. past pointing. Dysmetria results in incoordination of movements, which is called ataxia.

2 *Failure of progression of voluntary movements.* This results in:

   (a) *Dysdiadochokinesia*—the inability to perform rapid successive alternating movements, e.g. repeated supination and pronation of the forearm.

   (b) *Dysarthria*—defective speech. Articulation is jerky and explosive. Syllables of words are separated from one another (scanning speech).

3 *Kinetic or intention tremors.* These are coarse, rhythmic, involuntary movements, which occur during voluntary movements but disappear at rest and during sleep. They occur due to the absence of the damping function of the cerebellum.

4 *Nystagmus.* This is a tremor of the eyeball, which occurs when the patient attempts to fix his/her gaze on an object to the side of his/her head (horizontal nystagmus). It is also due to absence of the damping function.

5 *Rebound phenomenon.* This is elicited by asking the patient to flex his/her forearm against resistance. When the resistance is suddenly removed, the limb overshoots the normal range (e.g. the forearm will fly quickly to strike the patient's face). This is due to the loss of the braking effect of the cerebellum.

6 *Hypotonia.* This is due to the loss of the facilitatory effect of the cerebellum on the stretch reflex. When the knee jerk is elicited, it is reduced and pendular. Sometimes hypotonia is the first sign of cerebellar disease.

7 *Decomposition of movements.* This is the inability to perform successive components of a complex motor act. It is tested by the heel–knee test.

8 *Rough movements.* Delicate movements, such as threading a needle or buttoning of a shirt, become very difficult.

9 *Disturbance of posture and gait.* The head is tilted to the side of the lesion. The gait is unsteady and the patient walks with a wide base in a drunken fashion and tends to fall to the side of the lesion.

Control of voluntary movement

At this point in the discussion, it seems useful to try to describe the functional organization of the motor system and the control of voluntary movement. Commands for voluntary movement arise in the cortical association areas (see Fig. 16.74). According to the command, movements are then planned in various areas of the brain, including the motor and premotor cortex and also the basal ganglia and the lateral cerebellum (corticocerebellum). The basal ganglia and corticocerebellum deliver their information to the motor and premotor cortex via the thalamus. The plans are coded in terms of movements rather than individual muscle contractions. Impulses then pass via the corticospinal tract and other pathways to the spinal and cranial motor neurons, which activate motor nerves.

When muscle contraction occurs, it stimulates the receptors in muscles, tendons, joints and the skin, which send feedback information (via sensory tracts) directly to the motor cortex and to the intermediate portions of the cerebellum (spinocerebellum). The output from the latter goes both to the motor cortex, to adjust and smooth the move-

Table 16.13 Various levels of lesions which can result in disturbed motor function.

Level of lesion	Examples of disorders
Muscular level	Familial periodic paralysis
Neuromuscular junction	Myasthenia gravis
Lower motor neuron	Poliomyelitis
Cerebellum	Medulloblastoma
Extrapyramidal system	Parkinsonism
Pyramidal system (upper motor neuron)	Cerebrovascular accident in the internal capsule
Cerebral cortex	Apraxia (i.e. inability to carry out a movement although the patient understands its purpose and the muscles are not paralysed)

ment, and to motor neurons (via brain stem pathways), to adjust posture continuously during movement.

Table 16.13 shows examples of disorders of motor function, resulting from lesions at different levels of the motor system.

The thalamus

The thalamus is the gate for essentially all sensory signals on their way to the cerebral cortex, with the single exception of those from the olfactory system. It is thus the highest subcortical sensory centre.

The thalamus is made up of a number of nuclei, which can be functionally divided into:

1 Nuclei which project to the whole cerebral cortex (i.e. non-specific projection nuclei).

2 Nuclei which project to specific areas of the cerebral cortex and limbic system (i.e. specific projection nuclei).

Non-specific projection nuclei

The non-specific projection nuclei constitute the midline and intralaminar nuclei. They receive signals from the reticular activating system and project to all areas of the cerebral cortex.

Specific projection nuclei

These can be divided into:

1 *Nuclei relaying specific sensory information.* These include the **medial** and **lateral geniculate bodies**, which relay auditory and visual information to the auditory and visual cortices, respectively. They also include the **postero-ventral nuclei** (ventrobasal nuclei), which relay somatic sensations to the sensory area (postcentral gyrus) of the cerebral cortex.

2 *Nuclei relaying motor information.* These are the **lateral ventral nuclei** which relay impulses from the basal ganglia and cerebellum to the cerebral cortex.

3 *Nuclei concerned with recent memory and emotions.* These are the **anterior thalamic nuclei**. They are stimulated by signals from the mammillary bodies of the hypothalamus, and discharge to the cortical part of the limbic system.

4 *Nuclei concerned with higher integrative functions.* These are the **dorsolateral nuclei**, concerned with higher functions of the cerebral cortex, e.g. language. They project to the cortical association areas.

Functions of the thalamus

The thalamus is a relay station for all types of sensations—fine and crude somatic sensations, pain, temperature, visual and auditory sensations—on their way to their respective centres in the cerebral cortex. Besides relaying, the thalamus is a major centre in perceiving pain, and its intralaminar nuclei may be one of several important sites at which the analgesic system of the brain can inhibit pain transmission. As far as motor function is concerned, the thalamus also relays signals from the basal ganglia and cerebellum to the motor areas of the cerebral cortex. Moreover, it relays autonomic signals and others related to emotional reactions, due to its connections with the hypothalamus and limbic system, respectively. The thalamus may also play an important role in coding, storing and recalling memories.

The thalamic syndrome

The thalamic syndrome is a condition caused by thrombosis of the thalamostriate artery. As a result, there is damage to the **posterior thalamic nuclei**, leaving the medial and anterior groups of nuclei intact. In other words, some pathways through the thalamus are destroyed while others are left intact. The patient presents with loss of almost all sensations on the contralateral side of the body. There is ataxia due to the loss of fibres relaying position and *kinaesthetic* sensations (i.e. rate of movement sense). The pain threshold is raised but, when the threshold for perception is reached, even minor stimuli can produce a peculiarly unpleasant, severe and prolonged pain, which might become difficult to tolerate. This is an example of secondary hyperalgesia, which occurs due to facilitation of the **medial nuclei**, which relay impulses of the slow, chronic type of pain. As a result, impulses along the nerve fibre on the afferent pain pathway pass through more easily. The patient may also suffer from emotional disturbances. Partial recovery of sensations may occur after some time.

Fig. 16.75 Hypothalamic control centres and functions. GI, gastrointestinal. (Reproduced with permission from Guyton, A.C. (1987) *Textbook of Medical Physiology*, 7th edn. Saunders, Philadelphia.)

The hypothalamus

The hypothalamus is situated at the base of the brain, just rostral of the brain stem. It is an important centre for the integration of visceral reflexes, so as to maintain the constancy of the internal environment.

Control centres of the hypothalamus

Figure 16.75 shows division of the hypothalamus into various centres, each of which constitutes a number of nuclei or areas. The anterior centres include the supraoptic and paraventricular nuclei, the medial and posterior preoptic area and the anterior hypothalamic area. Medial centres include the dorsomedial and ventromedial nuclei. Lateral centres constitute the lateral hypothalamic area and the posterior centres include the posterior hypothalamus, the perifornical nucleus, the mammillary body and the arcuate and periventricular zone.

For the hypothalamic centres to be able to perform their function of homoeostasis, numerous to-and-fro connections between it and various areas of the brain must exist. The hypothalamus receives afferents from the preolfactory area, the limbic lobe, the amygdala, the hippocampus, the non-specific thalamic nuclei and the globus pallidus, and collaterals from the sensory ascending tracts. It sends efferents to the neurohypophysis, the anterior thalamic nuclei and the brain stem reticular formation.

Functions of the hypothalamus

Many visceral, behavioural and emotional reactions are reflexly regulated by the hypothalamus:

1 *Autonomic functions.* Almost all autonomic functions are modified by the hypothalamus. Previously, the hypothalamus was called 'the head ganglion of the autonomic nervous system'. Stimulation of the anterior hypothalamic centres produces parasympathetic effects, while stimulation of the posterior dorsomedial and lateral hypothalamic centres produces sympathetic effects.

2 *Temperature regulation.* Homothermic animals subjected to transection just below the hypothalamus become poikilothermic. The reflex responses activated by cold (e.g. cutaneous vasoconstriction, shivering) are controlled by the posterior hypothalamus. Heat-losing mechanisms (e.g. cutaneous vasodilatation, sweating) are controlled by the anterior hypothalamus.

3 *Body-water regulation.* Electrical stimulation of particular areas—the drinking centre—in the hypothalamus of an animal makes it drink, whereas its destruction abolishes the sensation of thirst. Injection of hypertonic saline into the hypothalamus causes polydipsia. The thirst centre is located in the supraoptic region of the hypothalamus.

4 *Food intake regulation.* Food intake is regulated by a balance between two centres. The *feeding centre* is located in the lateral hypothalamus and, when stimulated, leads to extreme hunger, a voracious appetite and an intense desire to search for food. Continuous stimulation leads eventually to obesity. However, damage to this area produces severe loss of appetite, known as *anorexia*. The other centre, called the *satiety centre*, is located in the ventromedial nucleus and, when stimulated, anorexia occurs. Damage to this area causes the hunger centre to become overactive, leading to hyperphagia and obesity, known as hypothalamic obesity.

5 *Control of sexual functions.* The hypothalamus, through its influence on the anterior pituitary, regulates sexual function. Oestrus, maternal behaviour and care of the young in lower animals are under direct hypothalamic control.

6 *Defence reactions.* As a component of the limbic system, the hypothalamus is part of the effector mechanism of emotional expression. It is involved in the expression of rage and fear.

7 *Wakefulness and sleep.* The hypothalamus is part of the reticular activating system, which is indispensable to the initiation and maintenance of the alert wakefulness of the healthy animal. Also, stimulation of the mediorostral suprachiasmal portion of the anterior hypothalamus is found to promote sleep, and lesions in the same area can sometimes cause such intense wakefulness that the animal actually dies of exhaustion.

8 *Relation of cyclic phenomena.* Lesions of the hypothalamus disrupt the circadian rhythm in the secretion of ACTH and melatonin. It therefore appears that the hypothalamus adjusts bodily rhythms to the 24-hour light–dark cycle.

9 *Behavioural functions.* The hypothalamus is part of the limbic system, which is concerned with the affective nature of sensations. Stimulation of certain regions of the hypothalamus pleases the animal, whereas stimulation of other parts causes terror, pain, fear and other types of aversion. However, the prefrontal lobe overrides the hypothalamus and limbic system in determining behaviour, including sexual, feeding and emotional reactions.

10 *Neuroendocrine functions.* The hypothalamus controls the posterior pituitary by a neural mechanism and the anterior pituitary by a humoral mechanism.

Antidiuretic hormone and oxytocin are produced in the supraoptic and paraventricular nuclei and transported to the posterior pituitary along the axons of the hypothalamohypophyseal tracts. The hypothalamus also produces

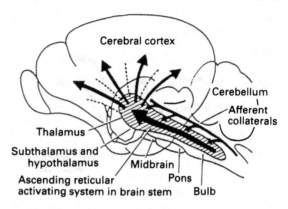

Fig. 16.76 Diagrammatic representation of ascending reticular system projected to the cerebral cortex in the cat brain. (Reproduced from Starzl, T.E., Taylor, C.W. & Magoun, H.M. (1951) Collateral afferent excitation of the reticular formation of the brain stem, *J. Neurophysiol.*, 14, 479, with permission from the American Physiological Society, Bethesda.)

at least nine chemicals, which are carried to the anterior pituitary by the hypothalamohypophyseal portal system. Most of these release anterior pituitary hormones, e.g. corticotrophin-releasing hormone (CRH) and growth hormone-releasing hormone (GHRH), while others inhibit the release of anterior pituitary hormones, e.g. prolactin inhibitory hormone (PIH) and somatostatin.

Arousal mechanisms, sleep, wakefulness and the electrical activity of the brain

The reticular activating system (RAS)

The RAS is a multisynaptic pathway located within the reticular formation of the brain stem (Fig. 16.76). It receives collaterals from the classical sensory pathways as they ascend to their respective relay nuclei in the thalamus, and sends ascending branches to all areas of the cerebral cortex. Some of these branches pass directly but most of them synapse in the non-specific nuclei of the thalamus (i.e. intralaminar and midline nuclei) before they pass to the cortex.

The RAS is activated to an equal degree by impulses from all the classical sensory pathways. This led to the use of the term 'non-specific or diffuse system' to distinguish it from the classical sensory pathways, which are specific in the sense that they are activated by only one sensory modality. While impulses arriving along sensory pathways determine activity in the RAS, the RAS determines the overall activity of the cerebral cortex.

Fig. 16.77 Stimulation (arrow) of median nerve giving evoked responses in contralateral sensory cortex. Upward wave is surface-negative. EP, evoked potential.

Fig. 16.78 Normal electroencephalogram. (Reproduced with permission from Guyton, A.C. (1987) *Textbook of Medical Physiology*, 7th edn. Saunders, Philadelphia.)

Evoked cortical responses

Electrical activity produced in the cortex in response to stimulation of a receptor can be monitored by electrodes placed on the surface of the cerebral cortex of an anaesthetized animal. Barbiturate anaesthesia is used to dampen the spontaneous electrical activity of the brain. The response consists of two positive waves, separated by a negative wave (Fig. 16.77). The first positive wave is called the *primary evoked potential (EP)*. It has a short latency of 5–12 ms and is only recorded from a specific localized area of the cortex (e.g. if the hand is stimulated, the wave is observed over the 'hand area' of the sensory cortex). The primary evoked potential is followed by a small negative wave due to hyperpolarization.

The second positive wave is called the *diffuse secondary response*. It is a large prolonged positive wave. It has a longer latent period of 20–80 ms. It is widespread over the cortex and other brain structures. This wave is probably evoked by stimulation of the non-specific thalamic nuclei. Its longer latency is due to the slower passage of impulses through multiple synapses in the RAS and also to the appearance of widespread reverberations in cortical pathways.

In clinical practice evoked responses can be recorded over the brain or the spinal cord while applying repeated stimuli (100–1000 times) to a specific receptor area. The recording is made possible by a computerized averaging technique, which summates the EPs and cancels interference. When somatosensory, auditory or visual stimuli are applied the evoked potentials are known as SSEP, AEP or VEP, respectively. This technique, especially VEP, has proved to be useful in the detection, localization and follow-up of lesions in the sensory pathways being investigated.

The electroencephalogram (EEG)

The EEG is a continuous record of the background activity of cortical neurons in unanaesthetized subjects or experimental animals. It can be recorded by applying electrodes on the scalp or by placing them directly on the surface of the brain. The electrical activity appears on a multichannel recorder as waves of variable intensity (0–200 μV) and frequency (1–50 Hz); the wave intensity and pattern depending on the degree of cerebral cortical activity.

Types of normal EEG waves

There are four types of normal EEG waves (Fig. 16.78):

1 *Alpha waves.* These are rhythmic waves occurring at a frequency of 8–13/s (8–13 Hz) with an amplitude of about 50–100 μV. They are most marked in the parieto-occipital region, but are sometimes observed in other locations. Alpha waves are recorded in all mentally and physically relaxed adults who are awake but with the eyes closed. Visual stimulation causes immediate replacement of the alpha waves by low-voltage, more frequent, beta waves.

2 *Beta waves.* These are observed in the frontal and parietal regions. They are of lower voltage than alpha waves but are faster, i.e. frequency of about 18–30 Hz. They occur during intense activation of the central nervous system or during tension.

3 *Theta waves.* These are large, 100 μV waves, having a frequency of 4–7 Hz. They occur in the parietal and temporal regions of normal children and in adults under emotional stress.

4 *Delta waves.* These are the slowest (1–3½ Hz, of high

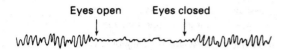

Fig. 16.79 Alpha rhythm replaced by asynchronous discharge on opening of the eyes. (Reproduced with permission from Guyton, A.C. (1987) *Textbook of Medical Physiology*, 7th edn. Saunders, Philadelphia.)

voltage). They occur in infancy and in deep sleep in both children and adults.

The **alpha rhythm** (or a similar rhythm) is observed in many mammalian species—a characteristic of the wakeful state at rest—although minor species variation may exist. Alpha waves are the result of spontaneous feedback activity in the RAS–thalamocortical system, whereas **delta waves** are due to activity within the cortical neurons independent of the reticular–thalamic discharge. Since the delta rhythm characterizes adult slow-wave sleep, it follows that during this type of sleep the cortex is released from the influence of the reticular–thalamic projection.

Theta and delta waves should not occur in an adult during the waking state. If they are recorded, they indicate an abnormality. Overbreathing or hyperventilation induces bilateral theta and delta waves.

Desynchronization or alpha block

The intensity (i.e. voltage) of brain waves is determined mainly by the number of neurons that discharge synchronously. Random non-synchronous firing of whatever number of neurons, however strongly they may discharge, will cancel each other and produce waves of weak voltage. Frequency of brain waves, on the other hand, is determined by the total level of cerebral activity. This can be clearly seen in Fig. 16.79. While the eyes are closed, synchronous discharge of many cerebral neurons produces the regular, relatively high-voltage, alpha waves (also called the *dominant rhythm*), but, when the eyes are opened these waves are immediately replaced by faster, low-voltage, irregular beta waves. The higher frequency is due to the increased brain activity (enhanced by visual stimuli), and the lower voltage is due to the break-up of the synchronous activity that produced the alpha waves. This is known as desynchronization, arousal or alerting response or 'alpha block'.

Alpha block can be produced by many forms of sensory stimuli besides visual (e.g. smell, auditory, etc.). The pathway of this response starts from the respective sensory pathway, then via collaterals to the RAS and from there to the intralaminar and non-specific thalamic projection system, which activates the cerebral cortex.

Factors affecting the activity of the RAS

The activity of the RAS is increased by impulses along collaterals from the specific sensory pathways. Proprioceptive and painful stimuli are particularly effective and can arouse a person from sleep. Descending impulses from the temporal lobe and certain areas of the frontal lobe of the cerebral cortex have a strong excitatory effect on RAS. Such impulses may be responsible for the alerting responses due to emotions and related psychic phenomena. Another important region in the cerebral cortex that activates the RAS is the motor cortex. This is probably the cause why voluntary movements help in keeping a person awake. Adrenaline and noradrenaline secreted from the adrenal medulla produce alerting responses. The effect is probably mediated by blood pressure, because increases in blood pressure increase the excitability of the reticular formation.

Activity in the RAS can be diminished (or inhibited) by many factors, which include:

1 Impulses from the sleep-producing centres.

2 Various lesions that damage cells of the brain stem, e.g. vascular lesions, poisons, brain tumours, prolonged hypoxia and infectious diseases. These disorders may lead to coma. Coma differs from sleep in that a person cannot be aroused by any stimulus. In some comatose patients, other areas in the brain are inactivated too. In such cases, the electrical activity of the brain stops and the brain waves are said to be 'flat'. This is known as brain death.

Clinical uses of the EEG

The EEG can be used clinically in:

1 *Localizing brain tumours*. If the tumour is large enough to block electrical activity from a given portion of the cerebral cortex, the voltage of the brain waves in the region of the tumour will be considerably reduced. On the other hand, the presence of a tumour can lead to very high-voltage waves in the EEG. The latter is more frequent and results from abnormal electrical excitation of the compressed areas surrounding the tumour.

2 *Diagnosis of different types of epilepsy*. Epilepsy is a condition characterized by uncontrolled excessive activity of either part or all of the nervous system. It can be divided into two major types:

(a) *Grand mal epilepsy*. In this type there is characteristically increased neuronal discharge from all areas of the brain and the lower reticular activating system. It is characterized by an aura, i.e. sensory hallucinations, followed by generalized tonic convulsions of the entire body, leading to clonic jerks. During the attack the person may bite his/her tongue, has difficulty breathing and

Grand mal epilepsy

Petit mal epilepsy

Fig. 16.80 Electroencephalograms in epilepsy. (Reproduced with permission from Guyton, A.C. (1987) *Textbook of Medical Physiology*, 7th edn. Saunders, Philadelphia.)

Alert wakefulness (beta waves)

Quiet wakefulness (alpha waves)

Stage 1 (low voltage and spindles)

Stages 2 and 3 (theta waves)

Stage 4 slow wave sleep (delta waves)

REM sleep (beta waves)

1 second

Fig. 16.81 Electroencephalogram during the different stages of sleep. (Reproduced with permission from Guyton, A.C. (1987) *Textbook of Medical Physiology*, 7th edn. Saunders, Philadelphia.)

may also urinate or defecate as the extreme signals reach the viscera. Grand mal seizures last from a few seconds to as long as 3–4 min and are followed by depression of the whole nervous system, during which the person remains in a state of stupor. The EEG shows characteristic high-voltage spikes, during the tonic phase, followed by slow waves during the clonic jerks. This pattern is seen all over the brain (Fig. 16.80).

(b) *Petit mal epilepsy*. This type is characterized by 3–30 s of unconsciousness, during which the patient may show several twitch-like contractions of muscles, usually in the head region, i.e. muscles of the corner of the eye, blinking. This is followed by return of consciousness or resumption of previous activity. Petit mal attacks may initiate grand mal attacks and they too almost certainly involve the reticular activating system. The EEG during the attack shows a characteristic spike-and-dome pattern all over the brain (3 Hz).

3 *Diagnosis of psychopathic disturbances*. This needs an experienced electroencephalographer and is useful in only certain types of psychopathic disturbances.

Sleep

Sleep is a state of loss of consciousness from which a subject can be aroused by appropriate stimuli. As a person falls asleep, different stages can be identified from an EEG recording (Fig. 16.81):

1 Alert wakefulness, characterized by high-frequency beta waves.

2 Quiet wakefulness, in which the person is relaxed and quiet with the eyes closed and which is associated with alpha waves.

3 Light sleep (stage 1), which is characterized by low-voltage waves, broken by sleep spindles, i.e. spindle-shaped bursts of alpha waves (12–14 Hz).

4 Slow-wave sleep (stages 2, 3 and 4), which is characterized by very low-frequency waves—theta waves in stages 2 and 3, and the slower delta waves (frequency 1–3 waves/second) in stage 4.

Types of sleep

During each night a person goes through stages of two different types of sleep, which alternate with each other. These are called:

1 *Slow-wave sleep*. This constitutes 75% of sleep time. It is exceedingly restful and is associated with a decrease in peripheral vascular tone, a 10–30% decrease in blood pressure and a decrease in respiratory and basal metabolic rate. The EEG pattern is typically theta and delta waves. Although slow-wave sleep is often called dreamless sleep, dreams do occur. But, unlike the other type of sleep, such dreams are not remembered, because they are not consolidated in memory.

2 *Rapid eye movement (REM) sleep*. This type occurs in episodes of 5–30 min, which recur about every 90 min. Tiredness shortens the duration of each episode, but, as the person becomes restful through the night, the duration greatly increases.

REM sleep is associated with active dreaming, which is remembered later. During this type of sleep, muscle tone is extremely depressed due to excitation of the reticular inhibitory centres, the heart and respiratory rates are irregular, there are rapid, roving movements of the eye and the person is more difficult to awaken during this period than during the slow-wave sleep.

This period is also characterized by occurrence of large phasic potentials, which originate in the pons and pass through the lateral geniculate body to the cortex: hence the name *ponto-geniculo-occipital* (PGO) spikes. PGO spikes stimulate the inhibitory reticular area and are therefore responsible for the hypotonia. The EEG pattern is similar to that of the alert wakeful state (i.e. beta waves), indicating a high level of activity in the brain during this period of sleep (Fig. 16.81). Thus, this type is often known as para-doxical sleep, because it is a paradox that a person can still be asleep despite the marked activity in the brain.

Mechanism of sleep

Sleep is an active process (not passive), in the sense that it is not merely absence of wakefulness but is actively pro-duced by inhibition of those parts of the RAS responsible for the alert conscious state of wakefulness. Stimulation of specific sites in the brain of a conscious animal were found to cause sleep and to produce the synchronized EEG pat-tern characteristic of the slow-wave type. These sites are located in:

1 *The diencephalon.* This includes the posterior hypo-thalamus, particularly the suprachiasmatic region, and parts of the diffuse nuclei of the thalamus.
2 *The medulla oblongata.* This includes some areas around the nucleus of the tractus solitarius.
3 *The basal forebrain*, especially the preoptic area.
These sites have substantial connections with each other and with the reticular area of the brain stem.

The mechanism producing REM sleep is located in the pontine reticular formation. Large cholinergic ponto-geniculo-occipital (PGO) spikes arise in this area and are thought to initiate REM sleep.

The role of neurotransmitters in producing sleep is still uncertain. While **serotonin** from the midbrain raphe was once considered the major transmitter associated with slow-wave sleep, it now appears that it contributes to wakefulness rather than sleep. In fact, serotonin agonists in humans suppress sleep, while its antagonist (*ritanserin*) increases slow-wave sleep. As for REM sleep, *nora-drenaline* from the pontine *locus ceruleus* was implicated. The view still holds that the origin of REM sleep is pontine, but it is triggered by cholinergic PGO spikes. Noradrener-gic discharge contributes to wakefulness instead. The list of substances related to sleep include a neural tissue peptide such as **muramyl peptide**, other putative peptides and **prostaglandins**, particularly prostaglandin D_2.

In summary, wakefulness is produced by activity in the RAS due to inputs from many sources, the most import-ant being the classical sensory pathways and the cerebral cortex. Sleep, on the other hand, is produced by discharge from the specific sites which actively inhibit the part of the RAS responsible for arousal. The most important of these sites are in the *diencephalon, medulla oblongata*, the *basal forebrain* and the *pontine reticular formation*. Various transmitters are involved in the wakefulness–sleep cycle; however, their specific roles are still unsettled.

Behaviour and the limbic system

Behaviour is a broad term, involving a number of different functions. However, the limbic system is responsible for those special types of behaviour associated with emotions, subconscious motor and sensory drives and the feelings of punishment, pleasure or reward.

Anatomically, the limbic system consists of a ring of cor-tex on the medial side of each hemisphere which surrounds the corpus callosum, known as the allocortex, and another ring, the juxtacortex, lying between the allocortex and the non-limbic, well-developed, cortical tissue, the neo-cortex. Subcortical nuclei of the limbic system include the septum, the paraolfactory area, the epithalamus, the anterior nuclei of the thalamus, portions of the basal ganglia, the hippocampus and the amygdala (Fig. 16.82). The hypothalamus occupies a central position among the structures of the limbic system. The reticular formation and allied regions of the brain stem also function in close association.

There are important routes of communication between the components of the limbic system and also between the limbic system and the neocortex. The limbic system cir-cuits are characterized by prolonged after-discharge. This probably explains the fact that emotional responses are generally prolonged and continue long after the stimuli that initiate them.

Functions of the limbic system

Olfaction

The limbic system was earlier called the rhinencephalon, due to its role in olfaction.

Autonomic responses and feeding behaviour

The limbic system produces the autonomic responses that accompany emotional states and behaviours. It is also asso-ciated with activities related to feeding, such as movements of the mouth. Lesions of the amygdala cause overeating, which can involve all kinds of food.

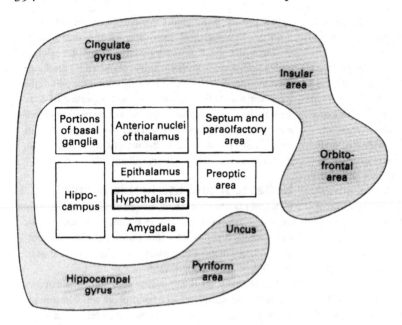

Fig. 16.82 Diagrammatic representation of the different components of the limbic system. (Reproduced with permission from Guyton, A.C. (1987) *Textbook of Medical Physiology*, 7th edn. Saunders, Philadelphia.)

Sexual behaviour

Sexual intercourse, or coitus, is basically reflexive in nature, but the components of behaviour that lead to it are regulated by the limbic system and hypothalamus. In animals, sexual behaviour depends to a great extent on the gonads and their hormonal output. Human sexual behaviour, however, is more complex and is far from being purely instinctual or hormonal. The complexity is due to the modification of sexual functions and behaviours by higher cerebral functions, such as learning, and by social and psychic factors. Damage of the limbic system would be expected to affect sexual behaviour.

Fear and rage

Fear and rage are two related phenomena which are instinctive and protective against threats of the environment. Fear, often called the fleeing or avoidance reaction, occurs when an animal is threatened, and rage, often called the fighting or attack reaction, occurs when the animal is threatened and cornered.

Besides the mental component, fear has external manifestations, such as sweating, pupillary dilatation, tachycardia, dryness of the mouth and escape reactions. The fear reaction can be produced by stimulation of some areas of the hypothalamus and amygdaloid nuclei and can disappear in lesions of the amygdala.

Normality in animals and humans is attained by a balance between *rage* and its opposite *placidity*. However, some lesions may tip the balance. When this occurs, trivial stimuli provoke violent episodes of rage, or the reverse, i.e. the most provoking stimuli do not disturb the animal's placidity. Either state would obviously depend on the site of the lesion. The rage reaction can be produced by removal of the neocortex or after lesions involving the ventromedial hypothalamic nuclei and septal nuclei while the neocortex is left intact. Placidity, on the other hand, can be produced after bilateral destruction of the amygdaloid nuclei.

Motivation

The limbic system also contains some areas whose stimulation gives a *rewarding* sensation and other areas whose stimulation gives the sense of *punishment* or avoidance. The former include points located in a medial band of tissue passing from the frontal cortex through the hypothalamus to the midbrain tegmentum. The greatest sense of reward is obtained from stimulation of points in the medial forebrain bundle, the tegmentum and the septal nuclei. The points where stimulation gives a sensation of punishment include the lateral portion of the posterior hypothalamus, the dorsal midbrain and the entorhinal cortex.

The sensations of reward and punishment are important in motivating our behaviour, i.e. we continue to do things that are rewarding and avoid those that result in punishment. They also play an equally important role in the learning process, e.g. a sensory experience causing neither reward nor punishment is not remembered very well because the animal or human being gets habituated to the stimulus. However, if the stimulus causes either reward or punishment, the cortical response becomes more intense (reinforcement).

Administration of some tranquillizers, such as chlorpromazine, inhibits both the reward and punishment centres, whereby the affective reactivity of the subject is greatly reduced. It is thus presumed that tranquillizers function in psychotic states by suppressing many of the behavioural areas in the central nervous system.

Some neurotransmitters are implicated in the pathways generating motivational behaviour and emotions. The most important of these are **noradrenaline**, **dopamine** and **serotonin**. Abnormalities in the levels of these substances are consistently found responsible for recognized mental disorders.

Higher functions of the nervous system

Memory

Memory is concerned with the storage and recall of information at the conscious or unconscious level. Formation and recall of a memory involve at least four stages:

1 Reception of the information.
2 Formation of a memory trace.
3 Consolidation of the memory trace.
4 Recall (or retrieval) of the memory trace.

Information is received and interpreted in the sensory areas of the cerebral cortex, and the memory trace is the neuronal change through which this information is stored. Various theories attempt to explain the nature of this change, but almost all accept that it involves either facilitation of transmission across pre-existing synapses or growth of new synapses. There is no single brain area reserved for memory traces, but they are located in several regions, including the prefrontal and other cortical areas, the limbic system, the cerebellum and the temporal lobes. Penfield reported that stimulation of portions of the temporal lobes in humans evokes detailed memories of events that occurred in the remote past.

Consolidation of the memory trace is the process that encodes the memory and makes it remarkably resistant to erasing. About 5–10 minutes are needed for minimum consolidation, and an hour or more for maximum consolidation. Before this process and during it the memory trace is vulnerable, and following it there is a stable resistant

memory engram. Experiments in which rats were taught to run through a maze showed that, if given a large electric shock soon after running through the maze, they forgot what they had learnt. If the shock was given a few hours later, the memory was not affected. The process of consolidation involves the hippocampus and its connections. Damage to this region causes defects of recent memory in humans, and recent memory loss in alcoholic patients correlates with the presence of pathological changes in the mammillary bodies. This area has afferent and efferent connections with the hippocampus.

Consolidation is enhanced by: (i) rehearsal of information repeatedly in the mind—significant and interesting new information is naturally better rehearsed than less important information; and (ii) codification of new information into different classes, comparing it with stored information and then storing it with a similar class. Storage includes not only the new information but also details of the results of the comparisons. This facilitates the process of searching inside the memory stores and therefore retrieval. There is evidence from educational psychology suggesting that highly emotional experiences have a marked facilitatory effect on the consolidation of memory.

Types of memory

There are three types of memory:

1 *Sensory memory*. This is the ability to retain sensory signals in the sensory areas of the brain for an extremely short period of time (several hundred milliseconds) following the actual sensory experience. The information can be further processed, i.e. it is scanned to pick out important points. Sensory memory forms the initial stage of the memory process.

2 *Primary memory (short-term memory)*. This is the memory of a few facts, words, numbers, letters or other information for seconds to hours. This type of memory is limited to about seven bits of information (e.g. telephone numbers, car plate numbers, recall of a visual scene, etc.). It is characterized by the fact that information in this memory store is instantaneously available, i.e. a person does not have to search through his/her mind for it. Because of the limited capacity of primary memory stores, old information is easily displaced when new bits of information are introduced, e.g. a newly learnt telephone number is forgotten if another number is learnt.

3 *Secondary memory (long-term memory)*. This is the storage of information that can be recalled days or even years later. This type is also known as fixed or permanent memory.

Fig. 16.83 Schematic diagram to show the flow of newly received information along the different memory stores.

Information in this memory store is not instantaneously available, due to large storage capacity, except when the memory is deeply ingrained. Memory can be ingrained deeply by the sudden impact of important events (e.g. death of a close relative) or by repeated learning (e.g. days of the week, number and times of prayers).

Reflexive memory is another type, concerned with learning motor skills (e.g. sports). It is largely an unconscious type which depends on active practice of the task over and over again. The basal ganglia and the circuitry of the cerebellum are responsible for consolidation of this type. Conscious memory of a certain task (e.g. knitting or driving a car) can be converted to reflexive by constant repetition.

Mechanisms of memory

The flow of newly received information is from the sensory memory in the sensory areas of the cortex to the primary memory store. Due to the limited storage capacity there, the delivered information undergoes either of two fates: either it is lost, i.e. 'forgotten', or it is passed over to the larger

secondary memory store, where it is fixed against erasing (Fig. 16.83).

Mechanisms of primary memory

1 *Presynaptic inhibition and presynaptic facilitation.* These are the theories behind two forms of simple primary memory: **habituation** and **sensitization**, respectively.

Habituation is the decreased response to a repeated stimulus which is neutral, i.e. does not arouse a sense of reward or punishment. In this way, the brain learns to ignore insignificant stimuli and give priority to others of more importance. The effect of habituation occurs due to progressive closure of Ca^{2+} channels in the membrane of the presynaptic terminal. Ca^{2+} influx is decreased and consequently the amount of transmitter released from the presynaptic neuron to activate the postsynaptic neuron is decreased (Fig. 16.84). The result is reduced responsiveness of the postsynaptic neuron to stimulation for up to several hours. This is a 'negative' type of memory in the sense that it teaches the brain to ignore rather than recall information.

In the same way, **sensitization** may be described as a 'positive' type of memory. It is the increased response to a stimulus applied previously once or more in association with a strong or noxious stimulus. Sensitization pathways have synapses lying at the terminal endings of presynaptic fibres (i.e. presynaptic synapses) before these fibres end on postsynaptic neurons (Fig. 16.84). Simultaneous stimulation of the presynaptic synapse causes release of **serotonin**, which acts on receptors on the presynaptic fibre and activates the adenyl cyclase/cyclic adenosine monophosphate (AMP) system there. The consequent phosphorylation blocks K^+ channels in the membrane of the presynaptic neuron. K^+ efflux needed for normal repolarization is inhibited, and so the action potential is prolonged. This facilitates Ca^{2+} entry into the presynaptic terminal, with a subsequent increase in transmitter release and stronger prolonged response of the postsynaptic neuron, i.e. sensitization.

2 *Post-tetanic facilitation.* This is a type of memory which occurs due to accumulation of Ca^{2+} within the presynaptic terminal (following repetitive stimulation), in excess of what the mitochondria and endoplasmic reticulum can absorb and what the calcium pump can move out of the neuron. The excess Ca^{2+} causes prolonged release of transmitter from the presynaptic fibre.

3 *Long-term potentiation (LTP).* LTP is caused by accumulation of Ca^{2+} in the postsynaptic neuron after brief repetitive stimulation of the presynaptic neuron. It is a more prolonged facilitation of synaptic pathways than any of

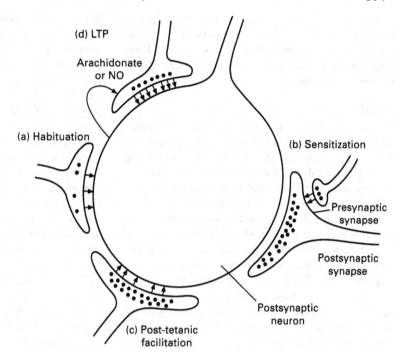

Fig. 16.84 Mechanisms of primary memory: (a) Habituation (presynaptic inhibition). (b) Sensitization (presynaptic facilitation). (c) Post-tetanic facilitation. (d) LTP, long-term potentiation.

the previously described mechanisms, with effects lasting up to many weeks. The proposed neural circuitry for LTP works as follows (Fig. 16.84). Stimulation of the sensory presynaptic neuron causes firing of the postsynaptic neuron. Ca^{2+} channels in the latter open and the influx of Ca^{2+} stimulates it to release a second messenger, which diffuses back to the presynaptic neuron, causing prolonged release of a larger quantity of transmitter. This keeps up the memory. It has been suggested that the messenger released from the postsynaptic fibre is **arachidonate** or **nitric oxide (NO)** and the transmitter released from the presynaptic neuron is **glutamate**.

Since information in the primary memory store is stored as continuous electrical activity, reverberating circuit after discharge was posed as another possible explanation for primary memory (see 'The reflex arc' in this chapter and Fig. 16.28). As the reverberating circuit fatigues or as new signals interfere with reverberations, the memory fades away.

Mechanisms of secondary memory. The process of consolidation necessary for the establishment of secondary memory (Fig. 16.83) is associated with definite structural changes. Various changes have been suggested: (i) an increase in the number of presynaptic terminals with a subsequent increase in new synaptic contacts; and (ii) an

increase in the number of synaptic vesicles, in the amount of transmitter within each vesicle and in the number of release sites and receptor sites. Irrespective of the nature of the change, all would call for enhancement of protein synthesis. Indeed, drugs that inhibit protein synthesis (i.e. puromycin) are associated in some cases with reduced learning ability. A group of genes known as **immediate early genes (IEGs)** are proposed to be involved in the consolidation process and a special protein called cAMP-responsive element-binding protein (CREB) which binds to DNA and alters the transcription of genes.

Abnormalities of memory

Loss of memory, called amnesia, can occur due to various lesions. Two types are:

1 *Anterograde amnesia.* This is the inability to retain information, particularly the symbolic types in the secondary memory store or even in the primary store, except for a few moments. There is therefore a specific problem of consolidation. Such patients usually suffer from learning disabilities. Anterograde amnesia results from bilateral lesions in the hippocampus.

2 *Retrograde amnesia.* This is the inability to recall information stored before the time of the lesion (i.e. from the past). Loss of recently stored memories is greater than loss of that of the remote past. This commonly occurs following

concussion, e.g. following an accident or electroconvulsive therapy. Hippocampal lesions might cause an element of retrograde amnesia along with the anterograde type. However, damage to some thalamic areas is associated with pure retrograde amnesia.

Learning

Learning is defined as the alteration of behaviour or modification of innate responses by experience and training. It involves many levels; the most advanced types of learning are largely cortical phenomena but the brain stem and even the spinal cord are also involved in these processes.

Conditioned reflexes are an important type of learning. A conditioned reflex is acquired by repeated association of two stimuli: one which produces an inborn reflex and one which does not. After some time, the latter stimulus alone (the conditioned stimulus) will produce the inborn response. In the classical experiments of Pavlov, placing meat in the dog's mouth (unconditioned stimulus) produced salivation (unconditioned response). But, when the unconditioned stimulus was immediately preceded by the ringing of a bell (conditioned stimulus) on several different occasions, the animal would eventually salivate when the bell was rung, without providing any meat. It should be noted that a vast number of somatic, visceral and other neural changes can be made to occur as conditioned reflex responses. The essential feature of conditioned reflexes is the formation of new functional connections in the nervous system (e.g. in Pavlov's experiment, a connection was made between the bell ringing and salivation—in other words, between the auditory pathway and the autonomic centres responsible for salivation).

The limbic system is very much involved in the process of learning. Events with a strong emotional content (i.e. pleasant or unpleasant) are most easily remembered, and damage to the hippocampus—one important component of the limbic system—seriously impairs the learning ability.

In operant conditioning, an animal learns to do something in order to get a reward or avoid punishment. The conditioned stimulus is a signal that alerts the animal to perform the task, and the unconditioned stimulus is the rewarding event. For example, a bell rings and the animal presses a lever and is rewarded by getting food. With repetition, this will condition the animal to perform the task (i.e. press the lever) whenever the stimulus (i.e. bell ringing) is presented. Alternatively, the stimulus may precede the punishing event, e.g. a bell rings and the animal gets an electric shock. In time, the animal is conditioned to take an avoiding reaction, such as jumping away, whenever the stimulus (e.g. bell ringing) is presented.

Speech and language

Speech is the conveying of thoughts and feelings by means of spoken (or written) symbols. It is produced by complex neuromechanical activity that requires the integration of various inputs (e.g. respiratory, articulatory, etc.). Language is the set of symbols used in the conveyance of thoughts and feelings. It involves faculties such as comprehension and expression. Language is the product of the meaning of words, their sound and the rules of grammar.

Various areas in the neocortex subserve the complex function of speech. The primary visual cortex in the occipital lobe and the primary auditory cortex in the temporal lobe enable a person to see visual images (e.g. written words) and to hear spoken words, respectively. Further analysis and interpretation of the incoming visual and auditory sensations are the function of the secondary sensory areas. Thus, damage of the secondary visual area results in word blindness or **dyslexia**, in which there is inability to read or write, due to problems in understanding the meaning of written words. Likewise, lesions in the secondary auditory area result in word deafness. In such a condition, the person fails to understand sounds or spoken words, even though they are heard.

A region in the posterior part of the superior temporal lobe, called Wernicke's area, is an area of confluence where the secondary somatic, visual and auditory areas meet. It is also known as the general interpretative area, due to its global importance in the higher levels of brain function. Wernicke's area is more highly developed in one cerebral hemisphere than the other, usually the left in the vast majority of the population. There it plays the final role of interpreting visual, auditory and other sensory information and *integrating* them together to formulate logically connected thoughts. Furthermore, it is also responsible for the *selection of words* to express these thoughts. Lesions in Wernicke's area do not prevent a patient from hearing different words or reading them, but they make him/her incapable of understanding the meaning conveyed by the spoken or written words.

Immediately behind Wernicke's area and in front of the visual cortex is the angular gyrus. This region is concerned with the interpretation of information obtained from read words or from other visual scenes. Damage to this area interrupts the passage of signals from the visual cortex into Wernicke's area and results in dyslexia.

The dominant hemisphere

Language function depends more on one cerebral hemisphere than the other—a fact which led scientists to call the hemisphere that is concerned with categorization and language function, the categorical or dominant hemisphere. The other hemisphere, which is specialized in spatiotemporal relations (i.e. recognition of faces, identification of objects by form, understanding, and interpretation of music) is called the representational or non-dominant hemisphere.

The categorical hemisphere in 95% of the population is the left one. In the remaining 5%, either there is no obvious lateralization or the right hemisphere is the categorical hemisphere. Handedness is related to hemispheric specialization, because the area of hand skills is actually more developed in the categorical hemisphere; however, it does not necessarily parallel it. Right-handed individuals constitute only 91% of the human population.

Language disorders

It is important to emphasize again the importance of Wernicke's area as the centre in the 'mind' for interpreting sensory experiences, for formation of thoughts in response to that interpretation and for the selection of words to express thoughts. Wernicke's area (Fig. 16.62) projects via the arcuate fasciculus to Broca's area (area 44) of the categorical hemisphere (if expression is by speech) or to the area of hand skills in premotor area 6 (if expression is in writing). Broca's area processes the information received from Wernicke's area into a coordinated pattern of movement and then projects that pattern to the primary motor cortex. The latter initiates movement of the muscles of speech in the tongue, lips and larynx, via the corticobulbar fibres of the pyramidal tract. When writing, the information received from Wernicke's area is processed in the area of hand skills. The result is a coordinated pattern of muscle movements projected to the arm and hand region of the primary motor cortex, which initiates the necessary muscle movements in the hand and arm.

Increasing amounts of knowledge about speech areas and the pathways involved have come from brain images obtained by positron emission tomography (PET). This is a new non-invasive technique which measures blood flows in specific regions of the brain. It involves injection of positron-emitting tracers and then detecting the gamma radiation produced when positrons collide with electrons in the circulating blood. The level of gamma energy in a specific brain area indicates the amount of blood flow there. Several of the areas tested during the process of speech are reconstructed, using computer programs, into images of blood flow. Since blood flow increases when a brain area is more active, increased gamma energy in a specific speech area is taken to indicate increased neuronal activity. Besides identification of the normal speech areas, the technique is

Table 16.14 Some characteristic forms of naming errors given by patients with different types of aphasia when the stimulus is a picture of a chair.*

Naming error	Type of aphasia	Site of lesion
'Tssair'	Motor	Broca's area
'Stool' or 'chossl'	Sensory	Wernicke's area
'I know what that is . . . I have some'	Anomic	Angular gyrus
'Flair . . . no, swair . . . tair'	Conduction	Arcuate fasciculus

* Based on Goodglass, H. (1980) Disorders of naming following brain injury. *American Scientist* **68**, 647.

used as a diagnostic tool in the different types of aphasia. PET also has other uses in the diagnosis and study of brain pathophysiology.

Aphasias are abnormalities of language functions due to injury of language centres in the cerebral cortex. This usually follows thrombosis or embolism of cerebral vessels, and the patient presents with impairment of either comprehension or expression or both. Aphasia can be classified as follows:

1 *Broca's aphasia (motor aphasia)*. Damage to Broca's area does not affect comprehension of written or spoken words, but the patient's speech is poorly articulated, produced slowly and with great effort, and abnormal in rhythm. The patient omits small words and endings and in severe cases the whole vocabulary may be limited to two to three words. This is also known as non-fluent aphasia.

2 *Wernicke's aphasia (sensory aphasia)*. The effects of lesions in Wernicke's area are different from those of the motor type in that the patient's comprehension of spoken and written language is impaired. Speech is fluent, of normal rhythm and articulation, but it is full of words that are incorrect and meaningless. The patient also tends to use neologisms (i.e. words he/she formulates) (Table 16.14). Wernicke's aphasia is often called 'fluent aphasia' referring to the 'meaningless and excessive talk' characteristic of these patients.

3 *Conduction aphasia*. The lesion affects the nerve fibres of the arcuate fasciculus, thus disconnecting Wernicke's from Broca's area. The patient's comprehension of speech or written material is normal, but repetition (e.g. of the words of the examining doctor) is most severely affected. As in Wernicke's aphasia, their own speech is fluent but full of words that make no sense.

4 *Anomic aphasia*. The lesion damages the angular gyrus in the categorical hemisphere, leaving Wernicke's and

Table 16.15 Summary classification of cortical aphasias.

Type of aphasia	Fluency	Comprehension	Repetition	Object naming	Writing
Broca's aphasia	Non-fluent	Good	Poor	Poor	Impaired
Wernicke's aphasia	Fluent	Poor	Poor	Poor	Impaired
Conduction aphasia	Fluent	Good	Poor	Poor	Impaired
Anomic aphasia	Fluent	Good	Good	Poor	Impaired
Global aphasia	Non-fluent	Poor	Poor	Poor	Impaired

Broca's areas intact. In these cases, there are no difficulties of speech and auditory comprehension, but visual
comprehension is abnormal. This arises due to the fact
that visual information is not processed and transmitted
to Wernicke's area. In addition, the patient finds difficulty
in naming objects (see Table 16.14); however, *anomia*
may be found in other types of aphasia.

5 *Global aphasia.* This occurs when there is widespread
destruction of both Wernicke's and Broca's areas, e.g. after
a severe stroke. In global aphasia, there is inability to comprehend or speak.

Table 16.15 gives a simple classification of cortical
aphasias. It is important to note that all types of aphasia are
associated with deficits in writing.

Further reading

1 Carpenter, R.H.S. (1996) *Neurophysiology*, 3rd edn. Edward
  Arnold, Sevenoaks, Kent.
2 Guyton, A.C. & Hall, J.E. (1991) Organisation of NS: The
  nervous system. In: *Textbook of Medical Physiology*, 9th edn,
  pp. 565–767. Saunders, Philadelphia.

17 / The Special Senses

Smell and taste

Introduction

Smell (**olfaction**) and taste (**gustation**) are specialized chemical senses. They are closely related, as evidenced by the common observation that the common cold not only depresses the sense of smell but also alters the sense of

Objectives

On completion of the study of this chapter, the student should be able to:

1 Understand the mechanisms involved in the chemical sensations of taste and smell.

2 Comprehend the visual pathways so as to recognize the manifestations of various lesions.

3 Explain the optical aspects of image formation on the retina.

4 Understand the nature and function of visual pigments.

5 Explain the mechanisms of colour vision.

6 Appreciate the visual explanation of perception of distance and three-dimensional characteristics of objects.

7 Understand the properties of sound so as to explain the mechanisms of auditory receptors.

8 Understand the mechanisms of hearing so as to explain the perception of pitch and loudness.

9 Develop an awareness of some clinical applications of the knowledge of the special senses.

10 Become aware of some commonly used clinical tests of vision and hearing.

taste. The two senses are related to food intake: if the smell and taste of a food are agreeable, the food is ingested; but it is rejected if either or both its smell and taste are unacceptable. The combined effect of the smell and taste of a food is included under the term *flavour*. There are, however, differences between the two senses. While smell receptors are **telereceptors** (distance receivers), i.e. the sensation is coming from a distance outside the body and is projected to the environment, taste is entirely confined to the mouth. Smell pathways do not relay in the thalamus and do not reach the sensory cortex at the postcentral gyrus. Instead, they end in the part of the brain referred to previously as the rhinencephalon but now considered as part of the limbic system. Taste pathways, on the other hand, relay in the thalamus and are finally projected to the postcentral gyrus.

Smell

The sense of smell is developed in some animals, such as the dog and rabbit, which are referred to as macrosmatic, but is greatly reduced in primates, including humans, which are referred to as microsmatic.

The olfactory mucosa in humans is located in the roof of

Fig. 17.1 Olfactory receptor and support cells. (Reproduced from Bray, J.J., Cragg, P.A., Macknight, A.D.C., Mills, R.G. & Taylor, D.W. (1989) *Lecture Notes in Physiology*, 2nd edn. Blackwell Scientific Publications, Oxford.)

the nasal cavity near the septum; it has a yellowish-brown colour. Its total area on both sides is about 5 cm². As air enters the nose, it is warmed by the lining epithelium, and convection or eddy currents arise from the airstream, passing through the lower part of the nose to reach the olfactory receptors in the roof.

The olfactory receptors are bipolar neurons (Fig. 17.1), which are about 10–20 million in number. Their dendritic zone is expanded into **olfactory rods**, which end in cilia. Between the receptor neurons there are supporting cells; these end in microvilli and secrete mucus, which overlies the mucosa. The axons of the receptor neurons are unmyelinated and collected in bundles called **fila olfactoria**, which go through the holes in the cribriform plate of the ethmoid bone to enter the olfactory bulb (Fig. 17.2). The receptor axons synapse with **mitral** and **tufted cells** in the **glomeruli** of the bulbs. A great deal of spatial summation occurs at this step, with over 20 000 receptors synapsing with tens of mitral and tufted cells. From the mitral cells arise the lateral and intermediate **olfactory stria**, which end, respectively, in the ipsilateral **olfactory cortex** and **uncus** and the **olfactory tubercle**. The medial olfactory stria arise from the tufted cells and cross the midline in the anterior commissure to end on granular cells in the opposite bulb. These commissural fibres are concerned with the transfer of olfactory memories from one side to the other.

Physiology of olfaction

Molecules of substances to be smelled dissolve in the mucous layer overlying the olfactory epithelium and combine with receptors on the cilia of the olfactory rods. The receptor cell is stimulated by means of a specific **G pro-**

Fig. 17.2 The olfactory pathway. (From Keele, C.A., Neil, E. & Joels, N. (eds) (1982) *Samson Wright's Applied Physiology*, 13th edn, kindly supplied by Professor E.W. Walls. Reproduced by permission of Oxford University Press, Oxford.)

tein (Golf). Adenylate cyclase is activated, thus increasing intracellular cyclic adenosine monophosphate (cAMP). The latter causes opening of Na^+ channels and an influx of Na^+. This is followed by a receptor potential. The receptor potential depolarizes the first segment of the axon, which leads to action potentials in the olfactory pathways.

There is no generally accepted classification of the basic types of smells recognized by humans. The sense of smell can be very sensitive, sensing minute concentrations of some substances in air. There is also no consistent correlation between strong smell and chemical structure, but substances with strong smells seem to be either highly water-soluble or lipid-soluble. Discrimination within a certain smell is poor, requiring a change in concentration of at least 30% before a difference can be detected.

Humans can distinguish about 10 000 different odours. There is considerable individual variation in the acuity of the sense of smell and, in general, women have a keener sense of smell than men. Smell is related to sexual function and in women it becomes more acute during ovulation. Adaptation can occur to pleasant as well as nasty smells and is specific for the odour being smelt. Adaptation in smell is partly central and partly due to changes in the receptors.

Clinical considerations

Loss of the sense of smell is called **anosmia** and its alteration is referred to as **parosmia** or **dysosmia**. **Hyperosmia** refers to an increased and hyposmia to a decreased acuity in the sense of smell.

Damage to the olfactory epithelium or pathways by trauma or disease may lead to anosmia or parosmia. Patients with adrenal insufficiency develop a more acute sense of taste and especially of smell. **Hyposmia** occurs in vitamin A deficiency and hypogonadism.

Taste

Gustatory receptors are found in the **taste buds**. These number about 10 000 in humans and are found on the tongue, epiglottis, soft palate and pharynx. On the tongue, taste buds are found in the **fungiform, foliate** and **vallate papillae**. They are absent in the small **filiform papillae** in the mid-dorsum of the tongue; consequently, the mid-dorsum of the tongue is insensitive to taste.

In the taste buds (Fig. 17.3) the receptor cells end in cilia, which project through the taste pore. Supporting cells are found between the receptors. Nerve fibres probably start as minute filaments within the receptors and form a plexus beneath the basement membrane before they emerge. Taste fibres from the anterior two-thirds of the tongue at first run

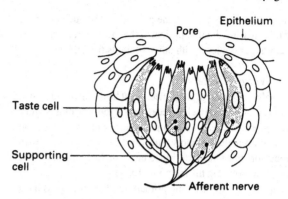

Fig. 17.3 Structure of the taste buds. (Reproduced from Bray, J.J., Cragg, P.A., Macknight, A.D.C., Mills, R.G. & Taylor, D.W. (1989) *Lecture Notes in Physiology*, 2nd edn. Blackwell Scientific Publications, Oxford.)

Fig. 17.4 The taste pathway. NTS, nucleus of tractus solitarius; ML, medial lemniscus; TR, thalamic radiation.

with the fibres subserving touch, pain and temperature in the *lingual nerve*. They then separate to join the *chorda tympani* nerve, which enters the medulla as part of the *facial nerve* (Fig. 17.4). Fibres from the posterior one-third of the tongue run in the *glossopharyngeal nerve* and those from the epiglottis, palate and pharynx travel in the *vagus nerve*. The taste fibres in the three cranial nerves form the **tractus solitarius**, whose nucleus lies in the medulla. After synapse in the nucleus of the tractus solitarius, second-order neurons arise and cross the midline to ascend in the medial lemniscus to the thalamus. Third-order neurons arise after the synapse in the posteroventral nucleus of the **thalamus** and, finally, project to the lower part of the post-central gyrus, along with other afferents from the face.

Physiology of taste

In order to be tasted, substances must be dissolved in saliva. Their molecules attach to receptors on the cilia of gustatory receptor cells, leading to a generator potential and action potentials in the gustatory pathways. The combination with receptors must be weak, since taste can be abolished quite easily by washing the mouth with water.

In the case of taste, the primary modalities (types) have been identified. They are **sour**, **salt**, **sweet** and **bitter**. All other tastes are produced by various combinations of these four primary modalities.

The mechanisms of stimulation of specific taste receptors are as follows. Sour is detected when acids containing H^+ block K^+ channels. Salt probably acts by depolarization of salt receptors due to influx of Na^+. Bitter stimuli act by a G protein (Go), which activates phospholipase C, leading to an increase of intracellular inositol triphosphate (IP_3), leading to Ca^{2+} release from the endoplasmic reticulum. Sweet stimuli work through a G protein (Gs), which activates adenylate cyclase, thus increasing cAMP, which leads to decreased K^+ conductance.

Each of the primary taste modalities is sensed maximally in a specific area of the tongue; thus, sweet is best appreciated at the tip, bitter at the back, sour along the edges and salt on the dorsum anteriorly near the edge. In addition, sour and bitter substances are tasted on the palate, and all four taste modalities are sensed on the pharynx and epiglottis.

Taste is generally less sensitive than smell. There is also individual variation, and acuity of taste declines in old age. Discrimination is as poor as in smell, similarly requiring a 30% change. Adaptation occurs with taste and, in humans, is due entirely to the receptors.

Relationship of chemical structure to taste

Some sapid (taste-producing) substances combine taste modalities but many substances have a taste belonging to one of the primary types.

A **sour taste** is given by acids, whether organic or inorganic. For any acid, sourness is directly proportional to the hydrogen ion concentration, thereby providing a definite link between chemical structure and the taste sensation. The reference acid is HCl, with a normal threshold of pH 3.5.

The **salt taste** is typically given by NaCl, which is used as the reference substance, with a threshold of 0.02 mol/litre. In the case of NaCl, the taste is due to the sodium ion but, in salts with other elements or metals, both the cation and the anion contribute and other tastes may be combined with the salty taste.

Many substances, organic and inorganic, are **bitter**. The reference substance is quinine sulphate, at a threshold of 0.000008 mol/litre. Urea, caffeine, nicotine, strychnine hydrochloride and morphine are bitter. The inorganic salts of magnesium, ammonium and calcium are also bitter and no definite chemical structure can be assigned to the bitter taste.

The most pleasant taste modality, **sweet**, is given by a variety of substances. The reference substance is sucrose, at a threshold of 0.01 mol/l. Other sugars are sweet, including lactose, glucose and fructose; polysaccharides, glycerol, some alcohols (not ethanol), aldehydes and ketones are also sweet. Chloroform is sweet. The amides of aspartic acid and some recently discovered proteins are sweet, as are the inorganic salts of lead and beryllium. Artificial sweetening substances are used by diabetics and in reducing diets; they include saccharin, dulcin, cyclamates and aspartame.

Clinical considerations

Complete taste blindness is termed **ageusia** and disturbed taste sensation is **dysgeusia**. Some diseases cause **hypogeusia**. **Hypergeusia** occurs in patients with adrenal insufficiency. Administration of drugs that have sulph-hydryl groups in their structure, such as penicillamine, may cause temporary ageusia.

Inability to taste phenylthiocarbamide (PTC) in dilute threshold concentrations is a defect which is inherited as an autosomal recessive factor and may be used in human genetic studies.

Vision

Anatomical considerations

The eyeball has a diameter of about 2.5 cm. It is basically composed of three layers, which are, from without inwards, the **sclera**, the **choroid** and the **retina** (Fig. 17.5).

The sclera consists of connective tissue, which is opaque, except anteriorly where it is modified by becoming transparent and more curved to form the **cornea**. The choroid is a pigmented layer with numerous blood-vessels. It is modified anteriorly to give the **ciliary body** and the **iris**. The ciliary body is a circular structure consisting of the **ciliary glands** and **smooth muscle**. The ciliary muscle consists of circular fibres and longitudinal fibres, which are inserted near the corneoscleral junction. Suspensory ligaments from the ciliary muscle are joined to the **zonule** or

Fig. 17.5 Horizontal section of the eye. (Reproduced from Bray, J.J., Cragg, P.A., Macknight, A.D.C., Mills, R.G. & Taylor, D.W. (1989) *Lecture Notes in Physiology*, 2nd edn. Blackwell Scientific Publications, Oxford.)

lens ligament. The lens is crystalline and biconvex, consisting of concentric laminae of elongated epithelial cells and surrounded by a capsule. The iris is the coloured part of the eye, with the aperture or **pupil** in its centre. It has circular smooth-muscle fibres, which constrict the pupil when they contract, and **radial** or **longitudinal fibres**, which dilate the pupil, in this way varying the amount of light that enters the eye. The circular fibres are supplied by *parasympathetic cholinergic nerves*, while the longitudinal fibres are innervated by *sympathetic adrenergic nerves*. Clinically, the pupil is usually dilated by instilling drops of atropine-like drugs into the eye, which paralyse the parasympathetic nerves. The retina lines the posterior two-thirds of the choroid and contains the receptors for light, the **rods** and **cones**. Medial or nasal to the anteroposterior axis of the eyeball is the spot where the optic nerve fibres leave the eye, called the **optic disc**, which measures about 1.5 mm in diameter. About 3 mm lateral or temporal to the optic disc and very close to the anteroposterior axis is the **macula lutea** (yellow spot), at the centre of which is a depression called the **fovea centralis**.

The space between the retina and the lens is filled with a transparent gelatinous material, called the **vitreous humour** or body. The space between the cornea anteriorly and the iris and lens posteriorly is called the anterior chamber. The posterior chamber is the narrow circular space bounded anteriorly by the iris and posteriorly by the ciliary body and lens. Both the anterior and posterior chambers are filled with **aqueous humour**. This is a fluid similar in composition to the plasma without the proteins,

but it has lower glucose and urea concentrations than in the plasma. The lens is avascular and metabolizes glucose taken from the aqueous humour. Aqueous humour is produced in the ciliary glands through active transport and diffusion. The primary event is active transport of Na^+, followed by Cl^- and HCO_3^- to maintain electrical neutrality; water follows the osmotic gradient created. Several nutrients, such as glucose and amino acids, move into the aqueous humour by carrier-mediated transport. The aqueous humour moves forward in the posterior chamber, going between the lens and the iris into the anterior chamber, and moves on to the iridocorneal angle, between the cornea and iris and through trabeculae or vacuoles in the lining endothelial cells, to drain into the sinus venosus sclerae or **canal of Schlemm**. This continuous production and drainage into venous blood of aqueous humour maintains intraocular pressure at 10–20 mmHg. A rise of pressure above 20 mmHg results in **glaucoma**, one cause of which is blockage of the canal of Schlemm. Glaucoma may result in blindness because the increased pressure compresses the optic nerve fibres and also the retinal artery at the optic disc.

External protection of the eye

The eye is protected by the bony orbit and by the eyelids, which have lashes on their edges and are lined on the inside by conjunctiva. Tear fluid is produced by **lacrimal glands**, which are located in the upper and outer part of the orbit. This fluid normally drains through the **nasolacrimal duct** into the nose. It is an isotonic solution of Na^+, Cl^-

Pigment
epithelium

Rod and cone

Outer segments

Inner segments

Outer nuclear
layer

Outer plexiform
layer

Inner nuclear
layer

Inner plexiform
layer

Ganglion cell
layer

Optic nerve fibres

Fig. 17.6 The neural structure of the retina. A, amacrine cell; C, cones; DG, diffuse ganglion cell; FB, flat bipolar cell; H, horizontal cell; MB, midget bipolar cell; MG, midget ganglion cell; R, rods; RB, rod bipolar cell. Note that the axon of the horizontal cell makes no synapses with the cone. These axons in mammals only synapse with the rods. (Reproduced with permission from Dowling, J.E. & Boycott, B.B. (1966) *Proceedings of the Royal Society (Series B)* **166**, 80.)

and HCO_3^-, with a low protein content and a bactericidal enzyme called *lysozyme*. There is normally a film of tear fluid lining the conjunctiva and cornea. Blinking, occurring spontaneously at the rate of about 20 times/min, is responsible for renewing this film. Blinking also occurs when the front of the eye is touched, when bright light is shone into the eye and in the case of a suddenly approaching object. In the case of irritation and when a foreign body enters the conjunctiva, the rate of tear secretion is increased, through a nervous reflex involving efferent *parasympathetic* fibres, in order to wash out the foreign body or irritant. Drainage capacity may be exceeded, in which case tear fluid spills

over and runs on the cheeks; this is termed lacrimation (weeping). Lacrimation may also occur under emotional circumstances.

The retina

The retina has 10 layers (Fig. 17.6). The arrangement of these layers can be appreciated when it is realized that the light receptors, the rods and cones, face the pigment layer towards the outer side of the eyeball, and that the rods and cones synapse with **bipolar neurons**, which synapse in turn with **ganglion cells**, the axons of which constitute the optic nerve fibres. The 10th layer is an internal **limiting**

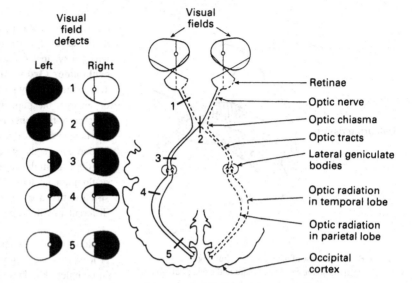

Fig. 17.7 The visual pathway and the effect of various lesions, 1–5. (Reproduced from Macleod, J. (ed.) (1974) *Davidson's Principles and Practice of Medicine*, 11th edn. With permission from Churchill Livingstone, Edinburgh.)

membrane. Horizontal cells make synaptic connections with and between receptors, while **amacrine cells**, having no axons but numerous processes, make horizontal connections between ganglion cells.

Each eye has about 120 million rods and 6 million cones. Each rod and cone has an outer segment, consisting of discs or saccules of membrane that contain a photosensitive pigment, an inner segment, which is rich in mitochondria and includes the nucleus, and a synaptic terminal. The numerous mitochondria signify high metabolic activity, which is manifested by the presence of Na^+, K^+ adenosine triphosphatase (ATPase) in the membrane of the inner segments. Rods are extremely sensitive to light and operate under *dim light* conditions. Cones have a higher threshold and operate under *bright light* conditions.

There are no rods or cones on the optic disc, which is consequently blind (the **blind spot**). The fovea centralis contains only cones. At the fovea, the blood-vessels and retinal neurons are displaced to the sides, so that light rays pass directly to the cones. The density of cones falls sharply in the periphery of the retina. The density of rods increases from outside the fovea towards the periphery of the retina. The fovea centralis is the spot with the highest acuity of vision: details of objects are distinguished and colour is appreciated. To see an object clearly, the head and eyes may be turned to face the object so that light reflected from it falls on the fovea centralis.

The **ophthalmoscope** is basically an instrument that illuminates the interior of the eye and the examiner, in effect, uses the eye lens of the subject as a magnifying glass to see the fundus. The optic disc is easily recognized, with retinal

blood-vessels emerging from it; about two disc diameters laterally is the slightly darkish macula lutea, which is not crossed by blood-vessels. Examination of the fundus may reveal conditions like *optic* **atrophy**, **papilloedema** and **retinal detachment**. In addition, viewing of the retinal blood-vessels constitutes the only opportunity to directly examine blood-vessels clinically. Examination of the fundus is therefore important in all diseases that may affect blood-vessels, particularly **hypertension** and **diabetes mellitus**. The retinal vessels supply the bipolar and ganglion cells of the retina. However, the receptor cells are nourished mainly from the capillary plexuses present in the **choroid**. Therefore, retinal detachment is damaging to the receptor cells.

There are 1.2 million fibres in the optic nerve. With 126 million receptors, one would expect converging connections of rods and cones with optic nerve fibres. Actually, one *foveal cone* synapses with one bipolar neuron and one ganglion cell, but about 10 *cones* in the periphery of the retina synapse with one bipolar neuron and one ganglion cell. In the case of *rods*, about 300 of them synapse with one bipolar cell and one ganglion neuron.

The visual pathways (Fig. 17.7)

Since light travels in straight lines, the right half of the retina views the left half of the field of vision and the upper half of the retina looks at the lower half of the visual field, and vice versa. It is noteworthy that, in the study of vision, the terms temporal and nasal are preferred to lateral and medial, respectively. The optic nerves emerge from the eyes to meet in the **optic chiasma**, where decussation of

Calcarine fissure

Fig. 17.8 Medial view of occipital lobe showing location of the visual areas on the calcarine fissure of the occipital lobe. 1, projection area for peripheral retina; 2, area for upper macula; 3, area for lower macula. Note that the projection of the macula occupies the largest part of the visual cortex.

fibres occurs in a regular pattern: fibres from the temporal half of the retina on each side proceed on the same side, while fibres from each of the nasal halves of the retinae cross to the opposite side. Fibres from the macula on each side behave in exactly the same way. The **optic tracts** carry fibres from the retinal and macular halves of the same side, i.e. the right optic tract carries fibres from the right halves of both retinae and maculae, and fibres from the left halves of the retinae and maculae are carried in the left optic tract. For the **field of vision**, the directions are reversed, e.g. the left optic tract carries impulses coming from the right half of each field of vision. Optic tract fibres synapse in the **lateral geniculate body** of the thalamus. The grey matter of the lateral geniculate body has six layers; contralateral fibres end in layers 1, 4 and 6, while fibres from equivalent spots on the ipsilateral side of the retina end in layers 2, 3 and 5. Fibres arising from the lateral geniculate body ascend in the optic radiation to the **occipital cortex**. The **primary cortical visual area** for the same-side halves of the field of vision are projected to the inner side of the opposite hemisphere above and below the **calcarine fissure** (Brodman's area 17; see Fig. 17.8). The macula is represented by a much larger area than the periphery of the retina, which is represented by small forward areas above and below the calcarine fissure. Nearby, areas 18 and 19 are visual association areas, where recognition of objects and other cognitive functions associated with vision are performed.

Some fibres branch off from the optic tract just before entering the lateral geniculate body; they go to the **pretectal area** of the superior colliculus of the midbrain, where a synapse occurs and new fibres arise to go to the **oculomotor (3rd cranial nerve) nucleus** on both sides. This is the pathway for the *light reflex*: when light is shone on an eye, the pupil constricts; the opposite pupil also constricts—the **consensual light reflex**. The consensual reaction is due to the fact that illumination of the retina in one eye sends impulses in both optic tracts and that the fibres from the superior colliculus go bilaterally to the oculomotor nucleus. The pathway for the pupillary constriction that accompanies **accommodation** is somewhat different, as will be explained below.

Lesions of the visual pathways (Fig. 17.7)
A lesion interrupting the whole of the *optic nerve* results in complete blindness in the corresponding eye. Beyond the optic nerve, lesions may result in blindness in half the field on each side; this is termed **hemianopia**. When the same sides are affected, the hemianopia is homonymous; when opposite sides are affected it is heteronymous. The terms temporal and nasal, as well as right and left, are also used.

If a lesion affects the central part of the *optic chiasma*, such as by pressure from a pituitary tumour, fibres from the nasal halves of both retinae are interrupted, leading to bitemporal hemianopia, which is heteronymous. A lesion pressing on the lateral sides of the chiasma would interrupt the fibres from the temporal halves of both retinae and would lead to binasal hemianopia, which is also heteronymous. Thus, chiasmal lesions lead to **heteronymous hemianopia**.

Lesions of the *optic tracts*, optic radiation or one complete side of the occipital cortex, i.e. retrochiasmal, lead to **homonymous hemianopia**. There are, however, two special characteristics of *cortical lesions*. First, since the macula is represented by a much larger area than the periphery of the retina, a lesion may not destroy all macular representation, resulting in macular sparing in the field of vision. Secondly, since fibres from the upper and lower quarters of both sides of the retinae and maculae travelling in the optic radiations in the parietal and temporal lobes project to the occipital cortex, respectively, above and below the calcarine fissure, a lesion interrupting the optic radiation in either lobe may result in *quadrantic* visual field defects (4 in Fig. 17.7). A cortical lesion acting entirely above or below the calcarine fissure would also result in quadrantic defects in the field of vision.

An important clue as to the location of the lesion in

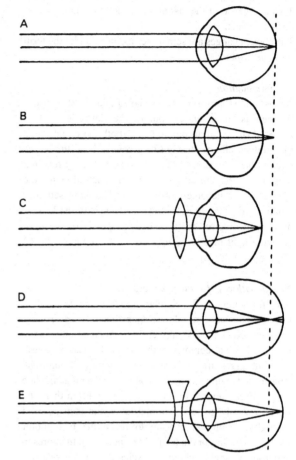

Fig. 17.9 Light refraction by lenses. A: Biconvex lens; B: biconvex lens of greater strength than A; C: same lens as A showing the refraction of light rays coming from a near point; D: biconcave lens. The line in the middle is the principal axis and F is the principal focus.

the visual pathways may be obtained by trying to elicit the **light reflex**. If light is shone on the blind half of the retina and the pupil constricts, it means that the pathway for the light reflex is intact; therefore, the lesion must be beyond the point where fibres leave the optic tract, just before the lateral geniculate body. If the light reflex is absent, the lesion must be in the optic nerve, chiasma or tracts before the fibres branch off.

Optics of the eye

Light rays coming from a distance greater than 6 m are considered *parallel*; those coming from less than 6 m away are considered *diverging*. When light passes from one medium to another medium of different density, it is **refracted** unless it strikes the interface between the two media perpendicularly. A biconvex lens converges parallel rays to a principal focus behind it, while a biconcave lens diverges parallel light rays, which may be extrapolated to give a **principal focus** in front (Fig. 17.9). The more curved the lens, the more it will bend the light and the shorter will be the focal length. The power of a lens (positive in the case of convex and negative in the case of concave) is measured in **dioptres (D)**. The dioptric power of a lens is the reciprocal of the focal length in metres. Thus, a lens with a focal length of 25 cm has a power of 1/0.25 m or 4 dioptres, while a lens with a focal length of 10 cm has a power of 10 dioptres.

The optically normal eye is termed **emmetropic**. In such an eye, parallel rays of light are refracted first by the cornea and then by the lens to be focused on the retina (Fig. 17.10A). When a normal individual is looking at the horizon, light is coming in parallel rays, the **ciliary muscle**

Fig. 17.10 Correction of common defects of refraction. (Reproduced from Emslie-Smith, D., Paterson, C.R., Scratcherd, T. & Read, N.W. (eds) (1988) *BDS Textbook of Physiology*, 11th edn. With permission from Churchill Livingstone, Edinburgh.)

is *relaxed* and the lens is under tension, so that it is in its most flattened shape. The power of this resting eye is about 60 D, with the cornea accounting for about 40–45 D and the lens 15–20 D. While *more refraction occurs at the cornea*, the advantage of the lens is, as will be explained, its ability to become more convex and therefore increase its power.

When the gaze is transferred from a far object to a near object (from which light rays would be diverging), certain changes occur in the eye in order to focus the image of the near object on the retina. These changes are:

1 Increasing the convexity or power of the lens, a process referred to as **accommodation**.

2 **Pupillary constriction**, so that light is concentrated on the more powerful centre of the crystalline lens.

3 Convergence of the **visual axes**, such that they meet at the near object.

The above changes are sometimes included under the term the *near response*.

Accommodation

At rest, the **ciliary muscle** is relaxed and the suspensory ligament is under tension, pulling the elastic lens into a flattened shape. In accommodation, both the circular and longitudinal ciliary muscle fibres *contract* and the whole ciliary body moves inward and forward, thereby relaxing tension on the suspensory ligament and allowing the *elastic lens* to become more convex. The increased convexity occurs mainly in the anterior surface of the lens. A number of dioptres are added to the power of the lens, allowing light rays to be focused on the retina (up to 12 dioptres in children).

Neural pathways for the near response

The ciliary muscle, the circular muscle in the iris and the two medial rectus muscles (responsible for *convergence* of visual axes) are all supplied by the oculomotor nerve, i.e. it is the final common pathway for the near response. Afferent fibres travel in the optic nerves through the chiasma to the optic tracts, synapse in the lateral geniculate body and *continue to the occipital cortex*. From there the fibres probably go to the frontal lobes and then descend through the internal capsule to reach the oculomotor nucleus in the midbrain. It should be noted that the fibres to and from the cerebral cortex are exclusive to the neural pathways for the *near response*. On the other hand, the fibres branching from the optic tract to the superior colliculus and proceeding to the oculomotor nucleus are exclusive to the pathway of the *pupillary light reflex*. A lesion in the pretectal region may occur in **neurosyphilis**, interrupting the **light reflex** but leaving the pathway for the near response intact, and resulting in the *Argyll Robertson pupil*, i.e. absent or sluggish response to light but constricting when looking at a near object.

Amplitude of accommodation and presbyopia

If an object is brought gradually nearer and nearer to the eye, a point is reached when the object cannot be focused and appears blurred. The nearest point to the eye where an object can be clearly seen is called the **near point**. At the near point the dioptric power of the eye is maximal, being equal to the sum of the power of the eye at rest plus the number of dioptres added by increasing the convexity of the lens. These additional dioptres are the **amplitude of accommodation**, which can be obtained by subtracting

Table 17.1 Variation of near point and accommodation with age.

Age (years)	Near point (cm)	Amplitude of accommodation (dioptres)
10	9.0	11.0
20	10.0	10.0
30	12.5	8.0
40	18.0	5.5
50	50.0	2.0
60	83.0	1.2
70	100.0	1.0

the power of the eye at rest from the total power at the near point. If the resting dioptric power of the eye is taken as zero, the amplitude of accommodation in dioptres is given by the reciprocal of the distance of the near point from the eye in metres, e.g. if the near point is 10 cm away, the amplitude of accommodation would be 10 dioptres.

With advancing age, the lens gradually loses its elasticity and therefore its capacity to increase its convexity. Consequently, the near point recedes and the amplitude of accommodation decreases with advancing age—a process called **presbyopia**. This is clearly illustrated in Table 17.1. By the age of 40–45 years, the near point starts to recede at a faster rate and close work becomes increasingly difficult. Many people beyond the age of 40 years require glasses with convex lenses for close work.

The retinal image

The refractive index of each of the cornea, aqueous humour and vitreous humour is 1.33, i.e. about the same as water, while the lens has a refractive index of 1.42. Normally, light is refracted towards the normal by the cornea and by the anterior surface of the lens, and away from the normal by the posterior surface of the lens, to be focused on the retina. This process may be simplified by assuming that all refraction is occurring at the cornea, and by defining the optic centre or **nodal point** of the eye, as in the schematic or **reduced eye of Listing** (Fig. 17.11). Any light ray passing through the nodal point is not refracted, but rays passing through any other point are refracted to be focused on the retina. In humans, the distance of the nodal point from the retina is about 15 mm. For an object AB, the retinal image is represented by ab in Fig. 17.11. Thus, the retinal image is inverted and this inversion continues to the occipital cortex. From infancy, the brain is genetically programmed to reverse the inversion so that we see the world the right way up.

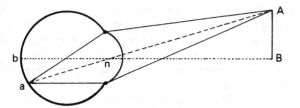

Fig. 17.11 Reduced or schematic eye showing the nodal point n. In this diagram it is assumed that all refraction takes place at the cornea. The refracted dotted lines converge on the retina to give an inverted image.

Triangles AnB and anb in Fig. 17.11 are similar and therefore:

$$\frac{AB}{ab} = \frac{Bn}{bn}$$

If the height of an object and its distance from the eye are known, and given that bn is equal to 15 mm, the size of the retinal image can be calculated.

Angle AnB is called the **visual angle**. It is the angle subtended by an object at the nodal point of the eye. Assessment of visual acuity, i.e. how well we can distinguish details in the field of vision, depends upon this angle. As long as two lines are separated by an arc of at least 1 minute and thus subtend a minimum visual angle of 1 minute at the nodal point, the distance between the two images on the retina will be 2 μm. In this case, two separate cones are stimulated by each point on the lines, leaving one unstimulated cone in between (the diameter of a cone is 1.5 μm). This means that the two lines are perceived as separate. Separation by an arc of less than 1 minute will stimulate two adjacent cones and the two lines will be perceived as a single line. Letters or symbols on charts which are used for assessing visual acuity are written so that the thickness of a line subtends a visual angle of 1 minute and the whole letter or symbol subtends an angle of 5 minutes at the nodal point. A subject stands at 6 m away from the chart and his/her visual acuity is given by the ratio d/D, where d is the distance from the chart (6 m) and D the distance indicated on the chart for the row that the subject has been able to read or identify correctly. Thus, normal visual acuity is 6/6, while a visual acuity of 6/12 is subnormal and indicates that the subject sees at 6 m what a normal subject can see at 12 m away.

Errors of refraction

Abnormalities of the length of the eyeball or its refractive power result in either **hypermetropia** (long-sightedness) or **myopia** (short-sightedness) (see Fig. 17.10). These abnormalities may be referred to as ametropia.

In **hypermetropia** the eyeball is too short and parallel rays of light are focused behind the retina. An affected individual has to employ some accommodation even for distant objects, leading to headaches and hypertrophy of the ciliary muscles from excessive use. The near point is further than the position in accordance with age so that glasses are required for close work at an earlier age. Glasses with convex lenses are used to correct the defect.

In **myopia** the eyeball is too long and parallel rays of light are brought to a focus in front of the retina. The far point becomes finite, i.e. the subject cannot see far, while the near point is too near for age and consequently the amplitude of accommodation is reduced. A myopic individual would not require glasses for close work, even in his/her old age. The defect is corrected by biconcave lenses.

Astigmatism. This is a condition in which the curvature of the cornea is not uniform; rarely, the lens may be affected. Light refracted by one meridian is focused differently from light refracted by another unequal meridian. Typically, an individual affected by astigmatism cannot focus vertical and horizontal lines on graph paper at the same time. The defect is corrected by *cylindrical lenses*, which focus light to a line, thus correcting the curvature in a certain meridian and ensuring the overall uniformity of curvature.

The duplicity theory

The visible spectrum extends from the 397 nm to the 723 nm wavelength of light. Within this range, the eye can function under two conditions of illumination: **dim light** and **bright light**. Vision in dim light is termed **scotopic vision** and in this type only the outline of objects in the field of vision can be distinguished; no details or colour can be appreciated. **Photopic vision** is employed in bright light and in it the details of objects, as well as their colour, can be distinguished. The presence of scotopic and photopic vision and the consequent double input from the eye to the central nervous system are the elements of the **duplicity theory**.

The scotopic visibility curve peaks at the 505 nm wavelength, while the photopic curve peaks at the 550 nm wavelength of light (Fig. 17.12). Scotopic vision is served by the rods, while photopic vision is due to the cones. This has been proved by the finding that the light absorbance of the rod pigment, rhodopsin, coincides almost exactly with the scotopic visibility curve, peaking at the 505 nm wavelength of light. The cones have three pigments, each

Fig. 17.12 Visibility curves for photopic (cones) and scotopic (rods) vision showing the wavelength range for each. The relative sensitivity has been equalized in this diagram. In reality, rod sensitivity is far greater.

most sensitive to one of the primary colours (see below). The light absorbance curve of a mixture of the three pigments also coincides with the photopic visibility curve, peaking at the 550 nm wavelength. It should be noted that

the Y axis in Fig. 17.12 is relative sensitivity, i.e. maximal sensitivity in both cases is taken as 100% and lesser sensitivities are expressed as a percentage. If absolute sensitivity values were employed, the curves would be of the same shape but the scotopic curve would be much higher than the photopic curve.

Figure 17.13 shows the range of luminance within which the eye may function. Note the great sensitivity of rod or scotopic vision and that there is a transition zone between rod vision and cone vision.

Photosensitive pigments

The pigments in the outer segments of rods and cones have two components: **retinene**, which is the aldehyde of vitamin A (retinol), and a protein called **opsin**. Retinene is the same in all the pigments; differences between the pigments are in the amino acid sequence of the opsin.

The opsin in **rhodopsin** is termed **scotopsin**. The amino acid sequence of scotopsin is determined by a gene on chromosome 3. Light bleaches rhodopsin or separates it into retinene and scotopsin. Recent work has shown that

Fig. 17.13 The range of luminance to which the human eye responds. The receptive mechanisms are indicated in the column on the right. (Reproduced from Emslie-Smith, D., Paterson, C.C., Scratcherd, T. & Read, N.W. (eds) (1989) *BDS Textbook of Physiology*, 11th edn. With permission from Churchill Livingstone, Edinburgh.)

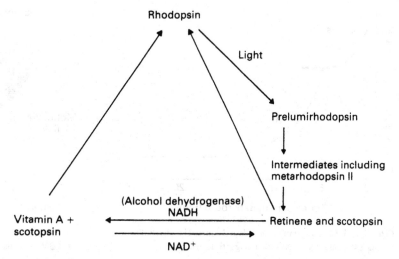

Fig. 17.14 The rhodopsin cycle in humans. NADH, NAD⁺, reduced and oxidized forms of nicotinamide adenine dinucleotide.

light actually acts only on retinene, changing its isomerism from the 11-*cis* form to the all-*trans* form. The shape of retinene is changed, giving rise to **prelumirhodopsin**, which subsequently changes to some intermediates, including metarhodopsin II, before being hydrolysed to retinene and scotopsin. Retinene and scotopsin may recombine to reconstitute rhodopsin. More slowly, retinene may be changed back to vitamin A, under the influence of the enzyme alcohol dehydrogenase, and vitamin A with scotopsin may regenerate rhodopsin. These changes are summarized in Fig. 17.14.

The action of light on the cone pigments is probably similar. The action of light on the photosensitive pigments in the outer segments of rods and cones results in the generation of receptor potentials, which lead to action potentials in the optic nerve fibres, as will be explained below.

The role played by vitamin A in rod function explains the fact that deficiency of this vitamin leads to impairment of the ability to see in dim light and may result in nightblindness or *nyctalopia*. With persistent vitamin A deficiency, cone function may also be affected.

The cone pigments and colour vision

The primary colours are red, green and blue. When red light (wavelength 723–647 nm), green light (575–429 nm) and blue light (492–450 nm) are mixed, white light or any spectral colour may be obtained. The **Young–Helmholtz** theory explaining colour vision in humans is now widely accepted. According to this theory, there are three types of cones, each containing a pigment most sensitive to one of the primary colours. Light entering the eye stimulates the cones in proportion to its spectral components and the differential discharge is coded and conveyed to the occipital cortex. Colour is sensed by cones in the fovea centralis and appreciated within photopic vision.

Human cone pigments have been named as follows:
- The red-sensitive or long-wave pigment.
- The green-sensitive or medium-wave pigment.
- The blue-sensitive or short-wave pigment.

Each of these pigments contains retinene and an opsin which differs among pigments in some of its amino acid sequence. The amino acid sequences of the opsins of the red- and green-sensitive pigments are very similar (96% homology), as they are both determined by adjacent genes on the X chromosome. The amino acid sequence of the opsin of the blue-sensitive pigment is determined by a gene on the autosomal chromosome 7 and has only 43% homology with each of the opsins of the red-sensitive and green-sensitive pigments. All the opsins of the cone pigments have 41% homology with the opsin of rhodopsin.

Colour-blindness

Colour-blindness may be due to weakness in detecting one of the primary colours, or to blindness to one or even two of the primary colours. Human beings may be divided into:

1 *Trichromats*. These include people who are normal in all respects in relation to colour perception, plus those with **weakness** in detecting **red, green or blue**, i.e. they need more of the affected primary colour to perceive colour normally.

2 *Dichromats*. These are **completely blind to red or green or blue** and they get their colour sensation by mixing only two of the primary colours.

Fig. 17.15 Dark adaptation for rods and cones. The threshold decreases as the subject stays for a longer time in the dark.

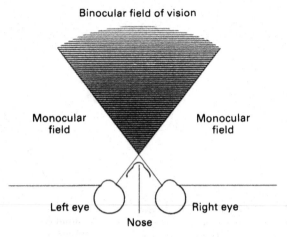

Fig. 17.16 Monocular and binocular fields of vision. The shaded area enclosed by the two fields is seen by both eyes (binocular vision).

3 *Monochromats.* These have only **one cone pigment**; to them the world is black and white and shades of grey.

Colour-blindness commonly affects red and green and in this case is usually inherited as a recessive factor on the X chromosome. As such, it affects men more than women and, although heterozygous women do not show the defect, they transmit it to half of their sons. In people of European stock, about 8% of males but only 0.4% of females are affected by colour defects in relation to red or green. Abnormalities in relation to blue are rare and are not sex-linked when inherited. Monochromats are extremely rare and they have other neurological defects. One of the convenient methods to test for colour-blindness is to use polychromatic plates (**Ishihara charts**). These indicate numbers or lines made of spots of certain colours against a background of confusing colours; a key gives the expected responses by normal people and by people affected by colour-blindness.

Dark adaptation

If a person is in brightly lit surroundings, he/she is using cones. If the light is suddenly switched off, at first nothing can be seen, but gradually the outline of objects in the field of vision starts to appear and the situation improves with time, reaching a maximum in about 20 minutes (Fig. 17.15). This is called **dark adaptation**, during which only the gross features of objects can be distinguished—not their details or colour.

It has been shown that, during the first 5 minutes, the threshold for cones decreases (or their sensitivity increases). From 5 to 20 minutes in the dark, a great increase occurs in the sensitivity of the rods, which thus account

for the greater share of dark adaptation. The main part of the time required for dark adaptation to reach its maximum is needed for *regeneration of rhodopsin* so that rods can function optimally. The changes that occur in the cones during the first 5 minutes are not fully understood. If light is switched on again, the rods are knocked out of action and the cones start to function, adjusting to the level of brightness within 5 minutes; this process may be called light adaptation.

Binocular vision

The field of vision for each eye may be mapped by using an instrument called the perimeter, the process being called perimetry. Basically, the subject looks with one eye at the point of fixation, while a target is moved along an arc at a certain meridian. The points where the target just enters into view for each meridian are marked on a chart. The field of vision for each eye is mapped on a separate chart. When in real life we use both eyes, the areas in the centre of the field of vision for the two eyes overlap and any object in this area will be seen by both eyes, i.e. the vision is **binocular**. At the temporal part of each field, vision is **monocular** (Fig. 17.16).

In binocular vision there would be two retinal images. The eyes are actually moved by the extraocular muscles in such a way as to ensure that the two retinal images fall on corresponding points on the retinae, the connections of these being organized so that the two images completely fuse at the cortical level. If one of the extraocular muscles is paralysed, e.g. the lateral rectus muscle, the affected eye is deviated inward as a result of the unopposed action of the medial rectus, and double vision or **diplopia** results, since the retinal image in the affected eye is not on the corresponding point.

Depth perception

Appreciation of depth in the field of vision is essentially monocular but is improved when using the two eyes. Two clues from the field of vision requiring only one eye are used to gauge depth: first, the relative sizes of objects—the further the object, the smaller it appears; secondly, *movement parallax*, by which near moving objects move right across the field of vision but distant moving objects appear to be almost stationary. Binocular vision contributes to depth perception through the process of *stereopsis*: a near object has its retinal image on the temporal part of the two retinae while the image of a far object falls to the nasal side towards the centre of the retina. This creates a kind of parallax in relation to location on the retina, which is, in turn, taken to the visual cortex and analysed.

Critical fusion frequency (CFF)

If a light source is interrupted regularly, as by a rotating notched disc, the light flickers. As the rate of interruption is increased, a frequency is reached when the flicker disappears and the light appears continuous. The frequency at which complete fusion of the successive flickering images just occurs to give an illusion of continuity is called the **critical fusion frequency (CFF)**. To ensure complete fusion, the light stimulus has to be delivered at a rate just exceeding the CFF. In motion pictures, frames are usually delivered at a rate of 24 per second, which is more than the CFF. If the projector slows down and the frequency of the frames drops to below the CFF, the picture on the screen starts to flicker.

Electrophysiology of vision

When light strikes the outer segments of rods and cones, it causes changes in the photosensitive pigments. These changes lead to receptor potentials, which are converted to action potentials in the optic nerve fibres.

There is Na^+, K^+ ATPase in the inner segment of rods. In the dark, Na^+ is pumped to the outside but it re-enters through sodium channels in the membranes of the outer segments and the synaptic zone, creating a continuous sodium current. When light strikes the outer segments, it changes the isomerism of retinene and produces several intermediates before complete bleaching of rhodopsin. One of the intermediates is **metarhodopsin II**, which leads to activation of transducin (a Gt protein). This causes activation of phosphodiesterase, which decreases intracellular

Light
↓
Change in photopigment isomerism
↓
Metarhodopsin II
↓
Activation of transducin
↓
Activation of Phosphodiesterase
↓
Decreased intracellular cyclic GMP
↓
Closure of sodium channels
↓
Hyperpolarization of receptor
↓
Potential change in bipolar cells and other neurones and ultimately action potentials in optic nerve fibres

Fig. 17.17 Possible linkage sequence between photopigment changes and electrical events in the retina.

cyclic guanosine monophosphate (cGMP) through converting it to 5'-GMP, and, as a result, closure of some of the sodium channels takes place in the membrane of the outer segments. This leads to less sodium entering and creates a negative potential. Thus, rods respond to light by *hyperpolarization* (Fig. 17.17). Cones also respond by hyperpolarization. While hyperpolarization in rods has a fast onset and slow offset, both processes are fast in cones.

A number of synaptic transmitters have been found in the retina, including acetylcholine, dopamine, serotonin, gamma-aminobutyric acid (GABA), substance P, somatostatin, vasoactive peptide (VIP), encephalin and other peptides. It seems that in the dark these transmitters are continuously released. By causing hyperpolarization in the receptors, light *decreases* the release of the transmitters, leading to electric potentials in **horizontal cells, bipolar neurons** and **amacrine cells**. The depolarizing potentials in amacrine cells have been identified as the **generator potentials** leading to action potential spikes in the **ganglion neurons** and optic nerve fibres.

Ganglion cells in the retina respond to light in the form of circles. One-half of the ganglion neurons discharge when the centre of the circular field is illuminated but are inhibited by illumination of the periphery of the field (**on-centre cells**). The other half discharges to illumination of the periphery but is inhibited by stimulation of the centre (**off-centre cells**). Cells in the **lateral geniculate body** and some neurons in cortical area 17 respond in a similar fashion. This type of response may be responsible for demarcating the edges of objects in the field of vision.

Two types of **cortical neurons** have been identified: simple cells, in area 17, and complex cells, mainly in the association areas 18 and 19 but also in area 17. Both respond to light in the form of lines. Simple cells respond according to the orientation of the line stimulus and neurons responding to the same orientation are arranged in vertical columns, called orientation columns, in the occipital cortex. Complex cells respond to the orientation of the light stimulus but discharge more when the line stimulus is moved and may thus be responsible for detecting form and movement. Most cortical neurons concerned with vision respond either to one eye or to the other. Neurons responding to the ipsilateral eye are arranged in vertical columns, alternating with columns of neurons responding to the contralateral eye; these are called **ocular dominance columns**. About half of the complex cells respond to stimuli from both eyes and may be concerned with stereopsis, which requires binocular vision.

Transmission of impulses along the visual pathways and cortical functions

Axons of retinal ganglion cells project a detailed spatial representation on the lateral geniculate body, which has six layers. Layers 1 and 2 contain large cells and receive impulses from large ganglion cells; this pathway is concerned with detection of movement, stereopsis and flicker. Layers 3–6 have small cells and receive impulses from small ganglion cells, and the pathway is concerned with colour vision, texture and shape of objects. The lateral geniculate body in turn projects a point-by-point representation on the visual cortex, which also has six layers. There are groups of cells in the visual cortex called *blobs* which are concerned with deciphering colour. Colour and visual detail are finally projected to association areas

in the anteroventral portion of the **occipital lobe** and the venteroposterior aspect of the **temporal lobe**. Form, three-dimensional position and movement are finally analysed at the superior portions of the **occipital lobe** and posterior **parietal lobe**.

Eye movements

The actions of the six extraocular muscles should be ascertained from an anatomy text. *Abduction* and *adduction* refer to rotation of the eyeball around the vertical axis, *elevation* and *depression* around the transverse horizontal axis and *intorsion* and *extorsion* around the horizontal anteroposterior axis. The nerve supply of the extraocular muscle may be conveniently remembered by referring to the following nonsensical formula: $LR_6(SO_4)_3$, i.e. the lateral rectus is supplied by the 6th or **abducent nerve**, the superior oblique is supplied by the 4th or **trochlear nerve**, and the rest are innervated by the 3rd or oculomotor nerve. The actions of extraocular muscles are highly coordinated in order to ensure that retinal images fall on corresponding points; otherwise, *diplopia* results.

There are four types of eye fixation movements which are related to visual function:

1 *Saccadic movements*. These are very rapid conjugate movements of the eyes, occurring when inspecting an object, when the gaze shifts from one object to another or during reading. Since they are present most of the time, they may be responsible for prevention of adaptation to the retinal image, which, if allowed, might lead to disappearance of objects under constant view! Sometimes eye movements responsible for preventing visual adaptation are referred to as **physiological nystagmus**.

2 *Smooth pursuit movements*. As the name implies, by these movements the eyes follow or track moving objects.

3 *Vergence movements*. **Convergence** occurs when the gaze is changed from a far to a near object or when fixing on an approaching object. **Divergence** of the visual axes occurs when the gaze is transferred from a near to a far object or when watching an object moving away.

4 *Vestibular movements*. These occur in order to maintain visual fixation when the head moves. During rotation the eyes move in the opposite direction in order to maintain fixation. When the limit is reached, the eyes snap back, and the process is repeated, leading to **nystagmus**.

All these movements are initiated in neural pathways related to their function, e.g. vestibular movements are initiated by stimuli in the semicircular canals and travel in the vestibular pathways, but the final common pathway is constituted by the nuclei of the 3rd, 4th and 6th cranial nerves, which innervate the extraocular muscles.

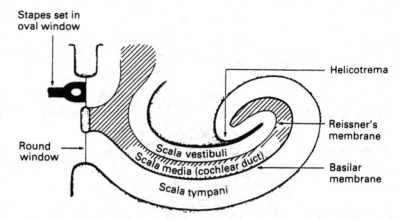

Stapes set in
oval window

Helicotrema

Reissner's
membrane

Round
window

Scala vestibuli

Scala media (cochlear duct)

Basilar
membrane

Scala tympani

Fig. 17.18 Diagram of the inner ear. (Reproduced from Bray, J.J., Cragg, P.A., Macknight, A.D.C., Mills, R.G. & Taylor, D.W. (eds) (1989) *Lecture Notes in Physiology*, 2nd edn. Blackwell Scientific Publications, Oxford.)

Hearing

Anatomical considerations

The ear consists of the outer, the middle and the inner ear. The **outer ear** consists of the pinna and the external auditory canal, directed medially and forwards to the eardrum or **tympanic membrane**. The tympanic membrane is shaped like a shallow funnel, with the tip of the funnel or umbo pointing inwards. It is lined by skin on the outside and mucous membrane on the inside. The **middle ear** is a cavity in the temporal bone filled with air and containing the three **ossicles**: the **malleus**, the **incus** and the **stapes**. The handle of the malleus (manubrium) is attached to the back of the tympanic membrane with its tip at the umbo; the head of the malleus articulates with the incus, the process of which articulates with the head of the stapes. The footplate of the stapes is attached to the wall of the **oval window** of the cochlea by an annular ligament, which is fixed firmly at a posterior point but is slightly loose otherwise, to allow for movement of the footplate.

The air in the cavity of the middle ear communicates with the nasopharynx through the **Eustachian** or **auditory tube** and then with the outside air. The opening of the auditory tube in the nasopharynx is normally closed but it opens during chewing, swallowing and yawning, to allow equalization of pressure between the middle ear and atmospheric pressure, i.e. on both sides of the tympanic membrane. A severe head cold may cause inflammation which closes off the auditory tube. The air trapped in the middle ear is partly absorbed, leading to atmospheric pressure pressing on the tympanic membrane and causing discomfort and reduced acuity of hearing.

There are two small striated muscles in the middle ear: (i) the **tensor tympani**, attached to the neck of the malleus;

when it contracts, it pulls the drum medially; and (ii) the **stapedius**, attached to the neck of the stapes; when it contracts, it tends to pull the footplate of the stapes out of the oval window. Simultaneous contraction of the two muscles reduces conduction of sound to the cochlea. Very loud sounds lead to reflex contraction of the tensor tympani and the stapedius, which thus reduces transmission of these loud sounds to the auditory receptors. This is termed the **tympanic reflex**, which is protective; however, it has a latent period of 40–160 ms, which makes it ineffective against brief sounds of high intensity.

The **inner ear** or labyrinth consists of the bony and membranous labyrinth. The bony part is a series of channels in the petrous part of the temporal bone, and membranes run inside the bony channels to form the **membranous labyrinth**. Between the bone and membranes is a fluid called **perilymph**, while inside the membranous labyrinth the fluid is **endolymph**; the two fluids do not mix. In the inner ear the **semicircular canals**, the **utricle** and the **saccule** are concerned with balance and are part of the vestibular system, which has been described in Chapter 16. The **cochlea** is concerned with hearing. In humans the cochlea is about 35 mm long; it is coiled spirally around a central bony pillar, called the modiolus, making two and three-quarter turns. Throughout its length it is divided into three chambers by two membranes: **Reissner's membrane** and the **basilar membrane** (Fig. 17.18). The upper chamber is called the **scala vestibuli**, which ends laterally at the oval window. The lower chamber is called the **scala tympani**, which ends laterally at the round window, which is closed by a **secondary tympanic membrane**. Between the two membranes is the **scala media** or **cochlear duct**, containing endolymph. Both the scala vestibuli and the scala tympani contain perilymph and communicate with each other at the apex of the cochlea (the helicotrema).

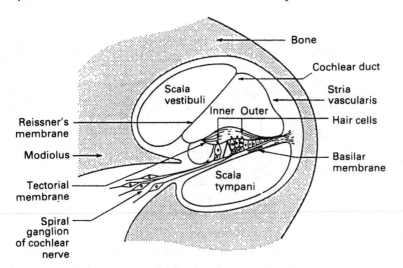

Fig. 17.19 Cross-section through the canals of the cochlea showing the organ of Corti (containing the hair cells) sitting on the basilar membrane. The inner and outer hair cells are separated by the tunnel of Corti. (Reproduced from Bray, J.J., Cragg, P.A., Macknight, A.D.C., Mills, R.G. & Taylor, D.W. (eds) (1989) *Lecture Notes in Physiology*, 2nd edn. Blackwell Scientific Publications, Oxford.)

The receptors for hearing are hair cells, which are found in the **organ of Corti** (Fig. 17.19). The organ of Corti sits on the basilar membrane and extends from the base to the apex of the cochlea. Between the rods of Corti is the tunnel of Corti, which contains perilymph. There is a single row of **inner hair cells** medial to the tunnel of Corti and numbering about 3500. Lateral to the tunnel of Corti are three rows of **outer hair cells**, numbering about 20 000. The hair cells have processes or **stereocilia** that pierce the tough reticular lamina. The processes of the outer, but not inner, hair cells are embedded in the elastic ribbon-like **tectorial membrane**. Nerve fibres, with cell bodies in the **spiral ganglion**, branch extensively around the bases of the hair cells. There are 28 000 fibres in the auditory nerve. About 90–95% innervate the inner hair cells, while only 5–10% supply the more numerous outer hair cells.

The auditory pathways

The axons of the neurons that innervate the hair cells constitute the cochlear division of the 8th nerve and synapse in the **dorsal** and **ventral cochlear nuclei** in the medulla (Fig. 17.20). Second-order neurons arise from these and go to synapse in the olive and trapezoid body of the same and opposite side, with slightly more fibres crossing to the opposite side than those proceeding ipsilaterally. Fibres then ascend in the lateral lemniscus. Some fibres synapse in the **nucleus of the lateral lemniscus** and most of the fibres then proceed to synapse bilaterally in the **inferior colliculi** and then in the **medial geniculate bodies** of the thalamus. Some collaterals from the lateral lemniscus go directly to the **medial geniculate body**, while other collaterals enter the **reticular formation**. From the medial

geniculate body, fibres are finally projected bilaterally to the **auditory cortex** Brodman's area 41, in the superior portion of the temporal lobe. There are auditory association areas adjacent to the primary auditory cortex. It should be noted that, once fibres leave the cochlear nuclei, they proceed *bilaterally* up to the cortex.

The auditory nerve also contains retrograde fibres which arise from the auditory cortex and reaches the cochlea through the superior olivary complex. These fibres are referred to as the **olivocochlear bundle**. The function of these retrograde or **centrifugal** signals is to inhibit specific areas of the organ of Corti and this sharpens attention to particular sounds, e.g. one instrument in an orchestra.

Sound

Sound, unlike light, requires a medium to travel in. It travels in air at the speed of 344 m/s and at a faster speed in water. Sound travels in the form of waves, which, in their simplest form, can be represented as sine waves (Fig. 17.21). There are two basic properties of sound waves: (i) **amplitude**, which determines the *intensity* of sound or its *loudness*—the higher the amplitude, the greater the intensity of sound; and (ii) **frequency**, or the number of cycles per second (Hz), which determines the *pitch* or tone of sound—the higher the frequency, the higher the pitch of sound. Intensity refers to the strength of the sound in physical terms, while loudness denotes appreciation of the sound intensity by the hearing apparatus. Loudness is affected by the frequency of sound (see Audibility below). Complex sounds with regularly repeating patterns are perceived as music, while sound waves of irregular frequency give a sensation of noise.

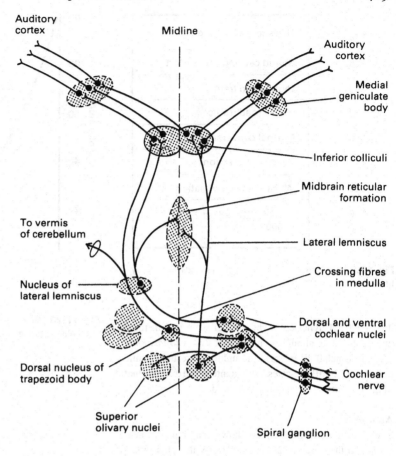

Fig. 17.20 Diagram of the main auditory pathways.

Fig. 17.21 Amplitude and frequency of sound waves. A: Record of a pure tone; B: same frequency (pitch) but lower amplitude (loudness) than A; C: same amplitude but greater frequency than B; D: shows a regularly repeated wave pattern, usually perceived as a musical sound; E: shows no regular wave pattern—this is perceived as noise.

Sound intensity may be measured in terms of energy, in microwatts or ergs per second, or pressure, in dynes/cm². The range in intensity between the threshold of sound and the loudest sound that can be tolerated is very large. It would therefore be inconvenient to employ a linear absolute scale to measure sound intensity in everyday life. A comparative logarithmic scale is employed, in which the basic unit is the bel (after A.G. Bell):

$$\text{bel} = \log \frac{\text{intensity of sound}}{\text{intensity of standard sound}}$$

Since intensity is directly proportional to the square of the sound pressure:

$$\text{bel} = 2 \log \frac{\text{pressure of sound}}{\text{pressure of standard sound}}$$

The bel is too large for everyday use and the decibel is used instead:

decibel (dB) = 0.1 bel

$$\text{Intensity of sound in decibels} = 20 \log \frac{\text{pressure of sound}}{\text{pressure of standard sound}}$$

The standard sound adopted as reference is the auditory threshold in healthy young people; in physical terms

Fig. 17.22 Scale (in decibels) for common sounds in everyday life.

Fig. 17.23 Part of the human audibility curve showing the threshold of hearing at different frequencies.

it is 0.000204 dynes/cm². The decibel scale is illustrated in Fig. 17.22. It should be noted that it is a *logarithmic scale*, in which 0 dB refers to the auditory threshold, while a sound of 120 dB indicates a sound intensity 10^6 times that of the intensity of the auditory threshold.

Audibility

The human **audibility curve** shows that humans hear sounds in the range of 20–20 000 Hz. Within this range, the threshold is lowest in the range 1000–4000 Hz and greater at lower and higher frequencies (Fig. 17.23). **Pitch discrimination** is best in the range 1000–3000 Hz. Human beings can distinguish up to 2000 pitches and training can even improve on this, as musicians do. In ordinary conversation the average male voice has a frequency of about 120 Hz while that of the female voice is about 250 Hz. Very loud sounds are felt as well as heard and are also partly conducted through the bones of the skull.

The mechanism of hearing

When sound waves strike the tympanic membrane, it vibrates with them but the vibration stops as soon as the sound ceases. Movement of the tympanic membrane is conducted through the ossicles to the oval window of the cochlea (Fig. 17.24). The ossicles constitute a system of levers which increases the force acting on the tympanic membrane by 1.3 times. Since the area of the tympanic membrane (about 50 mm²) is approximately 17 times that of the oval window of the cochlea (3 mm²), the pressure created by movement of the tympanic membrane is

Fig. 17.24 The movements of the bony ossicles and the oval window are converted into waves in the fluids of the inner ear. The waves die out at the round window. The tympanic membrane, bony ossicles, oval window and basilar membrane are indicated. (Reproduced from Passmore, R. & Robson, J.S. (eds) (1976) *Companion to Medical Studies*, 2nd edn, Vol. 1. Blackwell Scientific Publications, Oxford.)

Fig. 17.25 Displacement of various parts of the basilar membrane produced by waves in the cochlear fluids. The frequencies of the waves are shown at the top of each wave. It is seen that each part of the membrane shows maximal displacement at a different frequency, depending on the distance from the stapes. This gave rise to the place theory of the discrimination of pitch (frequency). (Reproduced from Bray, J.J., Cragg, P.A., Macknight, A.D.C., Mills, R.G. & Taylor, D.W. (eds) (1989) *Lecture Notes in Physiology*, 2nd edn. Blackwell Scientific Publications, Oxford.)

multiplied 17 times when it arrives at the oval window. This means that the force of sound vibration is multiplied 1.3×17 times or 22 times when it arrives at the oval window. Indeed, it has been calculated that about 60% of the sound energy is transmitted to the cochlea, which is a high efficiency when considering the inevitable loss due to resistance.

Sound may be conducted to the cochlea either by air or through bone. **Air conduction** constitutes the normal situation, when sound waves travelling in air cause vibration of the tympanic membrane, which is transmitted by the ossicles to the oval window of the cochlea. In **bone conduction** the sound causes vibration of the bones of the skull, directly transmitting the sound vibrations to the cochlea, e.g. when the base of a vibrating tuning-fork is put on the mastoid process or the forehead. Under normal circumstances, air conduction is more efficient than conduction through bone.

As indicated in Fig. 17.24, the footplate of the stapes rocks at the oval window like a hinged door fixed at a posterior point. This movement causes a pressure wave, which travels through the perilymph in the scala vestibuli and, through vibration of Reissner's membrane, to the endolymph of the scala media; this, in turn, conveys the wave to the perilymph of the scala tympani, through the vibration of the basilar membrane, and the wave eventually dies away at the round window of the cochlea. Normally the basilar membrane is not under tension. Stimulation of the hair cells is effected through vibration of the basilar membrane, on which the organ of Corti sits.

Like the arterial pulse wave, travelling waves in the cochlea reach a peak and then decline, to dissipate at the round window. High-frequency sounds reach a peak at the *base* of the cochlea, while low-frequency sounds peak at the *apex* of the cochlea, and medium frequencies

peak in betweem with displacement of the basilar membrane closely following this pattern (Fig. 17.25). Nerve fibres from each part of the basilar membrane are distinct and signal the place at which the wave has peaked to the auditory cortex. This is the main mechanism for **discrimination of pitch** or tone of sound and has been referred to as the **place principle**. However, this principle does not explain discrimination between sound frequencies below 2000 Hz. It has been found that, in addition to this, sound frequencies from 20 to 2000 Hz are also signalled to the cortex by having one burst of action potential synchronized with each sound wave, i.e. a **volley effect**. The place principle plus the volley effect has recently been referred to as the **duplex theory** of hearing.

Receptor potentials and the endocochlear potential

The hair cells are sitting on the basilar membrane with their upper ends fixed in the reticular lamina. Upper displacement of the basilar membrane moves the reticular lamina upwards and inward, while downward displacement of the basilar membrane moves the reticular lamina downward and outwards. The inward and outward movement of the reticular lamina causes a *shearing force* in relation to the tectorial membrane and bends the stereocilia of the outer hair cells. The stereocilia of the inner hair cells are bent by fluid movement under the tectorial membrane, to which they are not attached. Bending of the stereocilia of the hair cells alternately opens and closes cation channels at the tips of the stereocilia; entry of K^+ causes *depolarization*, while blocking K^+ entry causes hyperpolarization. The alternate depolarization and hyperpolarization constitute the hair cell **receptor potentials**, which thus change (transduce) the bending of the stereocilia into electrical energy. The receptor potential is directly proportional to the displacement of the basilar membrane and faithfully reproduces the characteristics of the sound. It probably releases a neurotransmitter that depolarizes the cochlear nerve endings, thus leading to action potentials in auditory nerve fibres.

Perilymph, which is formed mainly from plasma, has a composition similar to that of the extracellular fluid, with high Na^+ and low K^+ concentrations, while the composition of endolymph is nearer to that of the intracellular fluid, with low Na^+ and high K^+ concentrations. Endolymph is formed by the stria vascularis, which has a highly active Na^+, K^+ ATPase and an electrogenic K^+ pump. Studies with microelectrodes have shown that endolymph in the scala media has a positive potential (+80 mV) in relation to perilymph in either the scala vestibuli or the scala tympani; it is referred to as the *endocochlear potential*. Since the basilar membrane is relatively permeable to perilymph in the scala tympani, the tunnel of Corti and consequently the bases of the hair cells are bathed in perilymph; the stereocilia of the hair cells are bathed in endolymph. As the resting potential inside the hair cells is −60 mV, the potential difference across the tips of the stereocilia is 140 mV (60 mV + 80 mV). This high potential may be important for increasing the sensitivity of the hair cells to stimulation.

Function of the hair cells

It has recently been recognized that the inner and outer hair cells have somewhat different functions. The stereocilia of the inner hair cells are not embedded in the tectorial membrane and are actually bent by fluid movement under the tectorial membrane as explained above. It is now clear that the inner hair cells are the primary receptors for sound, transducing the fluid movement in the cochlea into action potentials in the auditory nerve. The outer hair cells, although far more numerous, stimulate only a small fraction of nerve fibres in the cochlear nerve. However, damage to these cells causes a significant loss of hearing. They seem to control the sensitivity of the inner hair cells. Retrograde (centrifugal) signals from the auditory cortex through the superior olivary nucleus to the proximity of the outer hair cells have been found to cause inhibition of their discharge and therefore to increase the sensitivity of adjacent hair cells to particular sound frequencies.

Pattern of impulse discharge in the auditory nerve and brain mechanisms

The pattern of the action potentials in the auditory nerve to the brain is responsible for the discrimination of pitch and loudness (intensity) of sound. At threshold sound intensity, an auditory nerve fibre discharges to one sound frequency,

depending upon the point in the basilar membrane being stimulated. As the intensity increases, the range of sound frequencies and area of basilar membrane stimulated widens; this increases the number of stimulated hair cells, causing spatial summation of impulses and increased spike rate of the action potentials. Thus, *impulse frequency* in the auditory nerve principally signals *loudness*. As previously explained, *pitch* is mainly determined by the place in the basilar membrane which is maximally displaced. Also low sound frequencies between 20 and 2000 Hz are signaled by a synchronous pattern of nerve impulse discharge (*the volley effect*).

The basilar membrane is represented on the auditory cortex with low tones anterolaterally and high tones posteromedially. The *auditory cortex* is also concerned with *sound localization*. The **auditory association areas**, adjacent to the primary auditory cortex are concerned with *interpreting* the meaning of the sound heard. In human beings a unilateral lesion affecting the primary auditory cortex will only slightly reduce hearing in the opposite ear because of the bilateral cortical connections of the auditory pathways.

Sound localization

The main mechanism for sound localization involves using the two ears. Differences in the time of arrival of the sound wave at the two ears (time-lag), as well as the differences in loudness, by which the nearer ear hears louder than the other, are employed as clues for localization. The time-lag mechanism works best for frequencies below 3000 Hz; the difference in the sound intensity mechanism is best for frequencies above 3000 Hz. For people deaf in one ear, some localization is possible by making use of a clue resulting from transformation of the sound wave front by the angle of the pinna.

Masking

The presence of a background sound affects the ability to hear another sound in the environment, i.e. background noise can mask the sound *wholly* or partly. Masking is due to the fact that some of the receptors are already stimulated and therefore refractory when the sound desired to be heard arrives. Masking is more effective when two sounds have similar rather than widely differing frequencies. Masking is present all the time in natural environments and is automatically taken into consideration, as when a speaker raises his/her voice in order to be heard.

Effect of noise on hearing

Modern industrial societies are noisy and noise pollution is another environmental hazard. Exposure to sound intensities above 80 dB may result in damage to the outer hair cells, depending upon the extent of the intensity and the duration of exposure. The damage usually starts at about 4000 Hz, and the subject is usually unaware of any deficit. Then it affects lower frequencies and, when it reaches frequencies below 1000 Hz, the ability to hear normal conversation is impaired, inducing the victim to seek medical advice.

Deafness

Deafness may be classified, according to its cause, into **conduction deafness** and **nerve** or **perceptive deafness**.

Conduction deafness is due to impairment of sound transmission through the external ear and middle ear. It may result from too much wax or a foreign body in the external auditory canal, repeated middle ear infections, a perforated drum, destruction of the ossicles or otosclerosis. Otosclerosis is a disease characterized by pathological fixation of the stapes in the oval window. Since the masking effect of background noise is greatly reduced, sounds are heard better by bone rather than by air conduction and sound frequencies are uniformly affected.

Nerve deafness may be congenital or may result from damage to the cochlea or auditory pathways. The cause may be toxic, e.g. administration of aminoglycoside antibiotics, such as streptomycin and gentamicin, or due to inflammation, e.g. cerebrospinal meningitis. Vascular lesions in the medulla or tumours, e.g. acoustic neuroma, may interrupt the auditory pathways and lead to some degree of deafness. In this connection, it should be remembered that the auditory pathways are characterized by bilateral representation and that, in contrast to vision, cortical lesions hardly ever result in deafness. In nerve deafness, hearing by both air and bone conduction is depressed.

Tests of hearing and audiometry

The audiometer is an instrument which is used to determine the auditory threshold for sound frequencies which may range from 50 Hz to 16 000 Hz. Pure tones are delivered through earphones (air conduction) or directly through a vibrating piece on the mastoid bone (bone conduction). The test is conducted in a soundproof, or at least very quiet, room. The responses are plotted on a chart (audiogram) where 0 dB is the normal threshold and any hearing loss in dB is indicated for each frequency. An audiogram gives a measure of the hearing loss, shows the frequencies affected and, by comparing air conduction with bone conduction,

gives an important clue as to whether the patient is suffering from conduction deafness or nerve deafness.

Before the audiometer became available, some simple tests using only a tuning-fork were used to differentiate between conduction and nerve deafness. These tests are still used by doctors as part of their examination of the ear.

Weber's test

The base of a vibrating tuning-fork is placed on the vertex of the skull. Normally, the sound should be heard equally well on both sides. In the case of unilateral *conduction deafness*, the sound is heard better (or lateralized) to the diseased side because of the absence of the masking effect of environmental noise on that side. In *nerve deafness* affecting one ear, the sound is lateralized to the normal side.

Rinne's test

The base of the vibrating tuning-fork is placed on the mastoid process until the subject cannot hear by bone conduction; then the prongs of the fork are held in the air near the ear. Normally, since air conduction is better than bone conduction, the subject will hear the vibration in the air after bone conduction is over, and this is referred to as a positive Rinne's test. If the subject does not hear the vibration in the air, the test is repeated but reversing the sequence, i.e. starting with the tuning-fork near the ear and, after hearing the vibration in the air is over, the base of the tuning fork is placed on the mastoid process. Normally, the vibration should not be heard through bone after hearing by air has stopped. If it is, this means bone conduction is better than air conduction and Rinne's test is said to be negative in this case. A negative Rinne's test is thus indicative of *conduction deafness*. A positive Rinne's test with hearing loss is indicative of *nerve deafness*.

Further reading

1 Ganong, W.F. (1999) Vision. In: *Review of Medical Physiology*, 19th edn, pp. 142–183. Appleton & Lange, Stamford, Connecticut.
2 Ganong, W.F. (1999) Hearing and equilibrium. In: *Review of Medical Physiology*, 19th edn, pp. 154–64. Appleton & Lange, San Mateo, California.
3 Ganong, W.F. (1999) Smell and taste. In: *Review of Medical Physiology*, 19th edn. Appleton & Lange, San Mateo, California.
4 Guyton, A.C. (1996) The nervous system: B. The special senses. In: *Textbook of Medical Physiology*, 9th edn, pp. 621–682. Saunders, Philadelphia.

Appendix 1 / Ranges of Reference Values in Human Blood, Plasma and Serum

| Determination | Reference value (varies with procedure used) | |
	Traditional units	SI units
Acetoacetate (S)	< 1.0 mg/dl	< 0.1 mmol/l
Adrenocorticotrophin (ACTH) (P)	15–70 pg/ml	3.3–15.4 pmol/l
Aldosterone (P)	3–10 ng/dl	83–277 pmol/l
Alpha-amino nitrogen (P)	3.0–5.5 mg/dl	2.1–3.9 mmol/l
Ammonia (B)	12–55 µmol/litre	12–55 µmol/l
Amylase (S)	4–25 units/ml	
Ascorbic acid (B)	0.4–1.5 mg/dl (fasting)	23–85 µmol/l
Bilirubin (S)	Conjugated (direct): up to < 0.2 mg/dl	< 3.4 µmol/l
	Total (conjugated plus free): up to 1.0 mg/dl	up to 17 µmol/l
Blood volume (B)	8.5–9.0% of body-weight in kg	80–85 ml/kg
Calcitonin (S)	Male: 0–14 pg/ml	0–4.1 pmol/l
	Female: 0–28 pg/ml	0–8.2 pmol/l
Calcium (total) (S)	8.5–10.5 mg/dl	2.1–2.6 mmol/l
Carbon dioxide content (S)	24–30 mequiv/l	24–30 mmol/l
Carotenoids (S)	0.8–4.0 µg/ml	1.5–7.4 µmol/l
Ceruloplasmin (S)	27–37 mg/dl	1.8–2.5 µmol/l
Chloride (S)	100–106 mequiv/l	100–106 mmol/l
Cholesterol (S)	120–220 mg/dl	3.1–5.7 mmol/l
Cholesteryl esters (S)	60–75% of total cholesterol	
Copper (total) (S)	100–200 µg/dl	16–31 µmol/l
Cortisol (a.m.) (S)	5–25 µg/dl	140–690 nmol/l
Cortisol (p.m.) (S)	3–16 µg/dl	83–441 nmol/l
Creatinine (S)	0.6–1.5 µg/dl	53–133 µmol/l
Follicle-stimulating hormone (FSH) (S)	Male: 3–18 mU/ml	3–18 arb. unit
	Female: 4.6–22.4 mU/ml	4.6–22.4 arb. unit
Glucose (true) (B)	70–110 mg/dl	3.9–5.6 mmol/l
Growth hormone (S)	Male: < 5 ng/ml	< 233 pmol/l
	Female: 0–30 ng/ml	0–1395 pmol/l
Insulin (fasting) (S)	6–26 µunits/ml	43–187 pmol/l
Iodine, protein-bound (S)	3.5–8.0 µg/dl	0.28–0.63 µmol/l
Iron (S)	50–150 µg/dl	9.0–26.9 µmol/l
Lactic acid (B)	5.4–17.1 mg/dl	0.6–1.9 mmol/l
Lipase (S)	Up to 2 units/ml	4.5–10 g/l
Lipids, total (S)	450–1000 mg/dl	0.8–1.3 mmol/l
Luteinizing hormone (LH) (S)	Male: 3–18 mU/ml	3–18 arb. unit
	Female: 2.4–34.5 mU/ml	2.4–34.5 arb. unit
Magnesium (S)	1.5–2.0 mequiv/l	0.8–1.3 mmol/l
Non-protein nitrogen (S)	15–35 mg/dl	10.7–25.0 mmol/l
Osmolality (S)	280–296 mosmol/kg water	280–296 mmol/kg
P_{CO_2} (arterial) (B)	35–45 mmHg	4.7–6.0 kPa

Continued

Determination	Reference value (varies with procedure used)	
	Traditional units	SI units
Pepsinogen (P)	120–140 ng/ml	120–140 µg/l
pH (B)	7.35–7.45	
Phenylalanine (S)	0–2 mg/dl	0–120 µmol/l
Phosphatase, acid, total (S)	Male: 0.13–0.63 sigma units/ml	36–175 nmol.s^{-1}/l
	Female: 0.01–0.56 sigma units/ml	3–156 nmol.s^{-1}/l
Phosphatase, alkaline (S)	13–39 IU/l (adults)	0.22–0.65 µmol.s^{-1}/l
Phospholipids (S)	9–16 mg/dl as lipid phosphorus	2.9–5.2 mmol/l
Phosphorus, inorganic (S)	3.0–4.5 mg/dl (infants in first year, up to 6.0 mg/dl)	1–1.5 mmol/l
Po_2 (arterial) (B)	75–100 mmHg	10.0–13.3 kPa
Potassium	3.5–5.0 mequiv/l	3.5–5.0 mmol/l
Progesterone (S)	Male: < 1.0 ng/ml	< 3.2 nmol/l
	Female:	
	0.2–0.6 ng/ml (follicular phase)	0.6–1.9 nmol/l
	0.3–3.5 ng/ml (midcycle peak)	0.95–11 nmol/l
	6.5–32.2 ng/ml (postovulatory)	21–102 nmol/l
Prolactin (S)	2–15 ng/ml	0.08–6.0 nmol/l
Protein:		
Total (S)	6.0–8.4 g/dl	60–84 g/l
Albumin (S)	3.5–5.0 g/dl	35–50 g/l
Globulin (S)	2.3–3.5 g/dl	23–35 g/l
Pyruvic acid (P)	0–0.11 mequiv/l	0–110 µmol/l
Sodium (S)	135–145 mequiv/l	135–145 mmol/l
Sulphate (S)	2.9–3.5 mg/dl	0.3–0.36 mmol/l
Testosterone (P)	Male: 300–1100 ng/ml	10.4–38.1 nmol/l
	Female: 25–90 ng/ml	0.87–3.12 nmol/l
Thyroid-stimulating hormone (TSH) (S)	0.5–5.0 µU/ml	0.5–5.0 arb. unit
Total tri-iodothyronine (T_3) (S)	75–195 ng/dl	1.16–3.00 nmol/l
Total thyroxine (T_4) (S)	4–12 µg/dl	52–154 nmol/l
Transaminase (SGOT) (S)	7–27 U/l	0.12–0.45 µmol.s^{-1}/l
Triacylglycerol (fasting) (S)	40–150 mg/dl	0.4–1.5 mmol/l
Urea nitrogen (BUN) (B)	8–25 mg/dl	2.9–8.9 mmol/l
Uric acid (S)	3.0–7.0 mg/dl	0.18–0.42 mmol/l
Vitamin A (Retinol) (S)	0.15–0.6 µg/ml	0.5–2.1 µmol/l

Mainly drawn from Scully, R.E., McNeely, B.U. & Mark, E.J. (1986) Normal reference laboratory values. *N. Engl. J. Med.* **314**, 39.
B, whole blood; P, plasma; S, serum; arb., arbitrary; SGOT, serum glutamic oxaloacetic transaminase.

Appendix 2 / The SI Units

SI stands for the Système International d'Unités (International System of Units) used in scientific reporting. In accordance with the decision of several scientific societies to employ a universal system of metric nomenclature, the SI system of units has been introduced.

The fractions and multiples used in the SI system (and their abbreviations) are given below.

Fractions and multiples

deci-	(d) $= 10^{-1}$	kilo-	(k) $= 10^3$
centi-	(c) $= 10^{-2}$	mega-	(M) $= 10^6$
milli-	(m) $= 10^{-3}$	giga-	(G) $= 10^9$
micro-	(μ) $= 10^{-6}$	tera-	(T) $= 10^{12}$
nano-	(n) $= 10^{-9}$		
pico-	(p) $= 10^{-12}$		

Units of concentration

Physical and chemical properties and consequently the biological activity of substances depend on the number of molecules in a solution. In SI units molar concentrations, which are based on the number of molecules per litre of fluid, are used instead of concentrations based on weight per unit volume. Thus:

$$1 \text{ Mole of a substance} = \frac{\text{Mass (g)}}{\text{Molecular weight}}$$

Moles depend on the number of atoms. The larger the molecular weight, the lower the molar concentration. In the traditional system, blood glucose, urea and cholesterol concentrations were expressed as 100 mg/100 ml, 30 mg/100 ml and 200 mg/100 ml, respectively. When converted into SI units (i.e. mmol/litre) they all become 5 mmol/litre.

Units of volume

Litre	(l)	Centilitre	(cl)
Decilitre	(dl)	Millilitre	(ml)

Units of mass

Kilogram	(kg)
Gram	(g)
Milligram	(mg)

Units of pressure

The basic unit of pressure as expressed in SI units is the newton per square metre (N m^2). This unit is also known as the pascal (Pa), and is usually expressed in 1000 pascals or kilopascals. In clinical practice, however, blood pressure is usually measured using a mercury manometer and expressed in mm of mercury. As the pascal is too small for clinical use, the kilopascal is used. The relationship between the kilopascal and mmHg is as follows: 1 kPa = 7.5 mmHg (Table A2.1) and 0.133 kPa = 1.0 mmHg.

Units of energy

The traditional unit of heat and energy is the calorie and kilocalorie (kcal). In SI units, the joule (J) is used to represent the unit of both heat and energy. Like the pascal, calories are too small for clinical use, and kilocalories are used. In the SI system they are converted to the kilojoule (kJ), corresponding to 1000 joules, and the megajoule (MJ), corresponding to 1 000 000 joules. In SI units: 1 kcal = 4.2 kJ.

Table A2.1 Relationship between the kilopascal and mm of mercury.

kPa	mmHg	kPa	mmHg
1	7.5	11	82.5
2	15.0	12	90.0
3	22.5	13	97.5
4	30.0	14	105.0
5	37.5	15	112.5
6	45.0	16	120.0
7	52.5	17	17.5
8	60.0	18	135.0
9	67.5	19	142.5
10	75.0	20	150.0

Bibliography

Brent, G.A. (1994) The molecular basis of thyroid nervous action. *N. Engl. J. Med.* **331**, 847.

Breziniski, A. (1997) Melatonin in humans. *N. Engl. J. Med.* **336**, 186.

Carpenter, R. (1996) *Neurophysiology*, 3rd edn. Edward Arnold, London.

Copstead, L.C. (1995) *Perspectives on Pathophysiology*, 1st edn. Saunders, Philadelphia.

Haslepp, C. *et al.* (eds) (1999) *Davidson's Principles and Practice of Medicine*, 18th edn. Churchill Livingstone, Edinburgh.

Fauci, A.S. *et al.* (1998) *Harrison's Principles of Internal Medicine*, 14th edn. McGraw-Hill, New York.

Firkin, F., Chesterman, C., Pennington, D. & Rush, B. (eds) (1989) *de Gruchy's Clinical Haematology in Clinical Practice*, 5th edn. Blackwell Scientific Publications, Oxford.

Ganong, W.F. (1999) *Review of Medical Physiology*, 19th edn. Appleton & Lange, Stamford, Connecticut.

Garrow, J.S. & James, W.P.T. (1993) *Human Nutrition and Dietetics*, 9th edn. Churchill Livingstone, Edinburgh.

Gillham, B., Papachristodoulu, D.K. & Hywel Thomas, J. (1997) *Will's Biochemical Basis of Medicine*, 3rd edn. Butterworth-Heinemann Ltd, Oxford.

Goyal, R.K. & Hirano, I. (1996) The enteric nervous system. *N. Engl. J. Med.* **334**, 1106.

Guyton, A.C. & Hall, J.E. (1996) *Textbook of Medical Physiology*, 9th edn. Saunders, Philadelphia.

Holmes, Oliver (1993) *Human Neurophysiology: A Student Text*, 2nd edn. Chapman & Hall Medical, London.

Johnson, L.R. *et al.* (eds) (1994) *Physiology of the Gastro-intestinal Tract*, 3rd edn. Raven Press, New York.

Knobil, E. & Neil, J.D. (eds) (1994) *The Physiology of Reproduction*, 2nd edn, 2 vols. Raven Press.

Patton, H.D., Fuchs, A.F., Hille, B., Scher, A.M. & Steiner, R. (1989) *Textbook of Physiology*, 21st edn. Saunders, Philadelphia.

Sherwood, L. (1997) *Human Physiology: From Cells to Systems*, 3rd edn. Wadsworth, Belmont, California.

Smith, A.F., Beckett, G.T., Walkin, S.W. & Rae, P.W.H. (1998) *Lecture Notes on Clinical Chemistry*, 6th edn. Blackwell Science Ltd, Oxford.

West, J.B. (1995) *Respiratory Physiology: The Essentials*, 5th edn. Williams & Wilkins, Baltimore.

Index